Common Malformations

COMMON MALFORMATIONS

LEWIS B. HOLMES, MD

Professor of Pediatrics
Harvard Medical School

Chief Emeritus
Genetics Unit
MassGeneral Hospital *for* Children

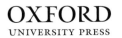

OXFORD
UNIVERSITY PRESS

OXFORD

UNIVERSITY PRESS

Oxford University Press, Inc., publishes works that further
Oxford University's objective of excellence
in research, scholarship, and education.

Oxford New York
Auckland   Cape Town   Dar es Salaam   Hong Kong   Karachi
Kuala Lumpur   Madrid   Melbourne   Mexico City   Nairobi
New Delhi   Shanghai   Taipei   Toronto

With offices in
Argentina   Austria   Brazil   Chile   Czech Republic   France   Greece
Guatemala   Hungary   Italy   Japan   Poland   Portugal   Singapore
South Korea   Switzerland   Thailand   Turkey   Ukraine   Vietnam

Published by Oxford University Press, Inc.
198 Madison Avenue, New York, New York 10016
www.oup.com

Library of Congress Cataloging-in-Publication Data

Holmes, Lewis B.
Common malformations / Lewis B. Holmes.
p. ; cm.
Includes bibliographical references.
ISBN 978-0-19-513602-9 (cloth : alk. paper) 1. Abnormalities, Human. I. Title.
[DNLM: 1. Congenital Abnormalities. QS 675 H751c 2011]
QM691.H65 2011
616'.042—dc22   2010009172

9 8 7 6 5 4 3 2 1

Printed in USA
on acid-free paper

Preface

═══════

One way to learn about congenital malformations is to examine a consecutive series of affected liveborn infants. With the help of a perinatal pathologist, the experience can be extended to stillborn infants and the findings at autopsy. Our evaluation of the malformed infants among 18,155 births over three years (February 16, 1972, to February 15, 1975) at the Boston Lying-In Hospital was that first learning experience. One recurrent theme was the amazing variation in both the patterns of physical features and the apparent causes in infants with common malformations.

During this three-year period, with the energetic and creative assistance of Catherine Cook and Cristina Cann, we examined, also, a systematic sample of 7,157 newborn infants for minor physical features (1). In addition, with the guidance of Joseph Alper, a pediatric dermatologist, we examined 4,641 of those infants for all types of birth marks. These examinations showed us the value of knowing about the range of normal for minor physical features and how to identify the common birth marks.

This project ended after three years. We were invited back in 1978 and resumed the Active Malformations Surveillance Program on January 1, 1979.

By the 1980s, the identification of malformations was being impacted significantly by the use of prenatal screening by ultrasound. We and others began to document the frequency of prenatal detection and the impact of the elective termination of the pregnancies with a malformed fetus (3–6).

Since the 1990s, there have been many publications on the prevalence rate and etiologic heterogeneity of common malformations by many research groups around the world. Within the past ten years, it has become possible to delineate "causative" developmental abnormalities, such as mutations, polymorphisms, and subtle deletions and duplications, which can cause common malformations. This has continued at a faster pace as the molecular technologies have improved.

We compile in this volume the observations and findings in many case series and population-based studies. Many of their findings have been quoted and compared. We congratulate these investigators and their staff members. This is an alphabetical listing of those whose findings have been used frequently in the descriptions of specific malformations: National Birth Defects Prevention Study of the Birth Defects Center, Centers for Disease Control, Atlanta, Baltimore-Washington Infant Study, California Birth Defects Monitoring Program, Slone Epidemiology Center, Patricia Baird, Mason Barr, Elisa Calzolari, John Carey, Edwardo E. Castilla and Iêda M. Orioli, Christina Chambers, Michael M. Cohen, Jr., Andrew Czeizel, Charlotte Ferencz, Matthew Forrester and Ruth Merz, John M. Graham, Jr., Muriel Harris, Terry Hassold, Diana Juriloff, Bengt Källén, Dagmar Kalousek, Brian Lowry, Kenneth Lyons Jones, Maria Luisa Martinez-Frias, Pierpaolo Mastroiacovo, Jeffrey Murray, Elizabeth Robert, Albert Schinzel, Roger Stevenson, Claude Stoll, Claudine Torfs, and David Weaver.

The identification of and diagnostic evaluation of all malformed infants born at Brigham and Women's Hospital, since 1972, has depended on the skill and knowledge of many nurses, pediatricians, surgeons, sonologists, cytogeneticists, and pathologists. The day-to-day conducting of the surveillance program has relied upon many individuals and their extra efforts. We thank, in particular: Leonard Atkins, Adi Ben-Yehuda, Frederick Bieber, Kathleen (Cote) Bowling, Kelly Brown, Cristina Cann, Tamsen Caruso, Kristine Church, Will Cochran, Catherine Cook, Shirley Driscoll, Paula Feldman, Wendy Fishbeck, Aleda Franz, David Genest, Caroline (McGuirk) Golden, Kerri Hirt-Armon, Kara Houde, Lisa Houde, Ellis Johnson, Celeste Krauss, Kathleen Leppig, Charles Limb, Angela Lin, Maria (Melenevsky) Livshin, Meredith Miller, Kathryn Nelson, Allyson Peller, Barbara Pober, Mary (Bebe) Poor, Sonja Rasmussen, John Rathjens, Nicole Rodier, Lisa Smeester, Julie Travitz, Leo Ungar, Susan Vincent, Martha Werler, Marie-Noel Westgate, Louise Wilkins-Haug, Mackensie Yore, Abigail Zavod, and Katherine Zuckerman. Louise Ryan and Brent Coull provided many biostatistical analyses.

Marie-Noel Westgate, Kara Houde and Katherine Zuckerman compiled many lists of infants with common malformations subdivided by apparent etiology. Their contributions were invaluable.

Photographs have been provided generously by Mason Barr, Frederick Bieber, John M. Graham, Jr., W. Hardy Hendren, and David Weaver.

Several drawings have been provided by Edith Tagrin, an accomplished medical illustrator. Meaghan Russell and Kathryn Rowan were very helpful in the organizing of the photographs.

The typing of the manuscript has been done primarily by Rosanna Greco, with assistance from Phyllis Dennehy, Sharon Kazlauskas, and Martha Furtek.

Marcie Rome obtained previously published prints and permissions from publishers and authors. Megan Clancy was very helpful in obtaining copies of many, many published articles. Maryann Ligotti was a very careful proofreader, who helped to improve many sentences.

REFERENCES

1. Leppig KA, Werler MM, Cann CI, Cook CA, Holmes LB. Predictive value of minor anomalies: I. Association with major malformations. *J Pediatr.* 1987;110:531–537.
2. Alper JC, Holmes LB. The incidence and significance of birthmarks in a cohort of 4,641 newborns. *Ped Dermatology.* 1983;1:58–68.
3. Limb CJ, Holmes LB. Anencephaly: changes in prenatal detection and birth status, 1972 through 1990. *Amer J Ob Gyn.* 1994;170:1333–1338.
4. Rasmussen SA, Bieber FR, Benacerraf BR, Lachman RS, Rimoin DL, Holmes LB. Epidemiology of osteochondrodysplasias: changing trends due to advances in prenatal diagnosis. *Am J Med Genet.* 1996;61:49–58.
5. Caruso TM, Westgate M-N, Holmes LB. Impact of prenatal screening on the birth status of fetuses with Down syndrome at an urban hospital, 1972–1994. *Genet Med.* 1998;1:22–28.
6. Peller AJ, Westgate M-N, Holmes LB. Trends in congenital malformations, 1974–1999: Effect of prenatal diagnosis and elective termination. *Obstet Gynecol.* 2004;104:957–964.

Contents

═══════

Common Malformations

Chapter 1

The Approach to the Malformed Newborn

Malformed infants are born usually as a complete surprise to healthy parents. Sometimes the moment of surprise is during prenatal sonography; at other times, it is in the delivery room. Regardless of the circumstances, the goal of the clinician is to help the parents to answer their overriding question: "Why did this happen?" The process of developing an answer starts ideally with an interview with both parents, a careful examination of the infant, a review of the findings in the diagnostic studies carried out, and a thorough discussion of the findings and the recommendations. This process is more effective when there are several meetings with the parents, so the clinician and each parent can become acquainted and achieve a level of mutual respect and trust. The final collation of the findings and the interpretation may only be possible after several days or weeks.

In reality, this process often occurs in brief snatches of time, and is complicated by fatigue, anxiety, or anger. It may not even be possible to meet with both parents at the same time.

Each step in this process is significant, so any shortcut is a calculated risk.

PREGNANCY HISTORY

The mothers of a malformed infant will usually review in detail the events that occurred during her pregnancy and look for potentially harmful fetal exposures. She will remember the cocktails drunk near the time of conception or the microwave oven near where she stood during pregnancy. Consider carefully each of her concerns, as well as the theories offered by her friends and relatives. For exposures that are potentially teratogenic (see Table 1-1), it can help for the clinician to review what is known and not known about that exposure's potential teratogenic effects. Some, but not all, parents

benefit from reading a published summary, such as those available in TERIS (1) or Reprotox (www.reprotox.org) (2). For exposures with debatable fetal effects, inviting a consultant to review the information available may be more effective. Be sure to warn the parents that many well-known resources, like the Physicians Desk Reference (PDR), do not provide accurate information about the fetal risks of drugs taken in pregnancy (3, 4). If the parents have been told that a drug taken in pregnancy is classified in the PDR as Category A, B, C, D or X, the information available should be reviewed. Describing an impressive-looking resource, like the Physicians Desk Reference, as inaccurate may be confusing. Good rapport and patience are needed.

Review the results of the all prenatal testing during the pregnancy to establish whether or not any findings are relevant. This discussion may identify findings the mother did not understand correctly, such as the significance of the thickness of the nuchal translucency or the levels of AFP or a finding by ultrasound, such as "echogenic bowel" or a choroid plexus cyst.

When evaluating an infant transferred from another hospital, request copies of the reports from the prenatal studies. Having the specific results can help to clarify the findings that are confusing to the mother and father.

With regard to exposures in pregnancy, experience has shown (5) that it is better to ask the mother about specific exposures, i.e., Do you have epilepsy . . . take an anticonvulsant drug? Do you take insulin to treat diabetes? If by contrast, a woman is asked if she takes any "drugs," she may assume this refers only to illicit drugs, such as cocaine or amphetamines.

The delivery itself can be relevant to the infant's physical features. For example:

a) Presentation of infant during birth process (6): the infant in face and brow presentation for a prolonged period can have deformations of the nose from pressure

TABLE 1-1 *Recognized Human Teratogens (2009)*

1. DRUGS
Aminopterin/amethopterin
Androgenic hormones
Angiotensin converting
enzyme(ACE) inhibitors
Busulfan
Carbamazepine
Cocaine
Cyclophosphamide
Cyclosporin
Diethylstilbestrol
Efavirenz
Etretinate
Fluconazole
Heroin/methadone
Iodide
Isotretinoin (13-cis-retinoic acid)
Lamotrigine
Lithium
Methimazole/Carbimazole
Mycophenolate mofetil
Paroxetine
Phenobarbital
Phenytoin
Propylthiouracil
Prostaglandin E_1 (misoprostol)

Tetracycline
Thalidomide
Trimethadione/paramethadione
Valproic acid
Warfarin

2. HEAVY METALS
Lead
Mercury

3. RADIATION
Cancer therapy

4. MATERNAL CONDITIONS
Alcohol
Insulin-dependent diabetes mellitus
Hypothyroidism
Iodide deficiency
Maternal phenylketonuria
Myasthenia gravis
Obesity, severe
Smoking cigarettes/marijuana
Systemic lupus erythematosus
Vitamin A deficiency
Vitamin K deficiency

5. INTRAUTERINE INFECTIONS
Cytomegalovirus
Herpes simplex

Parvovirus
Rubella
Syphilis
Toxoplasmosis
Varicella
Venezuelan equine encephalitis virus
West Nile virus

6. PROCEDURES/ASSISTED REPRODUCTION
Chorionic Villus Sampling (CVS)
Dilation and curettage (D&C)
Intracytoplasmic Sperm Injection (ICSI)

7. TRAUMA TO PLACENTA

8. OTHER EXPOSURES
Carbon monoxide poisoning
Gasoline fumes (excessive)
Heat
Hypoxia
Magnesium sulfate (high levels,
third trimester)
Methyl isocyanate
Methylene blue
Phthalates
Polychlorinated biphenyls
Toluene (excessive; glue sniffing)

against the uterus and a prominence of the occiput, the "star gazer" phenotype (Figures 1-1A and B); another example is the infant in breech presentation who has an increased risk for hip dislocation;

b) Unicornuate uterus: a potential cause of positional deformities (6);

c) Twins: monoamniotic, monochorionic twins are at risk for:

   i)   some malformations, like acardia (7), which occur only in such twin pairs;

   ii) many malformations (8), such as sirenomelia (9) and cloacal exstrophy (10), are more common in MZ twin pregnancies than in singleton pregnancies.

   iii) if one twin dies, and the pregnancy continues, tissue from the deceased and autolyzed twin can embolize to the living twin and produce abnormalities caused by obstructing an artery, such as bowel atresia, porencephaly, aplasia cutis, or amputations (11a).

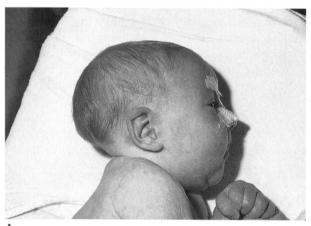
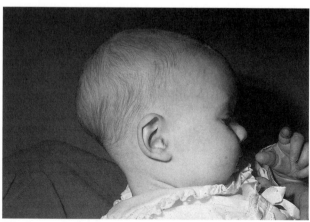

A   B

FIGURE 1.1   Shows deformations of posterior skull shape (Figure 1A) from a prolonged face and brow presentation: the "star gazer." More normal skull shape (Figure 1B) four months later, after no treatment.

MEDICAL HISTORY

Both the mother and the father should be interviewed about their medical histories. One focus will be on acute infections and chronic diseases in the mother, such as diabetes or hypertension. However, the father may be blaming himself for the child's problems because of past drug abuse. Ask him if he has any concerns and discuss their relevance, if any. Unfortunately, articles in the lay press often suggest that male exposures, such as those resulting from military service in Vietnam or the Persian Gulf, can be harmful to the fetus even though the scientific data available, to date, does not provide convincing evidence in humans (11b).

FAMILY HISTORY

Start with the immediate family: each parent and the infant's older sibling(s), aunts, uncles, and first cousins.

In reviewing the family history, if a reference is made to a distant relative with birth defects, keep that in mind. This reference could be pursued later, if it seems warranted by the findings in the affected infant.

The grandparents may be present for these initial discussions. Remember that they can be defensive about "our family." Asking for more information about a maternal or paternal relative can engender guilt; only do this, if necessary.

One instance in which a more extensive pedigree is needed is when the affected infant has an unbalanced chromosome translocation (12). In that situation personal discussions, using visual aids, with the persons at risk of carrying the balanced translocation are essential. However, this discussion is most effective after the medical status of the affected infant has stabilized and the family's attention can focus on the cause and the potential risks to other relatives.

PHYSICAL EXAMINATION

First, check with the infant's nurse to make sure this is a good time for you to examine the infant. She/he may prefer certain times.

Head and Body Size

Establish gestational age and use gestational age- and race-appropriate normal standards.

Definitions

i) use two standard deviations below the mean, i.e., 2 1/2 centile, for head circumference to define microcephaly and for length and weight to define growth restriction (13); some newborn nurseries provide growth curve standards in which the 10th percentile is the lowest curve shown; the infant whose head size is in the 10th percentile does not have microcephaly by this definition;

ii) each growth curve does not have the same trajectory, reflecting presumably differences between populations (14): select the standard that is most relevant to your geographic location; for example, a normal standard for Denver with a mile-high elevation, such as the Lubchenko charts (15), is not appropriate for an infant born at sea level.

Surface Exam

A quick head-to-toe surface exam will enable you to determine whether the infant has multiple major and minor dysmorphic features in several areas or a more localized abnormality;

Using the standard physical examination format, record the presence of each major and minor finding identified, starting with scalp, head, face, mouth, neck, chest, etc.—head to toe. If you use unfamiliar terms in your written report, provide an explanation or definition. (Many of these are provided by Aase in his book *Diagnostic Dysmorphology* (16) and in this book.)

If the parents are present, show them those features which you consider to be significant. You should expect that they won't readily understand why minor physical features matter. Explain how their presence can be relevant to the diagnosis and prognosis of their infant. It can help to point out that it is not uncommon for a parent and child to both have the same minor physical feature, such as a transverse palmar crease or syndactyly of toes 2-3, but uncommon for healthy relatives to have several minor physical features. Summarize the pattern of abnormalities you consider significant, including any effects on growth and any major malformations identified.

Examining Other Members of the Family

Decide when to examine the parents or sibs or other relatives. Family resemblance is always an important issue to consider. You can ask: Does he/she look like his/her older brother or sister did at birth? Or, whom does your mother say she/he resembles most? Ask the parents to bring in pictures of themselves or each older sib as an infant, so you can make the comparison yourself.

If the infant being evaluated has a large head size, the most common explanation is that one parent also has a large head (17). Measure each parent's head size and report the percentiles. The parent with a large head usually knows that it is big. Establishing this family resemblance helps to reassure the parents of this potentially benign reason for an infant to have a large head.

Some abnormalities present in a parent may not have been diagnosed previously. Two examples are: (1) hypertelorism and anosmia in the asymptomatic mother of a male infant with the telecanthus-hypospadias syndrome (Mendelian Inheritance in Man 313600) [18]; this finding in her suggests that she is mildly affected and will affect her risk for having another affected child; (2) coronal synostosis in the more mildly affected parent of a newborn with Crouzon's Disease (Mendelian Inheritance in Man #123500. Set a time to examine both parents (preferably together); tell them what you find and its significance, if any.

ESTABLISHING A DIAGNOSIS

Establish the Phenotype

Does the infant have primarily one major abnormality or is the infant dysmorphic with multiple major and minor anomalies? If there is a central, distinctive finding, the focus should be on that primary abnormality.

Are there any distinctive minor anomalies, like a single fifth finger crease (Figure 1-2) or sinus tracts (Figure 1-3)? These are unlikely to be familial and their presence makes it most likely that the infant is dysmorphic. The primary question is whether the infant is dysmorphic with multiple minor and major anomalies.

Decide whether growth restriction is another feature of the infant's phenotype. Assessments of size are best evaluated with measurements, which in turn require a normal standard. Preferably the reference source used makes possible a comparison based on gestational age, race, and sex, using two or more standard deviations from the mean as "significant." If this measurement is a distinctive finding, such as head size or length of fingers, it can be helpful to make the same measurement on each parent to confirm that the finding does not reflect family resemblance.

Associated Features

When an infant has a major malformation, there can be associated features to be looked for that could suggest a specific diagnosis. For example,

i) a branchial cleft sinus (Figure 1-3) in association with a preauricular tag or sinus can be a feature of the Branchio-oto-renal syndrome(MIM #113650);

ii) gum frenula (Figure 1-4) with clefts in the tip of the tongue, which occurs in the oral-facial digital syndromes;

iii) with absence of the superior head of the pectoralis major (Poland Anomaly), there can be abnormalities of the underlying rib, absence of the adjacent areola and nipple, or synbrachydactyly of the hand on that side.

iv) pits in the lower lip (Figure 1-5), a distinctive feature of the Van der Woude Syndrome (MIM #119300), an autosomal dominant mutation that can cause cleft lip or cleft palate.

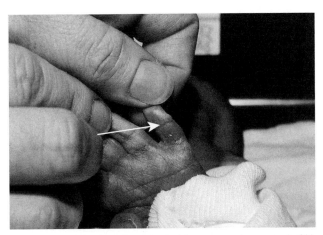

FIGURE 1.2   Distinctive minor physical features, such as a single fifth finger crease. (arrow)

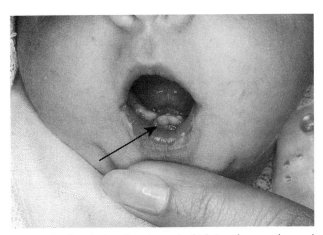

FIGURE 1.4   A gum frenulum (arrow) which is a feature of several malformation syndromes. (arrow)

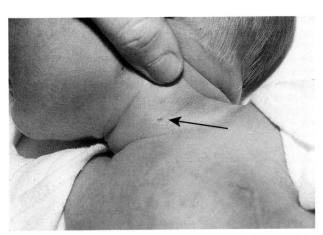

FIGURE 1.3   A branchial cleft sinus which can be a feature of the Branchio-Oto-Renal (BOR) Syndrome. (arrow)

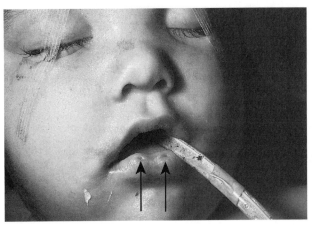

FIGURE 1.5   Lip pits (arrow) in the lower lip, a common feature of the Van der Woude Syndrome, in an infant being prepared for surgical repair of cleft palate (Courtesy of John Mulliken, M.D., Children's Hospital, Boston, MA).

Ranges of Severity

For most major malformations, there is, among several affected infants, a range of severity within the same phenotype. For example:

i) some infants with anencephaly have an associated open cervical spine, i.e., rachischisis;
ii) a mild unilateral cleft lip deformity at one end of the spectrum in comparison to a bilateral cleft deformity with a protruding premaxilla;
iii) asymptomatic unilateral renal agenesis in a continuum with bilateral renal agenesis/dysgenesis (19);
iv) absence of the fibula with five toes in comparison to absence of the fibula, with absence of toes 4 and 5 and shortening of the tibia (20).

However, there are also ranges of severity which represent significant differences. For example:
i) a skin-covered lumbosacral meningocele is a mild neural tube defect with a good prognosis, whereas a skin-covered meninocystocele with imperforate anus and bladder exstrophy are features of cloacal exstrophy, a much more complex and severe malformation.
ii) bilateral cleft lip and palate with absence of the premaxilla (Figure 1-6) is part of the spectrum of holoprosencephaly, whereas bilateral cleft lip and palate with the premaxilla present is typical of "isolated" cleft lip and palate;
iii) an isolated gastroschisis (Figure 1-7) is different from the syndrome of limb body wall defect in which gastroschisis, vertebral anomalies, and limb abnormalities occur.

Spectrum of a Phenotype

The so-called "isolated" major malformation occurs often in association with other structural abnormalities. For example, thumb hypoplasia is occasionally associated with both anencephaly and encephalocele [Figure 1-8] (21). Does this make the occurrence of encephalocele with thumb hypoplasia a specific multiple anomaly syndrome or just an occasional association? Family studies would determine whether or not there was an increased rate of occurrence of both the encephalocele and thumb hypoplasia in siblings. In considering these less common associated anomalies, it should be noted that animal studies of disorders similar to human abnormalities have shown in dissections of viscera and in the examination of fixed, stained, and cleared skeletons that additional abnormalities are common (22). Presumably the same "hidden" associations occur in humans, who appear to have "isolated" malformation.

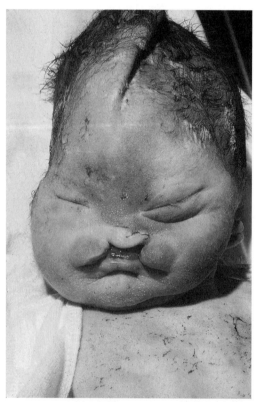

FIGURE 1.6   The cleft lip deformity with absence of the premaxilla portion of upper lip, a frequent facial feature of infants with holoprosencephaly.

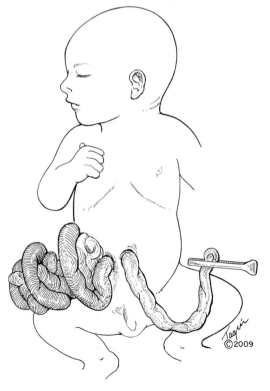

FIGURE 1.7   Gastroschisis, an abdominal wall defect which occurs typically to the right of the umbilical cord.

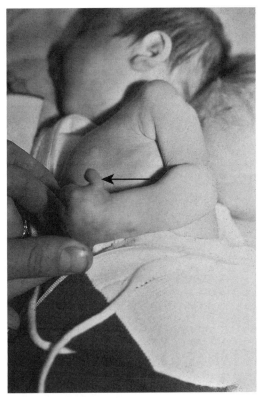

FIGURE 1.8 A hypoplastic thumb (arrow) in association with an occipital encephalocele.

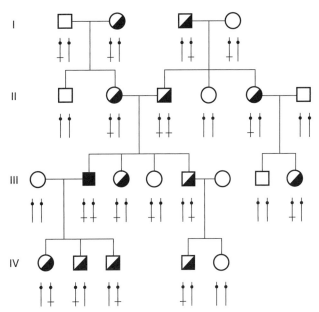

FIGURE 1.9 Pedigree which illustrates autosomal recessive inheritance; the horizontal bar indicates the mutation in one of two chromosomes in the heterozygote; there are four potential combinations for the children of parents who are heterozygous for the mutation; note that the affected (homozygous) individuals are in one generation.

Consider, as one example, the infant with "isolated" cleft lip deformity. Imaging studies have demonstrated an increased frequency of anomalies of the cervical vertebrae (23), the septum pellucidum (24), and brain morphology (25), which could be markers of cognitive dysfunction (26). These findings show that the phenotype can be more than the lip or palate deformity itself.

POTENTIAL CAUSES AND EXAMPLES

i)   malformations due to single mutant genes:
   a) autosomal recessive disorders, such as Jarcho-Levin Syndrome (MIM #277300); [Figure 1-9];
   b) autosomal dominant disorders, such as polycystic kidney disease, adult type: (MIM #173900); [Figure 1-10 A];
   c) X-linked recessive disorders, such as aqueductal stenosis (MIM #307000);
   d) X-linked dominant disorders, such as Melnick-Needles syndrome (MIM #309350). [Figure 1-10 B]
ii)   chromosome abnormalities:
   a) trisomies, such as trisomies 21 (Figure 1-11), 18 and 13;
   b) monosomies, such as 45, X Turner Syndrome;
   c) deletion in chromosomes, which cannot be identified in a Giemsa-stained karyotype (Figure 1-12 A&B);

   d) deletion identified in microarray or array CGH (comparative genomic hybridization [Figure 1-13 A&B] (27);
   e) uniparental disomy.
iii)   exposures to maternal diseases, such as diabetes mellitus;
iv)   exposures to medications, such as:
   anticonvulsant drugs, such as valproate (28) or phenobarbital;
   the anticoagulant coumadin or retinoic acid;
v)   vascular disruption, resulting in:
   amniotic band syndrome;
   Poland Anomaly and deficiencies of cranial nerves (29);
vi)   twinning process, that is an abnormality that occurs only in monochorionic, monoamniotic twins: acardia;

There are other postulated causes of structural abnormalities that are difficult to prove:

vii)   multifactorial inheritance (30, 31) of predisposing genetic differences with or without environmental exposures, such as:
   relative folate deficiency plus predisposing genetic deficiencies leading to the occurrence of spina bifida;
   Hirschsprung's aganglionosis, which can be associated with several different mutations (32).
viii)   digenic inheritance (33), in which there are mutations at two different gene loci which cause the abnormality;

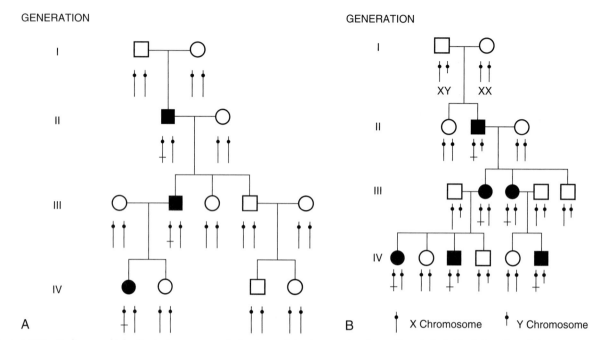

A

B | X Chromosome | Y Chromosome

FIGURE 1.10A Pedigree which illustrates autosomal dominant inheritance; the first affected individual is affected by a spontaneous mutation; note the parents are unaffected; each offspring has a 50% chance of inheriting the mutation; the individual who inherits the mutation will show its effects.

FIGURE 1.10B Pedigree for X-linked dominant inheritance. No male to male transmission. All daughters of affected men are affected. Can begin with spontaneous mutation.

Result : 47, XX, +21

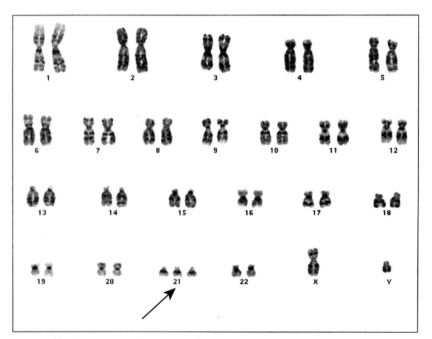

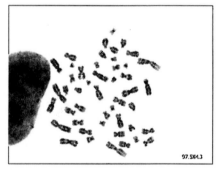

FIGURE 1.11 Giemsa-stained karyotype, showing trisomy 21. (arrow)

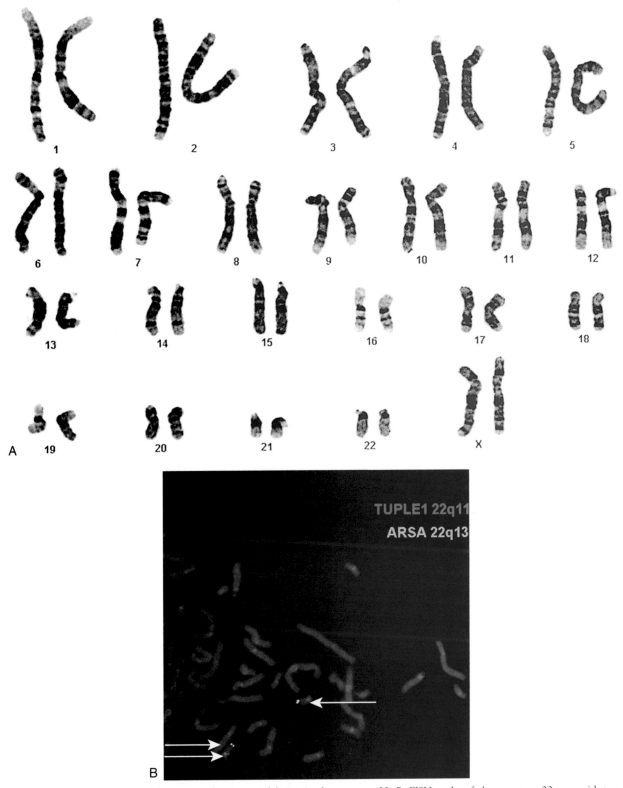

FIGURE 1.12   A: Giemsa-stained karyotype, showing no deletion in chromosome 22. B: FISH probe of chromosomes 22, one with two probes (arrows) and the other with only one (arrow), because of the deletion at 22q11.2.

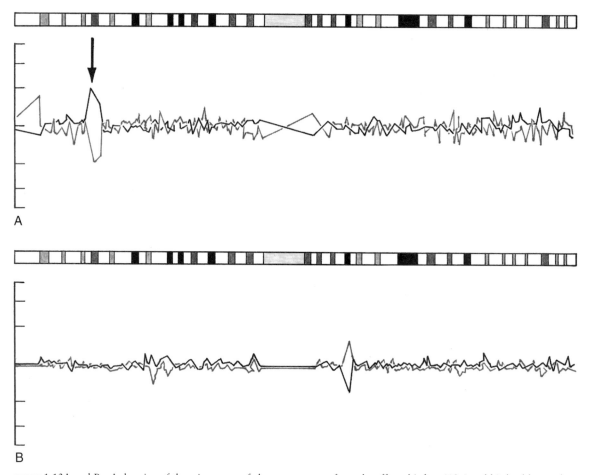

FIGURE 1.13A and B   A drawing of the microarray of chromosome one from the affected infant (13a) and his healthy mother. (13b) Adapted from figure in Kantarci S et al: *Am J Med Gen.* 2006;140A: 17–23. The ideogram of chromosome #1 is along top margin, showing the normal banding pattern. The arrow marks the region 1q41-1q42.12 with the de novo 5 megabase deletion, which caused the infant's multiple malformations. The mother and father did not have this deletion.

ix) triallelic inheritance (34); attributed to three mutations;

x) mosaicism in which there are two populations of cells, one mutant and causing an abnormality and the other normal (35–37);

xi) mitochondrial inheritance of genetic abnormalities, typically maternal (38), but theoretically paternal as well (39);

xii) other potential causes, not yet established, such as microsatellite instability (40)

DIAGNOSTIC TESTS

Having pointed out the physical features you consider significant, explain how their presence leads you to either consider specific clinical diagnoses or to suggest specific tests, such as chromosome analysis or mutation analysis or biochemical assays. If reference is made to a specific test, describe briefly what questions can and cannot be answered, such as what percentage of affected individuals are identified by the molecular testing

planned. Tell them when they should expect to receive the results.

One common misconception of parents is that the results of chromosome analysis determine whether a birth defect is "genetic" or not. Showing parents a karyotype can help in this discussion of visible changes, as opposed to point mutations.

If imaging studies showed an important finding, showing this along with a normal control can help in understanding the abnormality. An MRI image can provide a helpful two-dimensional view of a finding. Three-dimensional (3D) MRI imaging during pregnancy can help to visualize the extent of an abnormality.

For explaining heart defects, cardiologists have effectively used plastic models. Vivid diagrams are now available at several web sites, such as www.Nemours. org and www.KUMC.org.

The potential sources of information should be noted:

databases e.g. POSSUM (www.possum.net.au)
articles
books
abstracts

Online Mendelian Inheritance in Man (41) (http://www.3.ncbi.nlm.nih.gov/omim)
GeneTests & GeneClinics (www.genetests.org)

DISCUSSING THE CURRENT DIAGNOSIS OR DIAGNOSTIC POSSIBILITIES

One of the many difficulties for the parents and other relatives of a newborn infant with malformations (or other medical problems) is the time needed sometimes to establish the cause, the reason, the etiology of the problem. They ask: Isn't there a definitive test or a definitive opinion from an experienced clinician? It is difficult to have the findings tentative or the diagnosis to change as the results of additional tests become available.

Family meetings are helpful where the major findings and the interpretations of the principal consultants are reviewed. There should be a facilitator to coordinate the discussion. These are issues to consider for these discussions.

a) The setting: Is there enough space for each essential person to attend?
b) Who should be present: Invite everyone whom the parents wish to be present, including trusted friends of the family or grandparents or a minister.

    The medical team should include: the nurses who are daily care providers, nurse manager, social worker, residents, fellows, students involved, and the staff attending. The consultants who have been relied upon in establishing the diagnosis and prognosis should be there also.
c) How long should the meeting be? Allow enough time for the members of the family to ask their questions. Be realistic in the time commitment expected of consultants.
d) The discussion: Review the findings to date. Present the current thinking about the underlying problem. Outline the results which are pending, and explain why any conclusion is tentative.
e) Visual aides: Use whatever is essential to the diagnosis, such as diagram of a heart abnormality, or a karyotype to show the abnormality or a radiograph or other image to describe a finding.
f) The summing up:
    i)   outline the current findings and interpretations, including any differences of opinion;
    ii) describe when new information is expected and how this will be conveyed to the parents and by whom;
    iii) set the next meeting time.

COUNSELING

In addition to presenting the current diagnosis, there are related issues to anticipate or to bring up:

Guilt and Anger: The Reaction to the Birth of a Malformed Infant

Whether the diagnosis is made in the delivery room or during pregnancy, the parents describe it as a tough time. There is guilt over possibly having caused their infant's abnormality. This is particularly strong in those situations in which the parent has the same deformity or the mother is an insulin-dependent diabetic or the mother took a drug recommended to treat a medical condition.

The challenge for the clinicians, the nurses, and the physicians is to help identify these strains and make them realistic. If the mother is blaming herself for an exposure that is not realistic, this should be addressed thoroughly and repeatedly. It may help to review with the entire family the evidence against the exposure she blames for the problem.

When the parents appear to be overwhelmed with guilt, be supportive. This is a common reaction (42). Try to help them, slowly, to move on to discussions of the care of their infant.

Anger can also be a strong emotion in this reaction. If you have the opportunity, discuss with the angry parent whatever they are angry about. Sometimes the open discussion and recognition that they are angry helps to clarify the issues and decrease the intensity.

Whatever the parent's response, work with the team of nurses, social workers, and physicians to develop a coordinated response to help the family cope.

The negative family history can also provide false reassurance. For example, in evaluating a child with a cleft palate in association with lip pits, an apparent example of a new mutation for the autosomal dominant Van der Woude Syndrome (MIM #119300), we learned that the father had his lip pits removed as a teenager. Unfortunately, the plastic surgeon who removed the lip pits did not recognize their potential genetic significance.

The negative family history for an infant with a "genetic" abnormality

When dealing with a birth defect that is attributed to an underlying genetic abnormality, point out that most genetic conditions in newborn infants occur as a complete surprise to healthy, unaffected parents. Initiate this discussion, rather than waiting for parents (or grandparents) to ask. If they understand why the family history is often negative for an infant with a genetic disorder, this can help the family to accept the diagnosis. In this discussion, it can help to show an example of autosomal recessive inheritance (Figure 1-9), with the affected relatives typically in only one generation for a rare mutation and with no consanguinity. In illustrating autosomal dominant inheritance, show the occurrence in a previous generation of the presumed spontaneous mutation (Figure 1-10A).

Environmental Exposures

Usually the mother will have reviewed and re-reviewed all events during the pregnancy, often assuming that something she (or her infant's father) did "caused" her infant's malformation. Sometimes she is correct, but more often there is no scientific basis to attribute her infant's malformation to the inadvertent exposure(s) that occurred. Her concerns should be addressed thoroughly, possibly at a separate meeting. Bring to that meeting any clearly written documentation, if available, such as a reprint or pages from Friedman and Polifka's reference book, Teratogenic Effects of Drugs: A Resource for Clinicians (TERIS) [3] or the pages from the online database Reprotox (2). This effort shows her that you have heard her concerns and have searched for relevant information. Negative findings from systematic studies of the same exposure can help her to accept your statement that her exposures are not related to her infant's malformation.

Reliable sources, such as TERIS, Reprotox, and Shepard's Catalog of Teratogenic Agents (43) are essential for these discussions of potential environmental causes. Make sure your hospital subscribes to the MICROMEDIX Software, which includes the on-line TERIS (1), Reprotox (2) and Shepard's Catalog (43).

Other Sources: INTERNET, TV Shows and Friends

The parents of a malformed infant are eager to learn more about that abnormality. Many consult the Internet and obtain printouts of many related and unrelated medical articles that can cause more confusion than insight. They may receive unrequested comments from neighbors or acquaintances who report information they recall from a recent television program. Whatever the source, this new information should be reviewed respectfully in your discussions.

Encourage them to learn more about any relevant parent support group (44). These groups can provide very helpful information and valuable support.

FOLLOW-UP DISCUSSIONS

a) review all findings to date and their ramifications;
b) describe the role of second opinions; offer to facilitate these and to provide copies of crucial findings;
c) if the infant has a specific diagnosis, start the discussion of what is known about the natural history; tell the parents about the family support organizations available for that disorder.
d) provide reading material, if requested and available;
e) offer contacts with support groups (provide Web site and contact person) or another family with a similarly affected infant who has offered to talk to the parents (and whom you consider a reliable and accurate source of information);
f) start the process of discussing plans for meetings after discharge;
g) if the infant's condition is terminal, it is important to discuss the options they will have. Include in this a discussion of the value of a postmortem examination. Explain the potential added value of the autopsy. It may help to review another family's situation in which the postmortem changed the primary diagnosis and related options and changed significantly the parents' risks in future pregnancies.

REFERENCES

1. Friedman JM, Polifka JE. *Teratogenic effects of drugs: a resource for clinicians (TERIS)* 12th ed. Baltimore, MD: The Johns Hopkins University Press; 2000.
2. Scialli AR, Lione A, Boyle Palgett GK. *Reproductive Effects of Chemical, Physical, and Biologic Agents.* Baltimore, MD: The Johns Hopkins University Press; 1995. http://reprotox.org.
3. Friedman JM, Little BB, Brent RL, Cordero JF, Hanson JW, Shepard TH. Potential human teratogenicity of frequently prescribed drugs. *Obstet Gynecol.* 1990;75:594–599.
4. Lo WY, Friedman JM. Teratogenicity of recently introduced medications in human pregnancy. *Obstet Gynecol.* 2001;100: 465–473.
5. Mitchell AA, Cottler LB, Shapiro, S. Effect of questionnaire design on recall of drug exposure in pregnancy. *Am J Epidemiol.* 1986;123:670–676.
6. Graham JM Jr. *Smith's Recognizable Patterns of Human Deformation.* 3rd ed. Philadelphia: W.B. Saunders Company; 2007.
7. Stephens TD. Muscle abnormalities associated with the twin reversed-arterial-perfusion (TRAP) sequence (Acardia). *Teratology.* 1984;30:311–318.
8. Mastroiacovo P, Castilla EE, Arpino C, Botting B, Cocchi G, Gonjard J, Marinacci C, Merlob P, Metneki J, Mutchinick O, Ritvanen A, Rosano A. Congenital malformations in twins: an international study. *Am J Med Gen.* 1999;85:117–124.
9. Stevenson RE, Kelly JC, Aylesworth AS, Phelan MC. Vascular basis for neural tube defects: a hypothesis. *Pediatrics.* 1987; 80:102–106.
10. Keppler-Noreuil KM. OEIS Complex (omphalocele-exstrophy-imperforate anus-spinal defects): a review of 14 cases. *Amer J Med Genetics.* 2001;99:271–279.
11a. Schinzel AAGL, Smith DW, Miller JR. Monozygotic twinning and structural defects. *J Pediatric.* 1979;95:921–930.
11b. Trasler JM, Doerksen T. Teratogen Update: Paternal exposures—reproductive risks. *Teratology.* 1999;60:161–172.
12. Brackley KJ, Kilby MD, Morton J, Whittle MJ, Knight SJ, Flint J. A case of recurrent fetal anomalies associated with a familial subtelomeric translocation. *Prenatal Diagnosis.* 1999;19:570–574.
13. Hall JG, Gripp KW, Slavotinek AM, Allanson JE. *Handbook of Normal Physical Measurements.* 2nd ed. New York: Oxford University Press; 2007.
14. Raymond GV, Holmes LB. Head circumference standards in neonates. *J Child Neurol.* 1994;9:63–66.
15. Lubchenko LO, Hansman C, Boyd E. Intrauterine growth in length and head circumference as estimated from live births at gestational ages from 26 to 42 weeks. *Pediatrics.* 1966;37: 403–408.

16. Aase JM. *Diagnostic Dysmorphology.* New York: Kluwer Academic/Plenum Publishers; 1990.

17. Arbour L, Watters GV, Hall JG, Fraser FC. Multifactorial inheritance of non-syndromic macrocephaly. *Clin Genet.* 1996;60:57–62.

18. Cordero JF, Holmes LB. Phenotypic overlap of the BBB and G syndromes. *Am J Med Genet.* 1978;2:145–152.

19. Roodhooft AM, Birnholz JC, Holmes LB. Familial nature of congenital absence and severe dysgenesis of both kidneys. *N Engl J Med.* 1984;310:1341–1345.

20. Hootnick D, Boyd NA, Fixsen JA, Lloyd-Roberts GC. The natural history and management of congenital short tibia with dysplasia or absence of the fibula. *J Bone J Surg.* 1977;59-B: 267–271.

21. Huang T, Korson M, Krauss C, Holmes LB. Brief clinical report: four cases with hypoplastic thumbs and encephaloceles. *Am J Med Gen.* 2001;111:178–181.

22. Sillence DO, Ritchie HE, Selby PB. Skeletal anomalies in mice with cleidocranial dysplasia. *Am J Med Genet.* 1987;27: 75–85.

23. Sandham A. Cervical vertebral anomalies in cleft lip and palate. *Cleft Palate J.* 1986;23:206–214.

24. Nopoulos P, Berg S, Van Denmark D, Richman L, Canady J, Andreasen NC. Increased evidence of a midline brain anomaly in subjects with nonsyndromic clefts of the lip and/or palate. *J. Neuroimaging.* 2001;11:418–424.

25. Nopoulos P, Berg S, Canady J, Richman L, Van Denmark D, Andreasen NC. Structural brain abnormalities in adult males with clefts of the lip and/or palate. *Genet Med.* 2002;4:1–9.

26. Nopoulos P, Berg S, VanDemark D, Richman L, Canady J, Andreasen NC. Cognitive dysfunction in adult males with non-syndromic clefts of the lip and/or palate. *Neuropsychologia.* 2002;40:2178–2184.

27. Cheung SW, Shaw CA, Scott DA, Patel A, Sahoo T, Bacino CA et al. Microarray-based CGH detects chromosomal mosaicism not revealed by conventional cytogenetics. *Am J Mol Genet.* 2007;Part A 143A:1679–1686.

28. Wyszynski DF, Nambisan M, Surve T, Alsdorf RM, Smith CR, Holmes LB. Increased rate of major malformations in offspring exposed to valproate during pregnancy. *Neurology.* 2005;69: 961–965.

29. St Charles S, DiMario FJ Jr, Grunnet ML. Möbius sequence: further in vivo support for the Subclavian Artery Supply Disruption Sequence. *Am J Med Genet.* 1993;47:289–293.

30. Fraser FL. Evolution of a palatable multifactorial threshold model (The William Allan Memorial Award Address). *Am J Hum Genet.* 1986;32:796–813.

31. Conneally PM. The complexity of complex diseases. *Am J Hum Genet.* 2003;72:229–232.

32. Passarge E. Dissecting Hirschsprung disease. *Nature Genetics.* 2002;31:11–12.

33. Ming JE, Muenke M. Multiple hits during early embryonic development: digenic diseases and holoprosencephaly. *Am J Hum Genet.* 2002;71:1017–1032.

34. Katsanis N, Ansley SJ, Badano JL, Eichers ER, Lewis RA, Hoskins BE et al. Triallelic inheritance in Bardet-Biedl Syndrome, a Mendelian recessive disorder. *Science.* 2001;293: 2256–2259.

35. Happle R. Lethal genes surviving by mosaicism: a possible explanation for sporadic birth defects involving the skin. *J Am Acad Dermatol.* 1987;16:899–906.

36. Hyland VJ, Robertson SP, Flanagan S, Savarirayan R, Roscioli T, Masel J, Hayes M, Glass IA. Somatic and germline mosaicism for a R248C missense mutation in FGFR3, resulting in a skeletal dysplasia distinct from thanatophoric dysplasia. *Am J Med Genet.* 2003;120A:157–168.

37. Harvey RP. Patterning the vertebrate heart. *Nature Reviews.* 2002;3:544–556.

38. Elliott HR, Samuels DC, Eden JA, Relton CL, Chinnery PF. Pathogenic mitochondrial DNA mutations are common in the general population. *Am J Hum Gen.* 2008;83:254–260.

39. Schwartz M, Vissing J. Paternal inheritance of mitochondrial DNA. *N Engl J Med.* 2002;347:576–580.

40. de la Chapelle A. Microsatellite instability. *N Engl J Med.* 2003;349:209–211.

41. Boyadjiev SA, Jabs EW. Online Mendelian inheritance in Man (OMIM) as a knowledgebase for human developmental disorders. *Clin Genet.* 2000;57:253–266.

42. Nisell M, Öjmyr-Joelsson M, Frenckner B, Per-Anders R, Christensson K. How a family is affected when a child is born with anorectal malformation. Interviews with three patients and their parents. *J Pediatr Nursing.* 2003;18:423–432.

43. Shepard TH, Lemire RJ. *Catalog of Teratogenic Agents.* 12th ed. Baltimore, MD: The Johns Hopkins University Press; 2007.

44. International Directory of Genetic Advocacy Organizations and Related Resources. Tel: 1-800-336-GENE. www.genetic alliance.org

Chapter 2

Amniotic Bands

Definition

A localized disruption process during fetal development in which structural abnormalities and tissue deficiencies occur in structures that had been formed normally. The abnormalities include the amniotic band limb deformity, limb body wall defects and facial clefts. Associated deficiencies include distal tissue loss, constriction rings, scalp, defects, extra nodules, strands/ bands of tissue and crusted, denuded ends of digits, and syndactyly.

ICD-9:	759.801	(amniotic band sequence)
ICD-10:	Q79.8	(congenital constricting bands)
Mendelian Inheritance in Man:	%217100	(congenital constricting bands)

Historical Note

These phenotypes have been described by several individuals for at least three hundred years, as reported by Schwalbe in 1906 (1) and Keith in 1949 (2). For many years there were two conflicting theories of etiology: 1) the Streeter hypothesis (3) in 1930, in which he postulated that the amniotic bands represented developmental defects that occurred during the formation of the germinal disc; 2) the Torpin hypothesis, espoused in 1965 (4) and 1968 (5), in which he noted the amniotic strands attached to the limbs, head, and mouth and concluded that the tension of the strands produced secondary clefts and deformities. The Torpin hypothesis, i.e., the theory that the bands produced the defects, was prominent until the 1970s and 1980s when other hypotheses, like early

amnion rupture (6) and vascular disruption (7–9), were proposed as the primary underlying etiologic factor. The occurrence of internal anomalies in the affected infants argued against the Torpin hypothesis that the anomalies were caused by a mechanical effect of the bands (10, 11). In a re-analysis of the Streeter hypothesis (12), it was noted that the primary injury occurs prior to 26 days postconception, which would be prior to the existence of embryonic circulation.

More recent hypotheses have noted associated genetic polymorphisms and monogenic conditions (13, 14) in which the genetic abnormalities predispose to the occurrence of the process of vascular disruption. Many terms have been used to refer to this group of phenotypes, including ADAM (amniotic deformity, adhesions and mutilations), amniotic band disruption syndrome, limb body wall complex, amniotic band sequence, congenital constriction band syndrome, and amniotic adhesion malformation syndrome.

Appearance

The types of structural abnormalities produced by vascular disruption are determined by the time in gestation and the severity of the disruptive process. An early disruption has more extensive effects while a disruption during the fetal period will be more localized (7). There are several recognized clinical phenotypes, which could reflect different etiologic mechanisms (15, 16) or a common and broader spectrum of anomalies (17, 18).

a) Amniotic band limb deformity: the deformity of the hand or foot which includes loss of the distal portion of one or more of the central digits (primarily fingers 2, 3, and 4), some degree of syndactyly, often constriction rings and occasionally fibrous strands of tissue on the tip of or encircling one or more fingers (18–20). There can be extrusions or nodules

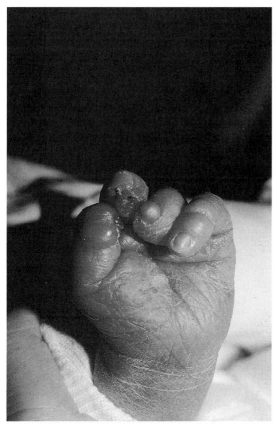

FIGURE 2.1   Affected hand, showing at birth thumb and two fingers tethered together.

of subcutaneous tissue at or near the ends of affected digits (Figures 2-1 & 2-2).

b) Terminal transverse limb deficiency: this appears to be an "amputation" of an arm, leg, or digit, sometimes in association with constriction rings.

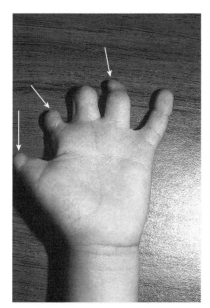

FIGURE 2.2   Hand of same infant after surgery, when older, with constriction rings on thumb, index and fourth fingers.

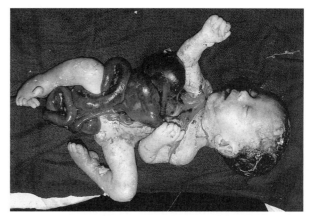

FIGURE 2.3   Limb-body-wall defect, lethal in newborn infant.

Sometimes a deep constriction ring is present on the lower leg in association with a club foot deformity.

c) Limb-body-wall defect (6, 8, 9, 15, 17): there is a ventral defect in the chest and/or abdomen with extrusion of intestines (Figure 2-3). There is a marked curvature of the spine, in association with abnormalities of the ribs and vertebrae. Some affected infants have associated limb deficiencies, preaxial polydactyly (21) [Figure 2-4] and extra bands of skin (22) [Figure 2-5].

d) Brain and facial clefts (6, 8, 9, 16, 23–25): there is absence of portions of the scalp and cranium with abnormal brain development and sometimes adherence to the placenta, disfiguring midfacial clefts and components of the other three phenotypes (Figure 2-6).

e) Subclavian artery supply disruption sequence (26, 27), interruption of the blood supply in the distribution of the subclavian and/or vertebral arteries can produce absence of the pectoralis muscle on the same side (Poland Anomaly), anomalies of cervical vertebrae (Klippel-Feil Syndrome), hypoplasia of cranial nerves (Möebius Syndrome), and terminal limb defects.

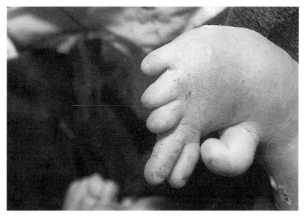

FIGURE 2.4   Preaxial polydactyly of first toe in this infant.

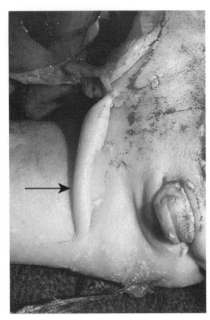

FIGURE 2.5 Extra band (arrow) of tissue on abdomen and upper leg in this infant.

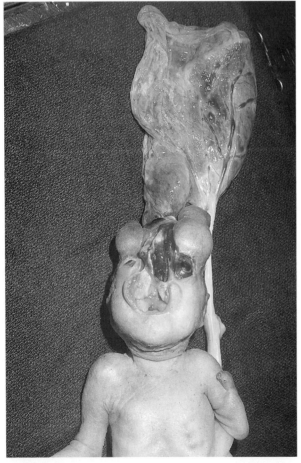

FIGURE 2.6 Severe brain malformations and facial clefts in infant with adherence of brain to placenta. Terminal transverse defect of left arm.

Associated Malformations

The amnion shows a distinctive change in association with amnion rupture: the loss of the layer of epithelial cells (16, 28, 29). The bands are made up of amniotic cells with a fibrous core (30).

No distinctive pattern of associated internal or external anomalies has been identified in infants with the amniotic band limb deformity. However, constriction rings and hypoplasia of digits occurs in either of the phenotypes, as well as anomalies, such as anencephaly (11).

In association with the limb body wall complex, there is a high frequency of anomalies of the heart, diaphragm, kidneys, vertebrae, and limbs (6, 8–12).

With the craniofacial anomalies, many of the facial clefts are atypical in not adhering to the points of tissue fusion in normal embryonic development (16, 24, 25). The more "typical" lateral cleft lip deformity occurs, also (31).

Developmental Defects

Several different hypotheses have been proposed:

a) vascular disruption: a process in which hypoperfusion leads to hypoxia, endothelial cell damage, hemorrhage, and tissue loss (7);
b) mechanical disruption (Torpin hypothesis) [4, 5]:
c) germ disc disruption (Streeter hypothesis) [12];
d) early amnion rupture (6);
e) amnion rupture and adherence of parts of the embryo to the sticky exocoelomic material (30);
f) genetic disruption: genetic factors in the mother and/or the fetus that predispose to defective coagulation or thrombophilia and the consequences of thrombosis and embolization; the specific mutations or polymorphisms have not been identified.

Regarding the severity of the physical abnormalities, the earlier the disruption, such as before 45 days of gestation, the more severe the anatomic defects (6, 25).

An animal model of atypical facial clefts was developed by applying nylon sutures at day 65 of the normal 140-day gestation (32). When the synthetic constricting bands were excised in utero, the repair occurred without scarring.

Knockout mice deficient in the *Tcfap2a* gene, which encodes the AP-2α protein, have a ventral body wall closure defect, suggestive of the thoracoabdominal schisis type of amniotic band deformity (33). Mouse knockouts, deficient for tumor necrosis factor alpha (TNF-α-/-), have excessive amount of apoptosis and craniofacial, trunk and limb reduction anomalies. This is another experimental model of vascular disruption defects (34).

Prevalence

Estimates of the prevalence of the amniotic band syndrome in population-based studies of live born infants have been between 1:5,000 to 1:10,000 (35, 38). A much higher prevalence was identified among 629 stillbirths (1983–1988) in Wisconsin, 0.6 to 1.4% of which were attributed to amnion disruption/limb-body wall disruption (37). Among 1,010 miscarriages (9 to 20 weeks gestation) evaluated in an embryopathology laboratory in Vancouver (1979–1986), 1% were considered to have amnion rupture sequence (36). The distribution of amniotic band phenotypes was: 61% (11/18) had limb constrictions and deficiencies and 39% (7/18) had disruptions of craniofacial-structures and abdominal defects.

A study of all 110 limb reduction defects identified among 161,252 liveborn and stillborn infants and elective terminations for fetal anomalies surveyed at Brigham and Women's Hospital in Boston showed that 0.22 per 1,000 (or 1 in 4,545) had a limb defect that was attributable to the vascular disruption process and 1 in 12,500 had the amniotic band limb deformity (39). This study did not include infants with amniotic band phenotypes without limb reduction defects, so it would be a minimal estimate.

Race/Ethnicity

An increased prevalence of amniotic band defects among infants born to young (less than 20) black multigravida women was noted in Atlanta (1968–1982) in comparison to older, black multigravida women and white women (35). In another study (41) of 73 infants with amniotic rupture sequence and 11 with body wall complex born in 1976 to 1998, the mothers were more likely to be black than non-black.

Birth Status

Many infants with more severe amniotic band phenotypes are born prematurely. An increased frequency among spontaneous abortuses (36) and stillborn infants (24, 37) has been reported.

Sex Ratio

In a population-based study in Atlanta (1968 to 1982), there were more affected female infants (0.14/1,000) than males (0.09/1,000) [35]. In two other population-based studies in Australia (38) and Hungary (19) in the 1980s, there were an equal number of affected males and females.

Sidedness

There was no significant asymmetry among the 134 affected infants identified in a population-based study in Hungary (1975–1984) [20].

Parental Age

A higher frequency of affected infants among mothers less than 20 or 25 years of age has been reported in several studies (35, 38, and 40).

Twinning

In a review of 14 sets of twins in which at least one had the amniotic band syndrome (41), it was noted that all 11 for whom placentation was recorded were monochorionic placentas, suggesting monozygous twinning (MZ). 4 (36%) of the apparent MZ twins were concordant for the amniotic band syndrome deformities. It was suggested, also, that amniotic band syndrome is much more common in MZ than in dizygous twin pregnancies.

Among the identical twin pairs with amniotic band syndrome described in case reports, several have been discordant: 1) in one set (42), the affected infant had absence of the right arm below the elbow; there was an amniotic band on the monochorionic-diamniotic placenta and absence of the amnion on the adjacent chorion; 2) in another set of monochorionic diamniotic twins (43), the affected twin had severe facial clefts, encephalocele, constriction rings, and distal deficiency of one finger; 3) in a third set (44), one twin had absence of the middle fingers on each hand, constriction rings, and clubfoot deformity.

Genetic Factors

Families in which several members have had defects attributable to vascular disruption, but no known etiologic factor, have been reported (45–49).

No molecular testing has been developed to screen for evidence of a genetic predisposition. However, several candidate genes have been identified in studies of limb deficiencies (50, 51) and gastroschisis, an abdominal wall defect attributed to vascular disruption (52). Those candidate genes included: NPPA (atrial natriuretic peptide), ADD1 (alpha adducing1), NOS3 (endothelial nitric oxide synthase), and TNF-α (tumor necrosis factor-alpha).

Environmental Factors

Several exposures during pregnancy have been shown to cause vascular disruption.

a) ergotamine—exposure to one or more doses of this vasoconstricting compound have produced paraplegia, constriction rings, and arthrogryposis (53, 54);
b) misoprostol (prostaglandin E_1 analogue): exposure at 6 to 8 weeks gestation by mouth or by vagina, as an illegal abortifacient, has been associated with the occurrence of amniotic band-type of hand deformities,

amyoplasia, arthrogryposis (often only in the lower half of the body), club foot deformity, cranial nerve deficiency (as in Möebius Syndrome), and occasionally hydrocephalus with water-shed vascular lesions involving the cranial nerve nuclei (55–57);

c) chorionic villus sampling (CVS): this occasional complication of this prenatal diagnosis procedure is more common the earlier in gestation, such as 7 to 8 weeks gestation, is performed (58 59); the distinctive limb defect is absence of the distal portion of the middle finger with tapering and stiffness of this finger and the adjacent 2nd and 4th fingers (60, 61); other effects include:

   i) fusion of two fingers or toes 2-3 with loss of distal structures, syndactyly tissue loss, and constriction rings (62);

   ii) terminal transverse limb defects more often in the hands than in the feet (63);

d) placental trauma (64-66);

e) hypoperfusion, caused by significant, prolonged hypotension during pregnancy;

f) reduction of multiple gestation (67);

g) dilation and curettage (D+C), the operative procedure; the described phenotypes include extensive facial clefts, scalp defects, and brain malformations after the procedure at 6 to 8 weeks of gestation (68); arthrogryposis after the procedure at 8 to 10 weeks of gestation (69).

h) twin-twin embolization after the death of a co-twin in monozygous twin pregnancies (70).

Treatment and Prognosis

Treatments in utero at 23 weeks gestation, using either fetoscopic laser release (71) or an endoscopic surgical release (72), have been successful on arms and legs with decreased perfusion from constriction rings. The surgical repair, after birth, of structures affected by constriction rings often requires a staged release to avoid problems of decreased blood flow (73). In general, the anatomy of the structure is normal, as it had formed normally before the disruptive event occurred (74).

The correction of the oral clefts, syndactyly, and other structural abnormalities is determined on an individual basis.

Genetic Counseling

The first question for the examining clinician is whether the phenotype of the affected infant is consistent with one of the five amniotic band syndrome phenotypes described above. Or, are the features more consistent with those of a rare disorder that shares some of the clinical features, such as constriction rings or tapered, shortened digits with no nail.

Examples are:

a) Adams-Oliver Syndrome (MIM %100300): an autosomal dominant condition that includes terminal transverse limb defects, scalp defects, and often heart defects;

b) Cornelia de Lange Syndrome (MIM #122470): associated with mutation or deletion in the NIPBL protein, whose features include growth restriction, distinctive facial features, absence of digits, hirsutism, and mental retardation;

c) Patterson-Stevenson-Fontaine Syndrome: an autosomal dominant disorder, whose features include hypoplastic toes, malar hypoplasia, and hearing loss (75);

d) Verloes-Koulischer-Oro-Acral Syndrome: absence of premaxillary teeth and gum, reduced or absent toes, some with constriction rings (76);

e) The phenotype of cleft lip and palate, amniotic bands, and polydactyly (77).

Each rare genetic disorder will have its own empiric recurrence risk in the sibling or offspring of an affected individual.

If the infant has the phenotype of one of the more common types of amniotic band syndrome, there is a very low likelihood of a recurrence in a subsequent sib or offspring of the affected individual. A few instances of affected siblings or close relatives have been reported (45-48). In one of the few analyses of a large number of relatives of 134 index cases with amniotic band syndrome, none (0%) of the 415 first-degree relatives was affected (19).

The accuracy of prenatal screening by ultrasound in confirming the absence of the features of amniotic band syndrome has not been established. Band structures can be identified during pregnancy without the occurrence of the amniotic band syndrome in the "exposed" fetus (78). A diagnosis of anencephaly prenatally by ultrasound can be shown at autopsy to be cranial destruction secondary to amniotic bands, with significantly different consequences in genetic counseling, including no established benefit from periconceptional folic acid supplementation and a much lower empiric recurrence risk.

REFERENCES

1. Schwalbe E. Allgemeine Missbildungslehre (Teratologie). Eine Einführung in das Studium der abnormen Entwick lung. In: Schwalbe E, (ed.). *Die Morphologie der Missbildungen des Menschen under der Tiere. Teil I.* Gena: Fischer; 1906.

2. Keith A. Concerning the origins and nature of certain malformation of the face, head, and foot. *Brit J Surg.* 1940;28:173–192.

3. Streeter GL. Focal deficiencies in fetal tissues and their relation to intrauterine amputation. *Contrib Embryol Carnegie Inst.* 1930; 22:1–44.

4. Torpin R. Amniochorionic mesoblastic fibrous strings and amniotic bands: Associated constricting fetal malformations of fetal death. *Am J Obstet Gynecol.* 1965;91: 65–75.

5. Torpin R. *Fetal Malformations Caused by Amnion Rupture during Gestation*. Springfield, IL: CC Thomas, 1968.

6. Higginbottom MC, Jones KL, Hall BD, Smith DW. The amniotic band disruption complex: timing of amniotic rupture and variable spectra of consequent defects. *J Pediatr*. 1979;95:544–549.

7. Van Allen MI. Structural anomalies resulting from vascular disruption. *Pediatr Clin N Amer*. 1992;39(2):255–277.

8. Van Allen MI, Curry C, Gallagher L. Limb body wall complex. I. Pathogenesis. *Am J Med Genet*. 1987;28:529–548.

9. Van Allen MI, Curry C, Walden CE, Gallagher L, Patten RM. Limb body wall complex. II. Limb and spine defects. *Am J Med Genet*. 1987;28:549–565.

10. Pagon RA, Stephens TD, McGillivray B, Siebert JR, Wright VJ, Hsu LL, Poland BJ, Emanuel I, Hall JG. Body wall defects with reduction limb anomalies: a report of fifteen cases. *Birth Defects*. 1979; Original Article Series XV (5A):171–185.

11. Hunter AGW, Carpenter BF. Implications of malformations not due to amniotic bands in the amniotic band sequence. *Am J Med Genet*. 1986;24:691–700.

12. Bamforth JS. Amniotic band sequence: Streeter's hypothesis reexamined. *Am J Med Genet*. 1992;44:280–287.

13. Robin NH, Abbadi N, McCandless SE, Nadeau JH. Disorganization in mice and humans and its relation to sporadic birth defects. *Am J Med Genet*. 1997;73:425–436.

14. Lee YM, Jeong C-H, Koo S-Y, Son MJ, Song HS, Bae S-K, Raleigh JA, Chung H-Y, Yoo M-A, Kim K-W. Determination of hypoxic region by hypoxia marker in developing mouse embryos in vivo: a possible signal for vessel development. *Developmental Dynamics*. 2001;220:175–186.

15. Moerman P, Fryns J-P, Vandenberghe K, Lauweryns JM. Constrictive amniotic bands, amniotic adhesions and limb body wall complex: discrete disruption sequences with pathogenetic overlap. *Am J Med Genet*. 1992;42:470–479.

16. Martinez-Frias ML, Bermejo E, Rodriguez-Padilla E. Body stalk defects, body wall defects, amniotic bands with and without body wall defects, and gastroschisis: Comparative epidemiology. *Am J Med Genet*. 2000;92:13–18.

17. Vanthay L, Mazzitelli N, Rittler M. Patterns of severe abdominal wall defects: Insights into pathogenesis, delineation, and nomenclature. *Birth Def Res (Part A): Clin Mol Teratol*. 2007;79: 211–220.

18. Light TR, Ogden JA. Congenital constriction band syndrome: pathophysiology and treatment. *Yale J Biol Med*. 1993;66: 143–155.

19. Czeizel AE, Vitéz M, Kodaj I, Lenz W. Study of isolated apparent amniogenic limb deficiency in Hungary, 1975–1984. *Am J Med Genet*. 1993;46:372–378.

20. Ribeiro MG, Castilla EE, Orioli IM. Can amputated digits point to clues about etiology? *Am J Med Genet*. 2004;128A:93–94.

21. Graham JM Jr, Higginbottom, MC, Smith DW. Preaxial polydactyly of the foot associated with early amnion rupture: evidence for mechanical teratogenesis? *J Pediatr*. 1981;98:943–945.

22. Nakamura K, Nanjyo B. Congenital skin tube pedicle associated with the constriction band syndrome. *Plast Reconstr Surg*. 1992;89:746–750.

23. Jones KL, Smith DW, Hall BD, Hall JG, Ebbin AJ, Massoud H, Golbus MS. A pattern of craniofacial and limb defects secondary to aberrant tissue bands. *J Pediatr*. 1974;84:90–95.

24. Keller H, Neuhauser G, Durkin-Stamm, MV, Kaveggia EG, Schaaff A, Sitzmann F. "ADAM" Complex (amniotic deformity, adhesions, mutilations) – a pattern of craniofacial and limb defects. *Am J Med Genet*. 1978;2:81–98.

25. Eppley BL, David L, Li M, Moore CA, Sadove AM. Amniotic band facies. *J Craniofac Surg*. 1998;9:360–365.

26. Bavinck JN, Weaver DD. Subclavian artery supply disruption sequence: hypothesis of a vascular etiology for Poland, Klippel-Feil and Möbius anomalies. *Am J Med Genet*. 1986;23:903–918.

27. St. Charles S, DiMarco FJ Jr, Grunnet ML. Möbius Sequence: further in vivo support for the subclavian artery supply disruption sequence. *Am J Med Genet*. 1993;47:289–293.

28. Herva R, Karkinen-Jääskeläinen M. Amniotic adhesion malformation syndrome: fetal and placental pathology. *Teratology*. 1984;29:11–19.

29. Genest DR, DiSalvo D, Rosenblatt M-J, Holmes LB. Terminal transverse limb defects with tethering and omphalocele in a 17 week fetus following first trimester misoprostol exposure. *Clin Dysmorph*. 1999;8:53–58.

30. Shepard TH. Amniotic bands and exocelomic stickiness. *Birth Def Res (part A): Clin Mol Teratol*. 2004;70:153.

31. Taub PJ, Bradley JP, Setoguchi Y, Schimmenti L, Kawamoto HK Jr. Typical facial clefting and constriction band anomalies: an unusual association in three unrelated patients. *Am J Med Genet*. 2003;120A:256–260.

32. Stelnicki EJ, Hoffman W, Foster R, Lopoo J, Longaker M. The *in utero* repair of Tessier Number 7 lateral facial clefts created by amniotic band-like compression. *J Craniofacial Surg*. 1998;9: 557–563.

33. Schorle H, Meier P, Buchert M, Jaemisch R, Mitchell PJ. Transcription factor AP-2 essential for cranial closure and craniofacial development. *Nature*. 1996;381:235–238.

34. Torchinsky A, Shepshelovich J, Orenstein H, Zaslavsky Z, Savion S, Carp H et al. TNF-α protects embryos exposed to developmental toxicants. *Am J Reprod Immunol*. 2003;49: 159–168.

35. Garza A, Cordero JF, Mulinare J. Epidemiology of the early amnion rupture spectrum of defects. *Am J Dis Child*. 1988;142: 541–544.

36. Kalousek DK, Bamforth S. Amnion rupture sequence in previable fetuses. *Am J Med Genet*. 1988;31:63–73.

37. Luebke HJ, Reiser CA, Pauli RM. Fetal disruptions: assessment of frequency, heterogeneity, and embryologic mechanisms in a population referred to a community-based stillbirth assessment program. *Am J Med Genet*. 1990;36:56–72.

38. Bower C, Norwood F, Knowles S, Chambers H, Haan E, Chan A. Amniotic band syndrome: a population-based study in two Australian states. *Paed Perinatal Epidemiol*. 1993;7: 395–403.

39. McGuirk CK, Westgate M-N, Holmes LB. Limb deficiencies in newborn infants. *Pediatrics*. 2001;108:e64–71 (http://www. pediatrics.org/cgi/content/full/108/4/e64).

40. Werler MM, Louik C, Mitchell AA. Epidemiologic analysis of maternal factors and amniotic band defects. *Birth Defects Res (Part A): Clin Mol Teratol*. 2003;67:68–72.

41. Lockwood C, Ghidini A, Romero R. Amniotic band syndrome in monozygotic twins: prenatal diagnosis and pathogenesis. *Obstet Gynecol*. 1988;71:1012–1016.

42. Kancherla PL, Untawale VG, Gabriel JB, Chauhan PM. Intrauterine amputation in one monozygotic twin associated with amniotic band: a case report. *Am J Ob Gyn*. 1981;140: 347–348.

43. Donnenfeld AE, Dunn LK, Rose NC. Discordant amniotic band sequence in monozygotic twins. *Am J Med Genet*. 1985;20: 685–694.

44. Métneki J, Czeizel AE, Evans JA. Congenital limb reduction defects in twins. *Eur J Pediatr*. 1996;155:483–490.

45. Etches PC, Stewart AR, Ives EJ. Familial congenital amputations. *J Pediatr*. 1982;101:448–449.

46. Lubinsky M, Sujansky E, Sanger W, Salyards P, Severn C. Familial amniotic bands. *Am J Med Genet*. 1983;14:81–87.

47. Soltan HC, Holmes LB. Familial occurrence of malformations possibly attributable to vascular abnormalities. *J Pediatr*. 1986; 108:112–114.

48. Hennekam RC, Hofstee N. Familial liability to intrauterine vascular impairments. *Pediatrics*. 1990;86:326–327.

49. Levy R, Lacombe D, Rougier Y, Camus E. Limb body wall complex and amniotic band sequence in situ. *Am J Med Genet.* 2007;Part A 143A:2682–2687.

50. Hunter AG. A pilot study of the possible role of familial defects in anticoagulation as a cause for terminal limb reduction malformations. *Clin Genet.* 2000;57:197–204.

51. Carmichael SL, Shaw GM, Iovannisci DM, Yang W, Finnell RH, Cheng S, Lammer EJ. Risks of human limb deficiency anomalies associated with 29 SNPs of genes involved in homocysteine metabolism, coagulation cell-cell interactions, inflammatory response, and blood pressure regulation. *Am J Med Genet.* 2006;Part A 140A:2433–2440.

52. Torfs CP, Christianson RE, Iovanisci DM, Shaw GM, Lammer EJ. Selected gene polymorphisms and the interaction with maternal smoking, as risk factors of gastroschisis. *Birth Def Res (Part A): Clin Mol Teratol.* 2006;76:723–730.

53. Verloes A, Emonts P, Dubois M, Rigo J, Senterre J. Paraplegia and arthrogryposis multiplex of the lower extremities after intrauterine exposure to ergotamine. *J Med Genet.* 1990;27:213–214.

54. Raymond GV. Teratogen update: ergot and ergotamine. *Teratology.* 1995;51:344–347.

55. Gonzalez CH, Marques-Dias M-J, Kim CA, Sugayama SMM, DaPaz JA, Huson SM, Holmes LB. Congenital abnormalities in Brazilian children associated with misoprostol misuse in first trimester of pregnancy. *Lancet.* 1998;351:1624–1627.

56. Pastuszak AL, Schüler L, Speck-Martins CE, Coelho K-EFA, Cordello SM, Vargas F, Brunoni D, Schwarz IVD, Larran da buru M, Safattle H, Meloni VFA, Koren G. Use of misoprostol during pregnancy and Möbius Syndrome in infants. *N Engl J Med.* 1998;338:1881–1885.

57. Marques-Dias MJ, Gonzalez CH, Rosemberg S. Möbius sequence in children exposed *in utero* to misoprostol: neuropathological study of three cases. *Birth Def Res (Part A): Clin Mol Teratol.* 2003;67:1002–1007.

58. Firth HV, Boyd PA, Chamberlain P, MacKenzie IZ, Lindenbaum RH, Huson SM. Severe limb abnormalities after chorion villus sampling at 56-66 days' gestation. *Lancet.* 1991;337:762–763.

59. Botto LD, Olney RS, Mastroiacovo P, et al. Chorionic villus sampling and transverse digital deficiencies: evidence for anatomic and gestational-age specificity of the digital deficiencies in two studies. *Am J Med Genet.* 1996;62:173–178.

60. Burton BK, Schulz CJ, Burd LI. Spectrum of limb disruption defects associated with chorionic villus sampling. *Pediatrics.* 1993;91:989–993.

61. Golden CM, Ryan LM, Holmes LB. Chorionic villus sampling: a distinctive teratogenic effect on fingers? *Birth Def Res (Part A): Clin Mol Teratol.* 2003;67:557–562.

62. Planteydt HT, van de Vooren MJ, Verweij H. Amniotic bands and malformations in child born after pregnancy screened by chorionic villus biopsy. *Lancet.* 1986;ii:756–757.

63. Los FJ, Brandenburg H, Niermeijer MF. Vascular disruptive syndromes after exposure to misoprostol or chorionic villus sampling. *Lancet.* 1999;353:843–844.

64. Ossipoff V, Hall BD. Etiologic factors in the amniotic band syndrome: a study of 24 patients. *Birth Defects: Original Article Series XIII.* 1977;(3D):117–132.

65. Viljoen DL. Porencephaly and transverse limb defects following severe maternal trauma in early pregnancy. *Clin Dysmorph.* 1995;4:75–78.

66. Webster WS, Lipson AH, Brown-Woodman PD. Uterine trauma and limb defects. *Teratology.* 1987;35:253–260.

67. Roze JM, Tschupp MJ, Arvis PL, et al. Interruption selective de grossesses et malformations embryonnaires des extremites. *J Gynecol Obstet Biol Reprod.* 1989;18:673–677.

68. Holmes LB. Possible fetal effects of cervical dilation and uterine curettage during the first trimester of pregnancy. *J Pediatr.* 1995;126:131–134.

69. Hall JG. Arthrogryposis associated with unsuccessful attempts at termination of pregnancy. *Am J Med Genet.* 1996;63:293–300.

70. VanAllen MI, Siegel-Bartelt J, Dixon J, Zuker RM, Clarke HM, Toi A. Constriction bands and limb reduction defects in two newborns with fetal ultrasound evidence for vascular disruption. *Am J Med Genet.* 1992;44:598–604.

71. Keswani SG, Johnson MP, Adzick NS, Hori S, et al. In utero limb salvage: fetoscopic release of amniotic bands for threatened limb amputation. *J Pediatr Surg.* 2003;38:848–851.

72. Ronderos-Dumit D, Briceño F, Navarro H, Sanchez N. Endoscopic release of limb constriction rings in utero. *Fetal Diagn Ther.* 2006;21:256–258.

73. Light TR, Ogden JA. Congenital constriction band syndrome pathophysiology and treatment. *Yale J Biol Med.* 1993;66:143–155.

74. Upton J III. Management disorders of Separation—Syndactyly. In: Mathes SJ (ed.), Henz VR (ed., Hand Surgery Volumes). *Plastic Surgery*, 2nd ed., vol. VIII, *The Hand and Upper Limb*, Part 2. Saunders Elsevier; 2006: chap. 204, 139–150.

75. Wilkie AOM, Goodacre TEE. Patterson-Stevenson-Fontaine Syndrome: a 30-year follow-up and clinical details of a further affected case. *Am J Med Genet.* 1997;69:433–434.

76. da Silva DC, Verloes A. Further delineation of the Verloes-Koulischer-Oro-Acral Syndrome. *Am J Med Genet.* 1998;80:535–537.

77. Robin NH, Franklin J, Prucka S, Ryan AB, Grant AH. Clefting, amniotic bands, and polydactyly: a distinct phenotype that supports an intrinsic mechanism for amniotic band sequence. *Am J Med Genet.* 2005;137A:298–301.

78. Mahony BS, Filly RA, Collen PW, Golbus MS. The amniotic band syndrome: antenatal sonographic diagnosis and potential pitfalls. *Am J Obst Gynecol.* 1985;152:63–68.

Chapter 3

Bowel Atresias

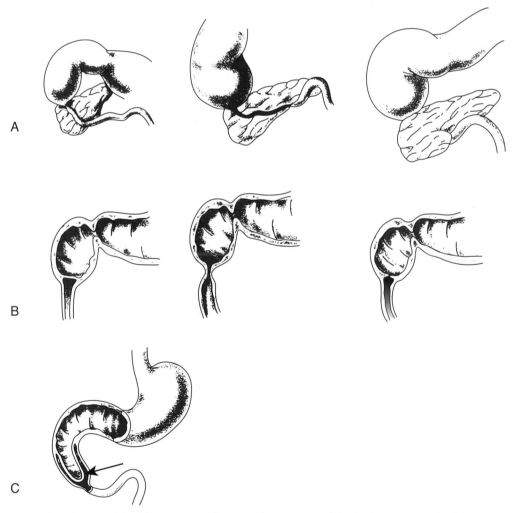

FIGURE 3.1   Diagram of the different causes of congenital obstruction of the duodenum. A: atresia of duodenum at level of pancreas. B: incomplete obstruction. C: obstruction by thin web (arrow), referred to as "windsock". (From Millar AIW et al. In: Ashcraft KW, Holcomb GW, Murphy JP, eds. *Pediatric Surgery* 4th ed. Philadelphia: Elsevier Saunders; 2005: 418.)

DUODENAL ATRESIA

Definition

Atresia of the small intestine at the level of the duodenum is one of the causes of congenital duodenal obstruction. The other causes are duodenal stenosis and obstruction by a membrane or diaphragm.

ICD-9:	751.100	(stenosis or absence of duodenum)
ICD-10:	Q41	(congenital absence, atresia and stenosis of duodenum)
Mendelian Inheritance in Man:	223400	(duodenal atresia)

Appearance

In a review of 503 infants with congenital duodenal obstruction (1957–1967) [1], 49% had duodenal atresia, 41% a diaphragm or membrane, and 10% stenosis. The relative frequencies of the different types of duodenal obstruction have been confirmed and extended in several subsequent case series (2–8). The atresia is most often (80%) in the second part of the duodenum distal to the duodenal papilla (8–10). Three types of congenital duodenal obstruction have been delineated (Figure 3-1):

1) type I, the duodenum is obstructed completely by a membrane or partially by a fenestrated membrane; there can also be an apparent obstruction by a "windsock" membrane; 2) in type II, there is a fibrous cord that connects the dilated proximal of the duodenum and the distal segment; 3) in type III, there is complete discontinuity or a gap between the proximal and distal segments of the duodenum.

Membranous duodenal stenosis is usually located in the first or second part of the duodenum and not distal to the ampulla of Vater. This condition is diagnosed later than duodenal atresia. The symptoms of duodenal stenosis after birth are vomiting and failure to thrive, but not bile-stained vomiting (11, 12). The residual barrier may be incomplete, which affects the pattern of the symptoms. The orifice in the duodenal membrane can be a single central, eccentric orifice or multiple orifices with varying size.

Associated Malformations

Half of the infants with duodenal atresia have associated abnormalities, such as malrotation, other bowel atresias, i.e., esophageal atresia and imperforate anus, heart defects, anomalies of the bile ducts, annular pancreas, and Down Syndrome. In the series of 118 infants in Cape Town, South Africa (8), 32% had Down Syndrome, 16% had heart defects, 7% had esophageal and anorectal anomalies.

In a case series of 103 infants in Indianapolis (1972–1997) [13], 54% had associated anomalies, including heart defects in 35%, Down Syndrome in 31%, malrotation in 37%, annular pancreas in 37%, anterior portal vein in 4%, and a second web in 3%. The anomalous biliary ducts provide communication between the proximal and distal segments of the duodenum (14), and, thereby, air will be present in the distal bowel. This can delay the recognition of duodenal atresia as the primary abnormality.

Infants with duodenal atresia often have anomalies of the bile and pancreatic ducts. The abnormalities include stenosis of the common bile duct, abnormal branching of the biliary tree, ectopic orifices, biliary atresia, agenesis of the gall bladder, and choledochal cysts (14, 15).

Malrotation of the midgut occurred in 11% of 17 patients in one series (16). However, it was not possible to detect accurately the presence of malrotation by upper gastrointestinal barium study.

In one case series (17), subglottic stenosis occurred in one (1) of 120 infants with duodenal atresia. In one of two brothers with duodenal atresia, one had a small glottis and larynx, which made intubation difficult and was associated with postoperative studies.

The association of duodenal atresia with Down Syndrome is well established. About 30% of individuals with duodenal atresia have Down syndrome; 5% of individuals with Down syndrome have duodenal atresia. In a survey of 2,894 infants with Down Syndrome in comparison to 2,490,437 births, the rate of occurrence of duodenal atresia was 46/1,000 in the infants with Down Syndrome in comparison to 0.17/1,000 in the unaffected children. This difference was a Risk Ratio of 264.9 (18). The risk ratio for annular pancreas among the infants with Down Syndrome in comparison to unaffected children was even higher, 430.3.

Developmental Defect

The duodenum begins to develop from the foregut and the midgut in the fourth week post fertilization. The junction of the two parts of the duodenum is just distal to the origin of the common bile duct. During the fifth to seventh weeks, the lumen is obliterated temporarily by the proliferation of its epithelial cells. The duodenum is recanalized by a coalescence of vacuoles by the end of the embryonic period (19, 20).

Duodenal atresia and stenosis have been attributed to a failure of recanalization of the duodenum. The duodenal diaphragm has been considered due to incomplete recanalization of the duodenum, and, thereby, a mild form of atresia (21).

The annular pancreas develops because of a failure of the normal process of emigration of the ventral pancreas and bile duct to the area behind the duodenum. This leaves pancreas tissue encircling the second portion of the duodenum as a nondistensible ring, which produces obstruction (9).

Gene knockout studies of the gene fibroblast growth factor receptor 2b (Fgfr2b) have produced in the developing mouse fetuses a range of duodenal changes from atresia to a mucosal web to normal (22). This is an experimental model of autosomal recessive duodenal atresia.

Prevalence

The prevalence of duodenal atresia in population-based studies was 0.13/1,000 in Hawaii (1986–2000) [7] and 0.11/1,000 in Central-East France (1976–1992) [4].

Race/Ethnicity

In the multiracial Hawaii islands, there were no significant differences in the rate of occurrence of duodenal atresia among infants of Caucasian and Asian ethnicity (7). In Atlanta in the Metropolitan Atlanta Congenital Defects Program (1968–1989), the prevalence rate for white singletons was 0.11/1,000 and 0.13/1,000 for black singletons (23). No differences were identified in the prevalence rates for duodenal atresia between non-Hispanic Caucasians and Vietnamese in California (24).

Birth Status

An increased frequency of both premature birth and low birth weight has been observed for infants with duodenal atresia (4, 13) and in infants with duodenal obstruction caused by duodenal membranes (12). 45% of 103 affected infants evaluated in Indianapolis (1972–1991) were born prematurely (13). In central-east France, 35% of the affected infants were born before 37 weeks gestational age (4); birth weight was less than 2,500 grams in 60% of the 69 infants with duodenal atresia.

Sex Ratio

Several case series have shown an excess of females among infants with congenital duodenal atresia and stenosis: 53% of the 503 infants born in 65 hospitals 1957–1967 (1), 57% of 138 affected neonates in Indianapolis (5), and 57% of 49 affected infants in Dublin (25). However, a small excess of males was noted in two other series: in Hawaii (7) 55% of 38 infants were males and in central-east France (4), 52% of 170 infants were males.

Parental Age

In a series of 49 infants with congenital duodenal obstruction in Dublin (1986–1989) [25], the mean age of the mother was 33 years. Among these mothers, the mean age of those with infants with Down Syndrome, the mean age was 34; the mean age of the other mothers was 26 years.

In Hawaii, 1986–2000, the frequency of infants with duodenal atresia in women 35–39 was twice that of women 25–29, a difference due to the associated chromosome abnormalities, specifically Down Syndrome [7].

Twinning

The rate of twinning was 4% in two case series of infants with duodenal atresia: the 170 affected infants in central-east France (4) and the 71 infants in metropolitan Atlanta (23).

Concordance of both monozygous (26) and dizygous twins (27) has been reported.

Genetic Factors

Most affected infants have no affected sibs or parents. The empiric recurrence risk was 5% in the families of 503 affected infants (1). Duodenal atresia has been reported in siblings with unaffected parents (28–31) and in one affected parent and child (32). The sites and types of obstruction at the duodenum have varied in the affected siblings: 1) duodenal web in one sibling and duodenal atresia with annular pancreas in the other (30); 2) in a second family (17), one male infant had atresia of the fist portion of the duodenum associated with partial annual pancreas, complete nonrotation and nonfixation of the intestines, and a congenitally small glottis; his affected older brother had a duodenal web in the fourth part of the duodenum; 3) two affected sisters had atresia distal to the ampulla of Vater (28). No distinctive features have been identified in the infants born to related parents with apparent autosomal recessive inheritance (31, 33).

Environmental Factors

Intestinal atresias were part of the teratogenic effect of thalidomide which Smithells (34) described among 154 children whom he considered to have the thalidomide embryopathy. 3 (2%) of the 154 affected children had duodenal atresia and died in the perinatal period. Smithells noted that one of these infants with duodenal atresia had, also, phocomelia of both arms and both legs.

Injections of methylene blue during amniocentesis, to distinguish between the amniotic sacs of monozygous twins, has caused an increased frequency of intestinal atresia (35), but not duodenal atresia, by producing constriction and hypoxia of the blood supply to the intestine.

Treatment and Prognosis

One challenge is the management of the dilated duodenum, which is always present after repair of duodenal atresia. Pleating of this section, as in Kimura's diamond-shaped anastomosis, will reduce the risk for late-onset megaduodenum (36, 37).

Surgical repair of duodenal atresia due to annular pancreas and malrotation has been carried out by laparoscopy (38).

Volvulus of the intestine, which occurs in most infants with malrotation, rarely occurs in infants with duodenal atresia (39). This has been attributed to the lack of distension and peristalsis of the small intestine. 12% of the 169 infants in one series had additional abdominal surgeries, such as fundoplication and lysis of adhesions (40).

A late mortality rate of 6% has been reported in case series of infants with duodenal atresia, usually reflecting the complications of associated heart defects (40).

Genetic Counseling

Many infants with congenital duodenal obstruction are diagnosed prenatally, because of the associated polyhydramnios. Prenatal detection as early as 12 weeks has also been reported (41). Because of the high frequency of associated chromosome abnormalities, 28.6% in one study (42), amniocentesis is very helpful in establishing the underlying diagnosis for the fetus with apparent duodenal atresia.

Associated malformations of the gastrointestinal tract, biliary system, and heart are common in infants with duodenal atresia, duodenal membrane, and duodenal stenosis.

Duodenal atresia and other types of congenital duodenal obstruction occur in several different rare Mendelian syndromes, such as:

1) the autosomal dominant Feingold syndrome of microcephaly, esophageal and duodenal atresia, thumb hypoplasia, syndactyly, and learning disabilities (MIM# 164280);
2) abdominal *situs inversus*, congenital duodenal obstruction, heart defects, and spleen anomalies (43), for which autosomal recessive inheritance has been postulated;
3) Duodeno-jejunal atresia with volvulus, absent dorsal mesentery, and absent superior mesenteric, a familial phenotype distinct from the apple peel small bowel syndrome (44).

Autosomal recessive inheritance is assumed if the affected infant is born to unaffected, but related, parents (1, 31, 33).

If the parents are not related, the empiric recurrence risk in the next pregnancy after the birth of an infant with "isolated" duodenal atresia was 5% in one large case series (1).

ESOPHAGEAL ATRESIA

Definition

The esophagus ends blindly at the level of the thoracic vertebrae 4 or 5, and above the bifurcation of the trachea.

ICD-9:

	750.300	(esophageal atresia without mention of tracheoesophageal [T-E] fistula)
	750.310	(esophageal atresia with mention of T-E fistula)
	750.320	(tracheoesophageal fistula without mention of esophageal atresia)
	750.325	(tracheoesophageal fistula – "H" type)
	750.330	(bronchoesophageal fistula with or without mention of esophageal atresia)
	750.340	(stenosis or stricture of esophagus)

	750.350	(esophageal web)
	750.380	(other tracheoesophageal anomalies)
ICD-10:	Q39.0	(atresia of esophagus without fistula)
	Q39.1	(atresia of esophagus with tracheo-esophageal fistula)
Mendelian Inheritance in Man:	189960	(tracheoesophageal fistula with or without esophageal atresia)

Appearance

The many published case series have provided descriptions of this abnormality (45–56). Almost all affected infants have a proximal pouch of the esophagus that ends blindly above the level of the bifurcation of the trachea. The pouch is often hypertrophied and dilated from filling by amniotic fluid swallowed before the infant's birth.

Five different types of esophageal atresia have been described, referred to as types A, B, C, D, and E (Figure 3-2).

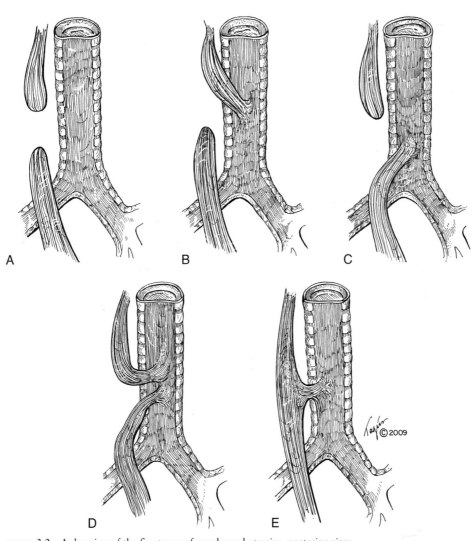

FIGURE 3.2   A drawing of the five types of esophageal atresias, posterior view.

Type C is the most common type (80%); the esophagus ends blindly and a tracheoesophageal fistula extends from just above the bifurcation of the trachea to the stomach. About 8% of infants have type A, in which there is only esophageal atresia and no fistula. Infants with type B esophageal atresia have a proximal tracheoesophageal (TE) fistula; this accounts for 1% of cases. In type D, also 1% of affected infants, there are two fistulas, one proximal and the other distal. 4% have the "H type" tracheoesophageal fistula, but no esophageal atresia; this is type E.

Associated Malformations

Many infants with esophageal atresia have associated malformations; some have specific malformation syndromes (58, 59) [Table 3-1, Figures 3-3 and 3-4].

Population-based studies have shown that the frequency of associated malformations was 55% in two samples: 1) among the 149 affected infants among 534,834 consecutive live births in British Columbia (1966–1980) [49] and 2) among the 345 infants with esophageal atresia born in the southwest of England (1942–1973).

In a survey of the radiographs of 44 patients with esophageal atresia, there was a high frequency of excessive vertebral segmentation, including either 13 or more thoracic vertebrae and 6 or more lumbar vertebrae (59). In another case series of 83 infants with tracheoesophageal atresia, including those with chromosome abnormalities, radiographs showed that hypersegmentation was the most common abnormality in thoracic or lumbar vertebrae. Butterfly vertebrae and hemivertebrae were the other common findings (59).

The most common associated malformations are one or more of the malformations of the VACTERL Syndrome or Association (V=vertebrae; A=anus; C=heart; TE=tracheoesophageal; R=renal and L=limb), with heart defects, anomalies of vertebrae, and imperforate anus the most common (45, 47, 54, 55, 57).

Several other less common associations with no identified mutations have been described:

1. esophageal atresia, holoprosencephaly, mid-gut rotation, and imperforate anus (61);
2. esophageal atresia, congenital diaphragmatic hernia, and lung hypoplasia (62); the affected infants are often stillborn or die soon after birth;
3. esophageal atresia, duodenal atresia, and lung agenesis (63, 64); the second part of the duodenum is the most common site of the duodenal obstruction.
4. tracheoesophageal fistula, duodenal atresia, biliary atresia, hypoplastic pancreas, hypospadias, and low birth weight; the first two affected sibs were born to consanguineous parents (65)
5. bilateral microphthalmia, esophageal atresia, and cryptorchidism (66);

TABLE 3-1 *Esophageal Atresia*: Etiologic and phenotypic heterogeneity.*

	Non-Transfers	
	Isolated	Multiple Anomalies
1. Mendelian inheritance (3.1%):		
a) Fanconi Anemia		1
b) Treacher Collins Syndrome		1
2. Chromosome abnormalities (12.3%):		
a) trisomy 21		3
b) trisomy 21 mosaic		1
c) trisomy 18		4
3. Exposures (9.2%):		
a) Infants of diabetic mothers		5
b) Carbamazepine		1
4. Twinning (9.2%):		
a) Zygosity not known:	2	4
5. Unknown etiology:		
a) Esophageal atresia (EA) alone (36.9%)	24	
b) EA + components of VACTERL Association (24.6%)		16
c) Other phenotypes		
holoprosencephaly (1.5%)		1
renal agenesis/ dysgenesis (3.1%)		2
	26	39 Total 65* (1: 3,173)

*These affected infants were identified in the Active Malformations Surveillance Program at Brigham and Women's Hospital (BWH) in Boston among 206,244 liveborn and stillborn infants and elective terminations because of fetal anomalies in the years 1972–1974, 1979–2000. "Non transfers" refers to the fact that the mother had always planned to deliver at BWH. Mothers whose infant's anomalies were identified were identified elsewhere by prenatal studies, and were transferred to BWH for care because of those findings, were not included.

Two well-known multiple anomaly syndromes in which esophageal atresia is an occasional associated abnormality are:

6. oculo-auriculo-vertebral spectrum (MIM %164210), or hemifacial microsomia [67];
7. Fryns Syndrome (MIM 229850) of congenital diaphragmatic hernia, lung hypoplasia, heart defects, distal digit hypoplasia, and genitourinary anomalies [68].

Developmental Defects

There continues to be debate about the embryogenesis of anomalies of the esophagus (69, 70). It is agreed that

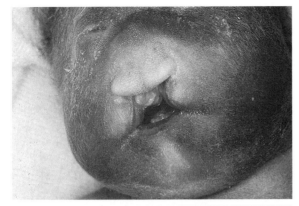

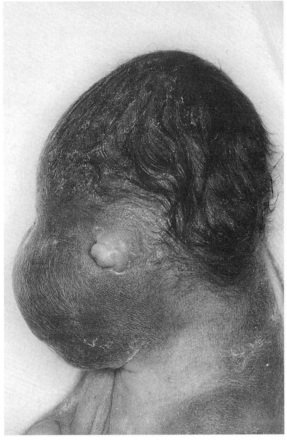

FIGURES 3.3 & 3.4 Infantile with holoprosencephaly, median cleft lip (Figure 3.3), esophageal atresia, anophthalmic and microtia (Figure 3.4), a specific, but rare, phenotype.

the esophagus develops from the foregut just below the pharynx. The developing esophagus is partitioned from the trachea. It has been postulated that the atresia of the esophagus represents failure of recanalization of the esophagus during the eighth week of development (71). The fistula that often develops has been attributed to an abnormal epithelial connection between the trachea and the esophagus (72). In a rat model, anomalies of the trachea and esophagus were attributed to disturbances in either epithelial proliferation or apoptosis (73).

Mutations that "cause" isolated esophageal atresia have not been identified. However, mouse knockout models, including Sonic Hedge Hog (Shh $^{-/-}$; chromosome 7q36), Gli2 $^{-/-}$ (2q14), Gli3 $^{+/-}$ (7p13) and Foxf1 $^{+/-}$ (16q24), have esophageal atresia plus other anomalies (74, 58). Other mouse mutants, such as those in TBX4 (17q21-q22), produce tracheoesophageal fistula, but not esophageal atresia (74).

Exposure of rat fetuses to adriamycin on embryonic day 10 has produced abnormalities of the notochord and esophageal atresia, possibly mediated by ectopic expression of Shh (75). Treatment of mouse embryos at embryonic days 7.5 and 8.5 produced an undivided foregut at embryonic day 11.5, possibly from an alteration of Shh expression (76). Dietary vitamin A deficiency in rats has produced (74) in the exposed pups multiple anomalies of the respiratory tract, cardiovascular system, urogenital system, diaphragm and eyes. Vitamin A exerts its effects through the family of retinoic acid receptors (RARα, β and γ and Rα, β and γ). In double-knockout mice, such as RARα$^{-/-}$ and RXR $^{-/-}$, the tracheo-esophageal septum is absent. This has been interpreted to show that vitamin A is essential to the morphogenesis of the foregut. RARα has been mapped to chromosome 17q21.1 in humans and RARβ to 3p24 (74).

Prevalence

1) 0.34/1,000: esophageal atresia, including those with other anomalies in southwest England (1942–1973) [45];
   0.18/1,000: isolated esophageal atresia (45);
2) 0.14/1,000: esophageal atresia, including those with other anomalies in Hungary: 1970–1977 [47];
   0.08/1,000: isolated esophageal atresia;
3) 0.22/1,000: esophageal atresia with and without other anomalies in Boston: 1972–1974, 1979–2000 (Table 3-1);
   0.11/1,000: isolated esophageal atresia.

Race/Ethnicity

In malformations surveillance in California (53), the prevalence rates in African Americans, Hispanics, and Asians were lower than among white Americans.

In a comparison of the associated malformations (1982–1998) in 48 Asian infants born in Hong Kong and 34 European infants born in the Netherlands, there was a significant difference in the frequency of associated malformations (77). 50% of the Asian infants and 74% of the European infants had associated anomalies (p = 0.04). The major difference was the frequency of urogenital anomalies, such as agenesis or dysplasia of one or both kidneys: 26% in Europe and 4% in Hong Kong.

Birth Status

An increased frequency of prematurity has been noted, with a much higher rate of associated anomalies among the lower birth weight infants (7, 12). Among 345 affected infants identified in southwest England between 1942 and 1973, 21 (6%) were stillborn (45).

Sex ratio

Several studies have shown a small excess of affected males, such as 186:159: M:F in southeast England (45). However, not all studies (47, 50) have shown a difference in sex ratio.

Parental age

A higher frequency of esophageal atresia has been observed among both younger and older mothers, which produces a U-shaped distribution in maternal age (45, 47). In Hungary, the U-shaped distribution was present only in unskilled and semiskilled workers (47); the basis for this correlation was not established. The higher frequency of esophageal atresia among older mothers could be due to the occurrence in infants with trisomies 21, 18, and 13, which are more common among older mothers.

Twinning

An association with twinning, including both monozygous and dizygous twins, has been observed. In a series of 1,215 infants with esophageal atresia, 50 (4%) were from a twin pregnancy (78). In a series of 45 infants with esophageal atresia in Boston (Table 3-1), 9.2% were a co-twin. All twin pairs were discordant for esophageal atresia. In another questionnaire-based survey of 579 families with a child with esophageal atresia, 25 sets of twins (18 like-sex and all discordant) were reported in comparison to 8 among 1,031 control families who responded (79).

Among the 50 sets of twins among 1,215 infants with esophageal atresia, both twins were affected only in 2 sets (78). In three case reports of twins: in one set (80) both of the monozygous twins had esophageal atresia and one had also the additional malformations of the VACTERL Association; in the other two sets of monozygous twins, both infants had esophageal atresia with tracheoesophageal fistula (81, 82).

Genetic Factors

The 1% occurrence of esophageal atresia, and no other anomalies, in a sibling of an affected child has been postulated to reflect multifactorial inheritance (83–85). However, the fact that the recurrence risk is only about

1% and the very low likelihood that both identical twins are affected has been interpreted to mean that genetic factors are uncommon (78).

Individual families with an affected aunt, parent and child have been reported (86). No distinctive features of the atresia have been described in these individuals. In one reported family (87), a female infant had esophageal atresia and a male first cousin had VACTERL with hydrocephalus.

The empiric recurrence risks have been studied in several populations, including Minnesota (84), Hungary (47), and England (85), all Caucasian populations. The occurrence of esophageal atresia in siblings of affected individuals was 1/347 sibs (0.3%) in Minnesota and 1/130 sibs (0.8%) in England. In the Minnesota study (84), five (1.4%) of the 347 sibs did not have esophageal atresia, but had malformations in the VACTERL spectrum, such as heart defects or vertebral anomalies. In Hungary (3), one (1%) of 128 brothers examined and none of 103 sisters had esophageal atresia.

The rate of occurrence in offspring of affected individuals was documented in the same studies: 1/41 offspring (2.4%) in Minnesota (the parent had esophageal atresia with a tracheoesophageal fistula and the affected child had esophageal atresia with fistula, heart defect, and a radial ray anomaly). In England (85), 15 affected individuals (born 1947–1959) had 28 children, one (3.6%) of whom had esophageal atresia (type C).

Family studies showed among 600 first degree relatives of individuals with esophageal atresia a significant increase in the occurrence of one or more of the VACTERL Association anomalies, gastro-esophageal reflux, recurrent respiratory infections, and autonomic dysfunction, in comparison to controls (79).

Gene linkage studies in four families with syndromic esophageal atresia showed linkage to chromosome 2p23-p24. This rare autosomal dominant syndrome, known as oculodigito-esophageoduodenal (ODED) syndrome or Feingold Syndrome (MIM #164280), includes atresia of the esophagus and duodenum, microcephaly, shortened fingers, and syndactyly. In one family with this syndrome, there was a submicroscopic deletion in the critical region (88). A more common finding has been mutations in exon 3 of the MYCN gene (89).

Mutations have also been identified in two other multiple anomaly syndromes associated with esophageal atresia:

1) the Rogers Syndrome or anophthalmia/microphthalmia and esophageal atresia [MIM #600992] which has been associated with mutations in SOX2, a developmental gene (90, 91);
2) the CHARGE Association (ocular coloboma (C), heart defects (H), choanal atresia (A), retarded growth(R), genital anomalies (G), and ear anomalies (E) [MIM #214800] has been shown, in several but not all

affected individuals, to be associated with mutations in CDH7, a gene in the chromodomain gene family (92).

Chromosome trisomies, especially 21 and 18, have been associated with esophageal atresia and other anomalies (Table 3-1). An interstitial deletion in 17q22-q23.3 has been associated with esophageal atresia in a few patients (93). Many of the affected children have been dysmorphic, had heart and skeletal anomalies (such as symphalangism), and moderate to severe developmental delay.

Environmental Factors

The most frequently observed environmental factor is insulin-dependent diabetes mellitus in the mother (Table 3-1).

Esophageal atresia is one of the multiple anomalies observed in some infants exposed during pregnancy to methimazole or carbimazole, medications used to treat hyperthyroidism (94). Exposure to excessive alcohol (95) intake during pregnancy, maternal phenylketonuria (57), and the immunosuppressive drug mycophenolate (96) have all been postulated also to occasionally cause esophageal atresia.

It has been proposed that esophageal atresia has occurred as a transgenerational effect of prenatal exposure to diethylstilbestrol (DES) [97]. The biologic plausibility of this hypothesis has not been established.

Treatment and Prognosis

The presence of major heart defects and the anomalies of the VACTERL Association are major risk factors for an affected infant's survival (54). In an analysis of the outcome of 134 infants with esophageal atresia at one hospital in Liverpool (1986–1997), the relative risk of death was 3.47 (95% CI:1.5 to 7.96) for infants with major heart defects and 2.54 (95% CI:1.14 to 4.86) for infants with the VACTERL Association (54).

Most infants with atresia of the esophagus develop esophageal dysmotility following the surgical repair. Recurrences of the tracheoesophageal fistula can occur also, especially at the site of the primary anastomosis.

Many affected infants develop also gastroesophageal reflux disease (GERD) [98]. More aggressive medical management has been used to reduce the need for fundoplication.

An initial repair of esophageal atresia and tracheoesophageal fistula has been carried out with thoracoscopic operations, instead of an approach through a thoracotomy. The results in 104 affected infants were comparable to those whose initial operation was performed through a thoracotomy (99). One significant advantage of repair via thoracoscopy was to avoid the musculoskeletal complications of thoracotomy, including "winged" scapula, a symmetry of thoracic wall secondary to atrophy of serratus anterior muscle, scoliosis of thoracic vertebrae, and abnormal development of one breast.

Genetic Counseling

Since infants with esophageal atresia may have one of several potential causes and associated malformations, establishing the clinical diagnosis is the first step in counseling. Chromosome analysis with microarray CGH is essential in a diagnostic evaluation of the affected infant with multiple anomalies. The frequency of chromosome duplications and deficiencies has not been determined.

Dysmorphic infants with multiple anomalies should be evaluated for having one of the several syndromes (same listed above) with associated esophageal atresia.

For infants with isolated esophageal atresia with or without an associated tracheoesophageal fistula, the empiric risk of occurrence in subsequent sibs or offspring appears to be very low, approximately 1 to 3%.

Prenatal screening by ultrasonography could focus on signs of esophageal pouch in the neck (101) and the potential associated anomalies of the heart, vertebrae, and limbs. The presence in affected infants of an extra pair of ribs, i.e., 13 pairs, has been associated with long gap atresia (59, 101).

The prognosis of infants identified prenatally has been worse than that of infants not diagnosed in utero, presumably because they have more associated malformations. The accuracy of prenatal detection in either early or late pregnancy has not been established.

IMPERFORATE ANUS

Definition

Absence of an opening of the anus.

ICD-9:   751.230   (imperforate anus
                          with fistula)
            751.240   (imperforate anus without
                          fistula)
ICD-10:   Q42.2   (imperforate anus with
                          fistula)
            Q42.3   (imperforate anus without
                          fistula)
Mendelian   207500   (imperforate anus)
Inheritance
in Man:
            301800   (imperforate anus;
                          X-linked)

Appearance

There are three variations of this abnormality: 1) imperforate anus or anal atresia; 2) anal stenosis; and 3) membranous atresia. The infant with imperforate anus has no anal opening. There is a prominent midline raphe that extends from the lower edge to the vagina in a female or the lower edge of the scrotum in males, posteriorly, past the normal site of the anus (Figure 3-5).

The raphe contains a disorganized cluster of skeletal muscle fibers, possibly representing rudiments of the external anal sphincter (102). The presence of a fistula between the rectum and the vagina (Figure 3-6) or perineum (Figure 3-7) is indicated by the extrusion of meconium in these areas after birth.

The clinical classification of anal atresia, suggested initially by Ladd and Gross (102), was two categories of severity: a) "low" anomalies, which are located at or below the levator (puborectal) muscle, and b) "high" anomalies, which are above the levator muscle (103, 104). The infants with the "high" anomalies are more likely to have associated malformations of the vertebrae and genitourinary structures (103–105).

The term anal stenosis refers to a narrow anal canal with the anal opening at the normal site of the anus.

The term membranous atresia of the anus refers to a thin layer of tissue that covers the anus, which is in the normal location. This membrane is thin and may be blue, reflecting the color of meconium behind it. The membrane will bulge with an increase in intra-abdominal pressure. Both anal stenosis and membranous atresia are considered "low" anomalies.

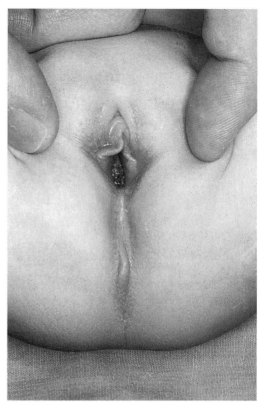

FIGURE 3.5 Prominent midline raphe in perineum of infant with imperforate anus. (Courtesy of W. Hardy Hendren, M.D., Massachusetts General Hospital, Boston, MA).

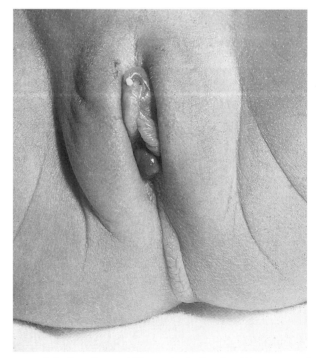

FIGURE 3.6 Prominent midline raphe in female with presence of black meconium in vagina, reflecting rectovaginal fistula. (Courtesy of W. Hardy Hendren, M.D., Massachusetts General Hospital, Boston, MA).

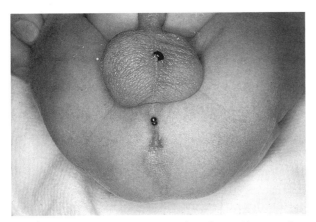

FIGURE 3.7 Imperforate anus in male infant with meconium coming from fistula to perineum below scrotum and in center of scrotum. (Courtesy of W. Hardy Hendren, M.D., Massachusetts General Hospital, Boston, MA).

Associated Malformations

The unselected consecutive case series, identified through malformations surveillance programs (105–111), have shown that many of the affected infants have only "isolated" imperforate anus, meaning no anomalies except in the related and adjacent structures ("regional anomalies"), such as vertebrae, sacrum, and urinary tract. The percentages of "isolated" cases in several studies were: 32% (106), 41% (107), 39–60% (108), 47% (109), 45% (110), and 23% (111). A similar rate of associated anomalies has been reported in follow-up studies by surgical groups in several case series (112, 113).

There are two groups of associated malformations: those in the same anatomic area ("regional") and those outside of that area ("non-regional"). For example, in British Columbia (1952–1983) [106], 21.9% of the 356 infants with imperforate anus had "regional" anomalies and 59.6% had "non-regional" anomalies (108). Urogenital anomalies have been the predominant "regional" anomaly, including urogenital fistulas into the vagina, urethra, bladder, or perineum. Hypospadias occurred in 5.5% of 638 affected children in France, Sweden, and California in 1970s and 1980s; 17.4% had severe renal anomalies (108).

The analysis of 304 affected infants in Spain (1976–1998) from a survey of 1,575,388 consecutive live births showed that the association of vertebral, renal/urinary tract, and genital defects was much more likely (70 times) in infants with imperforate anus than in infants with other anomalies (110).

A higher frequency of regional anomalies has been identified with magnetic resonance imaging (MRI) than by radiography: 30% of the infants with "low" atresia and 50% of those with "high" atresia had anomalies,

such as sacral agenesis, tethered spinal cord and genitourinary anomalies (113).

Many malformation syndromes are associated with imperforate anus, including persistence of the cloaca (114), urorectal sepectum malformation sequence (115), cloacal exstrophy, the VACTERL Association, and several monogenic disorders, such as the Jarcho-Levin Syndrome (MIM #277300) of spondylocostal dysplasia, the FG Syndrome (MIM #192350) [Table 3-2], of mental retardation, imperforate anus, large head and hypotonia; and the Currarino Syndrome (MIM #176450) of partial agenesis of sacrum, urogenital anomalies, and imperforate anus.

Developmental Defect

The outer or inferior one-third of the anal canal is ectodermal in origin and is derived from the proectoderm. The upper or superior two-thirds of the anal canal is derived from the hindgut and is endodermal in origin (104). In the infant with anorectal agenesis, the rectum

TABLE 3-2 *Etiologic and phenotype heterogeneity of infants with imperforate anus: Brigham and Women's Hospital, 1972–1974, 1979–2000*.

	Isolated	Multiple Anomalies
1. Mendelian disorders:		
Jarcho-Levin Syndrome (116)		1
FG Syndrome (117)		1
2. Chromosome abnormalities:		
Trisomy 21		5
Trisomy 18		1
3. Specific syndromes:		
Cloacal exstrophy/persistent cloaca		2
Renal agenesis/dysgenesis		3
VACTERL Association		5
4. Exposures:		
Infants of diabetic mothers		1
5. Twinning:		0
6. Unknown etiology:		
a) isolated	7	
b) multiple anomalies		14
	7	33 Total: 40* infants (1 in 5,156)

Legend: *The affected infants were identified by the Active Malformations Surveillance Program at Brigham and Women's Hospital in Boston among 206,224 livebirths, stillbirths and elective terminations for fetal anomalies. The mothers were "non-transfers", meaning that they had always planned to deliver at this hospital. Infants born to mothers, who had planned to deliver at another hospital, but who transferred their obstetrical care after the prenatal detection of the fetal anomalies, have been excluded.

usually ends blindly with formation of a fistula to the bladder or vagina. In reviewing serial sectionals of developing human embryos (118), it was suggested that the fistulae were ectopic anal orifices.

It has been suggested (104) that most anorectal anomalies arise from incomplete separation of the cloaca into urogenital and anorectal portions. However, serial sections of developing human embryos, the postulated down growth of the urorectal septum, and fusion of this septum with the cloacal membrane was not observed (118). Another mechanism was suggested: the cloacal membrane ruptures and a secondary occlusion of the anal orifice occurs. A failure of recanalization of the occluded anal orifice would be the theoretical cause of imperforate anus in this model.

In a porcine model of imperforate anus (122a), there was an association with hypospadias and persistence of the cloaca.

Experimental models of anorectal malformations have been developed. For example, mice homozygous for a targeted disruption of GLI2, which encodes a sonic hedgehog-responsive transcription factor, had imperforate anus and recto-urethral fistula (120).

All-trans retinoic acid, administered by gavage on day nine of gestation in ICR mice, produced anorectal malformations (121), with incomplete partitioning of the cloaca and formation of rectourethral and rectocloacal fistulas. These effects were attributed to disruption of the normal retinoid-mediated signaling pathway.

Prevalence

The rates of occurrence of anal atresia in several population-based studies have been similar: 0.39/1,000 or 1:2,524 in British Columbia (1964–1982) [106], 0.3/1,000 in Denmark (1964–1978) [107], 0.48/1,000 in France (1979–1995) [109] and 0.44/1,000 in Hawaii (1986–1999) [111].

Rate/Ethnicity

The prevalence rate in California was lower in African American infants than among white infants (108).

Birth Status

The pregnancies are often complicated by either oligo- or polyhydramnios (109). A higher rate of premature delivery before 38 weeks gestation and a lower birth weight have been noted in several case series. An increased rate of occurrence in the first pregnancy has been observed in some (108), but not all (109), birth defect registries.

In a study of isolated anal atresia among 4.6 million births in Europe, there was a reduced gestational age and mean birth weight among infants with anal atresia and persistent cloaca, but not for infants with isolated anal atresia (105).

Sex Ratio

A higher rate of affected males has been noted in several birth defects registries (105–111) and case series (112).

Parental Age

The maternal age group 25-29 years had the highest prevalence rate in Hawaii (1986–1999) [111]. In several European countries (1980–1994), the strongest correlation with increased maternal age (over 35) was among infants born with a "high" (supralevator) atresia and no fistula (105).

Twinning

No increase in the frequency of twinning has been reported among infants with anal atresia.

Three of four sets of like-sex twins in one series (108) were concordant for anal atresia, as part of multiple malformations.

Genetic Factors

There are rare reports of an affected parent and child with "isolated" imperforate anus (MIM: #207500). Affected sisters with unaffected parents have been reported (122b). Pedigrees consistent with X-linked inheritance (MIM: #301800) have been reported also. These apparent monogenic patterns of inheritance are uncommon. No distinctive phenotypic features have been identified in the affected close relatives, in comparison to those with "sporadic" imperforate anus.

No molecular abnormalities have been identified in individuals with "isolated" imperforate anus.

However, several observations have been made in individuals with imperforate anus and other anomalies. The Currarino Syndrome (MIM: #176450) is an autosomal dominant disorder that includes partial agenesis of the sacrum (S2 to S5), a presacral mass, urogenital anomalies, and imperforate anus (123). Mutations have been identified in the homeobox gene HLXB9 that encodes the nuclear protein HB9 (124). In studies of 72 individuals from nine families with Currarino Syndrome, those with mutations had low penetrance and highly variable phenotypes.

A second study of associated mutations was a systematic search in the human T (Brachyury) gene, a transcription factor essential for the development of posterior mesodermal structures, among 28 individuals with sacral agenesis and anorectal atresia (125). One of the 28 affected children and her mother had a rare C1013T variant in exon 7. A third example is the identification of a deletion in GLI3 (nucleotide 2188-2207) in a family with the apparent phenotype of polydactyly, imperforate anus, and vertebral anomalies (124). The delineation of a hypothalamic hamartoma showed that this phenotype was more similar to that of the Pallister-Hall Syndrome (MIM: 146510) than the VACTERL Association.

Among children with imperforate anus and other anomalies, there is also an increased frequency of chromosome abnormalities, including trisomy 21, trisomy 18, and several other abnormalities. The frequencies of chromosome abnormalities among all affected individuals identified in several malformations surveillance programs have been 8.1% (111), 4.4% (108), and 3.7% and 4.5% (106).

Clinical studies of infants with imperforate anus, iris coloboma, and other anomalies (127) led to the delineation of a distinctive pattern of anomalies that was referred to as the "cat-eye syndrome." There is an associated chromosome abnormality, most often a super numerary bisatellited chromosome 22, which is tetrasomy of the short arm of chromosome 22 from band 11 to the terminal end (22 pter->q11).

The frequency of anal atresia was higher (0.18% or 1 in 555) in a pig model of anal atresia than in humans (128). Using a complete genome search was microsatellite markers, two loci were identified; GLI2 was a candidate gene at one of these loci.

Environmental Factors

Maternal diabetes is associated with an increased frequency of infants with anorectal anomalies and vertebral anomalies (109, 129) (Table 3-2).

In a review of 154 individuals with the thalidomide embryopathy, nine had anomalies of the intestine, six had anal stenosis, and three had duodenal atresia (130).

Prevention

In one large study in China (131), a decreased frequency of imperforate anus was observed among the mothers of infants who had taken folic acid supplements in comparison to women who had not taken these supplements.

Treatment and Prognosis

At birth, the physical examination, imaging studies, and observation for 24 hours are needed to determine the presence of associated fistulas and other anomalies (132). Contrast studies are more informative after intraluminal pressure has increased, usually by 24 hours of age. The presence of meconium on the perineum (Figure 3-7) is evidence of a perineal fistula. Meconium in the urine means there is a rectourinary fistula.

X-rays or MRI are needed to identify anomalies of the vertebrae and sacrum. Ultrasound can be used to screen for hydronephrosis and hydrocolpos.

If the infant with imperforate anus has signs of a perineal fistula, an anoplasty without a protective colostomy can be performed (132). This can be done in the newborn period or delayed, with dilations of the fistula. If the infant has meconium in the urine with an abnormal sacrum, a colostomy is indicated. The primary repair will be delayed for a few weeks.

Most infants who have a repair of an anorectal malformation have some degree of functional difficulties with defecation. Careful follow-up and management are essential for the best outcome.

Genetic Counseling

For the infant with imperforate anus and other anomalies, the first priority is a diagnostic evaluation to establish the phenotype and to rule out specific syndromes of multiple anomalies. Chromosome analysis is also indicated because of the significant possibility that an abnormality will be identified.

A genetic relationship between imperforate anus and anteriorly placed anus (Figure 3-8) has not been established in family studies.

For unaffected parents of an infant with "isolated" imperforate anus, the empiric recurrence risk estimates have been 2.8% (108) and 2.4% (110) in two studies. The case reports of affected parent and child suggest that there is a "genetic risk," although this is a relatively infrequent occurrence. No distinctive phenotype features have been reported in the affected parents and children that could be used in counseling.

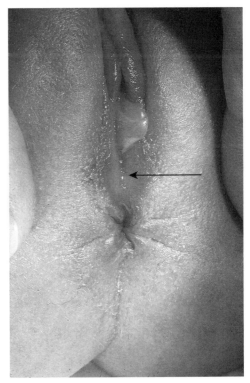

FIGURE 3.8 Anteriorly placed anus, just below labia (arrow), in female infant.

The anteriorly placed anus (Figure 3-8) is less severe than imperforate anus, but may require surgical repair. The genetic relationship, if any, between the anteriorly placed anus and imperforate anus has not been evaluated."

Prenatal screening by ultrasound could identify the affected fetus through the associated vertebral and other anomalies, even in the first trimester (133). However, its accuracy in detecting the fetus with isolated imperforate anus is probably low. Maternal serum AFP levels were below the tenth centile of normal in 4 of 7 infants with anal atresia in one study (134).

JEJUNOILEAL ATRESIA

Definition

Occlusion of the ileal or jejunal portion of the small intestine by either obstruction or absence of the bowel itself.

ICD-9:	751.190	(stenosis, atresia, or absence of small intestine)
	751.105	(stenosis, atresia, or absence of small intestine with fistula)
ICD-10:	Q41	(absence, atresia, and stenosis of small intestine)
Mendelian Inheritance in Man:	%243150	(multiple intestinal atresias)
	%243600	(jejunal atresia)

Appearance

Four types of ileal stenosis and atresia have been described:

Type I: obstruction by membrane of mucosa and submucosa (Figure 3-9);
Type II: fibrous band interrupts bowel;
Type III: atresia with proximal and distal ends of bowel ending blindly (Figure 3-10);
Type IV: multiple segments of atresia (Figure 3-11).

The frequencies of each type in a series of 277 neonates with jejunoileal obstruction were: 23%, type I; 27%, type II; 25%, type III; and 24%, type IV. Within type III, 18% had the V-shaped mesenteric defect and 7% had the "apple peel" atresia (Figure 3-12) (135).

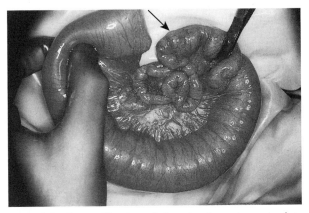

FIGURE 3.9 Shows dilated small intestine (arrow) proximal to region of ileal stenosis. (Courtesy of W. Hardy Hendren, M.D., Massachusetts General Hospital, Boston, MA).

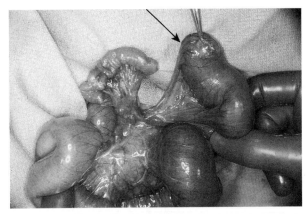

FIGURE 3.10 Shows dilated small intestine (arrow) that ends at gap in intestine, which is region of ileal atresia. (Courtesy of W. Hardy Hendren, M.D., Massachusetts General Hospital, Boston, MA).

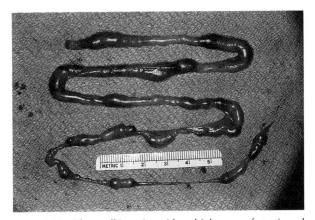

FIGURE 3.11 The small intestine with multiple areas of atresia and the appearance of a "string of sausage." (Courtesy of W. Hardy Hendren, M.D., Massachusetts General Hospital, Boston, MA).

Associated Malformations

Several case series (136–140) and population-based studies (141–145) of infants with jejunoileal, jejunal, and ileal atresia have been published from many different geographic areas. Several show that about half of the affected infants have no other malformations.

In a series of 35 infants with jejunoileal atresia in New Zealand (1979–1995) [138], the associated anomalies were malrotation of the intestine in 23%, heart defects (11%), and anomalies of the urinary tract (14%). In a series of 48 infants with jejunoileal atresia in Japan (1978–2004) (140), operative findings showed volvulus in 27.1%, intussusception in 25%, and constriction by abnormal bands in 8.3%.

Among 24 infants with ileal atresia identified in Atlanta, Georgia (1968–1989 [141]), 14 (58%) had no associated malformations, 2 (8%) had multiple unrelated anomalies, and 8 (33%) had specific phenotypes, such as gastroschisis, omphalocele, volvulus, and annular pancreas.

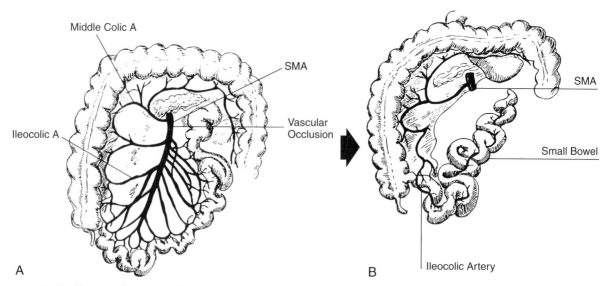

FIGURE 3.12   Shows a diagram of the "apple peel" syndrome: occlusion of the superior mesenteric artery causes absence of part of the jejunum; the distal small intestine is maintained by collateral vessels and has an appearance suggestive of an apple peeling. (From Seashore JH et al., *Pediatrics* 1987;80:540–544. Used with permission.).

Eighteen (54.6%) of 33 infants identified in the Spanish Collaborative Study of Congenital Malformations (ECEMC) from 1976–1998 had isolated ileal atresia (144).

The term apple peel atresia, introduced in 1961(146), refers to a high level jejunal atresia with a discontinuity of the small bowel and a wide gap in the mesentery (Figure 3-12). The distal ileum is shortened and coils around a retrograde perfusing vessel, suggestive of a coiled apple peel. This retrograde perfusing artery is compensating for the absence of most of the superior mesenteric artery, which is interrupted a short distance below its origin. The colon is small, but is not "typical microcolon" (147). The apple peel type of jejunal atresia has been associated with a high incidence of prematurity, malformation, and short bowel syndrome, and a high mortality rate (148).

The type IV multiple atresia phenotype has a distinctive appearance on radiographs: meconium peritonitis produces a distinctive "string of pearls" or "string of sausage" that is considered pathognomonic (146) (Figure 3-11).

Developmental Defects

The first theory as to the cause of intestinal atresia was the lack of recanalization of the intestine in the solid cord stage of its development (149).

The second major theory was the vascular hypothesis. This was suggested by the research of Professor Jannie Louw, a South African surgeon whose son had been born with atresia of the small intestine and had died in infancy just after World War II (150). Louw and Barnhard showed in 1955 (150, 151) the ligation of mesentery arteries in developing dog fetuses produced atresia of the small intestine. In his reviews of clinical cases, Louw had observed in many infants with atresia that the bowel below the obstruction contained meconium sometimes, including squamous epithelial cells and even bile. Since bile is not excreted until the eleventh week of fetal development, and the skin does not have squamous epithelium until the third month, these findings suggested that the obstruction occurred in the third month of gestation. Because of his research findings, he began to resect the proximal dilated portion of the dilated bowel, which improved significantly the survival rate of the infants with intestinal atresia.

The association of jejunoileal atresia with volvulus (151) is consistent with the vascular hypothesis of causation, as the twisting of the bowel would interrupt blood supply, cause necrosis of the affected bowel, and produce bowel atresia. In a series of 32 infants with single mid-and low jejunoileal atresia, 13 appeared to have had intrauterine volvulus and 12 had had intussusception as the primary event (151). The etiology of the intussusception was not determined.

Hypoxia and hypoperfusion have been postulated to occur in mesenteric arteries and lead to small bowel atresia following several types of intra-uterine events, including the prenatal diagnosis procedure chorionic villous sampling (CVS) [152], laser treatment of twin-twin transfusion (153), embolization of autolyzed tissue from a deceased co-twin (154), abnormal vasculature of the placenta (155), and inherited thrombophilias, such as the Factor V Leiden mutation and the R353Q polymorphism of the factor VII gene (156).

The mouse gene knockout model deficient in fibroblast growth factor receptor 2b (Fgtr2b-/-) is associated with intestinal atresia, primarily in the colon, and a constellation of additional developmental defects, such as microphthalmia and anophthalmia (157). Histologic studies showed an inhibition of epithelial proliferation and increased apoptosis. These findings were suggestive of another etiologic mechanism for intestinal atresia, rather than the vascular insufficiency mechanism.

Another experimental model is adriamycin, an anti-tumor agent, injected on days 6 to 9 of gestation in pregnant Sprague-Dawley rats. The exposed fetuses developed multiple intestinal atresias (158). The abnormal vascular anatomy was visible on days 12 and 13, but the cellular basis for the bowel atresia was not determined. Additional anomalies of the trachea, esophagus, kidney, anus, and skeleton were also produced.

An intriguing mechanism for producing intestinal atresia in calves was by palpating once a day the amniotic vesicle between days 32 and 41 of gestation (159). In one such study, 7 of the 12 calves were born with intestinal atresia.

Prevalence

The prevalence rates of jejunoileal atresia in population-based surveys have been: 0.042/1,000 (62% isolated) in Spain among 1,527,579 births (1976–1998) [110], 0.047/1,000 (76% isolated) in eight countries in South American among 1,896, 796 births (1967–1996) [144], and 0.08/1,000 in cental-east France among 1,443,418 births (1970–1992) [143].

Race/Ethnicity

In Atlanta (141), the prevalence rate was higher among black than white infants. In Hawaii (145), the prevalence rates were significantly higher among Asian and Pacific Islander infants than white infants.

Birth Status

Isolated atresias of the jejunum and ileum have been associated with low birth weight and decreased gestational age (139, 144, 145).

Sex Ratio

In many series, the sex ratio of affected females was equal. In Atlanta (141), there was a greater percentage of affected females than males among black and white infants with jejunal atresia, but not among those with ileal atresia.

Parental Age

In studies in France (143) and Hawaii (145), there was an increased frequency of intestinal atresia among the infants of mothers below age 20 in France and in Hawaii.

Twinning

An increased frequency of twinning in individuals with jejunoileal atresia has been observed in several populations: a seven-fold increase in Atlanta (141), a 3.8 fold increase in Hawaii (145), and an overall rate of 4.4% in France (143).

A potential confounder of the association with twinning is the use of methylene blue, injected to mark the sac entered in amniocentesis, in the prenatal diagnosis procedure (160). The twin exposed to methylene blue has a significant risk of developing atresia of the small intestine. The types of associated bowel atresia include jejunal atresia, ileal atresia, and multiple ileal atresias. The mechanism of this fetal effect of methylene blue was postulated to be ischemic damage in the small intestine.

There have been several case reports of identical twins with ileojejunal atresia, some of which were concordant (161), i.e., both affected, and others in which only one of the twins was affected (162).

In consanguineous families with intestinal atresia attributed to autosomal recessive inheritance, both twins are affected. However, each twin will not necessarily have the same type of jejunoileal atresia (163).

Genetic Factors

Three phenotypes of small bowel have occurred in siblings with unaffected parents: 1) ileal atresia; 2) apple peel jejunal atresia; 3) multiple small intestine atresias (146, 163–165). For the consanguineous families with affected male and female siblings, autosomal recessive inheritance has been postulated. However, the fact that identical twins have been discordant [162] (assuming that there was no exposure to methylene blue at amniocentesis), suggests that genetic mechanisms other than autosomal recessive inheritance could also be involved.

In case series (5) and population-based studies (166), an increased frequency of cystic fibrosis has been observed among infants with ileal or jejunoileal atresia. One hypothesis for the mechanism is that meconium ileus, an effect of cystic fibrosis in the fetus, can cause localized areas of bowel ischemia.

Among infants with Down Syndrome in California, there was a 142.2 fold increase in the frequency of atresia and stenosis of the small intestine, in addition to the common association with duodenal atresia (167).

Environmental Factors

Exposure during pregnancy to environmental factors, such as cocaine (168) and vasoactive compounds, like pseudoephedrine (169) in the first 10 weeks of pregnancy, have been postulated to cause intestinal atresia. The risk from the mother taking vasoactive compounds was increased among those who also smoked 20 or more cigarettes a day. The minimal exposure to vasoactive drugs in pregnancy that is associated with an increased risk of bowel atresia has not been determined.

An episode of anaphylactic shock at 10.5 weeks gestation, due to sensitivity to an antibiotic, was associated with the occurrence of type IV jejunal atresia in both identical twins (170).

The increased rate of occurrence of intestinal atresia in infants exposed to the prenatal diagnosis procedures chorionic villus sampling (CVS) has been attributed to blood loss following the procedure, hypotension, and ischemia. The vasculature in the developing digits, cranial nerves, and intestine are more vulnerable to the disruption of end-arteries, especially when performed before 10 weeks gestation.

Treatment and Prognosis

The surgeon's choice between primary anastomosis and creating a stoma depends on the extent of the abnormality and the degree of dilatation of the intestine proximal to the atresic segment. If the atresia is high jejunal or proximal ileal, primary anastomosis is the likely choice. If the degree of dilatation is severe, decompression of the intestine may be required. For infants with distal ileal atresia, establishing a stoma and closure later is usually the choice (171).

The survival of infants with jejunoileal atresia over the past 40 years has improved significantly (172). Critical factors have included the age of the infant at surgery, the confounding effect of prematurity, the type of surgical repair, improvements in anesthesia and postoperative care, parental nutrition, and the presence of other anomalies, such as malrotation.

Impaired motility of the intestine after surgical repair has been a major cause of morbidity. Staining the cells in the small intestine of affected human fetuses with neuronal markers, such as c-kit and glial fibrillary acidic protein (GFAP), showed that the maturation of the myenteric plexus was delayed significantly in the tissue below the area of the atresia (173). Treatment with minimal feeding by mouth was proposed as a way to stimulate peristalsis in the intestine below the atresia and, thereby, shorten recovery.

Treatment with recombinant growth hormone (174) has been shown to be a promising approach to the common complication of short bowel syndrome.

Genetic Counseling

The initial examination and evolution of the affected infant will establish whether or not the infant is dysmorphic or has multiple anomalies. Most infants with jejunoileal atresia have no associated malformations. The evaluation should include screening for having undiagnosed cystic fibrosis.

For the dysmorphic infant with associated anomalies, chromosome analysis and array CGH analysis are appropriate diagnostic tests.

If no chromosome abnormality is identified by chromosome analysis or array CHG, the clinician should consider specific multiple anomaly syndromes. Examples are:

1. Microcephaly, apple peel intestinal atresia and anomalies of the anterior segment of the eye (MIM 243605); the associated molecular abnormality has not been identified, but in one affected infant mutations in PAX6, FOXC1, PITX2 and MYCN were excluded (175).
2. Amyoplasia with intestinal atresia (176).

The counseling about the risk for recurrence for infants with "isolated," jejunoileal atresia, born to unaffected and unrelated parents, is uncertain. No extensive family studies have established the empiric recurrence risk.

Case series have shown that there are several families in which unaffected, unrelated parents have had two or more infants with either the apple peel jejunal atresia (148) or multiple atresias (177). The fact that in one set of identical twins (162) only one twin had apple peel atresia makes mendelian pattern of inheritance, such as autosomal recessive, less likely.

Intestinal atresia can be detected by prenatal sonography because of the associated dilated loops of the bowel and polyhydramnios. The fetuses detected prenatally tend to be those with more severe symptoms and whose recovery is longer. However, those diagnosed prenatally have the benefit of earlier surgery (178).

REFERENCES

1. Fonkalsrud EW, deLorimier AA, Hays DM. Congenital atresia and stenosis of the duodenum. *Pediatrics.* 1969;43:79–83.
2. Adeyemi SD. Duodenal obstruction in Nigerian newborns and infants. *Scand J Gastroenterol.* 1886;21(Suppl 124): 151–161.
3. Schier F, Schier C, Waldschmidt J, Grasemann S. Duodenal atresia: Experiments with 145 patients. *Zentralbl Chir.* 1990;115(3): 135–142.
4. Francannet C, Robert E. Etude épidémiologigue des atresia intestinales: Registre Centre-Est 1976–1992. *J Gynecol Obstet Biol Reprod.* 1996;25:485–494.
5. Dall Vecchia LK, Grosfeld JL, West KW, Rescorla F, Scherer LR, Engum SA. Intestinal atresia and stenosis: a 25-year experience with 277 cases. *Arch Surg.* 1998;113:490–497.
6. Murshed R, Nicholls G, Spitz L. Intrinsic duodenal obstruction: trends in management and outcome over 45 years (1951–1995) with relevance to prenatal counseling. *Brit J Obst Gynaecol.* 1999;106:1197–1199.
7. Forrester MB, Merz RD. Population-based study of small intestinal atresia and stenosis, Hawaii, 1986–2000. *Public Health* 2004;118:434–438.
8. Millar AJ, Rode H, Cywes S. Intestinal atresia and stenosis. In: Ashcraft KW, Holcomb GW III, Murphy JP, eds. *Pediatric*

Surgery. 4th ed. Philadelphia: Elsevier Saunders; 2005: 416–419.

9. Oldham KT, Columbani PM, Foglia R, Skinner MA, eds. *Principles and Practice of Pediatric Surgery.* Volume 2: Chapter 72. Stomach and Duodenum. Philadelphia: Lippincott Williams & Wilkins; 2005: 1163–1168.

10. _____. "Duodenal Obstruction." In: O'Neill Jr JA, Grosfeld JL, eds. *Principles of Pediatric Surgery.* 2nd ed. St. Louis: Mosby; 2004: 471–475.

11. Mikalesson C, Arnbjörnsson E, Kallendorff CM. Membranous duodenal stenosis. *Acta Paediatr.* 1997;86:953–955.

12. Huang F-C, Chaang J-H, Shieh C-S. Congenital duodenal membrane: a ten-year review. *Acta Paediatr Sin.* 1999;40: 70–74.

13. Grosfeld JL, Rescorla FJ. Duodenal atresia and stenosis: reassessment of treatment and outcome based on antenatal diagnosis, pathologic variance, and long-term follow-up. *World J Surg.* 1993;17:301–309.

14. Knechtle SJ, Filston H. Anomalous biliary ducts associated with duodenal atresia. *J Pediatr Surg.* 1990;25:1266–1269.

15. Shih H-S, Ko S-F, Chaung J-H. Is there an association between duodenal atresia and choledochal cyst? *J Pediatr Gastroent Natr.* 2005; 40:378–381.

16. Zerin JM, Polley TZ Jr. Malrotation in patients with duodenal atresia: a true association or an unexpected finding on postoperative upper gastrointestinal barium study? *Pediatr Radiol.* 1994; 24:170–172.

17. Baumgartner F, Moore TC. Atretic, obstructive proximal duodenal mass associated with annular pancreas and malrotation in a newborn male. *Eur J Pediatr Surg.* 1992;2:42–44.

18. Torfs CP, Christianson RE. Anomalies in Down Syndrome individuals in large population-based registry. *Am J Med Genet.* 1998;77:431–438.

19. Moore KL, Persaud TVN. *The Developing Human: Clinically oriented Embryology.* 7th ed. Philadelphia: WB Saunders Company; 1993:259–263.

20. O'Rahilly R, Müller F. *Human Embryology and Teratology.* 3rd ed. New York: Wiley-Liss; 2001:254–256.

21. Ando H, Kaneko K, Ito F, Seo T, Harada T, Watanabe Y. Embryogenesis of pancreaticobiliary maljunction inferred from development of duodenal atresia. *J Heptobiliary Pancreat Surg.* 1999;1:50–54.

22. Fairbanks TJ, Kanard R, DelMoral PM, Sala FC, DeLanghe S, Warburton D, Anderson KD, Bellusci S, Burns RC. Fibroblast growth factor receptor 2 IIIb invalidation—a potential cause of familial duodenal atresia. *J Pediatric Surg.* 2004; 39:872–874.

23. Cragan JD, Martin ML, Waters GD, Khoury MJ. Increased risk of small intestinal atresia among twins in the United States. *Arch Pediatr Adolesc Med.* 1994;148:733–739.

24. Shaw GM, Carmichael SL, Nelson V. Congenital malformations in offspring of Vietnamese Women in California 1985–1997. *Teratology* 2002;65:121–124.

25. Akhtar J, Guiney EJ. Congenital duodenal obstruction. *Br J Surg.* 1992;79:133–135.

26. Gahukamble DB, Adnan AR, AlGadi M. Distal foregut atresia in consecutive siblings and twins in the same family. *J Pediatr Surg.* 2003;19:288–292.

27. Yokoyama T, Ishizone S, Mamose Y, Terada M, Kitahara S, Kawasaki S. Duodenal atresia in dizygotic twins. *J Pediatr Surg.* 1997;32:1806–1808.

28. Gahukamble DB, Khamage AS, Shaheen AQ. Duodenal atresia: its occurrence in siblings. *J Ped Surg.* 1994;29:1599–1600.

29. Thepcharoennirund S. Familial duodenal atresia: a report of two siblings. *J Med Assoc Thai.* 2001;84:448–452.

30. Poki HO, Holland AJA, Pitkin J. Double bubble, double trouble. *Ped Surg Int.* 2005;21:428–431.

31. Best LG, Wiseman NE, Chudley AE. Familial duodenal atresia: a report of two families and review. *Am J Med Genet.* 1989;34: 442–444.

32. Mitchell CE, Marshall DG, Reid WD. Preampullary congenital duodenal obstruction in a father and son. *J Pediatr Surg.* 1993; 28:1582–1583.

33. Der Kaloustian VM, Slim MS, Mishlany HG. Familial congenital duodenal atresia. *Pediatrics.* 1974;54:118.

34. Smithells RW. Defects and disabilities of thalidomide children. *Brit Med J.* 1973;1:269–272.

35. Nicolini U. Intestinal obstruction in babies exposed in utero to methylene blue. *Lancet.* 1990;336:1258.

36. Kimura K, Makohara N, Nashijime E. Diamond-shaped anastomosis for duodenal atresia: an experience with 44 patients over 15 years. *J Pediatr Surg.* 1990;25:977–979.

37. Upadhyay V, Sakalkale R, Parashar, Mitra SK, Buick RG, Gornall P, Corkery JJ. Duodenal atresia: a comparison of three modes of treatment. *Eur J Pediatr Surg.* 1996;6:75–77.

38. Glüer S, Peterson C, Ure BM. Simultaneous correction of duodenal atresia due to annular pancreas and malrotation by laparoscopy. *Eur J Pediatr Surg.* 2002;12:423–425.

39. Samuel M, Wheeler RA, Mami AG. Does duodenal atresia and stenosis prevent midgut volvulus in malrotation? *Eur J Pediatr Surg.* 1997;7:11–12.

40. Escobar MA, Ladd AP, Grosfeld JL, Wet KW, Rescorla FJ, Scherer LR, Enguin SA, Rouse TM, Billmire DF. Duodenal atresia and stenosis: long-term follow-up over 30 years. *J Pediatric Surg.* 2004;39:867–871.

41. Dundas KC, Walker J, Laing IA. Oesophageal and duodenal atresia suspected at the 12-week booking scan. *Br J Obstet Gynec.* 2001;108:225–226.

42. Daniel A, Athayde N, Ogle R, George AM, Michael J, Pertile MD, Bryan J, Jammu V, Trudinger BJ. Prospective ranking of the sonographic markers for aneuploidy: data of 2143 prenatal cytogenetic diagnoses referred for abnormalities of ultrasound. *Aust N Zeal J Obst Gyn.* 2003;43:16–26.

43. Nawaz A, Malta H, Hamchou M, Jacobez A, Trad O, AlSalem AH. Situs inversus abdominus in association with congenital duodenal obstruction: a report of two cases and review of the literature. *Pediatr Surg Int.* 2005;21:589–592.

44. Pumberger W, Birnbacher R, Pomberger G, Dentinger J. Duodeno-jejunal atresia with volvulus, absent dorsal mesentery, and absent superior mesenteric artery: a hereditary compound structure in duodenal atresia? *Am J Med Genet.* 2002;109: 52–55.

45. David TJ, O'Callaghan SE. Oesophageal atresia in the South West of England. *J Med Genet.* 1975;12:1–11.

46. German JC, Mahour GH, Woolley MM. Esophageal atresia and associated anomalies. *J Pediatr.* 1976;11:299–306.

47. Szendrey T, Danyi G, Czeizel A. Etiological study on isolated esophageal atresia. *Hum Genet.* 1985; 70:51–58.

48. Holder TM, Ashcraft KW, Sharp RJ, Amoury RA. Care of infants with esophageal atresia, tracheoesophageal fistula and associated anomalies. *J Thorac Cardiovasc Surg.* 1987; 94:828–835.

49. Fraser C, Baird PA, Sadovnick AD. A comparison of incidence trends for esophageal atresia and tracheoesophageal fistula, and infectious disease. *Teratology.* 1987;36:363–369.

50. Sillén U, Hagberg S, Rubenson A, Werkmäster K. Management of esophageal atresia: review of 16 years' experience. *J Pediatr Surg.* 1988; 23:805–809.

51. Spitz L, Kiely EM, Morecroft JA, Drake DP. Oesophageal atresia: at-risk groups for the 1990s. *J Pediatr Surg.* 1994; 29:723–725.

52. Engum SA, Grosfeld JL, West KW, Resoria FJ, Scherer LR III. Analysis of morbidity and mortality in 227 cases of esophageal atresia and/or tracheoesophageal fistula over two decades. *Arch Surg.* 1995;130:502–508.

53. Torfs CP, Curry CJ, Bateson TF. Population-based study of tracheoesophageal fistula and esophageal atresia. *Teratology.* 1995;52(4):220–232.

54. Driver CP, Shankar KR, Jones MO, Larmont GA, Turnock RR, Lloyd DA, Losty PD. Phenotypic presentation and outcome of esophageal atresia in the era of the Spitz Classification. *J Pediatr Surg.* 2001;36:1419–1421.

55. Bianca S, Ettore G. Isolated esophageal atresia and perinatal risk factors. *Diseases of the Esophagus.* 2003;16:39–40.

56. Kalish RB, Chasen ST, Rosenzweig L, Chervenak FA. Esophageal atresia and tracheoesophageal fistula: the impact of prenatal suspicion on neonatal outcome in a tertiary care center. *J Perinat Med.* 2003;31:111–114.

57. Geneviève D, du Pontual L, Amiel J, Sarnacki S, Lyonnet S. An overview of isolated and syndromic oesophageal atresia. *Clin Genet.* 2007;71:392–399.

58. Brunner HG, Van Bokhoven H. Genetic players in esophageal atresia and tracheoesophageal fistula. *Current Opinion in Genetics & Development.* 2005;15:341–347.

59. Stevenson RE. Extra vertebrae associated with esophageal atresias and tracheoesophageal fistulas. *J Pediatr.* 1972;81: 1123–1129.

60. Weigel W, Kaufmann HJ. The frequency and types of other congenital anomalies in association with tracheoesophageal malformations. *Clin Ped.* 1976;15:819–834.

61. Cohen MM Jr. Perspectives on holoprosencephaly: Part I. Epidemiology, genetics, and syndromology. *Teratology.* 1989;40: 211–235.

62. Van Dooren M, Tibboel D, Torfs C. The co-occurrence of congenital diaphragmatic hernia, esophageal atresia/tracheoesophageal fistula, and lung hypoplasia. *Birth Def Res (Part A): Clin Mol Teratol.* 2005;73:53–57.

63. Sinha CK, Gangopadhyay AN, Sahoo SP, Gopal SC, Gupta DK, Sharma SP. A new variant of esophageal atresia with tracheoesophageal fistula and duodenal atresia: a diagnostic dilemma. *Pediatr Surg Int.* 1997;12:186–187.

64. Stark Z, Patel N, Clarnette T, Moody A. Triad of tracheoesophageal fistula-esophageal atresia, pulmonary hypoplasia, and duodenal atresia. *J Pediatr Surg.* 2007;42:1146–1148.

65. Martínez-Frías M-L, Frías JL, Galán E, Domingo R, Paisán L, Blanco M. Tracheoesophageal fistula, gastrointestinal abnormalities, hypospadias, and prenatal growth deficiency. *Am J Med Genet.* 1992;44:352–355.

66. Shah D, Jones R, Porter H, Turnpenny P. Bilateral microphthalmia, esophageal atresia, and cryptorchidism: the anophthalmia-esophageal-genital syndrome. *Am J Med Genet.* 1997;70:171–173.

67. Sutphen R, Galan-Gomez E, Cortada X, Newkirk PN, Kousseff BG. Tracheoesophageal anomalies in oculoauriculovertebral (Goldenhar) spectrum. *Clin Genet.* 1995;48:66–71.

68. Ayme S, Julian C, Gambarelli D, Mariotti B, Luciani A, Sudan N et al. Fryns Syndrome: report on 8 new cases. *Clin Genet.* 1989; 35:191–201.

69. Merei JM, Hutson JM. Embryogenesis of tracheoesophageal anomalies: a review. *Pediatr Surg Int.* 2002;18:319–326.

70. Kluth D, Fiegel H. The embryology of the foregut. *Sem Pediatr Surg.* 2003;12:3–9.

71. Moore KL, Persaud TVN. *The Developing Human: Clinically oriented embryology.* 7th ed. Philadelphia: W.B. Saunders Company; 2003: 256–257.

72. O'Rahilly R, Muller F. *Human Embryology and Teratology.* 3rd ed. New York: Wiley-Liss; 2001: 250–252.

73. Qi BQ, Beasley SW. Stages of normal tracheo-bronchial development in rat embryos: resolution of a controversy. *Dev Growth Differ.* 2000;42:145–153.

74. Felix JF, Keijzer R, Van Dooren MF, Rottier RJ, Tibboel D. Genetics and developmental biology of oesophageal atresia and tracheo-oesophageal fistula: lessons from mice relevant for paediatric surgeons. *Pediat Surg Int.* 2004;20:731–736.

75. Arsic D, Cameron V, Ellmers L, Quan QB, Keenan J, Beasley S. Adriamycin disruption of the Shh-Gli pathway is associated with abnormalities of foregut development. *J Pediatr Surg.* 2004;39: 1747–1753.

76. Ioannides AS, Henderson DJ, Spitz L, Copp AJ. Role of sonic hedgehog in the development of the trachea and oesophagus. *J Pediat Surg.* 2003;38:29–36.

77. van Heurn L WE, Cheng W, de Vries B, Saing H, Jansen NJG, Koostra G, Tam PKH. Anomalies associated with oesophageal atresia in Asians and Europeans. *Pediatric Surg Int.* 2002;18: 241–243.

78. Orford J, Glasson M, Beasley S, Shi E, Myers N, Cass D. Oesophageal atresia in twins. *Pediatr Surg Int.* 2000;16:541–545.

79. Brown AK, Roddam AW, Spitz L, Ward SJ. Oesophageal atresia, related malformations, and medical problems: a family study. *Am J Med Genet.* 1999;85:31–37.

80. King SL, Ladda RL, Shochat SJ. Monozygotic twins concordant for tracheoesophageal fistula and discordant for the VATER Association. *Acta Paediatr Scand.* 1977;66:783–785.

81. Blank RH, Prillaman PE Jr, Minor GR. Congenital esophageal atresia with tracheoesophageal fistula occurring in identical twins. *J Thorac Cardiovas Surg.* 1967;53:192–196.

82. Ohkuma R. Congenital esophageal atresia with tracheoesophageal fistula in identical twins. *J Pediatr Surg.* 1978;13:361–362.

83. Van Staey M, DeBie S, Matton MTh, DeRoose J. Familial congenital esophageal atresia: personal care report and review of the literature. *Hum Genet.* 1984;66:260–266.

84. McMullen KP, Karnes PS, Moir CR, Michels VV. Familial recurrence of tracheoesophageal fistula and associated malformations. *Am J Med Genet.* 1996;63:525–528.

85. Warren J, Evans K, Carter CO. Offspring of patients with tracheo-oesophageal fistula. *J Med Genet.* 1979;16:338–340.

86. Dennis NR, Nicholas JL, Kovar I. Oesophageal atresia: 3 cases in 2 generations. *Arch Dis Childh.* 1973;48:980–982.

87. Grech V, Fearne C, Parascandalo R, Soler P. VACTERL with hydrocephalus and isolated tracheo-oesophageal fistula in a first cousin. *Clin Dysmorphol.* 2000;9:145–146.

88. Celli J, Van Beusekom E, Hennekam RCM, Gallardo ME, Smeets DFCM, Rodríguez de Córdoba S, Innis JW et al. Familial syndromic esophageal atresia maps to 2p23-p24. *Am J Hum Genet.* 2000;66:436–444.

89. van Bokhoven H, Celli J, van Reeuwiji J, Rinne T, Glaudemans B, van Beusekom E et al. MYCN haploinsufficiency is associated with reduced brain size and intestinal atresias in Feingold syndrome. *Nature Genetics.* 2005;37:465–467.

90. Bardakjian TM, Schneider A. Association of anophthalmia and esophageal atresia: four new cases identified by the anophthalmia/microphthalmia clinical registry. *Am J Med Genet.* 2005; 132A:54–56.

91. Williamson KA, Hever AM, Rainger J, Rogers RC, Magee A, Fiedler Z, et al. Mutations in SOX2 cause anophthalmia-esophageal-genital (AEG) syndrome. *Hum Mol Genet.* 2006; 15:1413–1422.

92. Sanlaville D, Etchevers HC, Gonzalez M, Martinovic J, Clément-Ziza M, Delezoide AL et al. Phenotypic spectrum of CHARGE syndrome in fetuses with CHD7 truncating mutations correlates with expression during human development. *J Med Genet.* 2006; 43:211–217.

93. Marsh A, Wellesley D, Burge D, Ashton M, Browne C, Dennis NR, Temple KI. Interstitial deletion of chromosome 17 (del (17) (q22q23.3)) confirms a link to oesophageal atresia. *J Med Genet.* 2000; 37:701–704.

94. Foulds N, Walpole I, Elmslie F, Mansour S. Carbimazole embryopathy: an emerging phenotype. *Am J Med Genet A.* 2005;132(2):130–135.

95. Martínez-Frías M-L, Rodríguez-Pinilla E. Tracheosophageal and anal atresia in prenatal children exposed to a high dose of alcohol. *Am J Med Genet*. 1991;40:128.

96. Schoner K, Steinhard J, Figiel J, Rehder H. Severe facial clefts in acrofacial dysostosis: a consequence of prenatal exposure to mycophenolate mofetil? *Obstet Gynecol*. 2008;111:483–486.

97. Felix JF, Steegers-Theunissen RP, de Walle HE, de Klein A, Torfs CP, Tibboel D. Esophageal atresia and tracheoesophageal fistula in children of women exposed to diethylstilbestrol in utero. *Am J Obstet Gynecol*. 2007;197:38:e1–5.

98. Poenaru D, Laberge J-M, Neilson IR, Guttman FM. A new prognostic classification for esophageal atresia. *Surgery*. 1993;113:426–432.

99. Holcomb GW III, Rothenberg SS, Bax KMA, Martinez-Ferro M, Albanese CT, Ostlie DJ, van Der Zee DC, Yeung CK. Thoracoscopic repair of esophageal atresia and tracheoesophageal fistula. A multi-institutional analysis. *Ann Surg*. 2005;242:422–430.

100. Has R, Günay S, Topuz S. Pouch sign in prenatal diagnosis of esophageal atresia. *Ultrasound Obstet Gynecol*. 2004;23:523–526.

101. Kulkarni S, Rao RS, Oak S, Upadhyaya MA. 13 pairs of ribs- a predictor of long gap atresia in tracheoesophageal fistula. *J Pediatr Surg*. 1997;32:1453–1454.

102. Santulli TV, Kiesewetter WB, Bill AH Jr. Anorectal anomalies: a suggested international classification. *J Pediat Surg*. 1970;5:281–287.

103. O'Rahilly R, Müller F. *Human Embryology and Teratology*. 3rd ed. New York: Wiley Liss; 2001: 260–264.

104. Moore KL, Persaud TVN. *The Developing Human: Clinically Oriented Embryology*. 7th ed. Philadelphia: WB Saunders Co.; 2003: 279–285.

105. Cuschieri A, EUROCAT Working Group 2001. Descriptive epidemiology of isolated anal anomalies: a survey of 4.6 million births in Europe. *Am J Med Genet*. 2001;103: 207–215.

106. Spouge D, Baird PA. Imperforate anus in 700,000 consecutive liveborn infants. *Am J Med Genet Supp*. 1986;2: 151–161.

107. Christensen K, Madsen CM, Hauge M, Kock K. An epidemiological study of congenital anorectal malformations: 15 Danish birth cohorts followed for 7 years. *Paediatr Perinat Epidemiol*. 1990;4:269–275.

108. Harris J, Källén B, Robert E. Descriptive epidemiology of alimentary tract atresia. *Teratology*. 1995;52:15–29.

109. Stoll C, Alembik Y, Roth MP, Dott B. Risk factors in congenital anal atresias. *Ann Génét*. 1997;40:197–204.

110. Martínez-Frías ML, Bermejo E, Rodríguez-Pinilla E. Anal atresia, vertebral, genital, and urinary tract anomalies: a primary polytopic developmental field defect identified through an epidemiological analysis of associations. *Am J Med Genet*. 2000; 95:169–173.

111. Forrester MB, Merz RD. Descriptive epidemiology of anal atresia in Hawaii, 1986–1999. *Teratology*. 2002;66:S12–S16.

112. Mittal A, Airon RK, Magu S, Rattan KN, Ratan SK. Associated anomalies with anorectal malformation (ARM). *Indian J Pediatr*. 2004;71:509–514.

113. Heij HA, Nievelstein RA, de Zwart I, Verbeeten BW, Valk J, Vos A. Abnormal anatomy of the lumbosacral region imaged by magnetic resonance in children with anorectal malformations. *Arch Dis Childh*. 1996;74:441–444.

114. Wheeler PG, Weaver DD. Partial urorectal septum malformations sequence: a report of 25 cases. *Am J Med Genet*. 2001; 103:99–105.

115. Wheeler PG, Weaver DD, Obeime MO, Vance GH, Bull MJ, Escobar LF. Urorectal septum malformation sequence: report of thirteen additional cases and review of the literature. *Am J Med Genet*. 1997;73:456–462.

116. Poor MA, Alberti O Jr, Griscom NT, Driscol SG, Holmes LB. Non-skeletal malformations in one of three siblings with Jarcho-Levin syndrome of vertebral anomalies. *J Pediatr*. 1983; 103:270–272.

117. Bianchi DW. FG Syndrome in a premature male. *Am J Med Genet*. 1984;19:383–386.

118. Nievelstein RAJ, van der Werff JFA, Verbeek FJ, Valk J, Vermeij-Keers C. Normal and abnormal embryonic development of the anorectum in human embryos. *Teratology*. 1998;57:70–78.

119. Ross AJ, Ruiz-Perez V, Wang Y, Hagan DM, Scherer S, Lynch SA, Lindsay S, Custard E, Belloni E, Wilson DI, Wadey R, Goodman F, Orstavik KH, Monclair T, Robson S, Reardon W, Burn J, Scamber P, Strachan T. A homeobox gene, HLXB9, is the major locus for dominantly inherited sacral agenesis. *Nat Genet*. 1998;20:358–361.

120. Kimmel SG, Mo R, Hui CC, Kim PCW. New mouse models of congenital anorectal malformations. *J Pediatr Surg*. 1997;29: 211–216.

121. Bitoh Y, Shimotake T, Kubota Y, Kimura O, Iwai N. Impaired distribution of retinoic acid receptors in the hindgut-tailgut regions of murine embryos with anorectal malformations. *Ann Pediat Surg*. 2001;36:377–380.

122a. Finnigan DF, Fisher KRS, Vrablic O, Halina WG, Partlow GD. A proposed mechanism for intermediate atresia ani (AA), based on a porcine case of AA and hypospadias. *Birth Def Res (Part A): Clin Mol Teratol*. 2005;73:434–439.

122b. Winkler JM, Weinstein ED. Imperforate anus and heredity. *J Pediatr*. 1970; 5:555–558.

123. Lynch SA, Wang Y, Strachan T, Burn J, Lindsay S. Autosomal dominant sacral agenesis: Currarino Syndrome. *J Med Genet*. 2000;37:561–566.

124. Köochling J, Karbasiyan M, Reis A. Spectrum of mutations and genotype-phenotype analysis in Currarino syndrome. *Eur J Hum Gen*. 2001;9:599–605.

125. Papapetrou C, Drummond F, Reardon W, Winter R, Spitz L, Edwards YH. A genetic study of human T gene and its exclusion as a major candidate gene for sacral agenesis with anorectal atresia. *J Med Genet*. 1999;36:208–213.

126. Killoran CE, Abbott M, McKusick VA, Biesecker LG. Overlap of PIV syndrome, VACTERL and Pallister-Hall syndrome: clinical and molecular analysis. *Clin Genet*. 2000;58:28–30.

127. Frizzley JH, Stephan MJ, Lamb AN, Jonas PP, Hinson RM, Moffitt DR, Shkolny DL, McDermid HE. Ring 22 duplication/deletion mosaicism: clinical, cytogenetic, and molecular characterization. *J Med Gen*. 1999;36:237–241.

128. Cassini P, Montironi A, Botti S, Hori T, Okhawa H, Stella A, Anderson L, Giuffra E. Genetic analysis of anal stresia in pigs: evidence for segregation at two main loci. *Mammalian Genome*. 2005;16:164–170.

129. Martínez-Frías ML. Epidemiological analysis of outcomes of pregnancy in diabetic mothers: identification of the most characteristic and most frequent congenital anomalies. *Am J Med Genet*. 1994;51:108–113.

130. Smithells RW. Defects and disabilities of thalidomide children. *Brit Med J*. 1973;1:269–272.

131. Myers MF, Li S, Correa-Villasenor A, Li Z, Moore CA, Hong SX, Berry RJ. Folic acid supplementation and risk for imperforate anus in China. *Am J Epiderm*. 2001;154:1051–1056.

132. Levitt MA, Pena A. Outcomes from the correction of anorectal malformations. *Cur Opin Pediatr*. 2005;17:394–401.

133. Taipale P, Rovamo L, Hiilesmaa V. First-trimester diagnosis of imperforate anus. *Ultrasound Obstet Gynecol*. 2005;25: 187–188.

134. Run MV, Christaens GCML, Hagenaars AM, Visser GHA. Maternal serum alpha-fetoprotein in fetal anal atresia and other gastrointestinal obstructions. *Prenat Diagn*. 1998;18: 914–921.

135. Dalla Vecchia LK, Grosfeld JL, West KW, Rescoria FJ, Scherer LR, Engum SA. Intestinal atresia and stenosis: a 25-year experience with 277 cases. *Arch Surg*. 1998;133:490–497.

136. Danismend EN, Frank JD, Brown ST. Morbidity and mortality in small bowel atresia. Jejuno-ileal atresia. *Z Kinderchir*. 1987; 42:17–18.

137. Barrack SM, Kyambi JM, Ndungu J, Wachira N, Anangwe G, Safwat S. Intestinal atresia and stenosis as seen and treated at Kenyatta National Hospital, Nairobi. *East Afr Med J*. 1993;70: 558–564.

138. Kimble RM, Harding J, Kolbe A. Additional congenital anomalies in babies with gut atresia or stenosis: when to investigate and which investigation. *Pediat Surg Int*. 1997;12: 565–570.

139. Sweeney B, Surana R, Puri P. Jejuno ileal atresia and associated malformations: correlations with the timing of In utero insult. *J Ped Surg*. 2001;36:774–776.

140. Komuro H, Hori T, Amagai T, Hirai M, Yotsumoto K, Urita Y, Gotoh C, Kaneko M. The etiologic role of intrauterine volvulus and intussusception in jejunoileal atresia. *J Pediatr Surg*. 2004; 39:1812–1814.

141. Cragan JD, Martin ML, Moore CA, Khoury MJ. Descriptive epidemiology of small intestinal atresia, Atlanta, Georgia. *Teratology*. 1993;48:441–450.

142. Harris J, Källén B, Robert E. Descriptive epidemiology of alimentary tract atresia. *Teratology*. 1995;52:15–29.

143. Francannet C, Robert E. Etude épidémiologique des atresia intestinales: register Centre-Est 1976–1992. *J Gynecol Obstet Biol Reprod*. 1996;25:485–494.

144. Martinez-Frias ML, Castilla EE, Bermejo E, Prieto L, Orioli IM. Isolated small intestinal atresias in Latin America and Spain: epidemiological analysis. *Am J Med Gen*. 2000;93:355–359.

145. Forrester MB, Merz RD. Population-based study of small intestinal atresia and stenosis, Hawaii, 1986–2000. *Public Health*. 2004;118:434–438.

146. Santulli TV, Blanc WA. Congenital atresia of the intestine: pathogenesis and treatment. *Am Surg*. 1961;154:939–948.

147. Manning C, Strauss A, Gyepes MT. Jejunal atresia with "apple peel" deformity. A report of eight survivors. *J Perinatol*. xxxx; 9:281–286.

148. Seashore JH, Collins FS, Markowitz RI, Seashore MR. Familial apple peel jejunal atresia: surgical, genetic, and radiographic aspects. *Pediatrics*. 1987;80:540–544.

149. Tandler J. Zur Entwicklungsgeschichte de Menschilichen Duodenum in Fruhen Embruonalstadiem. *Morphol Jahrb*. 1900; 29:187–216.

150. Lloyd DA. From puppy dog to molecules: small-bowel atresia and short gut syndrome. *So Africa J Surgery*. 1999;37: 64–68.

151. Loux JH, Barnhard CV. Congenital intestinal atresia: observations on its origins. *Lancet*. 1955;2:1065–1071.

152. Luijsterburg AJ, van der Zee DC, Gaillard JL, Los FJ, Brandenburg H, van Haeringen A, Vermeij-Keers C. Chorionic villus sampling and end-artery disruption of the fetus. *Prenat Diagn*. 1997;17:71–76.

153. Arul GS, Carroll S, Kyle PW, Soothill PW, Spicer RD. Intestinal complications associated with twin-twin transfusion syndrome after antenatal laser treatment: report of two cases. *J Pediatr Surg*. 2001;36:301–302.

154. Schinzel AGL, Smith DW, Miller JR. Monozygotic twinning and structural defects. *J Pediatr*. 1979;95:921–930.

155. Komura H, Amagai T, Hori T, Hirai M, Matoba K, Watanabe M, Kaneko M. Placental vascular compromise in jejunoileal atresia. *J Pediatr Surg*. 2004;39:1701–1705.

156. Johnson SM, Meyers RL. Inherited thrombopilia: A possible cause of in utero vascular thrombosis with intestinal atresia. *J Pediatr Surg*. 2001;36:1146–1149.

157. Fairbanks TJ, Sala FG, Kanard R, Curtis JL, Del Moral PM, De Langhe S et al. The fibroblast growth factor pathway serves a regulatory role in proliferation and apoptosis in the pathogenesis of intestinal atresia. *J Pediatr Surg*. 2006; 41:132–136.

158. Merei JM. Embryogenesis of adriamycin-induced hindgut atresia in rats. *Pediatr Surg Int*. 2002;18:36–39.

159. Brenner J, Orgad U. Epidemiological investigations of an outbreak of intestinal atresia in two Israeli dairy herds. *J Vet Med Sci*. 2003;65:141:1143.

160. Cragan JD. Teratogen Update: Methylene blue. *Teratology*. 1999;60:42–48.

161. Matsumoto Y, Komatsu K, Tabata T. Jejuno-ileal atresia in identical twins: report of a case. *Surg Today*. 2000;30: 438–440.

162. Zerella JT, Martin LW. Jejunal atresia with absent mesentery and a helical ileum. *Surgery*. 1976;80:550–553.

163. Mishalany HG, Kaloustian VM. Familial multi-level intestinal atresias. Report of two siblings. *J Pediatr*. 1971;79:124–125.

164. Chiba T, Ohi R, Kamiyama T, Yoshida S. Ileal atresia with perforation in siblings. *Eur J Pediat Surg*. 1991; 1:51–53.

165. Herman TE, Siegel MJ. Neonatal radiology casebook. *J Perinat*. 1992;12:381–382.

166. Roberts HE, Cragan JD, Cono J, Khoury MJ, Weatherby MR, Moore CA. Increased frequency of cystic fibrosis among infants with jejunoileal atresia. *Am J Med Gen*. 1998;78:446–449.

167. Torfs CP, Christianson RE. Anomalies in Down syndrome individuals in a large population-based registry. *Am J Med Genet*. 1998;77:431–438.

168. Spinazzola R, Kenigsberg R, Usmani SS, Harper RG. Neonatal gastrointestinal complications of material cocaine abuse. *NY State J Med*. 1992;92:22–23.

169. Werler MM, Sheehan JE, Mitchell AA. Association of vasoconstrictive exposures with risks of gastroschisis and small intestinal atresia. *Epidemiology*. 2003;14:349–354.

170. Olson LM, Flom LS, Kierney CMP, Shermeta DW. Identical twins with rotation and type IV jejunal atresia. *J Ped Surg*. 1987;22:1015–1016.

171. Gornall P. Management of intestinal atresia complicating gastroschisis. *J Pediatr Surg*. 1989;24:522–524.

172. Smith GHH, Glasson M. Intestinal atresia: factors affecting survival. *Aust NJ J Surg*. 1989;59:151–156.

173. Khen N, Jaubert F, Sauvat F, Vourcade L, Jan D, Martinovic J et al. Fetal intestinal obstruction induces alteration of enteric nervous system development in human intestinal atresia. *Pediat Res*. 2004;56:975–980.

174. Velasco B, Lassaletta L, Gracia R, Tovar JA. Intestinal lengthening and growth hormone in extreme short bowel syndrome: a case report. *J Pediatr Surg*. 1999;34:1423–1424.

175. Van Bever Y, van Hest L, Wolfs R, Tibboel D, van den Hoonaard TL, Gischler SJ. Exclusion of a PAX6, FOXC1, PITX2 and MYCN mutation in another patient with apple peel intestinal atresia, ocular anomalies and microcephaly and review of the literature. *Am J Med Genet*. 2008;Part A 146A:500–504.

176. Shenoy MU, Marlow N, Stewart RJ. Amyoplasia congenita and intestinal atresia: a common etiology. *Acta Paediatr*. 1999;88: 1405–1412.

177. Puri P, Fujimoto T. New observations on the pathogenesis of multiple intestinal atresias. *J Pediatr Surg*. 1988;23:221–225.

178. Basu R, Burge DM. The effect of antenatal diagnosis on the management of small bowel atresia. *Pediatr Surg Int*. 2004; 20:177–179.

Chapter 4

Chromosome Abnormalities

INTRODUCTION

The estimates of the frequency of chromosome abnormalities vary with the gestational age of the embryo, fetus, or liveborn infant. The estimates have been from 37 to 62 % of spontaneous abortions, to 4 % of stillbirths and 0.3 to 0.8 % of liveborn infants (1–3).

The postulated origins of the aneuploidy have included the advanced age of the mother and for a small percentage, errors in the paternal contribution.

Several improvements in the methodology of chromosome analysis have occurred since identification of trisomy 21 in individuals with Down syndrome in 1959 by Jerome Lejeune. The initial karyotypes were unbanded (Figure 4-1), but could identify an apparent extra D group (chromosomes 13, 14, and 15) chromosome in an infant with the phenotype of trisomy 13. The advent of Giemsa staining made it possible to number each chromosome and to identify trisomies, as well as balanced and unbalanced translocations (Figure 4-2).

The advent of the FISH (fluorescent *in situ* hybridization) technology made it possible to identify specific deletions in what appeared to be a normal karyotype. One of the most common is the 22q11.2 deletion (Figure 4-3).

The chromosome microarray or aCGH (array-comparative genomic hybridization) has made it possible to identify more subtle deletions (Figure 4-3) and duplications, which were not suspected on the standard Giemsa-stained karyotype (4).

The common malformations have been shown to be associated frequently with abnormalities visible in the Giemsa-stained karyotype. Examples have been 10% of 212 fetuses with neural tube defects (5) and 33% of 60 infants with anophthalmia/microphthalmia (6).

Among the infants with common malformations and no visible chromosome abnormalities, the analysis by microarray will identify more significant deletions and duplications. This has occurred, for example, in infants

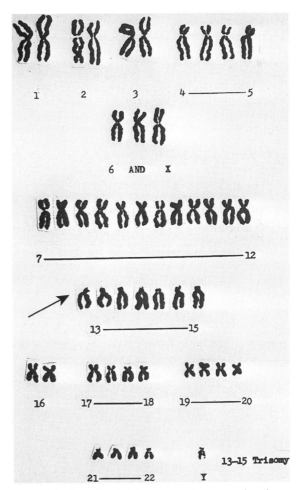

FIGURE 4.1 An unbanded chromosome karyotype that shows an extra chromosome in the "D group," chromosomes 13, 14, and 15. (arrow)

with congenital diaphragmatic hernia and multiple additional associated anomalies (7) [Figure 4-4]. We can look forward to more discoveries through this approach.

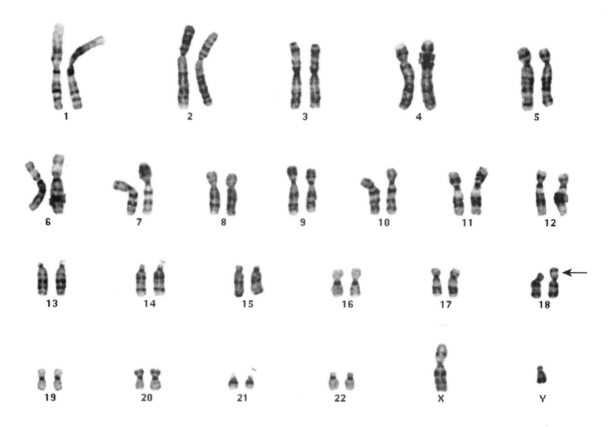

100.9X12.2

FIGURE 4.2   A Giemsa-stained karyotype that shows an unbalanced translocation, with "extra material" (arrow) on the short arm of one of the number 18 chromosomes (arrow).

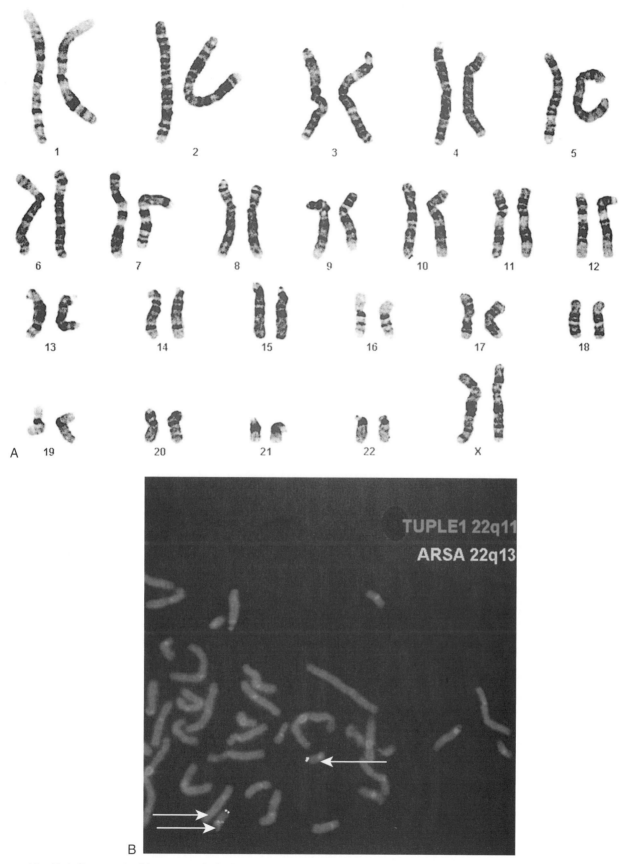

FIGURE 4.3 A) A Giemsa-stained karyotype which shows no abnormality. B) However, the use of fluorescent *in situ* hybridization shows the lack of one probe on one chromosome 22, reflecting the 22q11.2 deletion.

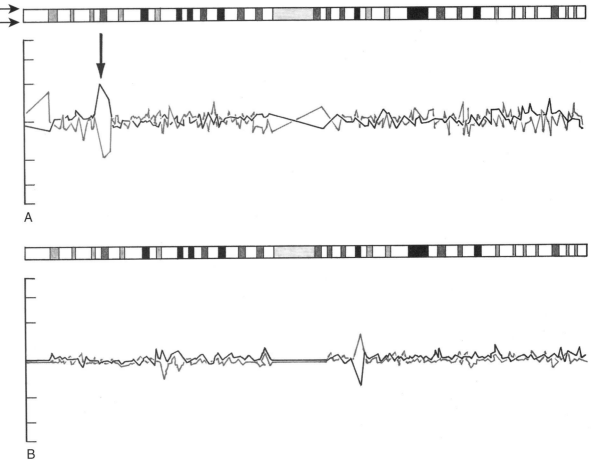

FIGURE 4.4a and b   The chromosome microarray of one chromosome number 1 that identified a deletion (arrow) in the region 1q 41-q 42.12 in an infant with a congenital diaphemagetic hernia (A). The bands on the normal chromosome are shown at the top of the figure (double arrow). The micro array of the infant's mother (B) shows no abnormality. Adapted from Kantarci's S et al.: *American Journal Med Gen.* 2006;140a: 17–23.

TRISOMY 21

Definition

The presence of an additional number 21 chromosome or that portion which is associated with the phenotype of trisomy 21.

ICD-9:	758.000	(trisomy 21)
ICD-10:	Q90.0	(trisomy 21, meiotic non-disjunction)
	Q90.1	(trisomy 21, mosaicism [mitotic non-disjunction])
	Q90.2	(trisomy 21, translocation)
	Q90.9	(Down Syndrome, unspecified)
Mendelian Inheritance in Man:	#190685:	Down Syndrome; trisomy 21
	*602917:	Down Syndrome Critical Region Gene 1; DSCR1
	*605296:	Down Syndrome Critical Region Gene 2; DSCR2 (gene map locus 21q22.3)
	*604829:	Down Syndrome Critical Region Gene B; DSCRB (gene map locus 21q22.2)
	*605298:	Down Syndrome Critical region Gene 3; DSCR3 (gene map locus 21q22.2)

Historical Note

Pictures and statues of individuals with Down Syndrome have been painted and published for thousands of years (12). In 1866, John Langdon Down, a British physician, published an article entitled "Observations of an ethnic classification of idiots" (13). He described some of the common associated physical features of individuals whom we now consider to have Down Syndrome: mental retardation, hypotonia, heart defects, abnormalities of the digestive tracts, congenital cataracts, and abnormalities of the face, hands, and feet. Two notable historical footnotes are the fact that Langdon Down's son, Reginald Langdon Down, was the first person to describe the classical pattern of palmar creases in individuals with Down Syndrome; in addition, his grandson John Langdon Down, Reginald's son, had Down Syndrome (14).

Several cytogeneticists, including first Lejeune (15), and, then, Book et al. (16), and Jacobs et al. (17), published the observation of the associated trisomy 21 in 1959. Later, the less common associations of translocation Down Syndrome and mosaicism, such as 47, XY, +21/46, XY, were described.

In 1961, leading scientists (18) urged that the term "mongolism" not be used, and suggested instead other terms, such as "Langdon-Down anomaly," "Down Syndrome or anomaly," "congenital acromilia," or "trisomy 21 anomaly." They expressed the hope that "agreement on a specific phrase would soon crystallize. . . ."

Studies of spontaneous abortions and stillbirths showed that 80% of the embryos and fetuses with trisomy 21 did not survive to become a term, liveborn infant (19).

In the decades of the 1980s, 1990s and since 2000, improvements were made in prenatal screening that led to the identification of more and more fetuses with trisomy 21 earlier and earlier in pregnancy among women of all ages (20). The techniques of prenatal screening included measuring the width of the nuchal translucency at 11 to 13 weeks of gestation (plus analytes), measuring more analytes in the mother's serum in the first and second trimester, and determining by ultrasound the absence of the normal degree of ossification of the nasal bone (21).

When the prenatal diagnosis was made at a gestational age when elective termination was an option, most couples chose to terminate the pregnancy (22–24).

The premature aging of individuals with Down Syndrome was also noted in the nineteenth century, long before the delineation of the entity of Alzheimer's disease (25). Later, one autosomal dominant gene for Alzheimer's disease was shown to be located on chromosome 21 (26). It was postulated that the occurrence of symptoms of Alzheimer's Disease in individuals with trisomy 21 would be due to over expression of these genes on their three number 21 chromosomes.

Cytogeneticists, analyzing unbalanced translocations involving chromosome 21, identified a specific region that appeared to produce the phenotype of Down Syndrome (27).

Appearance

Beginning with the observations of John Langdon Down (13), the clinical features of affected individuals have been described and tabulated by many clinicians (Table 4-1).

The examination of aborted embryos and stillborn fetuses with trisomy 21 (28) showed that the physical features that are used to identify the affected newborn, such as upward eye slant (Figure 4-5), epicanthus, shortened ear length (Figures 4-6 and 4-7) and increased space between toes 1 and 2 (Figure 4-8), cannot be relied upon to identify affected fetuses.

Many clinicians, notably Penrose in 1933 (29) and Walker in 1957 (30), developed lists of associated physical features, including dermal ridge patterns, that could be used to diagnose Down Syndrome. Preus (31), in a study of 174 individuals with Down Syndrome and 188 normal children, developed a diagnostic index of 12 features. She found that 82% of the suspected cases of Down Syndrome could be diagnosed as affected or unaffected with 99.9% confidence. The 12 features included primarily dermal ridge patterns on the fingers, palms, and great toe hallucal fifth fingers, as well as

TABLE 4-1 *Physical features of infants with Down Syndrome*

Physical Feature	Hall (32) Newborn infants	Lee and Jackson (33) Less than 1 year of age
brachydactyly	–	75.2%
flat profile of face	89%	88.2
upward eye slant	80	86.7
Brushfield spots (speckled iris)	42	34.7
overfolded helix of ear (Fig 4.6)	43	53
excess skin on back of neck (Fig 4.7)	81	60.3
clinodactyly of fifth finger (Fig 4.9)	32	42.9
transverse palmar crease (Fig 4.9)	53	60.3
muscle hypotonia	77	40.9
absence of Moro reflex	82	–
hyperflexibility of joints	77	51.4

Hall (1, 32) examined a sample of 57 newborns with Down Syndrome; Lee and Jackson (33) examined 88 children with Down Syndrome, 56% of whom were newborn infants or less than 1 year of age.

Brushfield spots in irides. She avoided features of a subjective nature.

Several clinicians have tabulated the frequency of physical features in individuals with Down Syndrome, including three that focused on newborn infants: Hall in 1964 (32), Lee and Jackson in 1972 (33) [Table 4-1]. All of these features were more subjective in nature. In addition to these well-known, common features, there ar e many distinctive features that have been observed in individuals with Down Syndrome, including: the speckling of the iris (Brushfield spots) which are more numerous and are located closer to the pupillary margin than those spots which occur in individuals without

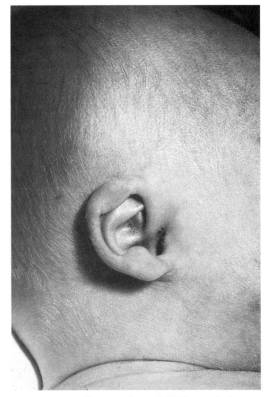

FIGURE 4.6   Small ears with overfolded upper helix.

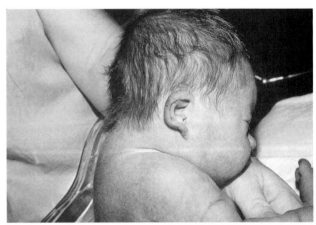

FIGURE 4.7   Fullness of soft tissue over neck and small ears.

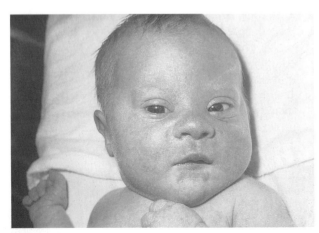

FIGURE 4.5   Upward eye slant.

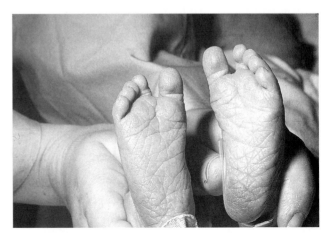

FIGURE 4.8   Increased space between toes 1 and 2.

Down Syndrome (34), a rosy red disc of the optic nerve with a large number of retinal vessels (35), abnormalities of the eustachian tube that could predispose to otitis media (36), a significantly shorter umbilical cord (37), labial folds which are shorter and wider than those of unaffected newborn females (38), and atlanto-axial instability of the cervical vertebrae (39).

Associated Malformations

Many major malformations are much more common in individuals with Down Syndrome than they are in unaffected infants. The amazingly wide range of frequencies identified in large population-based studies (40, 41), including, for example, in one a Risk Ratio (RR) of 108, which means a 108-fold increase in the frequency of atrioventricular canal, a well known association; a 5.3 fold increase for hypospadias; a 6.3 fold increase for cleft lip with/without cleft palate, and a 9.2 fold increase for polydactyly (Table 4-2). Not all malformations were more common in individuals with Down Syndrome. The exceptions included sirenomelia, cloacal exstrophy, anencephaly, spina bifida, and the limb body wall type of amniotic band syndrome.

Other population-based studies (42) and case-series from prenatal diagnosis centers (43) have confirmed that atrioventricular septal defect and ventricular septal defect are the most common heart defects detected

TABLE 4-2 *Increased frequency of major malformations* *in infants with Down Syndrome (33)*

MALFORMATION	INCREASED FREQUENCY (Risk ratio)
any cardiovascular abnormality	108.0**
atrioventricular (AV) canal	1009.1
hypoplastic left ventricle	47.1
coarctation of aorta	25.9
cleft palate without cleft lip	6.3
esophageal atresia	26.4
duodenal atresia	264.9
Hirschsprung Disease	101.8
annular pancreas	430.3
congenital hydrocephalus	10.1
cataract	54.3
clubfoot	7.9
polydactyly	9.2
syndactyly (Figure 4.10)	26.1
undescended testicle	37.7
hypospadias	5.3

*Findings among 2,894 infants with Down Syndrome in comparison to 2,490,437 non-Down Syndrome infants born in California 1983 to 1993 and surveyed by the California Birth Defect Monitoring Program (reference 33).

**A risk ratio of 108 for any cardio-vascular abnormality means that these abnormalities were 108 times more frequent in infants with Down Syndrome than the comparison infants who did not have Down Syndrome.

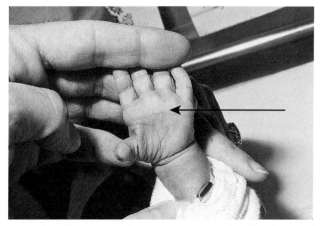

FIGURE 4.9 Transverse palmar crease (arrow) with clinodactyly of fifth finger.

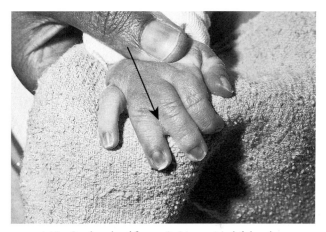

FIGURE 4.10 Syndactyly of fingers 3–4 (arrow) in left hand.

prenatally and postnatally in fetuses and infants with trisomy 21. Among 227 infants with Down Syndrome (42), 44% had congenital heart defects, 45% of which were atrioventricular septal defect (with or without other heart defects) and 35% were ventricular septal defects (with or without other heart defects), 8% were isolated secundum atrial septal defect, 7% isolated persistent patent ductus arteriosus, 4% isolated Tetralogy of Fallot, and 1% were other defects.

Developmental Defect

Trisomy of the distal third of chromosome 21, specifically band 21q22.1-q22.3, appears to be the cause of Down Syndrome (43–45). In one family (46), duplication of 4.3 Mb within 21q22.13-q22.2 was associated with Down Syndrome. One theory, the gene dosage hypothesis, states that the elevated expression of specific trisomic genes leads to the specific anatomic features of Down Syndrome. The competing theory is that the elevated activity of sets of genes leads to a decrease in genetic stability or homeostasis.

The parental origin and meiotic stage of nondisjunction have been determined in several case series (47, 48). These studies have shown consistently that the meiotic error is maternal in about 90% of the infants with trisomy 21 and paternal in 10%. Of the maternal cases in one study (47), 72% were due to meiosis I errors and 28% were due to meiosis II errors. Of the paternal cases, 45% reflected errors in meiosis I and 55% errors in meiosis II.

The increased risk of Alzheimer disease with dementia occurs in individuals with trisomy 21, but not in individuals with trisomies 13 and 18. The association between ApoE genotypes and the occurrence of Alzheimer's disease is true for individuals with Down Syndrome, as well as late-onset Alzheimer's disease in individuals with no chromosome abnormality (49). Shortening of the telomeres, a feature of individuals with Alzheimer's disease, has been shown to occur in older individuals with Down Syndrome and dementia (50, 51).

The examination of trisomy 21 embryos has shown that the formation of the atrioventricular (AV) node and the ventricular conduction system in fetuses with atrioventricular septal defect (AVSD) differs from the normal in weeks 5 to 16 of gestation (49). CRELD1 mutations, located on chromosome 3p25, appear to be genetic risk factors for arteriovenous septal defects (AVSD) on the genetic background of trisomy 21 (52).

Genetic markers have been looked for in the mothers of infants with Down Syndrome. For example, in one study (53) these mothers had a higher frequency of binucleated micronucleated cells in the peripheral lymphocytes than the control group. There was also a significant correlation between the presence of the binucleated micronucleated cells and the polymorphism 677C>T in MTHFR (methylenetetrahydrofolate reductase).

A mouse model of trisomy 21 has been established by manipulating mouse embryonic stem cells and achieving stable germ line transmission of almost complete human chromosome 21 (54, 55). The availability of this model will facilitate studies of the cellular effects of this aneuploidy. For example, Ts65Dn mice, a mouse model of Down Syndrome, have an excessive inhibition in the dentate nucleus, which compromised function. Chronic systemic treatment with GABA antagonists improved post-drug recovery of cognitive function (55).

Prevalence

Estimates of the prevalence rate at birth of a common chromosome abnormality are influenced by many confounding factors, including the frequency of older, more high-risk mothers in the population, the skill of the physicians examining the infants at birth, the frequency and sensitivity of the prenatal screening and testing in use, and whether the data included all pregnancies terminated electively after the prenatal diagnosis of Down Syndrome (56–60). For example, in 1933 the percentage of women 35 and older was 14.5%; by the 1970s it was about 5%; by 2002, it was back up to 13.8% (59). The 1 in 1,000 has been the approximate prevalence rate in racially diverse populations (56). More recent population-based estimates were higher: 1 in 800 (60).

Race/Ethnicity

Because of differences in the maternal ages of pregnant women and the utilization of prenatal screening and the choice of elective termination of pregnancy, it has been difficult to compare prevalence rates among different ethnic groups. No significant differences have been established with certainty (61). However, the likelihood of choosing elective termination is lower in some racial groups, which underscores the importance of including elective terminations. For example, in Atlanta (1990–1999), white women 35 and older were more likely to choose an elective termination than black women (62). Another potential confounder that can affect prevalence rates is an increase in the percentage of births among older women. This has occurred in Japan in association with an increase of the prevalence rate to 1.74 per 1,000 in the years 1990–1999 (63).

Birth Status

Many fetuses with an associated chromosome trisomy, specifically trisomies 21, 18, and 13, do not survive pregnancy (64–66). For example, in a study of 1,813 women with a fetus with either trisomy 21 or trisomy 18, 10.2% of those with trisomy 21 died at an average gestational age of 28.9 ± 1.3 weeks. 37.1% of the trisomy 21 fetuses died before 24 weeks gestational age (66).

Sex Ratio

A modest excess of males has been suggested in several studies, including fetuses diagnosed prenatally by amniocentesis and in spontaneous abortions. However, most studies of this issue have had serious limitations in the methodology used (67).

Parental Age

The correlation of the age of the mother with an increasing risk for having a newborn infant with trisomy 21 has been established in many studies. The prevalence rate increases from 1 in 625 at age 33 to 1 in 49 at age 43 (67). The correlation of this risk with the age of the father has not been established as well (69). In New York State (1983–1997), among the parents of 3,419 infants with Down Syndrome, the parental age had an effect only if the mother was 35 or older. If the mother was younger, there was no paternal age effect.

Twinning

Among identical (monozygous) twins, when one has trisomy, there are several reports (70, 71) of the other twin not having a chromosome abnormality. The reason for this discordance between presumed monozygous twins has not been established. One factor is the lack of molecular studies of discordant monochorionic diamniotic twins to confirm that they are identical. One potential explanation is that occasionally monochorionic diamniotic twins are dizygous (72).

In general, discordance for chromosome abnormalities among "identical" twins could reflect the more general observation that "most monozygotic twins are not identical" (73).

The frequency of twinning among newborns with Down Syndrome, in one study (74), was increased to 2.1 (± 0.6)% in comparison to 0.7 (± 0.3)% in the general population.

Genetic Factors

The empiric recurrence risk for trisomy 21 has been stated to be about 1% after the birth of one affected infant. The analysis of subsequent pregnancies monitored by prenatal diagnosis in North America (75) showed among mothers under age 30 that the rate of recurrence was 0.7% for trisomy 21 and 0.3% for other trisomies. A similar observation was made in Japan (74): 10 (1.29%) of 852 women with one previous fetus with trisomy 21 had a second fetus with trisomy 21. The recurrence risk was 1.1% (8/737) among women less than 35 years old and 2.6% (6/234) among women 35 and older. The rate of recurrence after the birth of an affected infant has been found to be higher than the age-related risks (75–77).

Some families have shown an increased risk for the same trisomy and others have an increased risk for a different trisomy. Studies of parents' lymphocytes, fibroblasts, and the mother's ovaries have identified mosaicism in specific individuals who have significantly elevated recurrence risks (76, 78). These extensive cytogenetic studies are indicated whenever parents have had two pregnancies with regular trisomy 21 or translocation trisomy 21.

There is a shared genetic susceptibility to Down Syndrome and Alzheimer's Disease. An association has been shown between polymorphisms of intron 8 of the presenilin—1 gene in mothers and the occurrence of trisomy 21 due to meiosis II errors (79).

Genetic differences in folate metabolism, such as polymorphisms in folate metabolism like methionine-synthase-reductase, methionine synthase, cystathionine-beta synthase, and methylene tetrahydrofolate reductase, have been postulated to be risk factors in the occurrence of Down Syndrome. Some, but not all, studies support this hypothesis (80, 88).

Environmental Factors

Mothers with a low socioeconomic status have an increased risk for having a fetus with Down Syndrome (82). The unidentified maternal exposures would be expected to affect trisomies that arise from maternal meiosis II errors, which occur at the time of ovulation. The responsible "exposures" have not been identified, but correlate with a lower maternal age, education level, income, and paternal occupation (83).

Treatment and Prognosis

The survival of individuals with Down Syndrome increased with more active treatment of surgical emergencies in the 1970s and 1980s, greater success in the surgical repair of heart defects, and in the treatment of associated leukemia. As a result, a dramatic increase in the median age at death increased from 25 years in 1983 to 49 years in 1997 (84). The increase is expected to increase in the future.

Follow-up studies have shown that several skeletal differences can create challenges in medical management: atlantoaxial instability causing compression of the spinal cord (38), hypoplasia of the first cervical vertebra (C-1) associated with spinal canal stenosis (85), and hip instability associated in adults with hip dysplasia and subluxation (86).

The economic burden of the management of the health care and non–health care costs of a child with Down Syndrome are an important aspect of the care of the affected children (87).

Genetic Counseling

The parents of a newborn infant will be expected to have different types of questions they focus on, first relating to the child: Why/how did this happen? Will he/she be mentally retarded? What additional medical problems may develop? Is there a treatment to improve his/her intelligence?

A practical aspect of the care of the newborn with Down Syndrome is to determine whether or not she/he has a significant heart defect. About half of the infants with Down Syndrome have a heart defect and atrioventricular septal defect is the most common heart defect (42, 43).

It is much better for the new parents of the infant with Down Syndrome to focus on being parents and not to take on the role of the manager of the infant's medical treatment and screening for potential problems. Since many pregnancies with fetuses with Down Syndrome diagnosed before 24 weeks gestational age are terminated electively, pediatricians and family practitioners trained since the 1980s have had less experience with "managing" the potential needs of the infant with Down Syndrome. Some recent publications provide practical advice (9, 10).

One challenge for the parents are periodic "new treatments" with the promise that this treatment will improve the intelligence of the infant with Down Syndrome (88). In the 1990s, treatment with either Piracetam, a nosotropic drug, or the use of megadoses of vitamins and minerals was advocated. A careful, systematic response was needed and was ultimately provided. Nevertheless, many parents were tempted to try expensive treatments with the logic: "Why not? It won't hurt." False hope is much worse than the innocuous treatments (89).

As for the next pregnancy, the risk of recurrence is higher than a woman's age-related risk. However, the precise risks have been elusive. As has been shown in North America (75) and Japan (76), the risk of recurrence is higher for the older mother than the younger mother. Some counselors compromise by simply adding 1% to the age-specific risk of occurrence. The most essential counseling message is that the mother with one previous affected fetus is a "high risk" individual. She should consider the more accurate and sensitive options of prenatal diagnosis by either chorionic villus sampling (CVS) or amniocentesis, rather than using less sensitive techniques of prenatal screening, such as measuring the nuchal translucency and maternal serum analytes. The procedure-related risks are an important issue in this discussion. The risk of losing the pregnancy is 0.2% (1 in 500) after amniocentesis and 1% after CVS. By contrast, there is no risk of losing the pregnancy after the ultrasound-based measurement of nuchal translucency, which appeals to many "high risk" women, in spite of its lower accuracy.

TRISOMY 18

Definition

The presence of an additional number 18 chromosome or that portion of an additional number 18 which is associated with the phenotype of trisomy 18.

ICD-9:	758.200	(Edwards syndrome, karyotype trisomy 18)
	758.295	(Edwards phenotype—normal karyotype)
ICD-10:	Q91.0	(trisomy 18, meiotic nondisjunction)
	Q91.1	(trisomy 18, mosaicism [mitotic nondisjunction])
	Q91.2	(trisomy, 18, translocation)
	Q91.3	(Edwards Syndrome, unspecified)
Mendelian Inheritance in Man:	601161:	Trisomy 18-like Syndrome
	#214150:	Cerebrooculofacioskeletal Syndrome (Pena-Shokeir Syndrome, type II)

Historical note

In 1960, Edwards, Harnden, Cemeron, Crosse, and Wolff (90) reported the first infant with trisomy 18, although they identified the extra chromosome in the unbanded karyotype as a number 17, not a number 18 (91). That infant's physical features included: "an odd-shaped skull, low-set and malformed ears, a triangular mouth with receding chin, webbing of the neck, a shield-like chest, short stubby fingers and toes with short nails, webbing of toes, ventricular septal defect, mental retardation, and neonatal hepatitis (Figure 4-11)."

Thereafter, trisomy 18 was referred to as "Edwards Syndrome" for many years. Anatomic dissections of infants with trisomy 18 showed, as did fetuses with trisomies 21 and 13, that there were structural differences

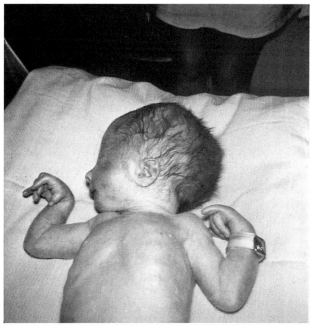

FIGURE 4.12   Side view shows prominence of occiput and flexion contractures of his hands.

throughout the body, well-demonstrated in arteries veins, nerves, and muscles (92, 93), as well as abnormalities of each organ or structure.

Unlike the phenotypes of trisomy 21 and trisomy 13, the infants with trisomy 18 had not been delineated by clinicians as a distinctive, recognizable phenotype. In hindsight, many of these infants had been considered to be small, prematurely born infants. Those with dramatic contractures of fingers, wrists, and other joints had been considered to have arthrogryposis (Figures 4-12 and 4-14).

Like trisomies 21 and 13, chromosome translocations were used to identify the critical part of chromosome 18, which in triplicate was associated with the trisomy 18 phenotype. In 1994 (94), the study of two children with duplication of part of chromosome 18 showed that duplication of the segment 18q12.1-qter was associated with the phenotype of Edwards Syndrome.

Studies of spontaneous abortions showed that 50% have an associated chromosome abnormality, with trisomy 18 a common finding. With the advent of routine prenatal sonography, fetuses were diagnosed as having the features of trisomy 18. Many affected fetuses were stillborn, and the true prevalence of trisomy 18 was much higher than would be predicted from the surveillance of liveborn infants.

With better identification of affected fetuses in elective terminations, stillborn infants, and affected liveborn infants who survived only a few hours, a more accurate natural history and rates of prevalence were established (95). Initially it seemed that all infants with trisomy 18 died in the newborn period or the first

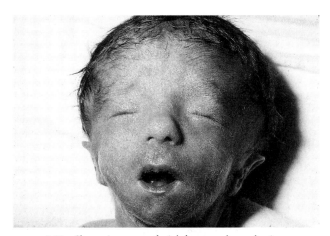

FIGURE 4.11   Shows immature facial features, hypoplastic supraorbital ridges, and telecanthus (increased intercanthal distance).

months of life. However, follow-up studies showed that a few affected children survived for many years, some for at least 20 years (96).

In the 1970s and 1980s there was more likelihood that surgical repair of major malformations would not be offered or recommended. Later, surgical repair began to be carried out (97). The debate continues over this issue (98).

The parents and health care professionals organized a support group SOFT (Support Organization for Trisomy 18, 13 and related disorders; www.trisomy.org), which has provided support for the families and an opportunity to learn more about the natural history of trisomy 18.

Appearance

The spectrum of the physical features of infants with trisomy 18 has been established in several case series (98–103; Table 4-3). The most common features were nonspecific: growth restriction, difficulty with feedings, developmental delay, and failure to thrive. In the physical examination, from head to toe, there are several common features: immature facial features (Figure 4-11),

telecanthus, a prominent occiput, small chin, webbed neck, short sternum (Figure 4-12 and 4-13), heart defects, hypoplastic fingernails with an excess of arch patterns (Figure 4-14), flexion contractures of the fingers, dorsiflexed first toes (Figure 4-15), a prominent heel (Figure 4-16), and "rocker bottom" feet. In one case series (99), it was noted that 33% (7/21) of the infants with trisomy 18 had a "cat-like cry," which illustrates the nonspecific nature of that finding which is often considered "pathognomonic" of the chromosome 5p- syndrome.

A trisomy 18 score was developed by Marion and colleagues (102), which identified correctly the presence or absence of trisomy 18 in a prospective series of 22 infants suspected clinically of having this diagnosis. No single physical feature was found to be pathognomonic. Only one feature, an arch pattern on more than five fingers, was never present in the infants suspected of having trisomy 18, but shown not to be affected. However, five or more fingers with arch patterns was not present in two (5.7%) of the 35 infants with trisomy 18. This finding occurs in several other disorders associated with hypoplasia of the distal phalanges, such as infants exposed to the anticonvulsant drug phenytoin.

TABLE 4-3 *Trisomy 18: Physical features present in newborn infants*

Physical features	Taylor AI et al (99) England (n = 27)	Hodes ME et al (101) Indianapolis (n = 29)	Lin H-Y et al (103) Taipei, Taiwan (n = 39)
Head			
pominent occiput	92%	91%	72%
microcephaly	8	77	56
telecanthus	80	–	33
narrow palpebral fissures	–	80	21
cornea opacity	–	–	13
Mouth			
high arched palate	–	88	38
Neck			
webbing	31	86	21
excess skin on nape	55	–	–
Chest			
short sternum	69	100	23
widely spaced nipples	–	100	10
Genitals			
hypospadias (males)	–	–	33
hypoplasia of labia majora (females)	–	100	13
Hands/feet			
clenched hand, crossed fingers	88	100	95
nail hypoplasia	63	–	13
simian crease	60	–	18
rocker bottom fat	–	87	90

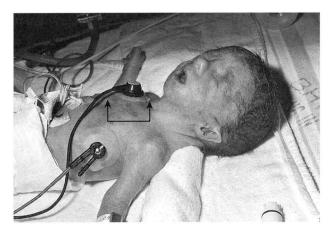

FIGURE 4.13   Shows short sternum (marked by arrows).

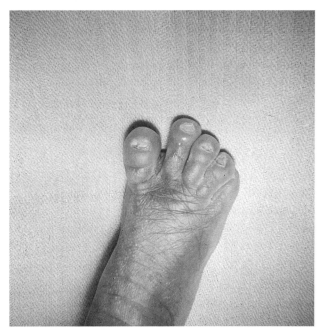

FIGURE 4.15   Dorsiflexed first toe.

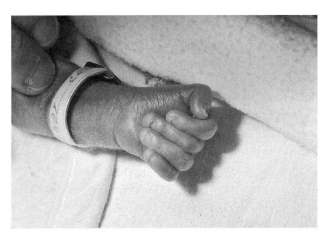

FIGURE 4.14   Clenched hand with hypoplastic fingernails.

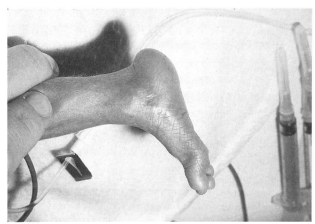

FIGURE 4.16   Prominence of heel.

Associated Malformations

Heart defects are one of the most common associated malformations (104–106). Based on prenatal echocardiography in a series of 255 fetuses with trisomy 18 (1999 to 2004 in London [106]), 73.5% had a cardiovascular abnormality. The most common defects were: ventricular septal defects, atrioventricular septal defects, hypoplastic left heart, and tetralogy of Fallot. In a series of infants evaluated postmortem (107), there were some different findings: almost all infants had dysplasia of one or more valves, that is polyvalvular disease, and a higher frequency of atrial and ventricular septal defect. The affected heart valves were redundant or had thick myxomatous leaflets, had long chordae tendinae and absent or hypoplastic papillary muscles. Polyvalvular disease is now considered a distinctive characteristic of the abnormalities present in a fetus or infant with trisomy 18. The valvular changes have been considered "fetal type" and are similar to those seen in very low birth weight infants at 25 weeks gestational age (107).

Malformations of the central nervous system were identified in 22.5% of 89 consecutive fetuses with

trisomy 18 in Taipei (1988–2004) [108]). The most common CNS abnormalities were holoprosencephaly, hypoplasia of the cerebellum, meningomyelocele, and occasionally anencephaly.

In that same series of 89 infants [109], 12 (13.5%) had an omphalocele and 4 (4.5%) had a congenital diaphragmatic hernia. Abnormalities of the umbilical cord, such as single umbilical artery, umbilical cord pseudocyst (110), and aneurysm of the umbilical artery (111), are another group of frequently associated abnormalities.

The contractures of the fingers with the index finger overlapping the third (Figures 4-12) are a distinctive finding looked for by the clinician examining the infant at birth, and by the sonologist in the second trimester of pregnancy. The detection of the contractures of the fingers is one feature that has led to the suspicion of clinical diagnosis of trisomy 18 in 67% of pregnancies (112). In three case series (92, 94, 96) [Table 4-3], the frequencies of clenched hands and flexed fingers were 88,100 and 95% respectively. The stiff, flexed fingers are also associated with the arch type of dermal ridge pattern on five or more fingers (102), instead of the usual occurrence in 5% of fingers. Less common digit anomalies include: preaxial polydactyl of the hand in 4.5% of 89 infants in one series (109) and absence of the thumb in 1% [111].

Several infants with trisomy 18 have had, in addition, the phenotypic features of malformations attributed to vascular disruption, such as limb-body-wall defects and craniorachischisis (114).

As evidence of the wide spectrum of anomalies of any anatomic structure, abnormalities of middle and inner ear structures (115) and the eyes (116) have been reported. In a series of 27 newborn infants with trisomy 15, one (3.7%) had a cleft lip deformity and three (11.1%) had a cleft palate (99).

Development Defect

In a series of 63 infants and their parents, DNA polymorphisms and microsatellites showed that 61 (96.8%) were of maternal origin and 3.2% were of paternal origin (117). Among the informative families, 31% of the meiotic errors were in meiosis I and 69% in meiosis II. Paternal meiosis errors were not identified. The two cases of paternal origin were due to mitotic errors, findings confirmed in other studies.

Studies of infants with unbalanced translocations have shown that the critical region for the trisomy 18 phenotype is 18q12.1-qter (94).

Multiple malformations similar to those present in affected liveborn infants have been the most common phenotypic features of fetuses with trisomy 18 that have been aborted spontaneously (118).

Cytogenetic studies of the placenta from liveborn infants or electively aborted fetuses with trisomy 18 and 13 (119) have shown that confined placental mosaicism is very common, that is both a trisomic cell line and a normal 46,XX or 46, XY cell line are present. (However, this is not found in infants with trisomy 21.)

The frequency of mosaicism for trisomy 18 in an affected fetus or newborn is quite rare, estimated at 1:70,000 livebirths (120).

Prevalence

The determination of the prevalence rate of trisomy 18 is affected by the extent of prenatal screening and prenatal diagnoses to detect affected fetuses that may not survive to term and whether chromosome analysis has been carried out on aborted fetuses, stillborn infants, and malformed infants who die soon after birth. For example, in the northern sector of the Northern and Yorkshire Heath Region in England in the period 1986–1992 (121), the prevalence rate of trisomy 18 among 18 week fetuses was 1 in 4,274 (0.24/1,000) and much less (1 in 8,333; 0.12/1,000) in livebirths. In Hawaii during the years 1986–1997, the prevalence rate was 0.47/1,000 (or 1 in 2,503) for livebirths and elective terminations combined (122).

Race/Ethnicity

No significant differences in prevalence rate among races have been established. Individual studies have suggested differences, such as the higher rate among Far Eastern Asians in Hawaii (122). In California, an increased rate of occurrence of trisomy 18 among Vietnamese liveborn and stillborn infants in comparison to non-Hispanic white infants was identified in 1985–1997 (123). In 11 states in the United States in the period 1999–2001, there were no differences in prevalence among non-Hispanic white, black, and Hispanic infants in a population-based surveillance program (124).

Population-based studies have shown that affected black infants survive longer than black males or infants from other racial groups, a factor which could affect estimates of prevalence rate (125).

Birth Status

Trisomies 21, 18, and 13 are more common among spontaneously aborted fetuses and stillborn infants than in liveborn infants. Among 106 fetuses with trisomy 18 diagnosed through prenatal screening in California, 32 were stillborn, with the average gestational age 28.9 ± 1.3 weeks (95).

Sex Ratio

At birth, there are more females with trisomy 18 than males. However, at the time of prenatal diagnosis, there is a similar number of affected males and females, a difference attributed to the lower survival rate of affected males (126, 127). For example, in the Trent region of England (127), among 88 infants with trisomy 18, the male: female ratio was 1.32 before 20 weeks gestation and 0.63 after 20 weeks. Among the 69 infants with trisomy 18 in Kanagawa prefecture in Japan (1991–2002), the sex ratio (M:F) was 10:3 in stillbirths, 10:7 in days 0 to 7 and 15:24 after seven days of age (128).

Parental Age

In the case series of 98 families with an infant with trisomy 18 in the United States, and who were members of SOFT (the parent support group), the mean maternal age was 31.2 years (range 18.1–44.9 years) in comparison to 26 years in the general population; the paternal age was 33.2 years (range 22.2–51.6 years) in comparison to 28.2 years in the general population (129). In Taipei, Taiwan, in the years 1988–2004, in a case series of 39 infants with trisomy 18 the mean maternal age was 29.4 years (range 20–46 years) and the paternal age was 31.4 years (range 22–46 years) [103].

Twinning

Some monozygous twins have been discordant for the presence of trisomy 18 (130, 132) and in others, both identical twins have had trisomy 18 (131). When both identical twins are affected, there can be significant differences in the associated major malformations (132).

Genetic Factors

The size of platelets have been a marker in the mothers of infants with trisomy 18 in comparison to normal controls (133). There was a correlation between the size of the platelets and in their fetuses with either trisomy 18 or 13, but not in fetuses with trisomy 21.

Empiric recurrence risk data has been published in three studies (129, 134, 135). Among 98 families with an infant with trisomy 18 in the American parent support group SOFT, the recurrence of trisomy 18 in a subsequent pregnancy was 0.55%. In a second study, none (0%) of 170 amniocenteses in subsequent pregnancies in Japan had a fetus with trisomy 18, although one fetus (0.6%) had a chromosome deletion (13p-). One explanation for the low recurrence risk could be the high rate of spontaneous abortion among fetuses with trisomy 18 (134).

Several infants with similarly affected siblings and no apparent chromosome abnormality have been identified. One group has been designated Pena-Shokeir Syndrome, type II (Mendelian Inheritance in Man: 21450). Clinically these infants have been indistinguishable from those with trisomy 18, until the normal results of chromosome analysis were available (136, 137).

Environmental Factors

None has been identified. However, the fact that the rate of occurrence of trisomy 21 is affected by socio-economic factors (138) makes it possible that the same could affect the occurrence of trisomy 18.

Treatment and Prognosis

The survival rates of fetuses and infants with trisomy 18 have been tabulated in several population-based studies (121, 125, 127) and case series (95, 129). Different ways have been developed for presenting the findings: a) in Scotland in the period 1974 to 1997 (121), among 84 infants with trisomy 18, the mean survival was six days, if an infant survived 48 hours, 58% of the infants survived for 1 week, 34% for 1 month and 3% for 1 year; b) in Switzerland (127) in the years 1964 to 2003, among 161 children with trisomy 18, 68% survived the first 24 hours, 40% survived one week, 22% the first month, 6% for the first year and 1% over 10 years.

Intensive treatment, such as the use of drugs to close the patent ductus arteriosus and heart surgery to repair defects, have been shown to increase survival significantly (139, 140).

Genetic Counseling

More and more affected fetuses with trisomy 18 are being identified through either prenatal genetic screening by ultrasound or diagnostic testing, such as chorionic villus sampling (CVS) or amniocentesis.

The sonologists identify the clenched hands, growth restriction, and a variety of associated malformations. In one retrospective review of the sonograms of 71 affected fetuses, the sensitivity for establishing the diagnosis was 91.5% (141).

Because of these diagnoses during pregnancy, the discussions of the diagnosis and the prognosis are occurring more often during pregnancy and with the sonologist, genetic counselor, and geneticist. The discussions often focus initially on whether or not to continue the pregnancy. Elective termination is the most common choice in North America and Europe. As with all such decisions, many factors influence the choices made (98, 126, 129, 139, 140).

When diagnosed later in pregnancy or if the pregnancy continues by choice, there are options for further testing, such as fetal echocardiography to look for the presence of an associated heart defect. Near the expected date of delivery, the parents and their doctors should discuss the high frequency of episodes of brachycardia and the option of an emergency cesarean section. Experience (121) has shown that half of the affected infants are born by cesarean section.

After the affected infant has been born, if there was no diagnosis by prenatal screening, the clinician can use the systematic "trisomy 18 score" developed by Marion and his associates (95). Rapid techniques can be used to shorten the time needed to process a sample of blood or bone marrow sample.

While waiting for the results of chromosome analysis, the clinician should consider whether the diagnosis could be "pseudotrisomy 18." The prognosis for infants with pseudotrisomy 18 and those with trisomy 18 are equally poor. Therefore, if this alternative diagnosis is a realistic possibility, the parents and the medical staff can make decisions about treatment or palliative care without the results of chromosome analysis being critical.

The physicians, nurses, social workers, and consultants should inform the parents about options in surgical treatment of malformations and aggressiveness in mechanical ventilation (139, 140). Greater information is available now on the success from surgical repair of the common malformations, such as heart defects (97).

The planning for discharge is complicated by the need to decide on whether or not apnea monitoring and resuscitation are needed. The parents should participate in developing the management plan. Membership in SOFT has been very helpful to the parents of the infant with long-term survival as a venue for discussions of longer-term care.

After the birth of the affected infant, the parents will ask the risk of recurrence of this and other chromosome abnormalities and options in prenatal diagnosis. While the risk of recurrence may be lower than for pregnancies after a fetus with trisomy 21, the parents will often use diagnostic studies, such as CVS and amniocentesis, for reassurance.

TRISOMY 13

Definition

The presence of an additional number 13 chromosome or that part of the additional number 13 which causes the trisomy 13 phenotype.

ICD 9:   758.1   (trisomy 13)

ICD10:   Q91.4   (trisomy 13, meiotic nondisjunction)
              Q91.5   (trisomy 13, mosaicism [mitotic nondisjunction])
              Q91.6   (trisomy 13, translocation)
              Q91.7   (Patau syndrome, unspecified)

Mendelian   None
Inheritance
in Man:

Historical Note

In 1960, Klaus Patau, David Smith, Eeva Therman, Stanley Inhorn, and H. P. Wagner (142) reported an infant with multiple anomalies in association with an extra chromosome in the D group, that is either number 13, 14, or 15. Dr. David Smith, the second author, had identified in this infant at age one month these anomalies: "apparent anophthalmia, hare lip, cleft palate and polydactyly of the left foot." Similarly affected infants had been described in medical reports long before chromosome analysis became available. In a review of early reports of infants with anophthalmia, Mette Warburg (143) predicted that an infant with no eyes, cleft lip, broad and oblong nose, six fingers on each hand and six toes on the left foot, reported by Bartolin in 1657, was an example of the trisomy 13 phenotype.

When chromosome analysis has been carried out on spontaneous abortions, it has been shown that trisomy 13 is much more common in spontaneous abortions than it is in liveborn infants (144).

Anatomic dissections (145) showed extensive variations, absences, and supernumerary elements in the muscles. Similar anatomic differences have been identified in each organ system examined in infants with trisomy 13.

As with trisomy 21 and trisomy 18, the study of infants with the phenotype of trisomy 13 in association with chromosome deletions and unbalanced translocations identified the "critical region" on chromosome 13 for this phenotype: 13q32 (146).

In view of the poor prognosis for survival and limited responsiveness to others, there has been debate over the management of the affected newborn infant. Recent reports show how aggressive treatment of heart lesions can increase the period of survival (147).

Appearance

The newborn infant with trisomy 13 is identified readily as having multiple malformations (148–152) [Table 4-4] in contrast to the infant with trisomy 18 whose physical abnormalities are more subtle. The notable facial features often include a keel-shaped brow, a cleft lip deformity (specifically absence of the premaxilla [Figure 4-17]), and microphthalmia (Figure 4-18) or anophthalmia. The most common limb anomaly is postaxial polydactyly (Figures 4-19 and 4-21). There are often several infantile hemangiomas on the face

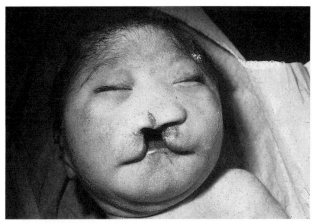

FIGURE 4.17 Newborn with trisomy 13 associated with absence of premaxilla (and associated holoprosencephaly).

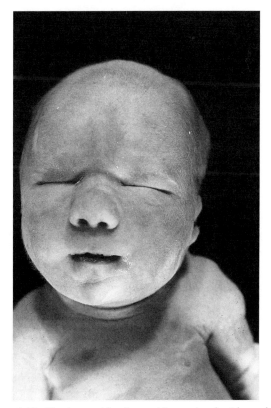

FIGURE 4.18 Newborn with trisomy 13 associated with no facial deformities; microphthalmia present.

(Figure 4-19), chest, and abdomen that develop within the first weeks after birth. A scalp defect on the crown of the head, which varies in size and number, is a common finding (Figure 4-20).

Associated Malformations

Several associated malformations are a common finding in the newborn infant with trisomy 13: heart defects, oral clefts, abdominal wall defects, limb defects (especially postaxial polydactyly [Figure 4-21]) and brain malformations (Table 4-4).

Heart defects are one of the most common malformations (152, 153). In a case series of 14 infants with trisomy 13 (153) in 1983–1988, the most common heart defects, identified by echocardiography in the first few days of life, were atrial septal defect (85%), patent ductus arteriosus (57%), ventricular septal defect (42%), and complex lesions. Valvular dysplasia was usually mild and most often involved the pulmonary valve.

Cleft lip occurred in 19.7% of infants in a consecutive series (1988–2002) of 4,698 liveborn infants with

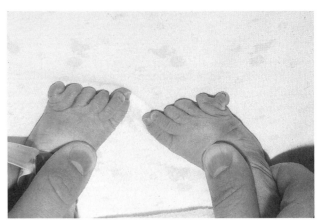

FIGURE 4.21   Postaxial polydactyly in both feet.

trisomy 13 (152). Both the common lateral cleft lip and absence of the central premaxilla (Figure 4-18) occur, the latter a feature of infants with holoprosencephaly.

Holoprosencephaly is, by far, the most common brain malformation. In the infants without holoprosencephaly, the most common CNS anomalies are abnormalities of the corpus callosum, hypoplasia of the hippocampus, hypoplasia of the olfactory bulbs and hypoplasia of the vermis, and dysplasia of the cortices of the cerebellum (154).

The most common gastrointestinal anomalies are: esophageal atresia, bowel atresia, omphalocele, and congenital diaphragmatic hernia.

The associated anomalies of the eye include microphthalmia, cataracts, coloboma of the iris (Figure 4-22)

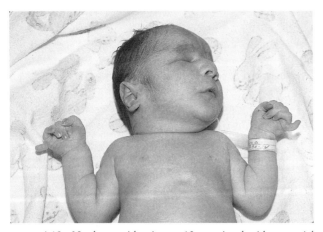

FIGURE 4.19   Newborn with trisomy 13 associated with postaxial polydactyly of each hand, and hemangiomas on eyelids and forehead, but no cleft lip deformity.

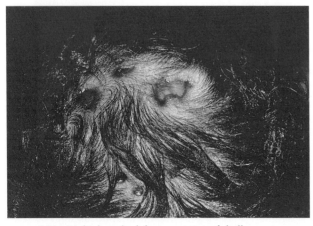

FIGURE 4.20   Multiple scalp defects on vertex of skull.

TABLE 4-4 *Common Associated Major Malformations in Infants with Trisomy 13*[*]

Defect	Increase in infants with trisomy 13 (Odds Ratio)
microcephaly	185.8
hydrocephalus	58.8
microphthalmia/anophthalmia	1210.9
microtia/anotia	105.3
heart defects	79.2
atrical septal defect	993.5
ventricular septal defect	1783.5
tetralogy of Fallot	724.9
cleft lip	1965.5
cleft palate	482.7
esophageal atresia	31.6
rectal/bowel atresia or stenosis	162.7
hypospadias	129.6
diaphragmatic hernia	125.0
omphalocele	80.2
polydactyly	1553.8

Legend: [*]From two large databases that included the occurrence of 39 common birth defects in 1,171 infants with trisomy 13 in comparison to unaffected newborn infants (152).

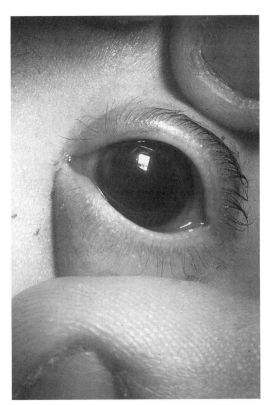

FIGURE 4.22 Iris coloboma.

and retina, persistent hyperplastic primary vitreous (PHPV), persistent tunica vasculosa lentis (PTVL), and dysplasia of the retina. The most distinctive eye anomalies in an infant with trisomy 13 are inferonasal coloboma of the iris and adjacent sectoral cataracts (155).

The analysis of the axial spine in fetuses with trisomy 13 at 14 to 19 weeks gestational age showed partial vertical clefting of the vertebral bodies of the lumbosacral and thoracic regions (156). In addition, there was a lack of ossification of the nasal bone. These findings are different from those present in the axial spine of fetuses with trisomies 18 and 21.

Developmental Defect

0.3% of liveborn infants have a chromosome abnormality with trisomies 21, 18, 13, and the extra sex chromosome syndromes (47,XXX, 47,XXY and 47,XYY) the most common. About 4% of fetal deaths between 20 weeks of gestation and term are associated with chromosome abnormalities, especially trisomies 21, 18, and 13. About 35% of spontaneous abortions between 6 weeks and 20 weeks gestation are associated with chromosome abnormalities, especially 45,X and trisomies 16, 21, and 22 (157).

As with trisomies 18 and 21, the extra number 13 chromosome in over 90% of the fetuses was from the mother and was due to an error in meiosis I (158). However, unlike trisomies 21 and 18, a significant portion of the errors in trisomy 13 were during meiosis II, specifically 37% in one study of 78 infants with trisomy 13 (158).

The cytogenetic analysis of the cytotrophoblasts in the placentas of liveborn infants or terminated pregnancies with trisomy 13 showed that all were mosaic (159). There was no mosaicism in the villous stroma, amnion, chorion, or the fetus/newborn. This confined placental mosaicism has been attributed to mutations that occurred in trophoblasts or extra embryonic progenitor cells during the morula or blastocyst stages.

Some infants with apparent trisomy 13 at birth, were initially mosaic and have lost the normal 46,XY or 46,XX cell line. The presence of a normal cell line in the placental cytotrophoblasts was thought to facilitate intrauterine survival of the trisomy 13 fetuses (159).

The "critical region" for the occurrence of the phenotype of trisomy 13 was suggested in 1993 (149) to be 13q32. Subsequent studies, using chromosome translocations, suggested that duplication of the 13q32→qter region produced the phenotype of trisomy 13 (160, 161).

Prevalence

Since a significant portion of fetuses with trisomy 13 occur as spontaneous abortions or stillborn infants, prevalence rates should reflect these occurrences. In the region of Trent in the United Kingdom for the period 1997–2001, the "birth-incidence date" was 1 in 9,522 (0.11/1,000) and the adjusted "birth-incidence rate" (including estimated abortions and stillbirths) was much higher: 1 in 5,263 (0.19/1,000) births (162). Elective terminations accounted for 38.3% of the fetuses with trisomy 13.

Race/Ethnicity

In a survey of common major malformations in 11 states in the United States (1999–2001), there was no significant difference in the rate of occurrence of trisomy 13 in white, black, or Hispanic infants (163). In Hawaii (164), the highest prevalence rate was among Far Eastern Asians.

Birth Status

The experience in five regional centers in England and Wales (1989–2003) with 411 fetuses diagnosed prenatally with trisomy 13 was that 49% ended in a miscarriage or stillbirth between 12 weeks of gestation and term (165). In the case series in Trent (162), in the United Kingdom (1997–2001), 7% of the affected fetuses were stillborn, 68% of the pregnancies were terminated by choice, and 18% of the affected infants were liveborn. In 14% of the affected infants, the diagnosis was not suspected until after the infant was born.

There was a much higher rate of births by cesarean section, breech presentation, and small for gestational age birth size (less than 10th centile) than among unaffected infants (166). Fetal distress and breech presentation were two common reasons for performing the cesarean section. In a review of delivery data provided by parents who were members of the parent support group SOFT (166), 19% of the infants with trisomy 13 were born at below 38 weeks gestation in comparison to 8% of normal infants. 38% had Apgar scores of 0–3 at 1 minute, 19% had scores of 0–3 at 5 minutes; in normal infants the scores respectively are 2 and 1.

Sex Ratio

Among liveborn infants in a large national (U.S.) database, there were slightly more female than male infants with trisomy 13: F:M = 53:47 (152). Among spontaneous abortions and stillbirths, there were more affected males than females (144, 157, 167).

In Atlanta, Georgia, black female infants with trisomy 13 survived longer than black male infants and infants from other racial groups (168).

Parental Age

The average age of the mothers was 31.3 years (range 31.7–40.8) and fathers 33.7 (range 25.3–42.5) in the parent support group SOFT (166) in comparison to 26 years and 28.2 years in the general population.

Twinning

Two sets of identical or monozygous twins have been reported in which both had trisomy 13 and very different associated malformations (169, 170).

In one set of monozygous twins, conceived by intracytoplasmic sperm injection (ICSI), only one twin had trisomy 13 (171).

Genetic Factors

Most affected newborn infants have trisomy 13. Mosaicism, 46,XX/47,XX+13, was present in 4.5% of infants in a case series of 44 infants with trisomy 13 (162).

The empiric recurrence risk, combining the medical experiences of parents in SOFT of infants with trisomy 13 (n=32) and trisomy 18 (n=98), was one recurrence in 181 pregnancies for a rate of 0.55% (95% CI: 0 to 1.63%) [166] in a study of the findings in Japan among 54 amniocenteses in the subsequent pregnancies of 46 women with a previous infant with trisomy 13, there were no (0%) occurrences of a second fetus with trisomy 13 or any other chromosome abnormality (172). The recurrence risk for trisomies 13 and 18

appears to be significantly lower than that for trisomy 21 (172, 173).

A 1.6 to 1.8-fold increase in the risk for a different viable trisomy was demonstrated for mothers whose previous child had either trisomy 13, 18, or 21. This observation came from the findings in the subsequent prenatal diagnoses that these women had (173).

An increase in the size of platelets in the mothers and their fetuses has been shown to be a biomarker of infants with trisomies 13 and 18, but not infants with trisomy 21, (174). There is also a decrease in total platelet count. This effect has been attributed to the aneuploidy, but the mechanism has not been identified.

Environmental Factors

No analyses have been reported. However, factors such as low socioeconomic status, in general, or poor dietary intake could be contributing factors, as they have been demonstrated in pregnancies with fetuses with trisomy 21 (175).

Treatment and Prognosis

Follow-up studies (176–178) have shown that most liveborn infants with trisomy 13 survive only for a few days. In a retrospective review of 32 infants with trisomy 13 born between 1974 and 1997 (177), the median survival was 8.5 days. They observed that 75% of the infants survived for one day. If they survived for two days, 76% survived for one week. If the infant was 14 days, 60% survived for one month. If the infant survived 30 days, 11% would reach 1 year of age.

A few infants with trisomy 13 have survived over 10 years, one to age 32 years (178).

Some parents have elected more aggressive treatments of the associated medical problems. These treatments can include pharmacologic interventions, such as indomethacin to facilitate closure of the patent ductus arteriosus, and surgical repair of heart defects and closure of abdominal wall defects (147, 179).

Developmental evaluations of the older surviving children have shown that they have severe to profound delays (180). However, they do show some psychomotor development. Some older children could use a walker, understand some words and phrases, crawl, follow simple commands, and recognize and interact with others.

Genetic Counseling

In the past 20 years an increasing portion of fetuses with chromosome abnormalities have been detected by different methods of prenatal screening. First-trimester screening has been developed at 11 to 13 weeks of gestation that utilizes the measurement of the nuchal translucency and the maternal serum levels of free beta-hCG and pregnancy-associated plasma protein-A (PAPP-A). The experience at the Harris Birthright Research Center for Fetal Medicine in London showed detection of 87% of the 61 fetuses with trisomy 13 in comparison to 90% of the 395 with trisomy 21 and 91% of the 122 fetuses with trisomy 18 (181).

Sonographic screening has been more sensitive than maternal serum screening to the detection of the physical features suggestive of trisomy 13. A retrospective review of 181 fetuses with trisomy 13 showed that 50.2% had one or more of these abnormalities: holoprosencephaly, omphalocele, or megacystis (182). 78% of the affected infants had a nuchal translucency above the 95th centile of normal. 71% had a rapid fetal heart rate, above the 95th centile of normal.

In pregnancies in which the mother has chosen to have prenatal screening, the first counseling encounter is during pregnancy. The challenges are to help the woman and the father of the baby to understand what trisomy 13 is and the prognosis for the affected infant.

Experience has shown that most couples choose to terminate the pregnancy after the diagnosis has been confirmed. However, a significant minority (10 to 15%) choose to continue the pregnancy.

For the occasional infant with trisomy 13 who is diagnosed after his/her birth, the counselor can show the parents the signs of the specific malformations present in the infant or identified in imaging studies.

While the chromosome studies on the infant with apparent trisomy 13 are pending, the clinician must consider, also, the possibility that has a phenotype that is very similar, but not associated with a visible chromosome abnormality. Two of these disorders are the holoprosencephaly-polydactyly syndrome or pseudotrisomy 13 syndrome (Mendelian Inheritance in Man 264480) and the Meckel-Gruber Syndrome (Mendelian Inheritance of Man #249000). The prognosis for an infant with trisomy 13 is similar to that for each of these similar disorders. However, as each is attributed to autosomal recessive inheritance, the recurrence risk in future pregnancies (25%) is much higher than for trisomy 13 (<1%). To establish the correct diagnosis, rapid cytogenetic studies on blood or bone marrow samples are essential.

The challenge in both prenatal and postnatal counseling is to make the discussion of the infant's prognosis balanced: the positive responses that the family may observe versus the limited prospects for a long-term, interactive relationship with his/her surroundings. There can be different perceptions of the comfort/discomfort level of the affected infant, particularly if the parents are not involved in the care of the infant in the intensive care unit (183).

Parent support group: SOFT (Support Organization for Trisomy 18, 13 and related disorders [SOFT]). Web site: www.trisomy.org.

REFERENCES

1. Nielsen J, Wohlert M. Chromosome abnormalities found among 34910 newborn children: results from a 13-year incidence study in Arhus, Denmark. *Hum Gen.* 1991;87:81–83, 1991.
2. Hassold T, Hunt P. To err (meiotically) is human: the genesis of human aneuploidy. *Nature Reviews: Genetics.* 2001;2:288–291.
3. Menasha J, Levy B, Hirschhorn K, Kardon XB. Incidence and spectrum of chromosome abnormalities in spontaneous abortions: new insights from a 12-year study. *Genet Med.* 2005;7:251–263.
4. Shearer BM, Thorland EC, Gonzales PR, Ketterling RP. Evaluation of a commercially available focused aCGH platform for the detection of constitutional chromosome anomalies. *Am J Med Genet.* 2007;Part A 143A:2357–2370.
5. Kennedy D, Chitayat D, Winsor EJT, Silver M, Toi A. Prenatally diagnosed neural tube defects: ultrasound, chromosome, and autopsy or postnatal findings in 212 cases. *Am J med Genet.* 1998;77:317–321.
6. Lowry RB, Kohat R, Sibbald B, Rouleau J. Anophthalmia and microphthalmia in the Alberta Congenital Surveillance System. *Can J Ophthalmol.* 2005;40:38–44.
7. Kantarci S, Casavant D, prada C, Russell M, Byrne J, Wilkins-Haug L et al. Findings from aCGH in patients with congenital diaphragmatic hernia (CDH): a possible locus for Fryns Syndrome. *Am J Med Genet.* 2006;140A:17–23.
8. Smith GF, Berg JM. *Down's Anomaly.* 2nd ed. New York: Churchill Livingstone; 1976.
9. Cohen WI, Nadel L, Madnick ME, eds. *Down Syndrome: Visions for the 21st Century.* New York: Wiley-Liss; 2002.
10. Matheis P, Eberly S, Van Dyke DC. *Williams J. Medical and surgical care for children with Down Syndrome: a guide for parents (Topics in Down syndrome).* Bethesda, MD: Woodbine House; 1995.
11. Soper KL, ed. *Mothers reflect on how children with Down Syndrome enrich their lives.* Bethesda, MD: Woodbine House; 2007.
12. Martinez-Frias ML. The real earliest historical evidence of Down Syndrome. *Am J Med Genet.* 2005;132A:231.
13. Down JL. Observations of an ethnic classification of idiots. *Clin Lect Rep London Hosp Rep.* 1866;3:259–262. Reprinted in *Ment Retard.* 1995;33:54–56.
14. Patterson D, Costa ACS. Down syndrome and genetics—a case of linked histories. *Nature Reviews/Genetics.* 2005;6:137–147.
15. Lejeune J, Le mongolisme. Primies exemple d'aberration autosomique humaine. *Ann Génét.* 1959;1:41–49.
16. Book JA, Fraccaro M, Lindsten J. Cytogenetical observations in Mongolism. *Acta Paediatr.* 1959;48:453–468.
17. Jacobs PA, Baikie AG, Court Brown WM, Strong JA. The somatic chromosomes in mongolism. *Lancet.* 1959;1:710.
18. Allen G, Nishimura H, Benda CE, Oster J, Böök JA, Penrose LS, Carter CO, Polani PE et al. Mongolism. *Lancet.* 1961;1:775.
19. Hook EB, Mutton DE, Ide R, Alberman E, Bobrow M. The natural history of Down Syndrome conceptuses diagnosed prenatally that are not electively terminated. *Am J Hum Genet.* 1995;57:875–881.
20. Wapner R, Thom E, Simpson JL, Pergament E, Silver R, Filkins K, et al. First-trimester screening for trisomies 21 and 18. *N Engl J Med.* 2003;349:1405–1413.
21. Cicero S, Sonek JD, McKenna DS, Croom CS, Johnson L, Nicolaides KH. Nasal bone hypoplasia in trisomy 21 at 15–22 weeks' gestation. *Ultrasound Obstet Gynecol.* 2003;21:15–18.
22. Forrester MB, Merz RD, Yoon PW. Impact of prenatal diagnosis and elective termination on the prevalence of selected birth defects in Hawaii. *Am J Epidemiol.* 1998;148:1206–1211.
23. Stoll C, Alembik Y, Dott B, Roth MP. Impact of prenatal diagnosis on livebirth prevalence of children with congenital anomalies. *Ann Génét.* 2002;45:115–121.

24. Caruso TM, Westgate M-N, Holmes LB. Impact of prenatal screening on the birth status of fetuses with Down Syndrome at an urban hospital, 1972–1994. *Genet Med.* 1998;1:22–28.

25. Jervis GA. Early senile dementia in mongoloid idiocy. *Am J Psychiatry.* 1948;105:102–106.

26. St George-Hyslop PH, Tanzi RE, Polinsky RJ, Haines JL, Nee L, Watkins PC, Myers RH, Feldman RG, Pollen D, Drachman D, et al. The genetic defect causing familial Alzheimer's disease maps on chromosome 21. *Science.* 1997;235:885–890.

27. Korenberg JR, Kawashima H, Pulst S-M, Ikeuchi T, Ogasawara N, Yamamoto K, et al. Molecular definition of a region of chromosome 21 that causes features of the Down Syndrome phenotype. *Am J Hum Genet.* 1990;47:236–246.

28. Stephens TD, Shepard TH. The Down Syndrome in the fetus. *Teratology.* 1980;22:37–41.

29. Penrose LS. *Mental Defect.* London: Sidqwick and Jackson; 1933.

30. Walker NF. The use of dermal configurations in the diagnosis of mongolism. *J Pediatr.* 1957;50:19–26.

31. Preus M. A diagnostic index for Down Syndrome. *Clinical Genetics.* 1977;12:47–55.

32. Hall B. Mongolism in newborn infants. An examination of the criteria for recognition and some speculations on the pathogenic activity of the chromosomal abnormality. *Clin Pediatr.* 1966;5: 4–12.

33. Lee LG, Jackson JF. Diagnosis of Down's syndrome: Clinical vs. laboratory. *Clin Pediatr.* 1972;11:353–356.

34. Donaldson DD. The significance of spotting of the iris in Mongoloids. *Arch Ophthalmol.* 1961;4:50–55.

35. Ahmad A, Pruett RC. The fundus in mongolism. *Arch Ophthalmol.* 1976;94:772–776.

36. Shibahara Y, Sando I. Congenital anomalies of the eustachian tube in Down Syndrome. *Ann Otol Rhinol Laryngol.* 1989;98: 543–547.

37. Moessinger AC, Mills JL, Harley EE, Rama Krishnan R, Berendes W, Blanc WA. Umbilical cord length in Down's Syndrome. *Am J Dis Ch.* 1986;140:1276–1277.

38. Iancu T. The "labial index" in Down's Syndrome. *Clinical Genetics.* 1975;8:81–84.

39. Morton RE, Khan MA, Murray-Leslie C, Elliott S. Atlantoaxial instability in Down's Syndrome: a five year follow up study. *Arch Dis Childh.* 1995;72:115–119.

40. Torfs CP, Christianson RE. Anomalies in Down Syndrome individuals in a large population-based registry. *Am J Med Genet.* 1998;77:431–438.

41. Cleves MA, Hobbs CA, Cleves PA, Tilford JM, Bird TM, Robbins JM. Congenital effects among liveborn infants with Down Syndrome. *Birth Def Res (Part A): Clin Mol Teratol.* 2007;79:657–663.

42. Freeman SB, Taft LF, Dooley KJ, Allran K, Sherman SL, Hassold TJ, Khoury MJ, Saker DM. Population-based study of congenital heart defects in Down Syndrome. *Am J Med Genet.* 1998;80:213–217.

43. Paladini D, Tartaglione A, Agangi A, Theodoro A, Forleo F, Borghese A, Martinelli P. The association between congenital heart disease and Down Syndrome in prenatal life. *Ultrasound Obstet Gynecol.* 2000;15:104–110.

44. Patterson D, Costa ACS. Down Syndrome and genetics—a case of linked histories. *Nature Review: Genetics.* 2005;6:137–147.

45. Antonarakis SE, Lyle R, Dermitzakis ET, Reymond A, Deutsch S. Chromosome 21 and Down Syndrome: From genomics to pathophysiology. *Nature Reviews: Genetics.* 2004;5:725–738.

46. Ronan A, Fagan K, Christie L, Conroy J, Nowak NJ, Turner G. Familial 4.3 Mb duplication of 21q22 sheds new light on the Down Syndrome critical region. *J Med Genet.* 2007;44: 448–451.

47. Antonarakis SE, Petersen MB, McInnis MG, Adelsberger PA, Schinzel AA, Brinkert F et al. The meiotic stage of non-disjunction in trisomy 21: determination by using DNA polymorphisms. *Am J Hum Genet.* 1992;50:544–550.

48. Ballesta F, Queralt R, Gómez D, Solsona E, Guitart M, Ezquerra M et al. Parental origin and meiotic stage of non-disjunction in 139 cases of trisomy 21. *Ann Genet.* 1999;42:11–15.

49. Rubinsztein DC, Hon J, Stevens F, Pyrah I, Tysoe C, Huppert FA, Easton DF, Holland AJ. Apo E genotypes and risk of dementia in Down Syndrome. *Am J Med Genet (Neuropsychiatric Genetics).* 1999;88:344–347.

50. Jenkins EC, Velinov MT, Ye L, Gu H, Li S, Jenkins EC Jr et al. Telomere shortening in T lymphocytes of older individuals with Down syndrome and dementia. *Neurobiol Aging.* 2006;27: 941–945.

51. Blom NA, Ottenkamp JAAP, Deruiter MC, Wenink ACG, Gittenberger-De Grott AC. Development of cardiac conduction system in atrioventricular septal defect in human trisomy 21. *Pediatr Res.* 2005;58:516–520.

52. Maslen CL, Babcock D, Robinson SW, Bean LJH, Dooley KJ, Willour VL, Sherman SL. CRELD1 mutations contribute to the occurrence of cardiac atrioventricular septal defects in Down syndrome. *Am J Med Genet. Part A.* 2006; 140A: 2501–2505.

53. Coppedè F, Colognato R, Bonelli A, Astrea G, Bargagna S, Siciliano G, Migliore L. Polymorphisms in folate and homocysteine metabolizing genes and chromosome damage in mothers of Down syndrome children. *Am J Med Genet. Part A.* 2007; 143A:2006–2015.

54. O'Doherty A, Ruf S, Mulligan C, Hildreth V, Errington ML, Cooke S et al. An aneuploid mouse strain carrying human chromosome 21 with Down Syndrome phenotypes. *Science.* 2005; 309:2033–2037.

55. Fernandez F, Morishita W, Zuniga E, Nguyen J, Blank M, Malenka RC, Garner CC. Pharmacotherapy for cognitive impairment in a mouse model of Down syndrome. *Nature Neurosci.* 2007;10:411–413.

56. Krivchenia E, Huether CA, Edmonds LD, May DS, Guckenberger S. Comparative epidemiology of Down Syndrome in two United States populations, 1970–1989. *Am J Epidemiol.* 1993;137: 815–828.

57. Bishop J, Huether CA, Torfs C, Lorey F, Deddens J. Epidemiologic study of Down Syndrome in a racially diverse California population, 1989–1991. *Am J Epidemiol.* 1997;145:134–147.

58. Carothers AD, Castilla EE, da Graca Dutra M, Hook EB. Search for ethnic, geographic, and other factors in the epidemiology of Down syndrome in South America: Analysis of data from the ECLAMC Project, 1967–1997. *Am J Med Genetics.* 2001;103: 149–156.

59. Resta RG. Changing demographics of advanced maternal age (AMA) and the impact on the predicted incidence of Down Syndrome in the United States: implications for prenatal screening and genetic counseling. *Am J Med Genet.* 2005;133A:31–36.

60. Canfield MA, Ramadhani TA, Yuskiv N, Davidoff MJ, Petrini JR, Hobbs CA et al. Improved national prevalence estimates for 18 selected major birth defects—United States, 1999–2001. *MMWR Morb Mortal Wkly Rep.* 2006;54:1301–1305.

61. Shaw GM, Carmichael SL, Nelson V. Congenital malformations in offspring of Vietnamese women in California, 1985–97. *Teratology.* 2003;65:121–124.

62. Siffel C, Correa A, Cragan J, Alverson CJ. Prenatal diagnosis, pregnancy terminations and prevalence of Down Syndrome in Atlanta. *Birth Def Res (Part A): Clin Mol Teratol.* 2004;70: 565–571.

63. Takeuchi A, Ehara H, Ohtani K, Maegaki Y, Nanba Y, Nagata I et al. Live birth prevalence of Down Syndrome in Tottori, Japan, 1980–1999. *Am J Med Genet. Part A.* 2008; 146A:1381–1386, 2008.

64. Halliday JL, Watson LF, Lumley J, Danks DM, Sheffield LJ. New estimates of Down Syndrome risks at chorionic villus sampling,

amniocentesis, and live birth in women of advanced maternal age from a uniquely defined population. *Prenat Diagn.* 1995;15: 455–465, 1995.

65. Hook EB, Muttan DE, Ide R, Alberman E, Bobrow M. The natural history of Down Syndrome conceptuses diagnosed prenatally that are not electively terminated. *Am J Hum Genet.* 1995;57: 875–881.

66. Won RH, Currier RJ, Lorey F, Towner DR. The timing of demise in fetuses with trisomy 21 and trisomy 18. *Prenatal Diagn.* 2005;25:608–611.

67. Huether CA. Epidemiologic aspects of Down Syndrome: sex ratio, incidence, and recent impact of prenatal diagnosis. In: H Kalter, ed., *Issues and Reviews in Teratology*, Vol 5. New York: Plenum Press; 1990: 238–316.

68. Hook EB. Chromosome abnormalities and spontaneous fetal death following amniocentesis: further data and associations with maternal age. *Am J Hum Genet.* 1983;35:110–116.

69. Fisch H, Hyun G, Golden R, Hensle TW, Olsson CA, Liberson GL. The influence of paternal age on Down Syndrome. *J Urol.* 2003;169:2275–2278.

70. Nieuwint A, Van Zalen-Sprock R, Hummel P, Pals G, Van Vugt J, Van Der Harten H, Heins Y, Madan K. 'Identical' twins with discordant karyotypes. *Prenat Diagn.* 1999;19:72–76.

71. O'Donnell CPF, Pertile MD, Sheffield LJ, Sampson A. Monozygotic twins with discordant karyotypes: a case report. *J Pediatr.* 2004;145:406–408.

72. Shalev SA, Shalev E, Pras E, Shneor Y, Gazit E, Yaron Y, Loewenthal R. Evidence for blood chimerism in dizygotic spontaneous twin pregnancy discordant for Down syndrome. *Prenat Diagn.* 2006; 26:782–784.

73. Machin GA. Some causes of genotypic and phenotypic discordance in monozygotic twin pairs. *Am J Med Genet.* 1996;61:216–228.

74. Bliumina MG, Lil'in ET, Patiutko RS. Multiple birth and Down Syndromic (in Russian). *Genetika.* 1975;11:153–154.

75. Warburton D, Dallarie L, Thangavelu M, Ross L, Levin B, Kline J. Trisomy recurrence: a reconsideration based on North American data. *Am J Hum Genet.* 2004;75:376–385.

76. Uehara S, Yaegashi N, Maeda T, Hoshi N, Fujimoto S, Fujimori S et al. Risk of recurrence of fetal chromosomal aberrations: analysis of trisomy 21, trisomy 18, trisomy 13, and 45,X in 1,076 Japanese mothers. *J Obstet Gynaecol Res.* 1999;25:373–379.

77. Morris JK, Mutton DE, Alberman E. Recurrences of free trisomy 21: analysis of data from the National Down Syndrome Cytogenetic Register. *Prenat Diagn.* 2005;25:1120–1128.

78. Sachs ES, Jahoda MGJ, Los FJ, Pijpers L, Wladimiroff JW. Trisomy 21 mosaicism in gonads with unexpectedly high recurrence risks. *Am J Med Genet Suppl.* 1990;7:186–188.

79. Peterson MB, Karadima G, Samaritaki M, Avramopoulos D, Vassilopoulos D, Mikkelsen M. Association between presenilin-1 polymorphism and maternal meiosis II errors in Down Syndrome. *Am J Med Genet.* 2000;93:366–372.

80. Scala I, Granese B, Sellitto M, Salomè S, Sammartino A, Pepe A, et al. Analysis of seven maternal polymorphisms of genes involved in homocysteine/folate metabolism and risk of Down Syndrome offspring. *Genet Med.* 2006;8:409–416.

81. Martinez-Frias M-L, Pérez B, Desviat LR, Castro M, Leal F, Rodríguez L, et al. Maternal polymorphisms 677C-T and 1298A-C of MTHFR and 66A-G MTRR genes: is there any relationship between polymorphism of the folate pathway, maternal homocysteine levels, and the risk for having a child with Down Syndrome? *Am J Med Genet (Part A).* 2006; 140A:987–997, 2006.

82. Christianson RE, Sherman SL, Torfs CP. Maternal meiosis II nondisjunction in trisomy 21 is associated with maternal low socioeconomic status. *Genet Med.* 2004;6:487–494.

83. Torfs CP, Christianson RE. Socioeconomic effects on the risk of having a recognized pregnancy with Down Syndrome. *Birth Defects Res (Part A): Clin Mol Teratol.* 2003;67:522–528.

84. Yang Q, Rasmussen SA, Friedman JM. Mortality associated with Down's Syndrome in the USA from 1983 to 1997: a population-based study. *Lancet.* 2002;359:1019–1025.

85. Sasaki H, Taketomi E et al. Occult spinal canal stenosis due to C-1 hypoplasia in children with Down syndrome. *J Neurosurg (6 Suppl Pediatrics).* 2007;107:457–459.

86. Hresko MT, McCarthy JC, Goldberg MJ. Hip disease in adults with Down syndrome. *J Bone Jt Surg.* 1993;75-B:604–607.

87. Chen Y, Qian X, Zhang J, Li J, Chu A, Schweitzer SO. Preliminary study into the economic burden of Down Syndrome in China. *Birth Def Res (Part A): Clin Mol Teratol.* 2008;82: 25–33.

88. Smith GF, Spiker D, Peterson CP, Cicchetti D, Justine P. Use of megadoses of vitamins with minerals in Down Syndrome. *J Pediatr.* 1984;105:228–234.

89. Holmes LB. Concern about Piracetam treatment for children with Down syndrome. *Pediatrics.* 1999;103:1978–1079.

90. Edwards JH, Harnden DG, Cameron AH, Crosse VM, Wolff OH. A new trisomic syndrome. *Lancet.* 1960;1: 787–789.

91. Smith DW, Patau K, Therman E, Inhorn SL. A new autosomal trisomy syndrome: multiple congenital anomalies caused by an extra chromosome. *J Pediatr.* 1960;57:338–345.

92. Bersu ET, Ramirez-Castro JL. Anatomical analysis of the developmental effects of aneuploidy in man—the 18-trisomy syndrome: I. Anomalies of the head and neck. *Am J Med Genet.* 1977;1:173–193.

93. Ramirez-Castro JL, Bersu ET. Anatomical analysis of the developmental effects of aneuploidy in man—the 18-trisomy syndrome: II. Anomalies of the upper and lower limbs. *Am J Med Genet.* 1978;2:285–306.

94. Boghosian-Sell L, Mewar R, Harrison W, Shapiro RM, Zackai EH, Carey J, Davis-Keppen L, Hudgins L, Overhauser J. Molecular mapping of the Edwards syndrome phenotype to two noncontiguous regions on chromosome 18. *Am J Hum Genet.* 1994;55:476–483.

95. Won RH, Currier RJ, Lorey F, Towner DR. The timing of demise in fetuses with trisomy 21 and trisomy 18. *Prenat Diagn.* 2005;25:608–611.

96. Shanske AL. Tisomy 18 in a second 20-year old woman. *Am J Med Genet Part A.* 2006;140A:966–967.

97. Graham EM, Bradley SM, Shirali GS, Hills CB, Atz AM. Effectiveness of cardiac surgery in trisomies 13 and 18 (from the Pediatric Cardiac Care Consortium). *Am J Cardiol.* 2004;93: 801–803.

98. Goc B, Walencka Z, Włoch A, Wojciechowska E, Więcek-Włodarska D, Krzystolik-Ładzińska J, Bober K, Świetliński J. Trisomy 18 in neonates: prenatal diagnosis, clinical features, therapeutic dilemmas and outcome. *J Appl Genet.* 2006;47: 165–170.

99. Taylor AI. Autosomal trisomy syndromes: a detailed study of 27 cases of Edwards; syndrome and 27 cases of Patau's syndrome. *J Med Genet.* 1968;5:227–252.

100. Emanuel I, Huang S-W, Chiang W-T, Yang C-P. Trisomy 18 syndrome in Chinese infants. Clinical findings and incidence. *J Med Genet.* 1970;7:138–141.

101. Hodes ME, Cole J, Palmer CG, Reed T. Clinical experience with trisomies 18 and 13. *J Med Genet.* 1978;15:48–60.

102. Marion RW, Chitayat D, Hutcheon RG, Neidich JA, Zackai EH, Singer LP, Warman M. Trisomy 18 score: a rapid, reliable diagnostic test for trisomy 18. *J Pediatr.* 1988;113: 45–48.

103. Lin H-Y, Lin S-P, Chen Y-J, Hung H-Y, Kao H-A, Hsu C-H et al. Clinical characteristics and survival of trisomy 18 in a medical center in Taipei, 1988–2004. *Am J Med Genet Part A.* 2006;140A:945–951.

104. Van Praagh S, Truman T, Firpo A, Bano-Rodrigo A, Fried R, McManus B, Engle MA, Van Praagh R. Cardiac malformations

in trisomy-18: a study of 41 postmortem cases. *J Am Coll Cardiol.* 1989;13:1586–1597.

105. Musewe NN, Alexander DJ, Teshima I, Smallhorn JF, Freedom RM. Echocardiographic evaluation of the spectrum of cardiac anomalies associated with trisomy 13 and trisomy 18. *J Am Coll Cardiol.* 1990;15:673–677.

106. Moyano D, Huggon IC, Allan LD. Fetal echocardiography in trisomy 18. *Arch Dis Child Fetal Neonatal Ed.* 2005;90: F520–F522.

107. Matsuoka R, Misugi K, Goto A, Gilbert EF, Ando M. Congenital heart anomalies in the trisomy 18 syndrome, with reference to congenital polyvalvular disease. *Am J Med Genet.* 1983;14: 657–668.

108. Chen C-P. Central nervous system anomalies associated with fetal trisomy 18. *Prenatal Diag.* 2005; 25:419–421.

109. Chen C-P. Aplasia and duplication of the thumb and facial clefts associated with fetal trisomy 18. *Am J Med Genet Part A.* 2006;140A:960–963.

110. Emura T, Kanamori Y, Ito M, Tanaka Y, Hashizume K, Marumo G, Goishi K. Omphalocele associated with a large multilobular umbilical cord pseudocyst. *Pediatr Surg Int.* 2004; 20:636–639.

111. Sepulveda W, Corral E, Kottmann C, Illanes S, Vasquez P, Monckeberg MJ. Umbilical artery aneurysm: prenatal identification in three fetuses with trisomy 18. *Ultrasound Obstet Gynecol.* 2003;21:292–296.

112. Carlson DE, Platt LD, Medearis AL. The ultrasound triad of fetal hydramnios, abnormal hand posturing, and any other anomaly predicts autosomal trisomy. *Obstet Gynecol.* 1992; 79:731–734.

113. Chen C-P. Aplasia and duplication of the thumb and facial clefts associated with fetal trisomy 18. *Am J Med Genet Part A.* 2006;140A:960–963.

114. Donaldson SJF, Wright CA, de Ravel TJL. Trisomy 18 with total cranio-rachischisis and thoraco-abdominoschisis. *Prenat Diagn.* 1999;19:580–582.

115. Miglets AW, Schuller D, Ruppert E, Lim DJ. Trisomy 18: a temporal bone report. *Arch Otolaryngol.* 102: 433–437.

116. Mullaney J. Ocular pathology in trisomy 18 (Edwards' Syndrome). *Am J Ophthal.* 1973;76:246–254.

117. Fisher JM, Harvey JF, Morton NE, Jacobs PA. Trisomy 18: studies of the parents and cell division of origin and the effect of aberrant recombination on nondisjunction. *Am J Hum Genet.* 1995;56:669–675.

118. Byrne J, Warburton D, Kline J, Blanc W, Stein Z. Morphology of early fetal deaths and their chromosomal characteristics. *Teratology.* 1985;32:297–315.

119. Kalousek DK, Barrett IJ, McGillvray BC. Placental mosaicism and intrauterine survival of trisomies 13 and 18. *Am J Hum Genet.* 1989;44:338–343.

120. Hsieh FJ, KO TM, Tseng LH, Chang LS, Pan MF, Chuang SM et al. Prenatal cytogenetic diagnosis in amniocentesis. *J Formosan Med Assoc.* 1992;91:276–282.

121. Embleton ND, Wyllie JP, Wright MJ, Burn J, Hunter S. Natural history of trisomy 18. *Arch Dis Child Fetal Neonatal Ed.* 1996;75:F38–41.

122. Forrester MB, Merz RD. Trisomies 13 and 18: prenatal diagnosis and epidemiologic studies in Hawaii, 1986–1997. *Genetic Testing.* 1999;3:335–340.

123. Shaw GM, Carmichael SL, Nelson V. Congenital malformations in offspring of Vietnamese women in California, 1985–97. *Teratology.* 2002;65:121–124.

124. Canfield MA, Honein MA, Yuskiv N, Xing J, Mai CT, Collins JS et al. National estimates and race/ethnic-specific variation of selected birth defects in the United States, 1999–2001. *Birth Def Res (Part A): Clin Mol Teratol.* 2006;76:747–756.

125. Rasmussen SA, Wong L-YC, Yang Q, May KM, Friedman JM. Population-based analyses of mortality in trisomy 13 and trisomy 18. *Pediatrics.* 2003;111:777–784.

126. Parker MJ, Budd JLS, Draper ES, Young ID. Trisomy 13 and trisomy 18 in a defined population: epidemiological, genetic and prenatal observations. *Prenat Diag.* 2003;23:856–860.

127. Niedrist D, Riegel M, Achermann J, Schinzel A. Survival with trisomy 18-data from Switzerland. *Am J Med Genet Part A.* 2006;140A:952–959.

128. Kurosawa K, Kuroki Y. No sex differences in 18 trisomy births in the Kanagawa Birth Defects Monitoring Program. *Congenital Anomalies.* 2004;44:97–98.

129. Baty BJ, Blackburn BL, Carey JC. Natural history of trisomy 18 and 13: I. Growth, physical assessment, medical histories, survival, and recurrence risk. *Am J Med Genet.* 1994;49: 175–188.

130. Schlessel JS, Brown WT, Lysikiewicz A, Schiff R, Zaslav AL. Monozygotic twins with trisomy 18: a case of discordant phenotype. *J Med Genet.* 1990;27:640–642.

131. Mulder AF, van Eyck J, Groenendaal F, Wladimiroff JW. Trisomy 18 in monozygotic twins. *Hum Genet.* 1989;83: 300–301.

132. Lee J-T, Chou H-C, Tsao P-N, Hsieh W-S, Hwu W-L. Trisomy 18 in monozygotic twins with discordant phenotypes. *J Formos Med Assoc.* 2004;103:314–316.

133. Thilaganathan B, Meher-Homji NJ, Nicolaides KH. Maternal platelet size as a marker for fetal trisomies 18 and 13. *Prenat Diagn.* 1995;15:605–608.

134. Ristic O, Fryns JP, Kleczowska A, Van Den Berghe H. On the recurrence risk of 18 trisomy. *Ann Genet.* 1991;34:47–48.

135. Uehara S, Yaegashi N, Maeda T, Hoshi N, Fujimori S et al. Risk of recurrence of fetal chromosomal aberrations: analysis of trisomy 21, trisomy 18, trisomy 13, and 45,X in 1,076 Japanese mothers. *J Obstet Gynaecol Res.* 1999;25:373–379.

136. Gershoni-Baruch R, Ludatscher RM, Lichtig C, Sujov P, Machoul I. Cerebro-oculo-facio-skeletal syndrome: further delineation. *Am J Med Genet.* 1991;41:74–77.

137. Lammer EJ, Donnelly S, Holmes LB. Pena-Shokeir phenotype in sibs with macrocephaly and without growth retardation. *Am J Med Genet.* 1989;32:478–481.

138. Torfs CP, Christianson RE. Socioeconomic effects on the risk of having a recognized pregnancy with Down Syndrome. *Birth Defects Res (Part A): Clin Mol Teratol.* 2003;67:522–528.

139. Kosho T, Nakamura T, Kawame H, Baba A, Tamura M, Fukushima Y. Neonatal management of trisomy 18: clinical details of 24 patients receiving intensive treatment. *Am J Med Genet Part A.* 2006;140A:937–944.

140. Kaneko Y, Kobayashi J, Yamamoto Y, Yode H, Kanetaka Y, Nakejima Y et al. Intensive cardiac management in patients with trisomy 13 or trisomy 18. *Am J Med Genet Part A.* 2008; 146A:1372–1380.

141. Viora E, Zamboni C, Mortara G, Stillavato S, Bastonero S, Errante G et al. Trisomy 18: fetal ultrasound findings at different gestational ages. *Am J Med Genet Part A.* 2007;143A: 553–557.

142. Patau K, Smith DW, Therman E, Inhorn SL, Wagner HP. Multiple congenital anomaly caused by an extra autosome. *Lancet.* 1960;1:790–793.

143. Warburg M. Anophthalmos complicated by mental retardation and cleft palate. *Acta Ophthalmol (Kbn).* 1960;38:394–404.

144. Parker MJ, Budd JL, Draper ES, Young ID. Trisomy 13 and trisomy 18 in a defined population: epidemiological, genetic and prenatal observations. *Prenat Diagn.* 2003;23:856–860.

145. Colacino SC, Pettersen JC. Analysis of the gross anatomical variations found in four cases of trisomy 13. *Am J Med Genet.* 1978;2:31–50.

146. Brown S, Gersen S, Anyane-Yeboa K, Warburton D. Preliminary definition of a "critical region" of chromosome 13 in q32: report of 14 cases with 13q deletions and review of the literature. *Am J Med Genet*. 1993;45:52–59.

147. Kaneko Y, Kobayashi J, Yamamoto Y, Yoda H, Kanetaka Y, Nakajima Y et al. Intensive cardiac management in patients with trisomy 13 or trisomy 18. *Am J Med Genet Part A*. 2008; 146A:1372–1380.

148. Taylor AI. Autosomal trisomy syndromes: a detailed study of 27 cases of Edwards' syndrome and 27 cases of Patau's syndrome. *J Med Genet*. 1968;5:227–242.

149. Magenis RE, Hecht F, Milham S Jr. Trisomy 13 (D₁) syndrome: studies on parental age, sex ratio and survival. *J Pediatr*. 1968; 73:222–228.

150. Hodes ME, Cole J, Palmer CG, Reed T. Clinical experience with trisomies 18 and 13. *J Med Genet*. 1978;15:48–60.

151. Rios A, Furdon SA, Adams D, Clark DA. Recognizing the clinical features of trisomy 13 syndrome. *Adv Neonatal Care*. 2004; 4:332–334.

152. Pont SJ, Robbins JM, Bird TM, Gibson JB, Cleves MA, Tilford JM, Aitken ME. Congenital malformations among liveborn infants with trisomies 18 and 13. *Am J Med Genet Part A*. 2006;140A:1749–1756.

153. Musewe NN, Alexander DJ, Teshima, Smallhorn JF, Freedom RM. Echocardiographic evaluation of the spectrum of cardiac anomalies associated with trisomy 13 and trisomy 18. *J Am Coll Cardiol*. 1990;15:673–677.

154. Sener RN. Bilateral, perisylvian and rolandic cortical dysplasia in trisomy 13 syndrome. *J Neuroradiol*. 1996;23:231–233.

155. Lueder GT. Clinical ocular abnormalities in infants with trisomy 13. *Am J Ophthalmol*. 2006;141:1057–1060.

156. Kjaer I, Keeling JW, Hansen BF. Pattern of malformations in the axial skeleton in human trisomy 13 fetuses. *Am J Med Genet*. 1997; 70:421–426.

157. Hassold T, Hunt P. To err (meiotically) is human: the genesis of human aneuploidy. *Nature Reviews: Genetics*. 2001;2:280–291.

158. Hall HE, Chan ER, Collins A, Judis L, Shirley S, Surti U et al. The origin of trisomy 13. *Am J Med Genet Part A*. 2007;143A:2242–2248.

159. Kalousek OK, Barrett IJ, McGillivray BC. Placental mosaicism and intrauterine survival of trisomies 13 and 18. *Am J Hum Genet*. 1989;44:338–343.

160. Ioan DM, Vermeesch J, Fryns JP. Terminal distal 13q trisomy due to de novo dup (13) (q32→qter). *Genet Couns*. 2005;16:435–436.

161. Chen C-P, Chern S-R, Hsu CY, Lee CC, Lee MS, Wang W. Prental diagnosis of de novo partial trisomy 13q (13q22→qter) and partial monsomy 8p (8p23.3→pter) associated with holoprosencephaly, premaxillary agenesis, hexadactyly, and a hypoplastic left heart. *Prental Diagn*. 2005;25:334–336.

162. Parker MJ, Budd JLS, Draper ES, Young ID. Trisomy 13 and trisomy 18 in a defined population: epidemiological, genetic and prenatal observations. *Prenat Diagn*. 2003;23:856–860.

163. Canfield MA, Honein MA, Yuskiv N, Xing J, Mai CT, Collins JS et al. National estimates and race/ethnic-specific variation of selected birth defects in the United States, 1999–2001. *Birth Defects Res (Part A): Clin Mol Teratol*. 2006; 76:747–756.

164. Forrester MB, Merz RD. Trisomies 13 and 18: prenatal diagnosis and epidemiologic studies in Hawaii, 1986–1997. *Genetic Testing*. 1999;4:335–340.

165. Morris JK, Savva GM. The risk of fetal loss following a prenatal diagnosis of trisomy 13 or trisomy 18. *Am J Med Genet Part A*. 2008;146A:827–832.

166. Baty BJ, Blackburn BL, Carey JC. Natural history of trisomy 18 and trisomy 13: I. Growth, physical assessment, medical histories, survival, and recurrence risk. *Am J Med Genet*. 1994; 49:175–188.

167. Huether CA, Martin RL, Stoppelman SM, D'Souza S, Bishop JK, Torfs CP et al. Sex ratios in fetuses and liveborn infants with autosomal aneuploidy. *Am J Med Genet*. 1996;14: 492–500.

168. Rasmussen SA, Wong L-YC, May KM, Friedman JM. Population-based analyses of mortality in trisomy 13 and trisomy 18. *Pediatrics*. 2003;111:777–784.

169. Loevy HT, Miller M, Rosenthal IM. Discordant monozygotic twins with trisomy 13. *Acta Genet Med Gemellol*. 1985;34: 185–188.

170. Naor N, Amir Y, Cohen T, Davidson S. Trisomy 13 in monozygotic twins discordant for major congenital anomalies. *J Med Genet*. 24:500–504, 1987.

171. Naylor CS, Tewari K, Asrat T. Tisomy 13 in one fetus from a twin gestation after intracytoplasmic sperm injection. A case report. *J Reprod Med*. 2001;46:497–498.

172. Uehara S, Yaegashi N, Maeda T, Hoshi N, Fujimoto S, Fujimori K et al. Risk of recurrence of fetal chromosomal aberrations: analysis of trisomy 21, trisomy 18, trisomy 13, and 45,X in 1,076 Japanese mothers. *J Obstet Gynaecol Res*. 1999; 25:373–379.

173. Warburton D, Dallaire L, Thangavelu M, Ross L, Levin B, Kline J. Trisomy recurrence: a reconsideration based on North American data. *Am J Hum Genet*. 2004;75:376–385.

174. Thilaganathan B, Meher-Homji NJ, Nicolaides KH. Maternal platelet size as a marker for fetal trisomies 18 and 13. *Prenat Diagn*. 1995;15:605–608.

175. Torfs CP, Christianson RE. Socioeconomic effects on the risk of having a recognized pregnancy with Down Syndrome. *Birth Defects Res (Part A): Clin Mol Teratol*. 2003;67: 522–528.

176. Wyllie JP, Wright MJ, Burn J, Hunter S. Natural history of trisomy 13. *Arch Dis Child*. 1994;71:343–345.

177. Brewer CM, Holloway SH, Stone DH, Carothers AD, Fitzpatrick DR. Survival in trisomy 13 and trisomy 18 cases ascertained from population based registers. *J Med Genet*. 2002;39:e54–56. http://www.jmedgenet.com/cgi/content/full/39/9/e54

178. Tunca Y, Kadandale JS, Pivnick EK. Long-term survival in Patau syndrome. *Clin Dysmorph*. 2001;10:149–150.

179. Graham EM, Bradley SM, Shirali GS, Hills CB, Atz AM. Effectiveness of cardiac surgery in trisomies 13 and 18 (from the Pediatric Cardiac Care consortium). *Am J Cardiol*. 2004;93:801–803.

180. Baty BJ, Jorde LB, Blackburn BL, Carey JC. Natural history of trisomy 18 and trisomy 13: II. Psychomotor development. *Am J Med Genet*. 1994;49:189–194.

181. Kagan KO, Wright D, Valencia C, Maiz N, Nicolaides KH. Screening for trisomies 21, 18 and 13 by maternal age, fetal nuchal translucency, fetal heart rate, free beta-hCG and pregnancy-associated plasma protein-A. *Hum Reprod*. 2008; 23:1968–1975.

182. Papageoghiou AT, Avgidou K, Spencer K, Nix B, Nicolaides KH. Sonographic screening for trisomy 13 at 11 to 13 (+6) weeks of gestation. *Am J Obstet Gynecol*. 2006;194:397–401.

183. Siegel LB. When staff and parents disagree: decision making for a baby with trisomy 13. *Mt Sinai J Med*. 2006;73:590–591. .figure 4.22 Iris coloboma.

Chapter 5

Cleft Lip and Palate

Definition

A lateral defect that extends from the upper lip part or all of the way up to the nostril. This includes the cleft lip "microform" in which there is a scar at birth in the same area as the frank cleft lip. This definition excludes absence of the premaxilla, the area just below the nasal septum, as that deformity is part of the spectrum of holoprosencephaly.

ICD-9:	749.1	(cleft lip, lateral)
	749.11	(cleft lip, lateral, left)
	749.12	(cleft lip, lateral, right)
	749.2	(cleft lip [lateral] and palate)
ICD-10:	Q36.0	(cleft lip, bilateral)
	Q 36.1	(cleft lip, medial)
	Q36.9	(cleft lip, unilateral)
	Q37.0	(cleft hard palate with cleft lip, bilateral)
	Q37.1	(cleft hard palate with cleft lip, unilateral)
	Q 37.2	(cleft soft palate with cleft lip, bilateral)
	Q 37.3	(cleft soft palate with cleft lip, unilateral)
	Q 37.4	(cleft hard and soft palate with cleft lip, bilateral)
	Q 37.5	(cleft hard and soft palate with cleft lip, unilateral)
Mendelian Inheritance in Man:	%199530:	orofacial cleft 1; OFC 1, non syndromic
	215900:	cleft lip with or without cleft palate

%602966: orofacial cleft 2; OFC2; cleft lip with or without cleft palate, nonsyndromic, 2); gene map locus 2p13;

%600757: orofacial cleft 3, OFC3; cleft lip with or without cleft palate, nonsyndromic, 3); gene map locus9q13;

%608371: orofacial cleft 4, OFC4; cleft lip with or without cleft palate non syndromic, 4; gene map locus 4q21-q31;

#608874: orofacial cleft 5, OFC 5; cleft lip with or without cleft palate, nonsyndromic, 5; gene map locus 4p16;

#608864: orofacial cleft 6, OFC6; cleft lip with or without cleft palate, nonsyndromic, 6; gene map locus 1q32-q41.

*600644: orofacial cleft 7, OFC 7; PVRL1 orofacial cleft; gene map locus 11q23-q24.

Appearance

The most common type of cleft lip is lateral to the center of the upper lip and just below the alae nasi of either nostril or both. The cleft is at the junction of the normal fusion between the maxillary process on each side of the face and the medial nasal process. The cleft is an opening of the labial groove, which normally fuses (3.4).

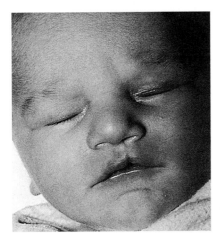

FIGURE 5.1 Shows "microform" or scar present at birth on upper lip.

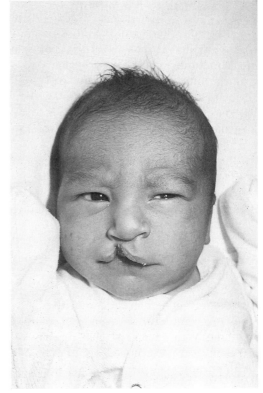

FIGURE 5.3 A more extensive unilateral cleft lip deformity.

The range of severity of the cleft lip (CL) is from a residual scar present at birth (5), referred to as a cleft lip "microform" (Figure 5-1), to a notch in the upper lip (Figure 5-2), to a more extensive cleft (Figure 5-3), to the bilateral cleft lip (Figure 5-4).

The typical cleft lip deformity is much more often unilateral, 72% in California (6), for example, than bilateral. Clefts of the lip, premaxilla, and palate are typically anterior to the incisive fossa; clefts of the secondary palate are posterior to the incisive fossa. Sometimes a bridge of tissue, referred to as Simonart's Band, joins the divided parts at the top of the cleft (7). Bilateral cleft lip is usually (85% of the time) associated with cleft palate (CLP) as well. When the cleft is through the lip and the alveolar part of the maxilla, the intermaxillary (central) part of the upper lip projects anteriorly (Figure 5-4).

The microform unilateral cleft lip (Figure 5-1) has been characterized by: 1) a notched mucosal margin; 2) a thin medial vermilion; 3) an elevated medial peak of cupid's bow; 4) furrowed philtral column; 5) hypoplastic orbicularis oris; 6) minor nasal deformity (8).

The orbicularis oris muscle, which is active in pursing the lips, is interrupted by the cleft lip deformity. This developmental defect, referred to as a subepithelial cleft in the orbicularis oris muscle, is considered a mild extension of the phenotype of the cleft lip deformity (9).

Because of the importance of recognizing a syndromic form of cleft lip/palate, the diagnostic evaluation should be an ongoing process throughout childhood.

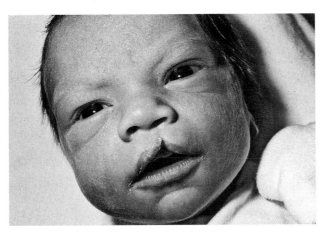

FIGURE 5.2 A mild unilateral cleft lip deformity.

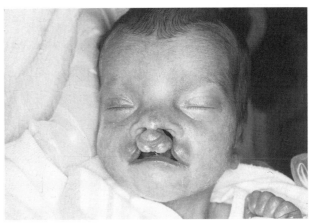

FIGURE 5.4 Bilateral cleft lip deformity with a protruding premaxilla.

Associated Malformations

As with other common malformations, some of the "associated" malformations are in adjacent or nearby anatomic structures and could conceivably be an effect of the same errors in the developmental process that led to the primary abnormality, i.e., cleft lip. Two examples of "adjacent" anomalies among infants with "isolated" cleft lip palate are anomalies of the cervical vertebrae and heart defects.

Regarding vertebral anomalies, an increased frequency (16 to19%) of posterior arch deficiency and fusion anomalies have been observed in the upper cervical vertebrae (C1 – C2) of children with both unilateral and bilateral cleft lip and palate in comparison to 7% in unaffected children (10).

The possible association of heart defects has been suggested in several case series: 6.7% (11), 9.5% (12), and 9.5% (13). These studies suggested that the heart defects are more common in children with oral clefts as part of a syndrome. The frequency of heart defects among infants with "isolated" cleft lip and cleft lip/palate remains to be determined in a population-based study with an appropriate comparison group without an oral cleft deformity.

There is also an increased frequency of associated major malformations involving other organ systems (14–17).

The rate is much higher for infants with cleft lip and palate than it is for infants with cleft lip only. The rate of occurrence has varied among studies (18), reflecting differences in the source of the information (personal examination vs. administrative sources), the severity of the cleft lip deformity, the skill and knowledge of the clinical examiner, the age of the child when evaluated, and whether or not diagnostic studies (such as chromosome analysis) had been carried out, and the racial/ethnic groups of the group being evaluated.

Determining that an infant has a specific associated syndrome has significant benefit in designing the follow-up evaluations needed, as well as for the genetic risks in a subsequent pregnancy. Some monogenic disorders and specific syndromes can be recognized at birth (Table 5-1).

In the affected infant who is stillborn or who does not survive the newborn period, it is important to identify the cleft lip with absent premaxilla, a sign of holoprosencephaly, and the cleft lip with pits in the lower lip (Figure 5-5) as a feature of the Van der Woude Syndrome (MIM #119300). Since many malformed infants who die do not have an autopsy, the clinician's observations in the delivery room can have special significance for subsequent discussions of potential causes and genetic risks.

In a survey of 334,262 births in 11 maternity hospitals in Strasbourg (1979–2003), including stillbirths and

TABLE 5-1 *Cleft lip with or without cleft palate: recognized etiologies*

	Spain* 1980–1985; (η = 382,390 births [25])		Brigham and Women's Hospital, Boston** 1972–74, 1979–2000 (η = 206,244)	
	Cleft lip alone (η = 80)	Cleft lip and palate (η = 248)	Cleft lip alone (η = 58)	Cleft lip and palate (η = 104)
I. *Single mutant gene*				
X-linked	0	2 (0.8%)	0	0
Autosomal recessive (AR)	1 (1.3%)	7 (2.8%)	0	1 (1%)
Autosomal dominant (AD)	4 (5.0%)	12 (4.8%)	2 (3.4%)	0
II. *Chromosome abnormalities*	1 (1.3%)	28 (11.3%)	3 (5.2 %)	22 (21%)
III. *Specific syndromes*			2 (3.4%)	7 (7 %)
IV. *Environmental factors*	3 (3.8%)	7 (2.8%)	2 (3.4%)	1 (1%)
V. *Twinning*				
MZ	0	0	0	0
DZ	0	0	2 (3.4 %)	0
Unknown zygosity	0	2 (0.8 %)	0	3*** (2.9%)
VI. *Unknown etiology*				
Isolated	65 (81.3 %)	155 (62.5 %)	44 (76%)	50 (48%)
Multiple anomalies	6 (7.5 %)	35 (14.1 %)	3 (5.2%)	20 (19%)
	80	248	58	104
	(1 in 4,800)	(1 in 1,542)	(1 in 3,556)	(1 in 1,983)

* Spain, 1980–1985, Newborn Malformations Program prior to legalization of elective terminations for fetal anomalies; courtesy of Maria Luisa Martinez-Frias, 2006.

** Brigham and Women's Hospital, Boston, identified in an Active Malformations Surveillance Program in years 1972–74, 1979–2000; surveyed 206,244 live births, stillborn and elective terminations for fetal anomalies; infants listed here were born to non-transferred mothers who had always planned to deliver at this hospital.

***Includes 2 of 4 quadruplets and 1 co-twin.

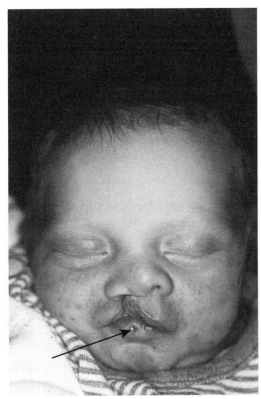

FIGURE 5.5 Unilateral cleft lip deformity with a pit in lower lip (arrow), a feature of the autosomal dominant Van der Woude Syndrome.

elective terminations for fetal anomalies, the apparent etiology was established in the period up to age 1 (17). 72% of the 390 affected infants had "isolated" CLP. Among the 28% with associated malformations, 9.2% had chromosome abnormalities, 1.8% had recognized nonchromosomal syndromes and the remainder had multiple anomalies.

In another consecutive sample of affected newborn infants identified in Japan among 701,181 births (1982–1994), 11.4% of the 362 infants with cleft lip had associated anomalies and 16.2% of 402 infants with cleft lip and palate had associated anomalies (15).

In an 18-year follow-up study of 616 live born infants with cleft lip and/or palate in Stockholm, Sweden, in the years 1975 to 1992 (14), the frequency of associated malformations varied by the severity of the cleft lip deformity: 8% in infants (η = 163) with unilateral cleft lip, 24% in infants (η = 177) with unilateral cleft lip and palate, and 35% in infants (η = 96) with bilateral cleft lip and palate. Some of the major malformations that were significantly more common were anophthalmia/microphthalmia, heart defects, bowel atresia and limb abnormalities, including polydactyly, syndactyly, and limb deficiency.

More specific syndromes are recognized when the child is older. For example, Jones (16), an experienced clinical geneticist, evaluated 574 children in medical follow-up and found that 86 (15%) had the cleft lip or cleft lip and palate as a single primary abnormality, while 14% had multiple malformation syndromes. Among the children with syndromic cleft lip deformity there were: chromosome abnormalities (like 22q11.2 deletion) (13%), monogenic disorders (like Van der Woude Syndrome [MIM #119300]) in 19%, teratogen-induced clefts (11%), and specific malformation syndromes (like CHARGE Association: MIM #214800) in 14%.

Developmental Defect

Major developmental changes occur simultaneously in the brain and the face of the developing human embryo (3, 19–21). Just before the neural folds fuse, ectodermal cells from the neural plate migrate into the underlying regions and become part of the mesenchyme. Neural crest cells form the skeletal and connective tissues of the face, including bone, cartilage, connective tissue and teeth, except for the enamel (3). By the end of the fourth week post-fertilization, the anterior neuropore has closed and the early elements that form the face are visible. Normally, the complex process of forming facial features involves differential growth of certain structures. The maxillary processes develop the medially directed palatal processes. The posterior nares migrate as the nasal septum grows downward. Mesenchyme from the maxillary processes migrate toward the midline. The tongue sinks below the level of the primitive palate, so the palate processes can become horizontal and fuse. The maxillary process grows to meet and fuse with the medial nasal process; failure of this fusion leads to the cleft lip deformity, which would be visible by six weeks (3). The fusion of the palate shelves occurs by 12 weeks in the human; failure will be apparent as cleft palate (19).

Serial sections of stage 17, 18, and 19 human embryos in Kyoto, Japan have confirmed the major growth processes involved (4). Embryos at stages 19, 20, and 22 with cleft lip showed reduced growth of the maxillary process and less fusion with the medial nasal process.

Many molecules have been identified that are essential for the growth, induction signals, and epithelial-mesenchyme interactions that are crucial for development of the upper lip, palate, and other face structures (19–21). These include extracellular matrix molecules and growth factors, which act as inductive signals, including sonic hedgehog (*Shh*), bone morphogenetic proteins (*Bmp*), fibroblast growth factors (*Fgf*), and members of the transforming growth factor β (*Tgfβ*) superfamily. *Shh* plays an important role in the early induction of facial primordial tissues in addition to expression in the palatal mesenchyne. *Bmp2* and *Bmp4*, on the other hand, are expressed more specifically within the epithelia and mesenchyme of the palatal shelves. The *Msx1* homeobox gene, which is also expressed in the facial primordial, is required for expression of *Bmp2* and *Bmp4* in the palatal mesenchyme and *Shh* in the mesenchyne. Epidermal growth factor (Egf) stimulates glycosaminoglycan production within the palatal shelves while *Tgfα*, expressed throughout the palatal mesenchyme and epithelia, stimulates extracellular matrix biosynthesis. Fibronectin and collagen III act as modulating factors on hyaluronate expansion during reorientation while collagen IX plays a critical role in signaling epithelial-mesenchymal interactions, appearing in the MEE cell surface just prior to shelf elevation. Transcription factors such as the *distal-less* (Dlx), HOX, GLI, and T-box families also play key roles in maxillary and mandibular specification and are regulated by *Shh*, *Bmps*, and *Fgf* signals. Epithelial-mesenchymal interactions are crucial in craniofacial development and specific sites of expression, such as the tooth buds, and may function as inductive signaling centers influencing palate morphogenesis.

The process of development that can lead to the occurrence of cleft lip and palate has also been studied in experimental animals, using mouse mutants, gene knockout models, and teratogens (22, 23). For example, the mouse strain AWySn has a cleft lip palate deformity that models the human non-syndromic CLP defect. The research studies have suggested that alleles of two different genes, that is, digenic inheritance, led to the occurrence of the cleft lip deformity (23). These findings in this mouse mutant show the relevance of the model of multiple genetic abnormalities contributing to the occurrence of non-syndromic CLP. Presumably the same mechanism will be identified in humans.

Prevalence

Both CL and CLP are heterogeneous in both etiology and phenotype (Table 5-1). The recognized etiologies include specific hereditary syndromes, chromosome abnormalities, environmental factors, and the conjoining of twins. These phenotypes subdivided into syndromic and non-syndromic or "isolated" CL or CLP. Prevalence rates are subdivided accordingly into "isolated" or nonsyndromic and syndromic CL or CLP.

Prevalence rates for infants with CL and CLP have been published primarily for infants followed through the first year of life, a follow-up that increases the identification of syndromic forms of CL and CLP. There are very few reports of the prevalence rates based on the findings at birth (24–26; Table 5-2).

The prevalence rate for CL alone has been consistently lower than the rate of CLP. In populations in Boston and in Spain the prevalence rates for CL were 0.23 and 0.21/1,000 respectively (Table 5-2) and for CLP were 0.43 and 0.65/1,000, respectively.

Combining CL and CLP, the prevalence rates among 220,927 newborn infants in eight South American countries (1967–1981) was 0.92/1,000 [27] and

TABLE 5-2 *Prevalence rates in newborn infants*

	Italy (24) (1981–1986) n = 220,927	Spain (25) (1980–1985) n = 382,340	Boston (26) (1972–74, 1979–2000) n = 206,244
Cleft lip alone			
"isolated"	Not provided	0.18/1,000 (n = 68)	0.23/1,000 (n = 52)
Total	Not provided	0.21/1,000 (n = 80)	0.29/1,000 (n = 65)
Cleft lip/palate			
"isolated"	0.7 (n = 154)	0.38/1,000 (n =147)	0.23/1,000 (n = 50)
Total	0.9 (n = 199)	0.65/1,000 (n = 248)	0.43/1,000 (n = 95)
Combined			
"isolated"	0.69/1,000 (n=154)	0.56/1,000 (n = 236)	0.46/1,000 (n =102)
Total	0.9/1,000 (n=199)	0.86/1,000 (n = 328)	0.72/1,000 (n = 160)

0.9/1,000 among 220,927 newborn infants in Italy (1981–1986) [24].

The percentage of infants with an "isolated" cleft deformity is higher in infants with CL than in those with CLP: 79% and 85%, respectively, for CL and 59% and 58% for CLP in Boston (26) and Spain (25), respectively (see Table 5-2).

There is, in addition, a very small rate of occurrence of other rare clefts, 2% in Italy (1981–1986) [24]. These include midface clefts (as in the amniotic band syndrome),

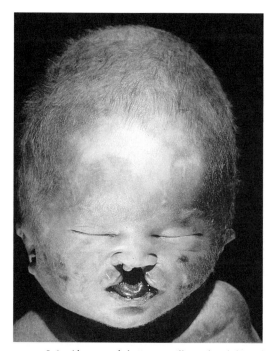

FIGURE 5.6 Absence of the premaxilla with a bilateral cleft lip, a feature of holoprosencephaly.

rare lateral clefts from the outer corners of the mouth and the midline cleft of the upper lip with absence of the premaxilla, which is a part of the spectrum of holoprosencephaly (Figure 5-6).

Race/Ethnicity

Major differences in prevalence of cleft lip with or without cleft palate have been identified between several race/ethnic groups. Rates are higher in Native American Indians [2.7/1,000] (28) and Japanese [1.1/1,000] (29) in comparison to white infants [0.8/1,000] (4). The rates in African Americans in the United States [0.5/1,000] (30) and Africans in Nigeria [0.4/1,000] (31) have been lower than in white infants in the United States. Restricting prevalence rates to nonsyndromic cleft lip with or without cleft palate, the rate was 1.6/1,000 in Madras, India (32), and 1.2/1,000 in Shanghai, China (33).

Birth Status

1,368 infants with CLP and 741 unaffected infants in eight countries in Latin America (27) showed that those with CLP had a lower birth weight. There was no increase in the frequency of premature births in infants with CLP in Hungary (34). In Atlanta, there was an increased frequency of prematurity among infants with CLP and other anomalies, but not among those with isolated CLP (35).

An overall increased frequency of neonatal death has also been observed in newborn infants with oral clefts (24).

A higher incidence of spontaneous abortion in previous pregnancies has been observed (36) also among the mothers of infants with CLP. There was also a correlation with the severity of the cleft deformity. One interpretation of this finding was that the fetal mortality in these sibships was a manifestation of an extreme liability to clefting in these families (35). However, this observation was not confirmed in the analysis of another population (37).

Sex Ratio

There have been more affected male than female infants in several studies. In the large study of 189 affected individuals in Denmark (38), the ratio of males:females was 2.88 for bilateral CLP, 2.23 for unilateral CLP, 2.06 for bilateral CL only, and 1.71 for unilateral cleft lip alone. In British Columbia (1952–1971) among 713,316 live births, there were twice as many males with cleft lip alone as females. The M:F ratio for CLP was 3.5:2.2 (28).

Among 18 infants with cleft lip "microform," 14 were males (5).

Sidedness

The left side is affected twice as often as the right (39).

Parental Age

A much higher rate of occurrence of nonsyndromic cleft lip and palate was observed among women 39 and older than in women 25–29 years old in California during the period 1983–1986 (40). However, in the state of Washington in 1987–1990, nonsyndromic CL ± CP was significantly more common among mothers less than 20 years of age (41).

In a study (42) of 1,920 children with nonsyndromic cleft lip with or without cleft palate in Denmark (1973–1996), there was a small increase in maternal age (odds ratio 1.21; 95CI 1.09–1.34) and paternal age (OR 1.12; 95 CI 1.03–1.2). The contribution of each parental age was dependent on the age of the other parent.

Twinning

Most studies have shown no difference in the frequency of oral clefts among multiple births compared to singletons (43). It has been suggested (10) that the frequency of CL, CLP, and CP along is higher among conjoined twins than in the general population.

The largest series of twins evaluated for concordance for CLP and CP was the 130 twin sets born in Denmark in the twentieth century. Among identical twins, both were affected 60% of the time, whereas the concordance rate was 10% for non-identical twins (44, 45). These rates were consistent for infants with either CL or CP.

Genetic Factors

Many common malformations, including cleft lip and palate, are caused by failure to meet one or more endpoints in the development process. Some of those processes are distributed continuously. Both genetic and environmental factors interact to affect these processes. The concept of multifactorial inheritance has been proposed to explain these abnormalities. There are several characteristics expected when an abnormal outcome is attributed to the process of multifactorial inheritance: 1) the frequency of occurrence in the first-degree relatives approximates the square root of the population frequency, 2) the frequency decreases with the decrease in the degree of relationship, the sex of the probands, and the severity of the defect in the index case; 3) the concordance rate in monozygotic twins is higher than in dizygotic twins, but not 100%, and 4) the recurrence risk is higher for unaffected parents with two affected children than the unaffected parents with one affected child. Some published data have been consistent with these characteristics. Other analyses of the pattern of inheritance of individuals with nonsyndromic CLP have led to many different conclusions. The alternative interpretations have included: autosomal recessive and autosomal dominant (46, 47).

An analysis of the recurrence risk has suggested that up to 14 interacting major gene loci may contribute to the occurrence of the cleft deformity (41, 46).

The transcription factors and induction signal molecules involved in the development of the palate and lip have been used in linkage and candidate gene associations in individuals with cleft lip and cleft palate. Linkage has been established in several different populations in several regions of the genome, such as chromosome 1q22.3 (region of IRF6), 2p13 (region of TFGA), 2q35-36, 6p21.3, 8p11-23, 17q12 and 18q21.1 (21, 47-53).

The presence of specific gene polymorphisms has been associated with an increased risk for nonsyndromic cleft lip and palate in two circumstances. Each involves polymorphisms in a gene that can be mutated to cause a syndromic type of cleft lip/palate: 1) the mutation in the gene interferon regulatory factor 6 (IRF6), which causes the rare Van der Woude Syndrome (MIM #119300) that is characterized by lower lip pits, cleft palate or lip, and hypodontia; 2) the mutation in the cell adhesion molecule PVRL1 (nectin-1), which causes an autosomal recessive CLP with ectodermal dysplasia (MIM *600644). Transmission disequilibrium testing of thousands of individuals with nonsyndromic cleft lip and palate showed that the presence of the single nucleotide polymorphisms V2741 in the gene IRF6 was a major risk factor among individuals with CLP in several populations (50, 53). Among individuals living on Margarita Island, north of Venezuela, being heterozygous for the W185X mutation in the PVRL1 gene has been a common risk factor for nonsyndromic CLP in the mainland of Venezuela (54).

Four other polymorphisms, the cystathionine beta-synthase c.844ins68 gene variant (55) and the C699T variant (56), the maternal methylene tetrahydrofolate reductase 2756AG (57) and methylenetetrahydrofolate dehydrogenase (MTHFD1 1958G→A) [58] have shown correlations with the occurrence of CLP in specific populations.

At this time, no commercial testing is available routinely for individuals with nonsyndromic CLP to identify causative mutations. When that becomes possible, two examples could be screening the MSX1 and FGFR1 genes. Mutations in MSX1 have been identified in families with autosomal dominant tooth agenesis, some of whom also have CLP or cleft palate (59). The analysis of one large cohort of individuals with CLP showed that 2% had mutations in MSX1 (60). Mutations in FGFR1 occur in individuals with autosomal dominant Kallmann Syndrome, the features of which are hypogonadotropic hypogonadism, anosmia, and often CLP (61). Genotyping of individuals with nonsyndromic CLP showed that 3 to 5% could be attributed to

polymorphisms in the fibroblast growth factor pathways, that is FGF1 to FGF10 (62).

Trasler (63) suggested that variation in the face shape of embryos in different strains of mice correlated with an increased susceptibility to developing cleft lip. Fraser and Pashayan (64) measured the facial features of the unaffected parents and siblings of children with clefts and confirmed Trasler's hypothesis for humans. Specific morphometric changes, such as a greater lower face height and increased interorbital distances, have been markers of the genetic predisposition in some parents and unaffected sibs, but not in all families studied. The many study designs and methods used have confirmed the complexity of the observations of Trasler and of Fraser and Pashayan (65, 66).

Environmental Factors

Several environmental exposures have been identified that are associated with an increased frequency of cleft lip and palate: the mother smoking cigarettes, taking certain anticonvulsant drugs, and drinking an excessive amount of alcohol.

Several, but not all, studies have shown that there is an increased frequency of cleft lip and palate among infants born to women who smoke cigarettes (67). A dose-response relationship has been shown.

Genetic susceptibility appears to be a confounding factor in the teratogenicity from the mother smoking cigarettes. When the fetus has the genetic polymorphisms 1088 and 1095, in N-acetyltransferace 1 (NAT1), the risk for cleft lip and palate, but not cleft palate alone, was increased significantly (68). This gene is involved in the biotransformation of toxic compounds derived from tobacco. In the same study, there was no positive correlation with the NAT2 status of the mother or the fetus and the risk for CLP. In another study (69), the presence in the fetus of the CYP variant 1A1*2C was associated with a significantly decreased risk of an oral cleft, if the mother smoked cigarettes. The CYP gene is involved in the metabolic pathway of cigarette smoke compounds.

The interaction between the pregnant woman smoking cigarettes and the presence of a rare TaqI polymorphism in the transforming growth factor alpha (TGFA) gene was significantly more common in fetuses with cleft lip and palate in one study in California (70), but not in another study of similar design in Denmark (71). A meta-analysis of 17 studies concluded that folic acid-containing supplements had a protective effect on the occurrence of oral clefts (72).

Mothers who take an anticonvulsant to prevent seizures or the symptoms of a mood disorder (or for any other medical condition) have an increased risk that the drug-exposed fetus will have major malformations, including CLP. This correlation is strongest for exposure during pregnancy to the anticonvulsant drugs phenobarbital (73) and lamotrigine (brand name Lamictal) (26) and carbamazepine (brand name Tegretol) [74], but inconsistently for exposure to phenytoin (brand name Dilantin) [73].

An increased frequency of CLP has been identified among fetuses exposed to alcohol during pregnancy (75).

Obese mothers with a BMI greater than 29 have been shown to have an increased risk for having an infant with an oral cleft deformity (76).

Prevention

Following the observation that a woman's diet and periconceptional supplementation with folic acid decreased the rate of occurrence of neural tube defects, Tolarova (77) tried the same approach for the recurrence risk for cleft lip with or without cleft palate. In 85 pregnancies supplemented with folic acid 10 mg for 3 months before and after conception, there was one recurrence (1%) in comparison to 15 (7.4%) recurrence in 212 control (unsupplemented) pregnancies, a very significant difference ($p = 0.023$; Fisher's exact test). A 65% decrease in the recurrence was observed in another case series in California (78) and in a case-control study in the Netherlands (1998–2000) [79]. Several prospective studies support this conclusion (72). These positive results underscore the potential value of folic acid supplementation in cereals and grains in the prevention of oral clefts as well as other common malformations, such as neural tube defects.

In developing countries, such as the Philippines, low levels of plasma zinc have been observed in the mothers of infants with nonsyndromic oral clefts (80). These nutritional factors in the Philippines could be relevant to the effect of migration of Filipinos to Hawaii and California: the highest prevalence rate of CLP is in the Philippines and the lowest is among Filipinos living in California (81). This observation suggests another supplementation in that setting which could be preventative. Further studies of this important observation are needed.

Treatment and Prognosis

The prenatal detection of the cleft lip deformity has been most successful after 24 weeks gestation (82), although earlier detection has been reported. Prenatal diagnosis has been very helpful in enabling the parents to learn about the problem and to prepare for the treatment needed. Experience has shown (83) that prenatal sonography can, in general, distinguish between the fetus with an isolated cleft lip and one with associated malformations. Whether or not the affected fetus has a syndromic form of CL is best established at birth and through subsequent re-evaluations.

While surgical repair in utero is not yet an option, experimental studies have shown that feto-endoscopic surgery offers the hope for scarless fetal wound healing (84).

Each cleft deformity must be treated individually. The surgical techniques being used, including diagramming, lengthening, rotation, and advancement tissue and Z-plasty, were developed in the 1950s and 1960s by several surgeons (85). The parents of an affected newborn can expect a much better cosmetic result than was obtained in the parent's generation.

Children with orofacial clefts often require special education services, such as help with speech and language (86). Among older children with "isolated" CL or CLP, the possible association of deficits in IQ and associated changes in brain imaging have been raised. Several studies (87–89) have shown an increased risk for IQ deficits, unrelated to associated problems, such as middle ear infections and hearing loss. The deficits are smaller in children with cleft lip alone than in children with cleft lip and palate. A correlation has been made between deficits in cognitive function and changes in brain imaging in one series of studies of adult men with cleft lip and/or palate deformity (90–92). These men were examined for associated physical features of specific syndromes; three had the Van der Woude Syndrome, but the remainder were considered to have isolated oral clefts.

Brain images of 34 adults with cleft lip and palate showed that 8% had an enlarged cavum septum pellucidum (CSP) in the midline (90) in comparison to 1% in healthy controls. The presence of the CSP and its size correlated inversely with the IQ of the affected individual (91). Quantitative analysis of magnetic resonance images showed other changes, including enlarged anterior regions of the cerebrum and decreased volume of the posterior cerebrum and cerebellum (92).

Genetic Counseling

The first step in the evaluation of an affected infant is to determine whether the cleft lip deformity is associated with cleft palate and whether there are other associated malformations or dysmorphic features. If there are associated dysmorphic features or other malformations, chromosome analysis should be carried out.

As the infant is followed, the issue of whether there are signs of a "syndromic" form of cleft lip should be reviewed periodically. In the preschool years, further testing for difficulties with learning should be considered.

When testing mutations in the several candidate genes becomes available commercially, that option should be discussed with the parents. Over time, there will be practical value for the parents and the affected child in knowing which mutations are present.

TABLE 5-3 *Empiric recurrence risks: cleft lip and palate*

I. Risk of affected sibling of affected newborn; parents unaffected

	Brothers and Sisters		Total	Reference
1. Caucasians				
a) one affected child				
proband male (η = 1,908)	3.9%			(93)
proband female (η = 1,008)	5.0%			(93)
	1st degree relatives			
b) one affected child (η = 1941)	4.0% ± 0.4			(94)
c) two affected children (η = 335)	9.0% ± 1.6			(94)
2. Japanese	1st degree relatives			
Proband male (η = 952)	2.1%			(95)
female (η = 753)	1.9%			(95)

II. One parent affected

	Sons & Daughters			
1. Caucasians – two studies (94, 96)				
a) affected parent (η = 247)	4.0 ± 1.2 %			(94)
b) affected father (η = 281)	3.9			(96)
affected mother (η = 159)	3.3			(96)
2. Japanese	Son	Daughter		
a) parent affected with cleft lip	1.9 %	2.8%	2.4 %	(95)
b) parents affected with cleft lip and palate	2.8	1.6	2.2	(95)

III. Severity of defect: two studies (89, 97)

1. one affected child, unaffected parent				
cleft lip only (η = 779) (left or right)			2.6%	(89)
cleft lip and palate (η = 1,696) (left or right)			4.1%	(89)
cleft lip and palate (η = 658) (bilateral)			5.6%	(89)
2. one affected child, unaffected parent				
a) cleft lip (CL)	0.5%			(97)
cleft lip and palate (CLP)	4.1			
b) unilateral CL	1.5			(98)
bilateral CL	5.8			
c) unilateral CL	1.6			
unilateral CLP	4.2			
bilateral CLP	6.6			

IV. Occurrence of isolated CLP in families, unselected populations

		Affected Relatives				
		1st Degree			2nd degree	3rd degree
	Affected Index cases	Fathers	Mothers	Sibs		
1. Italy (97) 1981–1986 (220,927) Consecutive births Rate 0.76/1,000	199	2.5%	1.2	4.6	0.5	
2. France (98) (126,087) Consecutive births Rate 0.82/1,000	468	Parents 2.1%	3		0.4	0.4

After the plans for the affected child's treatment have been made, the risk of another affected child in a future pregnancy should be discussed. The empiric risks identified in family studies are presented in Table 5-3.

In a future pregnancy, ultrasound imaging can be used reliably to detect the cleft lip deformity, but not cleft palate.

REFERENCES

I. General

1. Gorlin RJ, Cohen MM Jr., Levin LS. *Syndromes of the Head and Neck.* 3rd ed. New York: Oxford University Press; 2001.
2. Wyszynski DF, ed. *Cleft Lip and Palate: From Origin to Treatment.* New York: Oxford University Press; 2002.
3. O'Rahilly R, Müller F. *Human Embryology and Teratology.* New York: Wiley-Liss; 2001: 229–236.

II. Original articles

4. Diewert VM, Shiota K. Morphological observations in normal primary palate and cleft lip embryos in the Kyolo collection. *Teratology.* 1990;41:663–677.
5. Castilla EE, Martínez-Frías ML. Congenital healed cleft lip. *Am J Med Gen.* 1995;58:106–110.
6. Tolarová MM, Cervenka J. Classification and birth prevalence of orofacial clefts. *Am J Med Genet.* 1998;75:126–137.
7. Semb G, Shaw WC. Simonart's band and facial growth in unilateral clefts of the lip and palate. *Cleft palate Craniofac J.* 1991; 28:40–46.
8. Mulliken JB. Double unilimb Z-plastic repair of microform cleft lip. *Plast Reconstr Surg.* 2005;116:1623–1632.
9. Martin RA, Jones KL, Benirschke K. Extension of the cleft lip phenotype: the subepithelial cleft. *Am J Med Genet.* 1993;47: 744–747.
10. Horswell BB. The incidence and relationship of cervical spine anomalies in patients with cleft lip and/or palate. *J Oral Maxillofac Surg.* 1991;49:693–697.
11. Geis N, Seto B, Bartoshesky L, Lewis MB, Pashayan HM. The prevalence of congenital heart disease among the population of a metropolitan cleft lip and palate clinic. *Cleft Palate J.* 1981;18: 19–23.
12. Wyse RK, Mars M, Al-Mahdawi S, Russell-Eggitt IM, Blake KD. Congenital heart anomalies in patients with clefts of the lip and/ or palate. *Cleft Palate J.* 1990;27:258–264.
13. Barbosa MM, Rocha CMG, Katina T, Caldas M, Codorniz A, Medeiros C. Prevalence of congenital heart diseases in oral cleft patients. *Pediatr Cardiol.* 24:369–374, 2003.
14. Milerad J, Larson O, Hagberg C, Idelberg M. Associated malformations in infants with cleft lip and palate: a prospective, population-based study. *Pediatrics.* 1997;100:180–186.
15. Natsume N, Niimi T, Furukawa H, Kawai T, Ogi N, Suzaki Y, Kawai T. Survey of congenital anomalies associated with cleft lip and/or palate in 701,181 Japanese people. *Oral Surg Oral Med Oral Path Oral Radiol Endo.* 2001;91:157–161.
16. Jones MC. Facial clefting: etiology and developmental pathogenesis. *Clinics in Plastic Surgery.* 1993;20:599–606.
17. Stoll C, Alembik Y, Doll B, Roth M-P. Associated malformations in patients with oral clefts. *Am J Med Genet Part A.* 2007;143A: 2463–2465.
18. Wyszynski DF, Sárközi A, Czeizel AE. Oral clefts with associated anomalies: methodological issues. *Cleft Palate—Craniofac J.* 2006;43:1–6.
19. Richman JM, Lee S-H. About face: signals and genes controlling jaw patterning and identity in vertebrates. *Bio Essays.* 2003; 25:554–546.
20. Marazita ML, Mooney MP. Current concepts in the embryology and genetics of cleft lip and cleft palate. *Clin Plast Surg.* 2004; 31:125–140.
21. Stanier P, Moore GE. Genetics of cleft lip and palate: syndromic genes contribute to the incidence of non-syndromic clefts. *Hum Mol Genetics 13 (Review Issue 1).* 2004;R73–R81.
22. Juriloff DM, Harris MJ, Brown CJ. Unravelling the complex genetics of cleft lip in the mouse model. *Mamm Genome.* 2001; 12:426–435.
23. Juriloff DM, Harris MJ, Dewell SL. A digenic cause of cleft lip in A-strain mice and definition of candidate genes for the two loci. *Birth Def Res (Part A): Clin Mol Teratology.* 2004;70: 509–518.
24. Tenconi R, Cleminti M, Turolla L. Theoretical recurrence risks for cleft lip derived from a population of consecutive newborns. *J Med Genet.* 1988;25:243–246.
25. Maria-Luisa Martínez-Frías, Ph.D. Personal Communication, June 22, 2006.
26. Holmes LB, Baldwin EJ, Smith CR, Habecker E, Glassman L, Wong SL et al. Increased frequency of isolated cleft palate in infants exposed to lamotrigine during pregnancy. *Neurology.* 2008;70:2152–2158.
27. Menegotto BG, Salzano FM. Epidemiology of oral clefts in a large South American sample. *Cleft Palate-Craniofacial J.* 1991;28:373–376.
28. Lowry RB, Trimble BK. Incidence rates for cleft lip and palate in British Columbia 1952–1971 for North American Indian, Japanese, Chinese and total populations: secular trends over twenty years. *Teratology.* 1977;16:277–284.
29. Natsume N, Kawai T. Incidence of cleft lip and cleft palate in 39,696 Japanese babies born during 1983. *Int J Maxillofac Surg.* 1986;15:565–568.
30. Das SK, Runnels RS Jr., Smith JC, Cohley HH. Epidemiology of cleft lip and cleft palate in Mississippi. *So Med J.* 1995;88: 437–442.
31. Iregbulem LM. The incidence of cleft lip and palate in Nigeria. *Cleft Palate J.* 1982;19:201–205.
32. Nemana LJ, Marazita ML, Melnick M. Genetic analysis of cleft lip with or without cleft palate in Madras, India. *Am J Med Genet.* 1992;42:5–9.
33. Cooper ME, Stone RA, Liu Y-e, Hu D-N, Melnick M, Marazita ML. Descriptive epidemiology of nonsyndromic cleft lip with or without cleft palate in Shanghai, China, from 1980 to 1989. *Cleft Palate-Craniofacial J.* 2000;37:274–280.
34. Wyszynski DF, Sarkozi A, Vargha P, Czeizel AE. Birth weight and gestational age of newborns with cleft lip with or without cleft palate and with isolated cleft palate. *J Clin Ped Dent.* 2003;27: 185–190.
35. Rasmussen SA, Moore CA, Paulozzi LJ, Rhodenbiser EP. Risk for birth defects among premature infants: a population-based study. *J Pediatr.* 2001;138:668–673.
36. Shiota K. Maternal reproductive loss and cleft lip with or without cleft palate in human embryos. *Am J Med Genet.* 1984;19: 121–129.
37. Menegotto BG, Salzano FM. New study on the relationship between oral clefts and fetal loss. *Am J Med Genet.* 1990;37: 539–542.
38. Melnick M, Bixler D, Fogh-Andersen P, Conneally PM. Cleft lip ± cleft palate: an overview of the literature and an analysis of Danish cases born between 1941 and 1968. *Am J Med Gen.* 1980;6:83–97.
39. Derijcke A, Eerens A, Carels C. The incidence of oral clefts: a review. *Brit J Oral Maxillofac Surg.* 1996;34:488–494.

40. Shaw GM, Croen LA, Curry CJ. Isolated oral cleft malformations: associations with maternal and infant characteristics in a California population. *Teratology*. 1991;43:225–228.

41. DeRoo LA, Gaudino JA, Edmonds LD. Orofacial cleft malformations: associations with maternal and infant characteristics in Washington state. *Birth Def Res (Part A): Clin Mol Terat*. 2003; 67:637–642.

42. Bille C, Skytthe A, Vach W, Knudsen LB, Andersen A-MN, Murray JC, Christensen K. Parent's age and the risk of oral clefts. *Epidemiology*. 2005;16:311–316.

43. Robert E, Källén B, Harris J. The epidemiology of orofacial clefts. 1. Some general epidemiological characteristics. *J Craniofac Genet Dev Biol*. 1996;16:234–241.

44. Christensen K, Fogh-Andersen P. Cleft lip (± cleft palate) in Danish twins, 1970–1990. *Am J Med Genet*. 1993;47:910–916.

45. Christensen K, Fogh-Andersen P. Isolated cleft palate in Danish multiple births, 1970–1990. *Cleft Palate J*. 1993;30:469–474.

46. Marazita ML, Dan-Ning H, Spence MA, Liu Y-E, Melnick M. Cleft lip with or without cleft palate in Shanghai, China: evidence for autosomal major locus. *Am J Hum Genet*. 1992;51:648–653.

47. Beiraghi S, Nath SK, Gaines M, Mandhyan DD, Hutchings D, Ratnamala U et al. Autosomal dominant nonsyndromic cleft lip and palate: significant evidence of linkage of 18q21.1. *Am J Hum Genet*. 2007;81:180–188.

48. Schliekelman P, Slatkin M. Multiplex relative risks and estimating of the number of loci underlying an inherited disease. *Am J Hum Genet*. 2002;71:1369–1385.

49. Wyszynski DF, Albacha-Hejazi H, Aldirani M, Hammod M, Shkair H, Karam A, et al. A genome-wide scan for loci predisposing to non-syndromic cleft lip with or without cleft palate in two large Syrian families. *Am J Med Genet*. 2003;123A:140–147.

50. Marazita ML, Murray JM, Cooper M, Bailey-Wilson TJ, Albacha-Hejazi H, Lidral A, Moreno L, Arco-Burgos M, Beaty T. Meta-analysis of 11 genome scans for cleft lip with or without cleft palate. *Am J Hum Genet*. 2003;73:A79.

51. Zucchero T, Cooper M, Maher BS, Daack-Hirsch B, Nepomuceno B, Ribeino L, et al. Interferon Regulating Factor 6 (IRF6) gene variants and the risk of isolated cleft lip and palate. *N Engl J Med*. 2004;351:769–780.

52. Riley BM, Schultz RE, Cooper ME, Goldstein-McHenry T, Daack-Hirsch S et al. A Genome-wide linkage scan for cleft lip and cleft palate identifies a novel locus on 8p11-23. *Am J Med Gen Part A*. 2007;143A:846–852.

53. Park JW, McIntosh I, Hetmanski JB, Jabs EW, Vander Kolk CA, Wu-Chou Y-H et al. Association between IRF6 and nonsyndromic cleft lip with or without cleft palate in four populations. *Genetics in Medicine*. 2007;9:219–227.

54. Sozen MA, Suzuki K, Talavora MM, Bustos T, Fernandez Iglesia JE, Spritz RA. Mutation of PVRL1 is associated with sporadic, non-syndromic cleft lip/palate in Northern Venezuela. *Nat Genet*. 2001;29:141–142.

55. Rubini M, Brusati R, Garattini G, Magnani C, Liviero F, Bianchi F et al. Cystathionine beta-synthase c.844ins68 gene variant and non-syndromic cleft lip and palate. *Am J Med Genet Part A*. 2005; 136A:368–372.

56. Boyles AL, Wilcox AJ, Taylor JA, Meyer K, Fredriksen A, Ueland PM et al. Folate and one-carbon metabolism gene polymorphisms and their associations with oral facial clefts. *Am J Med Genet Part A*. 2008;146A:440–449.

57. Mostowska H, Hozyasz KK, Jagodzinski PP. Maternal MTR genotype contributes to the risk of non-syndromic cleft lip and palate in the Polish population. *Clin Genet*. 2006;69:512–517.

58. Mills JL, Molloy AM, Parle-McDermott A, Troendle JF, Brody LC, Conley MR et al. Folate-related gene polymorphisms as risk factors for cleft lip and cleft palate. *Birth Def Res (Part A): Clin Mol Teratol*. 2008;82:636–643.

59. Van den Boogaard M-JH, Dorland M, Beemer FA, Ploos van Amstel HK. MSX1 mutation is associated with orofacial clefting and tooth agensis in humans. *Nat Genet*. 2000;24:342–343.

60. Jezewski P, Vieira A, Schultz R, Machida J, Suzuki Y, Ludwig B et al. Mutations in MSX1 are associated with non-syndromic orofacial clefting. *J Med Genet*. 2003; 40:399–407.

61. Dodé C, Levilliers J, Dupont JM, DePaepe A, Le Dú N, Souss-Yanicostas N, et al. Loss-of-function mutations in FGFR1 cause autosomal dominant Kallmann Syndrome. *Nat Genet*. 2003;33: 436–465.

62. Riley BM, Mansilla MA, Ma J, Daack-Hirsch S, Maher BS, Raffensperger LM et al. Impaired FGF signaling contributes to cleft lip and palate. *Proc Nat'l Acad Sci USA*. 2007;104: 4512–4517.

63. Trasler DG. Pathogenesis of cleft lip and its relation to embryonic face shape in A-J and C57BL mice. *Teratology*. 1968;1:33–49.

64. Fraser FC, Pashayan J. Relation of face shape to susceptibility to congenital cleft lip. A preliminary report. *J Med Genet*. 1970; 7:112–117.

65. Ward RE, Moore ES, Hartsfield JK Jr. Morphometric characteristics of subjects with oral facial clefts and their relatives. In: Wyszynski DF, ed. *Cleft Lip and Palate: From Origin to Treatment*. New York: Oxford University Press, 2002: 66–86.

66. Weinberg SM, Neiswanger K, Richtsmeier JT, Maher BS, Mooney MP, Siegel MI, Marazita ML. Three-dimensional morphometric analysis of craniofacial shape in the unaffected relatives of individuals with nonsyndromic orofacial clefts: a possible marker for genetic susceptibility. *Am J Med Genet Part A*. 2008;146A:409–420.

67. Källén K. Material smoking and orofacial clefts. *Cleft Palate-Craniofacial J*. 1997;34:11–16.

68. Lammer EJ, Shaw GM, Iovannisci DM, Van Wacs J, Finnell RH. Maternal smoking and the risk of orofacial clefts. Susceptibility with NAT1 and NAT2 polymorphisms. *Epidemiology*. 2004;15: 150–156.

69. Chevrier C, Bahuau M, Perret C, Iovannisci DM, Nelva A, Herman C et al. Genetic susceptibilities in the association between maternal exposure to tobacco smoke and the risk of nonsyndromic oral cleft. *Am J Med Genet Part A*. 2008;146A: 2396–2406.

70. Shaw GM, Wasserman CR, Lammer EJ, O'Malley CD, Murray JC, Basart AM, Tolarova MM. Orofacial clefts, parental cigarette smoking, and transforming growth factor-alpha gene variants. *Am J Hum Genet*. 1996;58:551–561.

71. Kaare C, Olsen J, Norgaard-Pedersen B, Basso O, Stovring H, Milhollin-Johnson L, Murray JC. Oral clefts, transforming growth factor alpha gene variants, and maternal smoking: a population-based case-control study in Denmark 1991–1994. *Amer J Epid*. 1999;149:248–255.

72. Badovinac RL, Werler MM, Williams PL, Kelsey KT, Hayes C. Folic acid-containing supplement consumption during pregnancy and risk for oral clefts: a meta-analysis. *Birth Def Res (Part A): Clin Mol Teratol*. 2007;79:8–15.

73. Arpino C, Brescianini S, Robert E, Castilla EE, Cucchi G, Cornel MC et al. Teratogenic effects of antiepileptic drugs: use of an International Database on Malformations and Drug Exposure (MADRE). *Epilepsia*. 2000;41:1436–1443.

74. Hernandez-Diaz S, Smith CR, Wyszynski DF, Holmes LB. Major malformations among infants exposed to carbamazepine during pregnancy. *Birth Def Res (Part A): Clin Mol Teratol*. 2007;79: 357.

75. Werler MM, Lammer EJ, Rosenberg L, Mitchell AP. Maternal alcohol in use in relation to selected birth defects. *Am J Epid*. 1991;134:691–698.

76. Cedergen M, Källén B. Maternal obesity and the risk for orofacial clefts in the offspring. *Cleft Palate Craniofac J*. 2005;42: 367–371.

77. Tolarova M. Periconceptional supplementation with vitamins and folic acid to prevent recurrence of cleft lip. *Lancet*. 1982; ii:217.

78. Tolarova M, Harris J. Reduced recurrence of orofacial clefts after periconceptional supplementation with high-dose folic acid and multivitamins. *Teratology*. 1995;51:71–78.

79. van Rooij IA, Ocké MC, Straatman H, Zielhuis GA, Merkus HM, Steegers-Theunissen RP. Periconceptional folate intake by supplement and food reduces the risk of nonsyndromic cleft lip with or without cleft palate. *Prev Med*. 2004;39:689–694.

80. Tamura T, Munger RG, Corcoran C, Bacayao JY, Nepomuceno B, Solon F. Plasma zinc concentrations of mothers and the risk of nonsyndromic oral clefts in their children: a case-control study in the Philippines. *Birth Def Res (Part A): Clin Mol Teratol*. 2005; 73:612–616.

81. Croen LA, Shaw GM, Wasserman CR, Tolarova M. Racial and ethnic variations in the prevalence of orofacial clefts in California. *Am J Med Genet*. 1998;79:42–47.

82. Robinson JN, McElrath TF, Benson CB, Doubilet PM, Westgate M-N, Holmes LB et al. Prenatal ultrasonography and the diagnosis of fetal cleft lip. *J Ultrasound Med*. 2001;20:1165–1170.

83. Bergé SJ, Plath H, Van De Vondel PT, Appel T, Niederhagen B, Von Lindern JJ, Reich RH, Hansmann M. Fetal cleft lip and palate: sonographic diagnosis, chromosomal abnormalities, associated anomalies and postnatal outcome in 70 fetuses. *Ultrasound Obstet Gynecol*. 2001;18:422–431.

84. Papadopulos NA, Papadopulos MA, Kovacs L, Zeilhofer HF, Henke J, Boettcher P, Biemer E. Foetal surgery and cleft lip and palate: current status and new perspectives. *Brit J Plast Surg*. 2005;58:593–607.

85. Lewis MB. Unilateral cleft lip repair. *Clinics in Plastic Surgery*. 1991;20:647–657.

86. Yazdy MM, Autry AR, Honein MA, Frias JL. Use of special education services by children with orofacial clefts. *Birth Def Res (Part A): Clin Mol Teratol*. 2008;82:147–154.

87. Jocelyn LJ, Penko MA, Rode HL. Cognition, communication, and hearing in young children with cleft lip and palate and in control children: a longitudinal study. *Pediatrics*. 1996;97: 529–534.

88. Swanenburg de Veye HFN, Beemer FA, Mellenbergh GJ, Wolters WHG, Heineman-de Boer JA. An investigation of the relationships between associated congenital malformations and the mental and psychomotor development of children with clefts. *Cleft Palate-Craniofacial J*. 2003;41:257–303.

89. Laasmen M, Haapanen M-L, Mäenpää P, Pulkkimen J, Ranta R, Virsu V. Visual, auditory, and tactile temporal processing in children with oral clefts. *J Craniofac Surg*. 2004;15:510–518.

90. Nopoulos P, Berg S, Van Denmark D, Richman L, Canady J, Andreasen NC. Increased incidence of a midline brain anomaly in patients with nonsyndromic clefts of the lip and/or palate. *J Neuroimaging*. 2001;11:418–424.

91. Nopoulos P, Berg S, Van Demark D, Richman L, Canady J, Andreasen NC. Cognitive dysfunction in adult males with nonsyndromic clefts of the lip and/or palate. *Neuropsychologia*. 2002;40:2178–2184.

92. Nopoulos P, Berg S, Canady J, Richman L, Van Demark D, Andreasen NC. Structural brain abnormalities in adult males with clefts of the lip and/or palate. *Genetics in Medicine*. 2002;4:1–9.

93. Fraser FC. The genetics of cleft lip and cleft palate. *Amer J Hum Genet*. 1970;22:336–352.

94. Curtis EJ, Fraser FC, Warburton D. Congenital cleft lip and palate. *Am J Dis Ch*. 1961;102:851–857.

95. Koguchi H. Recurrence rate in offspring and siblings of patients with cleft lip and/or cleft palate. *Jap J Hum Genet*. 1975;20: 207–221.

96. Bixler D, Fogh-Andersen P, Conneally PM. Incidence of cleft lip and palate in the offspring of cleft parents. *Clin Genet*. 1971;2: 155–159.

97. Tenconi R, Clementi M, Turolla L. Theoretical recurrence risks for cleft lip derived from a population of consecutive newborns. *J Med Genet*. 1988;25:243–246.

98. Bonaiti C, Briard ML, Feingold J, Pavy B, Psaume J, Migne-Tufferaud G, Kaplan J. An epidemiological and genetic study of facial clefting in France. I. Epidemiology and frequency in relatives. *J Med Genet*. 1982;19:8–15.

Chapter 6

Cleft Palate

Definition

A partial or complete lack of fusion of the shelves of the palate. The cleft can involve the anterior portion only, the posterior hard and soft palate, or the entire length of the palate from uvula to the anterior teeth.

ICD-9:

	749.000	(cleft hard palate, unilateral)
	749.010	(cleft hard palate, bilateral)
	749.020	(cleft hard palate, central)
	749.030	(cleft hard palate, NOS)
	749.040	(cleft soft palate, alone unilateral)
	749.050	(cleft soft palate, alone bilateral)
	749.060	(cleft soft palate, alone central)
	749.070	(cleft soft palate, alone, NOS)
	749.080	(cleft uvula)

ICD-10:

	Q35.0	(cleft hard palate, bilateral)
	Q35.1	(cleft hard palate, unilateral)
	Q35.2	(cleft soft palate, bilateral)
	Q35.3	(cleft soft palate, unilateral)
	Q35.4	(cleft hard palate with cleft soft palate, bilateral)
	Q35.5	(cleft hard palate with cleft soft palate, unilateral)
	Q35.6	(cleft palate, medial)
	Q35.7	(cleft uvula)
	Q35.8	(cleft palate, unspecified, bilateral)
	Q35.9	(cleft palate, unspecified, unilateral)

Mendelian Inheritance in Man:

	#119540	(cleft palate, isolated; gene map locus 2q32)
	#303400	(cleft palate, X-linked (includes cleft palate with ankyloglossia) gene map locus Xq21.3)

Appearance

Cleft palate, reflecting the failure of the fusion process, sometimes occurs anteriorly, in front of the incisors. This anterior cleft is usually associated with a cleft lip (either unilateral or bilateral). More often, the cleft palate is in the posterior portion of the hard palate and extends through the soft palate and uvula. In a third type, the cleft extends from the anterior region throughout the entire palate (3, 4) [Figure 6-1].

Several classifications of cleft deformities have been proposed (5). Kernohan and Stark, proposed two groups: clefts of the primary palate, which considered to occur at 4 to 7 weeks of embryonic life and included clefts of the lip and premaxilla. Their second group was clefts of the secondary palate, which extend posterior to the incisive foramen. These clefts were said to have occurred at 7 to 12 weeks.

Cleft uvula occurs in an increased frequency among the close relatives of individuals with cleft palate and has been considered to be a microform of cleft palate (6, 7).

In a submucous cleft palate, there is a bony notch in the center of the posterior border of the hard palate, the soft palate is covered by skin, but the underlying muscle is divided (and palpable as such) and the uvula is bifid (8). The submucous cleft causes velopharyngeal

82

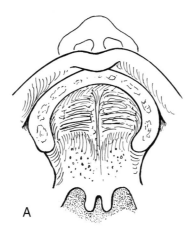

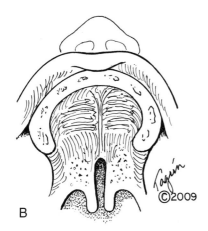

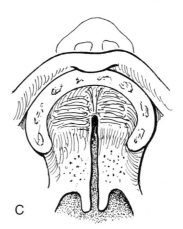

FIGURE 6.1   Diagrams of varying severity: A: cleft uvula (mild); B: cleft soft palate (moderate); and C: cleft hard and soft palate (severe).

incompetence, the symptoms of which are nasal emission of feedings and, in childhood, hypernasality of speech.

Associated Malformations

Anomalies are common in the adjacent structures. The eustachian tube (ET) cartilage is much smaller and the lumen is straighter than in controls, which contributes to ET dysfunction and predisposes to otitis media with effusion (9).

An increased frequency of anomalies of the cervical vertebrae, primarily posterior arch deficiency, has been reported (10). In an analysis (11) of lateral cephalographs of children ages 7 to 18 years with cleft palate (n=87) and submucous cleft palate (n=60), the frequencies of anomalies of upper and lower cervical vertebrae were 23/87 (26%) and 27/60 (45%), respectively. The frequency in the noncleft comparison group (n=100) was 7%.

An increased frequency of associated heart defects, an adjacent structure in early embryogenesis, has been noted in some studies (12, 13), but not others (14). This correlation may relate to syndromic cleft palate rather than to "isolated" cleft palate.

Population-based analyses in California (1983–1997) [15], Stockholm (1975–1992) [13], and Japan (1982–1994) [16] showed that infants with cleft palate often have associated major malformations. In Sweden (13), 52 (22%) of the 239 children with isolated cleft palate had associated malformations and in Japan (16), 20.7% of 188 affected children.

Imaging studies have shown an increased frequency of a midline brain anomaly, specifically an enlarged cavum septum pellucidum, in individuals with cleft palate (17). The presence of this finding correlated with the occurrence of deficits in cognitive function in this study. (17, 18). The adults with isolated cleft palate had deficits of 10 IQ points in full scale, performance, and verbal scales in comparison to controls.

In addition to these associated abnormalities in adjacent and nearby structures, cleft palate is a feature of many multiple anomaly syndromes (Table 6-1).

Over 300 disorders, which include cleft palate in the phenotype, are listed in Mendelian Inheritance in Man. Several experienced clinicians (19–23) have tabulated the diagnoses in the many affected children they have

TABLE 6-1 *Recognized etiologies of cleft palate*

	Isolated	Multiple anomalies
1. *Mendelian inheritance:*		
a) autosomal recessive		5
b) autosomal dominant		11
c) X-linked	1*	2**
2. *Chromosome abnormalities*		
a) trisomy 13		3
b) trisomy 18		3
c) 45,X		1
d) trisomy 9		1
e) translocations, unbalanced		2°
3. *Specific syndromes*		
"private syndrome"		1***
Anencephaly		6◊
4. *Environmental exposures*		
a) Infants of diabetic mothers		2
5. *Twinning*		(1)◊
6. *Unknown etiology*	40	17
Totals	41	54 = overall total 95
	(1:5,030)	(1:3,819) (1:2,170)
	(0.2/1,000)	(0.26/1,000) (0.46/1,000)

Legends: These infants were identified by the Active malformations Surveillance Program at Brigham and Women's Hospital in the years 1972–74, 79–2000 among 206, 244 liveborn and stillborn infants and elective terminations for fetal anomalies. Includes only infants born to women who had always planned to deliver at this hospital.
*Ref: Holmes LB. X-linked recessive cleft palate. *Pediatr Res.* 1975; 9: 360.
**Ref: Two separate X-linked syndromes:
1) Bianchi DW. FG Syndrome in a premature male. *Am J Med Genet* 1984;19:383–386.
2) Holmes LB, Schoene WC, Benacerraf BR. New syndrome: brain malformation, growth retardation, hypokinesia and polyhydramnios in two brothers. *Clin Dysmorphol.* 1997; 6:13–19.
°Translocations: 46,XX, der (18); t(8;18) (q22; q23) mat
            46,XX, -18, +der 18p (22q13.1; 18q22.2)
***Ref: Ment L, Alper J, Sirota RL, Holmes LB. Infant with abnormal pigmentation, malformations and immune deficiency. *Arch Dermatol.* 1978;114:1043–1044.
◊Includes one set of male twins: zygosity not known; one with anencephaly, rachischisis and cleft palate and the other healthy.

evaluated. In populations of consecutive newborns, 58% (19) and 47% (20), respectively, had associated malformations. Among older children and adults, the rates were similar, 55% (23), 42% (19), and 55% (20), but specific malformation syndromes and chromosome deletions, such as 22q11.2 deletion, were more likely to have been identified. The autosomal dominant Stickler Syndrome (MIM #108300) was the most common Mendelian condition. This disorder is often not diagnosed in a newborn infant with cleft palate and a small chin, unless examinations of the retina and molecular studies are carried out. The affected parent often will not have been diagnosed previously.

X-linked cleft palate due to a mutation in the transcription factor TBX22 was associated with ankyloglossia (tongue-tie) in 79% of affected males and 45% of carrier females in 13 unrelated families (24). There was a wide variation in the abnormality of the palate, including a complete cleft of the secondary palate, submucous cleft, bifid uvula, and a high vaulted palate. Ankyloglossia, but not cleft palate, was the only manifestation in 4% of the males with a TBX22 mutation.

Developmental Defects

The primary palate starts developing in the sixth week post-fertilization from the median palatine process (3, 4). The primary palate is the small anterior part of the hard palate in front of the incisors and forms the premaxillary part of the maxilla. The secondary palate, the most posterior portion of the hard palate and the soft palate, forms from the left and right palatal processes. The soft palate develops from the merging of the mesenchymal tissues. Before these processes can fuse, the tongue descends and the palate shelves become horizontal. Fusion of the shelves is a complex process that begins in the eighth week and includes cell death, loss of epithelium, and changes in the intracellular matrix. The fusion of the palate shelves is completed by 12 weeks or the failure to do so will be apparent as a cleft palate. The uvula becomes a single midline structure during the second trimester.

The developmental processes that lead to the formation of the cheeks, lips, nose, and palate involve many cell adhesion molecules, signaling molecules, growth factors and receptors, and transcription factors (25, 26). For palate development, several interactions between epithelial cells and mesenchymal cells are crucial. Epithelial growth factor (*Egf*) stimulates production of glycosaminoglycans within the palate shelves. Transforming growth factor alpha (*TGFα*) is expressed throughout the mesenchyme and epithelium of the palate and stimulates biosynthesis. Collagen III and fibronectin are factors that modulate hyaluronate expansion during the orientation of the palate shelves.

The transforming growth factor (*TGFβ*) and its three isoforms 1, 2, and 3 are all expressed during palate development. *TGFβ1* and 2 accelerate palate shelf fusion. *TGFβ3* may be crucial to the first adhesive interaction. Of note, the knockout mouse deficient in *TGFβ3* has isolated cleft palate due to failure of palate shelf fusion. Studies of this knockout mouse have shown that proteolytic degradation is essential for fusion of the palate shelves (27).

Many spontaneous mutations and gene knockouts have identified 50 genes in the mouse, which when altered, produce either nonsyndromic or syndromic cleft palate (28). These include genetic changes in signaling peptides, such as *Tgfβ3*, transcription factors (*Hoxa2*, *Dlx2*, *Msx1*, *Pax9*, *Tbx1*, and *p62*), and the vasoactive peptide ET1. For example, transforming growth factor beta (Tgf-β) is expressed in the developing palate.

These mutations have shown the importance in the development of cleft palate of several different factors and events, including size of palate shelves, timing of the elevation of the shelves, the lack of fusion of apposed shelves, head width, and lack of tongue movement. The human homologues of the mutant genes in the mouse are candidate genes for the many genetic differences postulated to be the basis for the occurrence of cleft palate in humans.

Prevalence

Many estimates of the prevalence rates of cleft palate have been published (29), but most rates are for infants evaluated through the first year of life and very few are for infants at birth (30, 31). The rate is subdivided usually into "isolated" cleft palate and "syndromic" cleft palate. Among newborn infants, the prevalence rates have been 0.5/1,000 for all infants with cleft palate, and 0.2 to 0.3/1,000 for isolated cleft palate (31, 32) [Table 6-1].

One potential limitation of the findings among newborn infants is the fact that cleft palate can be missed in the initial examinations. 25% were missed at birth in one follow-up study (33).

The bifid uvula is the end of the spectrum of cleft palate (Figure 6-1). It can be associated with submucous cleft palate and hypoplasia of the eustachian tube. 2.3% of 709 elementary school children had a cleft uvula; only 0.3% had a cleft of the full length of the uvula. The frequencies varied from 4.5% in Caucasian males and 2.7% of Caucasian females to 0.4% of black children. The rate was 11% among 944 Navajo Indian school children (34).

Race/Ethnicity

Marked differences have been observed in some studies in the prevalence rates for cleft palate among several racial/ethnic groups. Some of the lowest rates have been among African Americans in the United States: 0.34/1,000 in Mississippi (35) and 0.29/1,000 in California (36). Among Africans in Nigeria the rate was 0.05/1,000 in one study (37). Among Whites or Caucasians, the rates were 0.35/1,000 in California (36) and 0.5/1,000 in Denmark (37). The rate among Hispanics in California was 0.56/1,000 (36). The highest rates have been in Native American Indians (0.78/1,000) [39] and in Maori natives in New Zealand (1.87/1,000) [40], respectively.

Birth Status

An increased risk (OR 1.95; 95% CI 1.31–2.89) for low birth weight, but not preterm birth, was present among 582 infants with cleft palate alone who were born in Hungary between 1980 and 1986 (41). There was a shorter length at birth among Danish newborns with cleft palate in comparison to controls (p<.01) [38]. In metropolitan Atlanta (1989–1995), there was a significant risk (RR 2.4 [95% CI; 1.5–3.7]) for prematurity among all infants with cleft palate, but not those with isolated cleft palate (42).

Sex Ratio

Several studies have shown an excess of affected males (23, 29).

Parental Age

No increased risk has been correlated with the age of the mother. However, an association with increased age of the father has been reported (43).

Twinning

Population-based studies have shown that the frequency of clefting among twins is not increased in comparison to singletons (44, 45). Among monozygous twins in Finland and Denmark, there was a 33% to 55% likelihood that both would be affected (45, 46). Among nonidentical twins (dizygous), the likelihood that both were affected was much lower, usually less than 10%.

Genetic Factors

One prominent hypothesis is that nonsyndromic cleft palate is caused by both genetic and nongenetic factors, that is, the concept of multifactorial inheritance. However, analyses of the pattern of inheritance have not always confirmed that hypothesis (47).

Several different methods have been used to identify candidate genes that are associated with clefting: genome-wide linkage, association studies and animal studies with knockouts of specific genes, and chromosome deletions and balanced translocations (26, 46, 47). These studies have suggested that several genes on many chromosomes can affect the occurrence of palate. These include: *TGFA, MSX1, BCL3, RARA, MTHFR, CYP1A1, NAT1, NAT2, GSTT1, EPHX1* and *TCOF1*.

A few mutations that appear to "cause" cleft palate have been identified: a) Mutations in *interferon regulatory factor 6* (IRF6) cause the autosomal dominant Van der Woude Syndrome (MIM #119300). The phenotype of this disorder includes cleft palate or cleft lip in association pits in the lower lip (Figure 6-2). Variants in the *IRF6* gene have been shown also to correlate with the occurrence of nonsyndromic clefting (48); b) Mutations in *TBX22* are associated with X-linked cleft palate (MIM #303400) [Figure 6-3], which can be associated with ankyloglossia, as well (24). Changes in the *TBX22* gene appear to have a role in the occurrence of nonsyndromic cleft palate (49); c) Sequencing of *MSX1* in 917 individuals with nonsyndromic isolated cleft palate, as well as nonsyndromic cleft lip and palate, identified mutations in 16 (2%) [50].

Association studies have suggested that the *TCOF1* gene (51) and folate-related gene polymorphisms (52) could be risk factors in the occurrence of cleft palate.

Clinical testing for mutations associated with the occurrence of nonsyndromic cleft palate is not available yet. However, research studies have shown the relative frequency of some mutations in some of the candidate genes identified to date. For example, 4% of individuals with cleft palate, not selected because of pattern of inheritance or the presence of ankyloglossia, had mutations in the *TBX22* gene (25).

Chromosome deletions and balanced translocations have been another method for identifying gene loci that are associated with the occurrence of cleft palate. For example, the chromosome 2q32-q33 region is one in which haplo-insufficiency causes isolated cleft palate (53).

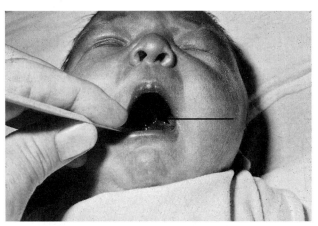

FIGURE 6.3   Cleft palate in newborn male (arrow) who is the nephew of man with cleft soft palate (presumed X-linked cleft palate).

SATB2, which belongs to the CUT superclass of homeodomain proteins and is expressed in the process of palate fusion, is a candidate gene in that region. However, no SATB2 pathogenic mutations were identified among 70 unrelated individuals with isolated cleft palate.

Empiric recurrence risks have been established for the offspring of affected individuals, as well as subsequent siblings born after the first affected child of unaffected parents (Table 6-2) [6, 54–56].

Environmental Factors

Several anticonvulsant drugs taken by the mother during pregnancy have been shown to be associated with an increased risk for the occurrence of major malformations, including oral clefts. The frequency of cleft palate has been shown to be increased significantly among infants exposed to lamotrigine (31), carbamazepine (57), valproate (58), and phenobarbital (59), each as monotherapy.

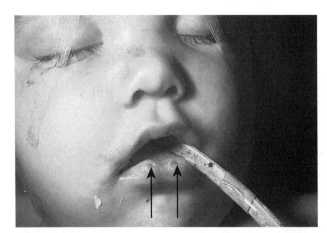

FIGURE 6.2   Picture of infant prepared for surgical repair of cleft palate. Note the pits in lower lip (arrows), a feature of the Van der Woude Syndrome (Courtesy of John Mulliken, M.D., Children's Hospital, Boston, MA).

TABLE 6-2 *Empiric recurrence risks for isolated cleft palate*

I. *Risk of Affected sibling of one affected newborn with unaffected parents:*
  1. Caucasians
    a) one affected child (n=1,034):   1.7 ± 0.4% (74)
    b) two affected children (n=106):   0.9 ± 0.9% (74)

II. *Risk of affected child if parent affected:*
  1. Caucasians
    a) offspring of affected parent (n=103): 5.8 (± 2.3)% (74)
    b) offspring of affected parent (n=150): 6.2 % (75)
       affected father (n=61):   6.3 % (75)
       affected mother (n=89):   6.1 % (75)
  2. Asian
    a) offspring of affected parent (n=50):   1.6 % (76)

Among infants of diabetic mothers, an increased frequency of cleft palate was identified in population-based surveillance programs (60).

Exposure during pregnancy to an excessive amount of alcohol can cause the fetal alcohol syndrome and an increased frequency of several major malformations, although there has been a lack of consistency in the association with specific malformations. In a study of exposure to three or fewer drinks per week (61), there was no association of an increased frequency of oral clefts with low alcohol consumption.

Smoking cigarettes during pregnancy has been associated with a doubling of the risk for oral clefts (62–65). An association between smoking and isolated cleft palate with the exposed fetus having a rare allele of transforming growth factor alpha (TGFA) was reported in one study in Maryland (63), but later not confirmed in two other studies in Maryland (64) and in Denmark (65). Analyses of polymorphisms in the CYP genes, which metabolize tobacco smoke compounds, have suggested that the presence of the CYP1A1*2C allele in the mother and the CYP2E1*5 allele in the fetus could reduce the risk for oral clefts, when the mother smokes cigarettes during pregnancy (66).

Obesity in the mothers, especially those with a BMI greater than 29, is associated with an increased risk for cleft lip (67).

Prevention

A decrease in the rate of occurrence of cleft palate alone was shown in two studies of women who had taken a multivitamin supplement that contained folic acid before conception and during early pregnancy: 50% reduction in California (68) and 60% reduction among malformed infants born in Boston, Philadelphia, and Toronto (69). A meta-analysis of 17 studies (70) concluded that, in aggregate, the findings support the hypothesis that taking a folic acid supplement decreases the risk for oral clefts.

An association of decreased socioeconomic status with the occurrence of a cleft palate has been attributed to some nutritional factors. For example, among Filipino women in the reproductive age group, those with a higher plasma zinc level had a lower risk for oral clefts in their children (71).

Treatment and Prognosis

Reflecting concern about speech development, there is a consensus that the surgical repair of the cleft palate should be completed before 18 months of age (73). However, there is no consensus on how early the surgery should be performed.

If the infant with isolated palate has a small chin, glossoptosis, and airway obstruction (the Pierre Robin Syndrome), the surgical repair will be adjusted to consider these additional risk factors.

The infant with a cleft palate should have regular evaluations by a speech pathologist to identify delays in receptive or expressive language. This evaluation should assess whether or not there is velopharyngeal insufficiency, which could prompt additional evaluations and treatments.

Genetic Counseling

The first step for the clinician is to determine whether or not the child has an isolated cleft palate or cleft palate as one of several malformations.

Recently it has been noted that an infant with an apparent isolated cleft palate could have discontinuities of the orbicularis oris muscle, which would indicate that the infant actually has an occult lip defect and not just a cleft palate (73). This occult defect in the orbicularis oris muscle, which facilitates puckering of the mouth, is identified by ultrasound.

When an infant has isolated cleft palate, at some point the parents will be interested in the risk of recurrence in a subsequent pregnancy. The information available is limited to only a few racial/ethnic groups (Table 6-2).

A diagnostic evaluation is indicated for the infant with cleft palate and other anomalies. Marked heterogeneity has been demonstrated in follow-up studies (77). Continued evaluations over time and screening tests, such as for the chromosome 22q11.2 deletion, are often needed to identify the underlying primary diagnosis.

The recurrence risk for a genetic disorder, which includes cleft palate, will be specific to that condition.

Prenatal screening by ultrasound is not reliable for detecting cleft palate. Three-dimensional imaging can identify the cleft palate, but its accuracy has not been established.

REFERENCES

I. General References

1. Gorlin RJ, Cohen MM Jr, Hennekan RCM. *Syndromes of the Head and Neck.* 4th ed. New York: Oxford University Press; 2001.
2. Wyszynski DF, ed. *Cleft Lip and Palate: From Origin to Treatment.* New York: Oxford University Press; 2002.
3. O'Rahilly R, Müller F. *Human Embryology and Teratology.* 3rd ed. New York: 2001: 229–235.
4. Moore KL, Persaud TVN. *The Developing Human: Clinically Oriented Embryology.* 7th ed. Philadelphia: WB Saunders; 2003: 230–235.
5. Millard DR Jr. *Cleft Craft: The Evolution of Its Surgery I. The Unilateral Deformity.* Boston: Little, Brown and Company; 1976: 41–55.

II. Articles

6. Fraser FC. The genetics of cleft lip and cleft palate. *Am J Hum Genet.* 1970;22:336–352.
7. Meskin LH, Gorlin RJ, Isaacson RJ. Abnormal morphology of the soft palate. II. The Genetics of Cleft Uvula. *Cleft Palate J.* 1965;2:40–45.

8. Sommerlad BC, Fenn C, Harland K, Sell D, Birch MJ, Dave R, Lees M, Barnett A. Submucous cleft palate: a grading system and review of 40 consecutive submuscous cleft palate repairs. *Cleft Palate-Craniofac J.* 2004;41:114–123.

9. Matsune S, Sando I, Takahashi H. Abnormalities of lateral cartilaginous lamina and lumen of eustachian tube in cases of cleft palate. *Ann Otol Rhinol Laryngol.* 1991;100:909–913.

10. Sandham A. Cervical vertebral anomalies in cleft lip and palate. *Cleft Plate J.* 1986;23:206–214.

11. Horswell BB. The incidence and relationship of cervical spine anomalies in patients with cleft lip and/or palate. *J Oral Maxillofac Surg.* 1991;49:693–697.

12. Uyse RK, Mars M, al-Mahdawi S, Russell-Eggitt IM, Blake KD. Congenital heart anomalies in patients with clefts of the lip and/or palate. *Cleft Palate J.* 1990;27:258–264.

13. Milerad J, Larson O, Hagberg C, Ideberg M. Associated malformations in infants with cleft lip and palate: a prospective, population-based study. *Pediatrics.* 1997;100:180–186.

14. Barbosa MM, Rocha CMG, Katina T, Caldas M, Codorniz A, Medeiros C. Prevalence of congenital heart diseases in oral cleft patients. *Pediatr Cardiol.* 2003;24:369–374.

15. Shaw GM, Carmichael SL, Yang Wei, Harris JA, Lammer EJ. Congenital malformations in births with orofacial clefts among 3.6 million California births, 1983–1997. *Am J Med Genet.* 2004;125A:250–256.

16. Natsume N, Niimi T, Furukawa H, Kawai T, Ogi N, Suzuki Y et al. Survey of congenital anomalies associated with cleft lip and/or palate in 701,181 Japanese people. *Oral Surg Oral Med Oral Pathol Oral Radiol Endod.* 2001;91:157–161.

17. Nopoulos P, Berg S, VanDemark D, Richman L, Canady J, Andreasen NC. Increased incidence of a midline brain anomaly in patients with nonsyndromic clefts of the lip and/or palate. *J Neuroimaging.* 2001;11:418–424.

18. Nopoulos P, Berg, VanDemark D, Richman L, Canady J, Andreasen NC. Cognitive dysfunction in adult males with non-syndromic clefts of the lip and/or palate. *Neuropsychologia.* 2002;40:2178–2184.

19. Shprintzen RJ, Siegel-Sadewitz VL, Amato J, Goldberg RB. Anomalies associated with cleft lip, cleft palate or both. *Am J Med Genet.* 1985;20:585–595.

20. Stoll C, Alembik Y, Dott B, Roth MP. Associated malformations in cases with oral clefts. *Cleft Palate Craniofac J.* 2000;37:41–47.

21. Jones MC. Etiology of facial clefts: prospective evaluation of 428 patients. *Cleft Palate J.* 1988;25:16–20.

22. Jones MC. Facial clefting: etiology and developmental pathogenesis. *Clinics Plastic Surgery.* 1993;20:599–606.

23. Saal HM. Classification and description of nonsyndromic clefts. In: Wyszynski DF, ed. *Cleft Lip and Palate: From Origin to Treatment.* New York: Oxford University Press; 2002: 47–52.

24. Marcano ACB, Doudney K, Braybrook C, Squires R, Patton MA, Lees MM et al. TBX22 mutations are a frequent cause of cleft palate. *J Med Genet.* 2004;41:68–74.

25. Stanier P, Moore GE. Genetics of cleft lip and palate: syndromic genes contribute to the incidence of non-syndromic clefts. *Hum Mol Genet.* 2004;13:R73–R81.

26. Juqessur A, Murray JC. Orofacial clefting: recent insights into a complex trait. *Current Opinion in Genetics & Development.* 2005;15:270–278.

27. Blavier L, Lazaryev A, Groffen J, Heisterkamp N, DeClerck YA, Kaartinen V. TGF-β3-induced palatogenesis requires matrix metalloproteinases. *Mol Biol Cell.* 2001;12:1457–1466.

28. Juriloff DM. Mapping studies in animal models. In: Wyszynski DF, ed. *Cleft Lip and Palate: From Origin to Treatment.* New York: Oxford University Press; 2002: 265–282.

29. Tolarova MM, Cervenka J. Classification and birth prevalence of orofacial clefts. *Am J Med Genet.* 1998;75:126–137.

30. Tenconi R, Cleminti M, Turolla L. Theoretical recurrence risks for cleft lip derived from a population of consecutive newborns. *J Med Genet.* 1988;25:243–246.

31. Holmes LB, Baldwin EJ, Smith CR, Habecker E, Glassman L, Wong SL, Wyszynski DF. Increased frequency of isolated cleft palate in infants exposed to lamotrigine during pregnancy. *Neurology.* 2008; 70:2152–2158.

32. Maria-Luisa Martínez-Frías, Ph.D. Personal Communication, June 22, 2006.

33. Habel A, Elhadi N, Sommerlad B, Powell J. Delayed detection of cleft palate: an audit of newborn examination. *Arch Dis Child.* 2006;91:238–240.

34. Wharton P, Mowrer DE. Prevalence of cleft uvula among school children in kindergarten through grade five. *Cleft Palate-Craniofac J.* 1992;29:10–14.

35. Das SK, Runnels RS Jr, Smith JC, Cohley HH. Epidemiology of cleft lip and cleft palate in Mississippi. *So Med J.* 1995;88:437–442.

36. Croen LA, Shaw GM, Wasserman CR, Tolarová MM. Racial and ethnic variations in the prevalence of orofacial clefts in California, 1983–1992. *Am J Med Genet.* 1998;79:42–47.

37. Iregbulem LM. The incidence of cleft lip and palate in Nigeria. *Cleft Palate J.* 1982;19:201–205.

38. Jensen BL, Kreiborg S, Dahl E, Fogh-Andersen P. Cleft lip and palate in Denmark, 1976–1981: epidemiology, variability, and early somatic development. *Cleft Palate J.* 1988;25:258–269.

39. Coddington DA, Hisnanick JJ. Midline congenital anomalies: the estimated occurrence among American Indian and Alaska Native infants. *Clin Genet.* 1996;50:74–77.

40. Chapman CJ. Ethnic differences in the incidence of cleft lip and/or cleft palate in Auckland, 1960–1976. *NZ Med J.* 1983;96:327–329.

41. Wyszynski DF, Sarkozi A, Vargha P, Czeizel AE. Birth weight and gestational age of newborns with cleft lip with or without cleft palate and with isolated cleft palate. *J Clinic Pediatr Dent.* 2003;27:185–190.

42. Rasmussen SA, Moore CA, Paulozzi LJ, Rhodenhiser EP. Risk for birth defects among premature infants: a population-based study. *J Pediatr.* 2001;138:668–673.

43. Bille C, Skytthe A, Vach W, Knudsen LB, Andersen A-MN, Murray JC, Christensen K. Parent's age and the risk of oral clefts. *Epidemiology.* 2005;16:311–316.

44. Eufinger H, Rand S, Scholz M, Machtens E. Clefts of the lip and palate in twins: use of DNA finger printing for zygosity determination. *Cleft Palate-Craniofac J.* 1993;30:564–568.

45. Nordström REA, Laatikainen T, Juvonen TO, Ranta RE. Cleft-twin sets in Finland 1948–1987. *Cleft Palate-Craniofac J.* 1996; 33:340–347.

46. Christensen K, Fogh-Andersen P. Isolated cleft palate in Danish multiple births, 1970–1990. *Cleft Palate-Craniofac J.* 1993;30:469–474.

47. Koillinen H, Lahermo P, Rautio J, Hukki J, Peyrard-Janvid M, Kere J. A genome-wide scan of non-syndromic cleft palate only (CPO) in Finnish multiplex families. *J Med Genet.* 2005;42:177–184.

48. Zucchero TM, Cooper ME, Maher BS, Daack-Hirsch S, Nepomuceno B, Riberio L et al. Interferon regulatory factor 6 (IRF6) gene variants and the risk of isolated cleft lip or palate. *N Engl J Med.* 2004;351:769–780.

49. Suphapeetiporn K, Tongkobpetch S, Siriwan P, Shotelersuk V. TBX22 mutations are a frequent cause of non-syndromic cleft palate in the Thai population. *Clin Genet.* 2007;72:478–483.

50. Jezewski PA, Vieira AR, Nishimura C, Ludwig B, Johnson M, O'Brien SE et al. Complete sequencing shows a role for MSX1 in non-syndromic cleft lip and palate. *J Med Genet.* 2003;40:399–407.

51. Sull JW, Liang K-Y, Hetmanski JB, Fallin MD, Ingersoll RG, Park JW et al. Excess maternal transmission of markers in TCOF1

among cleft palate case-parent trios from three populations. *Am J Med Genet Part A*. 2008;146A:2327–2331.

52. Mills JL, Molloy AM, Parke-McDermott A, Troendle JF, Brody LC, Conley MR et al. Folate-related gene polymorphisms as risk factors for cleft lip and cleft palate. *Birth Def Res (Part A): Clin Mol Teratol*. 2008;82:636–643.

53. Fitzpatrick DR, Carr IM, McLaren L, Leek JP, Wightman P, Williamson K, Gautier P, McGill N, Hayward C, Fink H, Markham AF, Fantes JA, Bonthron DT. Identification of SATB2 as the cleft palate gene on 2q32-q33. *Hum Mol Gen*. 2003; 12:2491–2501.

54. Christensen K, Mitchell LE. Familial recurrence—pattern analysis of nonsyndromic isolated cleft palate—a Danish Registry Study. *Am J Hum Genet*. 1996;58:182–190.

55. Koguchi H. Recurrence risk in offspring and siblings of patients with cleft lip and/or cleft palate. *Jap J Human Genet*. 1975; 20:207–221.

56. Curtis EJ, Fraser FC, Warburton D. Congenital cleft lip and palate. *Am J Dis Child*. 1961;102:853–857.

57. Hernandez-Diaz S, Smith CR, Wyszynski DF, Holmes LB. Risk of major malformations among infants exposed to carbamazepine during pregnancy. *Birth Def Res (Part A): Clin Mol Teratol*. 2007;79:357.

58. Wyszynski DF, Nambisan M, Surve T, Alsdorf RM, Smith CR, Holmes LB. Increased rate of major malformations in offspring exposed to valproate during pregnancy. *Neurology*. 2005;64: 961–965.

59. Holmes LB, Wyszynski DF, Lieberman E. The AED (antiepileptic drug) Pregnancy Registry: a 6-year experience. *Arch Neurol*. 2004;61:673–678.

60. Becerra JE, Khoury MJ, Cordero JF, Erickson JD. Diabetes mellitus during pregnancy and the risk for specific defects: a population-based case-control study. *Pediatrics*. 1990;85:1–9.

61. Meyer KA, Werler MM, Hayes C, Mitchell AA. Low material alcohol consumption during pregnancy and oral clefts in offspring. The Stone Birth Defects Study. *Birth Defects Res (Part A): Clin Mol Terat*. 2003;67:509–514.

62. Werler MM. Teratogen update: smoking and reproductive outcomes. *Teratology*. 1997;55:382–388.

63. Hwang S-J, Beaty TH, Panny SR. Association study of transforming growth factor alpha (TGFβ) Taq I polymorphism and oral clefts: indication of gene-environment interaction in a population-based sample of infants with birth defects. *Am J Epidemiol*. 1995;141:629–636.

64. Beaty TH, Maestri NE, Hetmanski JB, Wyszynski DF, Vanderkolk CA, Simpson JC, et al. Testing for interaction between maternal smoking and TGFA genotype among oral cleft cases born in Maryland 1992–1996. *Cleft Palate Craniofac J*. 1997;34:447–454.

65. Christensen K, Olsen J, Nørgaard-Pederson B, Basso O., Støvring H, Milhollin-Johnson L et al. Oral clefts, transforming growth factor alpha gene variants, and maternal smoking: a population-based case-control study in Denmark, 1991–1994. *Am J Epidemiol*. 1999;149:248–255.

66. Chevrier C, Bahuau M, Perret C, Iovannisci DM, Nelva A, Herman C et al. Genetic susceptibilities in the association between maternal exposure to tobacco smoke and the risk of nonsyndromic oral cleft. *Am J Med Genet Part A*. 2008;146A: 2396–2406.

67. Cedergen M, Källen B. Maternal obesity and the risk for orofacial clefts in the offspring. *Cleft Palate Craniofac J*. 2005;42: 367–371.

68. Shaw GM, Lammer EJ, Wasserman CR, O'Mally CD, Tolarova MM. Risks of orofacial clefts in children born to women using multivitamins containing folic acid periconceptionally. *Lancet*. 1995;345:393–396.

69. Werler MM, Hayes C, Louik L, Shapiro S, Mitchell AA. Multivitamin supplementation and risk of birth defects. *Am J Epidermiol*. 1999;150:675–682.

70. Badovinac RL, Werler MM, Williams PL, Kelsey KT, Hayes C. Folic acid-containing supplement consumption during pregnancy and risk for oral cleft: a meta-analysis. *Birth Def Res (Part A): Clin Mel Teratol*. 2007;79:8–15.

71. Tamura T, Munger RG, Corcoran C, Bacayao JY, Nepomuceno B, Solon F. Plasma zinc concentrations of mothers and the risk of nonsyndromic oral clefts in their children: a case-control study in the Philippines. *Birth Def Res (Part A): Clin Mol Terat*. 2005; 73:612–616.

72. Weinberg SM, Brandon CA, McHenry TH, Neiswanger K, Deleyiannis FWB, de Salamanca JE et al. Rethinking isolated cleft palate: evidence of occult lip defects in a subset of cases. *Am J Med Genet Part A*. 2008;146A:1670–1675.

73. Hopper RA, Cutting C, Grayson B. In: Thorne CH, Beasley RW, Aston SJ, Bartlett SP, Gurtner GC, Spear SL, eds. *Cleft Lip and Palate*. Chap. 23, *Grabb and Smith's Plastic Surgery*. 6th ed. Philadelphia: WoltersKluwer Health/Lippincott Williams & Wilkins; 2007: 216–219.

74. Curtis EJ, Fraser FC, Warburton D. Congenital cleft lip and palate. *Am J Dis Child*. 1961;102:853–857.

75. Bixler D, Fogh-Andersen P, Conneally PM. Incidence of cleft lip and palate in the offspring of cleft parents. *Clin Genet*. 1971; 2:155–159.

76. Koguchi H. Recurrence rate in offspring and siblings of patients with cleft lip and/or cleft palate. *Jap J Hum Genet*. 1975;20: 207–221.

77. Jones MC. Etiology of facial clefts: prospective evaluation of 428 patients. *Cleft Palate J*. 1988;25:16–20.

Chapter 7

Club Foot

Definitions

There are three types of "club foot":

a) talipes equinovarus: the forefoot is angled downward and inward; the heel is also an inward, adducted position (Figures 7-1, 7-2, and 7-3);

b) talipes calcaneovalgus: the forefoot is tilted upward and the sole of the foot is rotated outward; the heel is the most downward projection of the foot (Figure 7-1);

c) metatarsus adductus: the distal third of the foot deviates inward (Figure 7-1).

ICD-9:	754.51	(talipes equinovarus)
	754.53	(metatarsus adductus)
	754.62	(talipes calcaneovalgus)
ICD-10:	Q66.0	(talipes equinovarus)
	Q66.1	(talipes calcaneovarus)
	Q66.2	(metatarsus varus)
	Q66.4	(talipes calcaneovalgus)
Mendelian Inheritance in Man:	#119800	(club foot: talipes equinovarus)

Appearance

a) Talipes equinovarus (1, 2): with the true, not-positional deformity, the foot is shortened, the heel is in varus (toward the midline), the forefoot is adducted toward midline and supinated; there can be deep creases over the medial side of the ankle and no creases over the lateral side of the ankle.

b) Talipes calcaneovalgus (3, 4): marked dorsiflexion and valgus position of the foot in relation to the leg; has been referred to as "reverse club foot" (5). The deformity is present at birth. Often the foot appears small and there are associated findings: calcaneous deformity of the ankle, valgus deformity at the subtalar joint, and diminished or absent inversion of the foot (3, 4). The positional calcaneovalgus deformity is distinguished by its spontaneous improvement.

c) Metatarsus adductus: the essential feature is medial deviation of the forefoot (6). In addition, there is inversion of the forefoot (7). A high spontaneous rate of correction, 89% in one study (8), is to be expected.

Associated Malformations

Often club foot is an isolated finding. But the three types are frequently components of many malformation syndromes (9). Club foot is also a common secondary effect of conditions that produce paralysis of the legs, such as spina bifida.

There is a high frequency of vascular anomalies in the legs of individuals with a club foot. 85% have been estimated to have absence of the anterior tibial artery in comparison to 12% in the general population (10). Absence of the posterior tibial artery is a much less common finding. When anterior tibial is absent, it is important to protect the posterior tibial and its terminal branch, the lateral plantar artery. When the posterior tibial artery is absent, an embryonic precursor of the peroneal artery persists and provides the function of the posterior tibial artery.

The presence of the flexor digitorum accessorius longus muscle was identified at the time of surgical correction in 6.6% of 835 affected patients in Saint Louis between 1980 and 2000 (11). The children with this accessory muscle were much more likely to have affected relatives than those without: 23.4% vs. 4.5% (p<0.001).

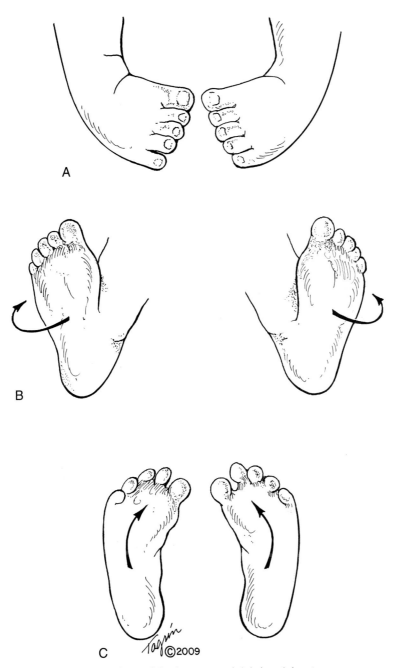

FIGURE 7.1   Shows the shape of the three types of club foot deformity:
A. talipes equinovarus
B. calcaneo valgus
C. metatarsus adductus

Developmental Defect

The primary sequence of events and underlying abnormalities remains speculative. In the many studies of fetuses, children, and adults with club foot deformity, some of the theories as to the primary problem have included: 1) a vascular deficiency (12), such as hypoplasia or premature termination of the anterior tibial and medial plantar arteries (13) and deficiency of the dorsalis pedis artery (14); 2) a disorder resembling fibromatosis that affects the ligaments in the third trimester of pregnancy (15); 3) a misshapen talus bone (16, 17); 4) anomalous muscles (18) and muscle imbalance (19).

Talipes calcaneovalgus was found in family studies by Ruth Wynne-Davies (1) to be more common in the firstborn children of young mothers, reflecting, she postulated, compression in a small, tight uterus.

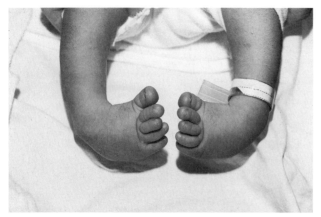

FIGURE 7.2   Shows bilateral talipes equinovarus.

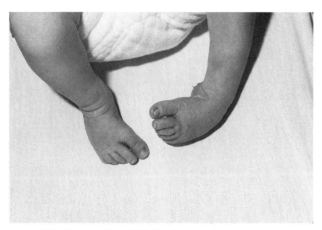

FIGURE 7.3   Shows unilateral (left) talipes equinovarus.

Prevalence; Race and Ethnicity

In the first family studies of this topic by Wynne-Davies in 1940–1961 among Caucasians in Exeter, England, the prevalence rate of talipes equinovarus was 1.2/1,000 (1). Marked differences in prevalence rates have been observed among several racial/ethnic groups. Among the 35,680 consecutive births evaluated in the National Collaborative Perinatal Project (1959–1964) [20], the prevalence rates for talipes equinovarus, talipes calcaneovalgus, and metatarsus varus per 1,000 infants were 2.3, 0.8, and 1.2/1,000 for white infants, respectively, and 1.2, 0.2, and 1.4/1,000 for black infants.

The prevalence of idiopathic talipes equinovarus club foot in Texas among blacks and U.S. and foreign-born Hispanics was comparable to that in whites (0.8/1,000 births [23]).

A low frequency rate has been observed in two Chinese populations: 0.3 and 0.4/1,000, respectively (21, 22).

High frequencies have been documented among the Maori native populations in New Zealand: 7/1,000 (24, 25); Aborigines in Australia: 3.5/1,000 (26);

African infants in South Africa: 3.5/1,000 (27); and Roma or gypsy infants in Hungary 3.4 ± 0.6/1,000 (28).

Birth Status

A significantly higher frequency of metatarsus adductus has been documented in twins compared to singletons and in premature infants compared to term infants (6). By age five years, the metatarsus adductus had resolved in the term infants, but in only 81% of the 484 premature infants (p< 0.05).

Sex Ration

All racial and ethnic groups have shown more affected males than females for each type of club foot deformity (1, 2, 6, 9, 20, 25).

Sidedness

50 to 60% of the affected children have only one affected leg, with the left leg affected more frequently than the right (1, 2, 25).

Parental Age

No consistent pattern of a significant increase or decrease in maternal or paternal age has been reported.

Twinning

In the one large series (29) of identical (MZ) and fraternal (DZ) twins, the concordance rates were 32.5% for MZ twins and 2.9% for DZ twins.

Both short stature in the mother and twin pregnancy have been identified as risk factors, presumably by causing intrauterine constraint (30).

Genetic Factors

Several families in which many relatives had specific types of club foot deformity have been reported. The clinical interpretation in these specific families has been either autosomal dominant (31) or autosomal recessive inheritance of a single gene mutation.

However, the findings in extensive family studies of 635 patients by Wynne-Davies in Scotland (1, 2) were interpreted as most consistent with multifactorial inheritance. The characteristics cited were: 1) the parents, sibs, and children of affected individuals have an increased likelihood of being affected; 2) with the frequency of talipes equinovarus in the general population being 1 in 1,000 (0.1%), the likelihood that the next child will be affected is 30 times greater or 3%; the chances of a second child having talipes calcaneovalgus or metatarsus adductus was 20 times higher; 3) all three types of club foot are more common in male than in female infants; the male relatives of the females with talipes equinovarus have an increased risk for being affected in comparison to the male relatives of affected males; 4) the concordance rate for identical twins was much higher than for fraternal twins (29).

The findings in family studies of the first-degree relatives of 174 children with talipes equinovarus club foot in Hungary were also interpreted as most consistent with the multifactorial threshold model (32).

Later, the segregation pattern in many families was interpreted as a "mixed model" and suggested a major gene affect, most likely a dominant gene (33).

More recent analyses using mathematical models, such as complex segregation analysis, have been interpreted as supporting most likely the single Mendelian gene hypothesis (34), specifically "the recessive mixed model with no differences based on ethnicity" (35).

The CASP10 gene, which encodes proteins that are regulators of apoptosis, is a candidate gene for the genetic susceptibility for idiopathic talipes equinovarus. Linkage with an allele of a variant in CASP10 was identified in parent-child trios (TDT; tandem disequilibrium test) in both white and Hispanic families with multiple affected individuals (36). Linkage analysis in a large family with 13 affected individuals and 41 unaffected members identified two regions of interest, but none with significant LOD scores (>3.0). The candidate genes in the regions on chromosome 3 were *Wnt7* and on chromosome 13, *LM07* (37). Mutations in the sulfate transporter genes *DTDST* were not identified in a study of 207 individuals with idiopathic talipes equinovarus club foot (38).

Elevated plasma levels of total homocysteine, an intermediary metabolite of methionine, have been found in the mothers of children with congenital idiopathic club foot in comparison to mothers of children with no congenital abnormalities in two studies (39, 40). In a study of 375 affected children-parent trials in the United Kingdom (1998–1999) [41], the child with the MTHFR C677T polymorphism, especially those homozygous (TT), had a lower risk for the club foot deformity. This association was not modified by the mother taking a folic acid supplement.

Empiric recurrence risks in subsequent sibs and offspring of affected individuals (Table 7-1) [1, 28] have shown that the recurrence risk is higher among the sibs of affected females (the less frequently affected sex). Theoretically, in the sibs of the more severely affected child, that is, with severe, bilateral club foot deformity, the risk will be higher than if the index case is affected mildly.

Environmental Factors

Three exposures during pregnancy have been associated with an increased risk for club foot: cigarette smoking, misoprostol, and "early" amniocentesis. Mothers who smoked cigarettes during pregnancy had a modest increase in their risk of having a child with a club foot deformity compared to women who did not smoke (42–46). A dose-response relationship was identified, as well as gender specific differences with the risk higher for the mothers of girls (45). Having a family history of club foot deformity, which implies the presence of one or more gene mutations that are risk factors for the occurrence of club foot, increased the risk of club foot among smoking pregnant women significantly in one study (44). The occurrence of the slow NAT2 acetylator could also be a risk factor for club foot in the infants of pregnant women who smoke (47).

TABLE 7-1 *Empiric Recurrence Risk Data*

Index Case			Affected Father	Affected Mother	Affected Brother	Affected Sister
1. Talipes equinovarus						
Male	a) England (1)	(η=97)	1/97 (1.%)	0/97 (0%)	4/115 (3.9%)	0/90 (0%)
	b) Hungary (28)	(η=118)	4/118 (3.3%)	3/118 (2.5%)	4/61 (6.6%)	1/60 (1.2%)
Female	a) England (1)	(η=47)	3/47 (6.8%)	0/47 (0%)	2/33 (6.0%)	2/34 (5.9%)
	b) Hungary (28)	(η=56)	1/56 (1.8%)	0/56 (0%)	2/29 (6.9%)	3/30 (10%)
2. Calcaneovalgus						
Male (1)		(η=26)	0/26	0/26	0/24	1/12 (8.3%)
Female (1)		(η=48)	0/48	0/48	1/20 (5%)	2/30 (6.7%)
3. Metatarsus Adductus						
Male (1)		(η=30)	0/30 (0%)	0/30 (0%)	0/26* (0%)	2/22 (9.1%
Female (1)		(η=42)	0/42	0/42	2/35**	1***/30
			(0%)	(0%)	(5.7%)	(3.3%)

*1 brother had talipes equinovarus
**2 brothers with equinovarus
***3 had talipes equinovarus in one foot and metatarsus varus in the other.

Exposure at 6 to 10 weeks of gestation to the synthetic prostaglandin E$_1$ analogue misoprostol, used as an abortifacient, produces intense uterine contractions. If the pregnancy continues, the fetus may exhibit signs of vascular disruption, common effects of which are the equinovarus club foot deformity and arthrogryposis affecting primarily both legs (48).

"Early" amniocentesis, performed at 11 to 14 weeks of gestation, has been associated with a 1% risk for club foot deformity (49). This risk is attributed to the fetal affects of decreasing the volume of amniotic fluid at that critical time in pregnancy.

Crowding of the fetus has been associated with an increased frequency of the equinovarus club foot deformity. The fact that the equinovarus club foot deformity is more common among firstborn infants has been attributed theoretically to the smaller intrauterine volume in the first pregnancy (1, 2, 34).

Seasonal variation, with a significant increase in the winter (December-March), has been observed in several studies (30, 50, 51). No cause of the seasonal increase has been established.

Experimental models of equinovarus club foot have been established in a paralyzed chick embryo (52) and by hyperthermia in pregnant guinea pigs (53).

Treatment and Prognosis

There is a consensus that the initial treatment of the congenital idiopathic club foot deformity should begin soon after birth and should be nonsurgical (6). The aggressive reduction method of Ponseti (54), which involves weekly stretching of the deformity followed by the application of long-leg casts, has been shown to correct all components of the deformity in almost all patients. 90% of the patients required five or fewer casts for correction. Most had a percutaneous tenotomy as part of the treatment. The time for correction in 157 patients (256 club feet) was 20 days (range 14–24) [55]. A 30-year follow up of children treated by the Ponseti method showed that 78% had an excellent or good outcome (56).

Occasionally serial casting is not successful and corrective surgery is needed to complete the correction.

The use of Botulinum A toxin to eliminate the function of the triceps surae muscle complex has been shown to be an effective adjunct to manipulation and casting, and as an alternative to Achilles tentomy (57).

After club foot surgery, ischemic necrosis is a rare complication (58). This has been attributed in those cases to a congenital deficiency of the anterior tibial and dorsalis pedis arteries.

Genetic Counseling

The unaffected parents of a child with idiopathic talipes equinovarus should be informed of their increased risk of having a second affected child (Table 7-1). If the first affected child is a female and severely affected, i.e., has a bilateral club foot deformity, the risk for a second affected child is higher. Empiric risk data has been published for only a few racial/ethnic groups. If there is no empiric data for the child's racial/ethnic group, but the prevalence rate is known, infants in racial groups with a higher prevalence rate will have higher empiric recurrence risks.

The parents in an at-risk pregnancy have the option of using prenatal screening by ultrasound to determine whether or not the fetus is affected (59–63).

Club foot is often a surprise finding in routine prenatal screening by ultrasound. Since club foot is a feature of many malformation syndromes, the specific etiology cannot be established until the infant has been examined at birth. There is also a significant risk for a false positive diagnosis. The rate of a false positive diagnosis of club foot was 11.8% in a study of 68 affected fetuses (59) and 6.4% in another study of 41 affected fetuses (60). The false positive rate was much higher (29%) for unilateral club foot (n=42) than for bilateral club foot deformity (7%) [n=45; p<0.5] in another study (62).

Chromosome analysis by amniocentesis should be considered, as the range of abnormalities detected has been wide, with the rates of 5.9% (59), 22% (60), 17.3% (61), and 30.6% (62) in different studies.

REFERENCES

1. Wynne-Davies R. Family studies and the cause of congenital club foot. *J Bone Jt Surg*. 1964;46-B:445–463.
2. Wynne-Davies R. Genetic and environmental factors in etiology of talipes equinovarus. *Clin Orthopaed Rel Res*. 1972;84:9–13.
3. Evans D. Calcaneovalgus deformity. *J Bone Jt Surg*. 1975;57-B:270–278.
4. Yu GV, Hladik J. Residual calcaneovalgus deformity: review of the literature and case study. *J Foot Ankle Surg*. 1994;33:228–238.
5. Edwards ER, Menelaus MB. Reverse club foot: rigid and recalcitrant talipes calcaneovalgus. *J Bone Jt Surg*. 1987;69-B:330–334.
6. Hunziker UA, Largo RH, Duc G. Neonatal metatarsus adductus, joint mobility, axis and rotation of the lower extremity in preterm and term children 0–5 years of age. *Eur J Pediatr*. 1988;148:19–23.
7. Reimann I, Werner HH. Congenital metatarsus varus. *Clin Orthopaed Rel Res*. 1975;110:223–226.
8. Ponseti IV, Becker JR. Congenital metatarsus adductus: the results of treatment. *J Bone Jt Surg*. 1966;48-A: 702–721.
9. Somppi E. Club foot. Review of the literature and an analysis of a series of 135 treated clubfeet. *Acta Orthopaedia Scandinavica*. 1984;55(Suppl 209):7–109.
10. Dobbs MB, Gordon JE, Schoenecker PL. Absent posterior tibial artery associated with idiopathic club foot. *J Bone Jt Surg*. 2004;86A:599–602.
11. Dobbs MB, Walton T, Gordon JE, Schoenecker PL, Gurnett CA. Flexor digitorum accessorius longus muscle is associated with familial idiopathic club foot. *J Pediatr Orthop*. 2005;25:357–359.
12. Atlas S, Saenz Menacho LC, Ures S. Some new aspects in the pathology of clubfoot. *Clin Orthopaed Rel Res*. 1980;149:224–228.
13. Sodre H, Bruschini S, Mestriner LA, Mirenda Jr F, Levinsohn EM, Packard Jr DS, Crider Jr RJ, Schwartz R, Hootnick DR.

Arterial abnormalities in talipes equinovarus as assessed by angiography and the Doppler technique. *J Pediatr Orthopaed*. 1990;10:101–104.

14. Katz DA, Albanese EL, Levinsohn EM, Hootnick DR, Packard Jr DS, Grant WD, Mann KA, Albanese SA. Pulsed color-flow Doppler analysis of arterial deficiency in idiopathic clubfoot. *J Ped Orthopaed*. 2003;23:84–87.

15. Fukahara K, Schollneier G, Uhthoff HK. The pathogenesis of clubfoot. A histomorphometric and immunohistochemical study of fetuses. *J Bone Jt Surg*. 1994;76–B:450–457.

16. Settle GW. The anatomy of congenital talipes equinovarus: sixteen dissected specimens. *J Bone Jt Surg*. 1963;45-A:1341–1354.

17. Ippolito E, Ponseti IV. Congenital club foot in the human fetus. *J Bone Jt Surg*. 1980;62–A:8–22.

18. Porter RW. An anomalous muscle in children with congenital talipes. *Clinical Anatomy*. 1996;9:25–27.

19. Feldbrin Z, Gilai AN, Ezra E, Khermosh O, Kramer U, Weintroub S. Muscle imbalance in the etiology of idiopathic club foot. *J Bone Jt Surg*. 1995;77B:596–601.

20. Chung CS, Myrianthopoulos NC, Yoshiaki H. Racial and prenatal factors in major congenital malformations. *Am J Hum Genet*. 1968;20:44–60.

21. Emanuel I, Huang S-W, Gutman LT, Yu F-C, Lin C-C. The incidence of congenital malformations in a Chinese population: the Taipei Collaborative Study. *Teratology*. 1972;5:159–170.

22. Ching GHS, Chung CS, Nemechek RW. Genetic and epidemiological studies of club foot in Hawaii: ascertainment and incidence. *Am J Hum Genet*. 1969;21:566–580.

23. Moorthi RN, Hashmi SS, Langois P, Canfield M, Waller DK, Hecht JT. Idiopathic talipes equinovarus (ITEV) (Clubfeet) in Texas. *Am J Med Genet*. 2005;132A:376–380.

24. Brougham DI, Nicol RO. Use of the Cincinnati incision in congenital talipes equinovarus. *J Pediatr Orthop*. 1988;8:696–698.

25. Cartlidge I. Observations on the epidemiology of club foot in Polynesian and Caucasian populations. *J Med Gen*. 1984;21:290–292.

26. Carey M, Bower C, Mylvananam A, Rouse I. Talipes equinovarus in Western Australia. *Paediatric Perinatal Epidem*. 2003;17:187–194.

27. Van Meerdervoort HFP. Congenital musculoskeletal malformation in South African blacks. A study of incidence. *SA Med J*. 1976;50:1853–1855.

28. Bellyei A, Czeizel A. A higher incidence of congenital structural talipes equinovarus in Gipsies. *Hum Hered*. 1983;33:58–59.

29. Idelberger K. Die Ergebnisse der Zwillingsforschung beim angeborenen Klumpfuss. *Brerh Dtsch Orthop Ges*. 1939;33:272–276.

30. Carey M, Mylvaganam A, Rouse I, Bower C. Risk factors for isolated talipes equinovarus in Western Australia, 1980–1994. *Paediatric Perinatal Epidem*. 2005;19:238–245.

31. Juberg RC, Touchstone WJ. Congenital metatarsus varus in four generations. *Clin Genet*. 1974;5:127–132.

32. Czeizel A, Bellyei Á, Kránicz J, Mocsai L, Tusnády G. Confirmation of the multifactorial threshold model for congenital structural talipes equinovarus. *J Med Genet*. 1981;18:99–100.

33. Wang J, Palmer RM, Chung CS. The role of major gene club foot. *Am J Hum Genet*. 1988;42:772–776.

34. Rebbeck TR, Dietz FR, Murray JC, Buetow KH. A single-gene explanation for the probability of having idiopathic talipes equinovarus. *Am J Hum Genet*. 1993;53:1051–1063.

35. de Andrade M, Barnholtz JS, Amos CI, Lochmiller CL, Scott A, Risman M, Hecht JT. Segregation analysis of idiopathic talipes equinovarus in a Texan population. *Am J Med Genet*. 79:97–102.

36. Heck AL, Bray MS, Scott A, Blanton SH, Hecht JT. Variation in CASP10 gene is associated with idiopathic talipes equinovarus. *J Pediatr Orthop*. 2005;25:598–602.

37. Dietz FR, Cole WG, Tosi LL, Carroll NC, Werner RD, Comstock D, Murray JC. A search for the gene(s) predisposing to idiopathic club foot. *Clin Genet*. 2005;67:361–362.

38. Bonafé L, Blanton SH, Scott A, Broussard S, Wise CA, Superti-Furga A, Hecht JT. DTDST mutations are not a frequent cause of idiopathic talipes equinovarus (club foot). *J Med Genet*. 2002;39:e20–22.

39. Volsett SM, Refsum H, Irgens LM. Plasma total homocysteine, pregnancy complications, and adverse pregnancy outcomes: the Hordaland homocysteine study. *Am J Clin Nutr*. 2000;71:962–968.

40. Karakurt L, Yilmaz E, Erhan Y, Serin E, Bektas B, Cikim G, Gürsu F. Plasma total homocysteine levels in mothers of children with club foot. *J Pediat Orthop*. 2003;23:658–660.

41. Sharp L, Miedzybrodzka Z, Cardy AH, Inglis J, Madrigal L, Barker S et al. The C677T polymorphism in the methylenetetrahydrofolate reductase gene (MTHFR), maternal use of folic acid supplements, and risks of isolated clubfoot: a case-parent-triad analysis. *Am J Epidemiol*. 2006;164:852–861.

42. VanDenEeden SK, Karagas MR, Daling JR, Vaushan TL. A case-control study of maternal smoking and congenital malformations. *Pediatr Perinat Epidemiol*. 1990;4:147–155.

43. Alderman BW, Takahashi ER, LeMier MK. Risk indicators for talipes equinovarus in Washington State, 1987–1989. *Epidemiology*. 1991;2:289–292.

44. Honein MA, Paulozzi LJ, Moore CA. Family history, maternal smoking, and clubfoot: an indication of a gene-environment interaction. *Am J Epid*. 2000;152:658–665.

45. Skelly AC, Holt VL, Mosca VS, Alderman BW. Talipes equinovarus and maternal smoking: a population-based case-control study in Washington State. *Teratology*. 2002;66:91–100.

46. Dickinson KC, Meyer RE, Kotch J. Maternal smoking and the risk for clubfoot in infants. *Birth Def Res (Part A): Clin Mol Teratol*. 2008;82:86–91.

47. Hecht JT, Ester A, Scott A, Wise CA, Iovannisci DM, Lammer EJ et al. NAT2 variation and idiopathic talipes equinovarus (clubfoot). *Am J Med Genet Part A*. 2007;143A:2285–2291.

48. Gonzalez CH, Marques-Dias MJ, Kim CA, Sugayama SMM, DaPaz JA, Huson SM, Holmes LB. Congenital abnormalities in Brazilian children associated with misoprostol misuse in first trimester of pregnancy. *Lancet*. 1998;351:1624–1627.

49. Farrell SA, Summers Am, Dallaire L, Singer J. Clubfoot, adverse outcome of early amniocentesis: disruption or deformation? *J Med Genet*. 1999;36:843–846.

50. Pryor GA, Villar RN, Ronen A, Scott PM. Seasonal variations in the incidence of congenital talipes equinovarus. *J Bone Joint Surg (Br)*. 1991;73:632–634.

51. Barker SL, Macnicol MF. Seasonal distribution of idiopathic congenital talipes equinovarus in Scotland. *J Pediatr Orthop B*. 2002;11:129–133.

52. Germiller JA, Lerner AL, Pacifico RJ, Loder RT, Hensinger RN. Muscle and tendon size relationships in a paralyzed chick embryo model of clubfoot. *J Ped Orthopaed*. 1998;18:314–318.

53. Edwards MJ. The experimental production of clubfoot in guinea-pigs by maternal hyperthermia during gestation. *J Path*. 1971;103:49–53.

54. Ponseti IV. *Congenital Clubfoot. Fundamentals of Treatment*. New York: Oxford University Press; 1996: 140.

55. Morcuende JA, Dolan LA, Dietz FR, Ponseti IV. Radical reduction in the rate of extensive corrective surgery for clubfoot using the Ponseti method. *Pediatrics*. 2004;113:376–380.

56. Cooper DM, Dirtz FR. Treatment of idiopathic club foot. A thirty-year follow-up note. *J Bone Joint Surg*. 1995;77-A:1477–1489.

57. Alvarez C, Tredwell SJ, Keenan SP, Beauchamp RD, Choit RL, Sawatzy BJ, DeVera MA. Treatment of idiopathic club foot utilizing Botulinum A toxin: a new method and its short term outcomes. *J Pediatric Orthop*. 2005;25:229–235.

58. Hootnick DR, Packard Jr DS, Levinsohn EM, Berkowitz SA, Aronsson DD, Crider Jr RJ. Ischemic necrosis following clubfoot surgery: the purple hallux sign. *J Pediatr Orthop*. 2004;13: 315–322.

59. Shipp TD, Benacerraf BR. The significance of prenatally identified isolated clubfoot: is amniocentesis indicated? *Am J Obstet Gynecol*. 1998;178:600–602.

60. Carroll SG, Lockyer H, Andrews H, Abdel-Fattah S, McMillan D, Kyle PM et al. Outcome of fetal talipes following in utero sonographic diagnosis. *Ultrasound in Obst Gynecol*. 2001; 18:437–440.

61. Bakalis S, Sairam S, Homfray T, Harrington K, Nicolaides K, Thilanganathan B. Outcome of antenatally diagnosed talipes equinovarus in an unselected obstetric population. *Ultrasound Obstet Gynecol*. 2002;20:226–229.

62. Mammen L, Benson CB. Outcome of fetuses with club feet diagnosed by prenatal sonography. *J Ultrasound Med*. 2004;23: 497–500.

63. Bar-On E, Mashiach R, Inbar O, Weigl D, Katz K, Meizner I. Prenatal ultrasound diagnosis of club foot: outcome and recommendations for counseling and follow-up. *J Bone Jt Surg*. 2005; 87:990–993.

Chapter 8

Congenital Diaphragmatic Hernia

Definition

Structural deficiencies in the diaphragm through which intestines and other viscera are herniated (Figure 8-1).

ICD-9 756.610 (anomalies of diaphragm)

	756.615	(Bochdalek hernia)
	756.616	(Morgagni hernia)
	756.620	(eventration of diaphragm)

ICD-10 Q79.0 (congenital diaphragmatic hernia)

Q79.1 (absence of diaphragm; congenital malformation of diaphragm NOS; eventration of diaphragm)

Mendelian Inheritance in Man: %142340 (Congenital diaphragmatic hernia I; DIH1)

%222400 (Diaphragmatic hernia 2; DIH2)

#610187 (Diaphragmatic hernia 3)

306950 (Hernia, anterior diaphragmatic; DIH3)

Appearance

Several types of congenital diaphragmatic hernias (CDH) have been delineated (1, 2):

a) Posterolateral hole or defect in the pleuroperitoneal membrane; foramen of Bochdalek; more common on left side (Figure 8-2); accounts for 80 to 90% of all congenital hernias of the diaphragm; usually hernia contains small intestine; frequently contains stomach, colon, and spleen; liver often present on right-sided Bochdalek hernias;

b) Parasternal hernia through foramen of Morgagni (Figure 8-2); usually occurs on right side of xiphoid process; hernia may contain liver, less often contains colon and stomach; accounts for 2% of all CDH.

c) defect in septum transversum (Figure 8-2); a rare defect of the central tendon of the diaphragm, which is derived from the septum transversum; this hernia is usually in the anterior portion of the diaphragm;

d) eventration of diaphragm; an area of thickness of diaphragm, but usually no open defect;

e) absence of the entire diaphragm on one or both sides; a rare abnormality.

Associated Malformations

Some abnormalities, such as lung hypoplasia, intestinal malrotation, and patent ductus arteriosus, are common and have been considered secondary effects of congenital diaphragmatic hernias.

In addition, there are genuine associated malformations, which have been documented in case series and population-based studies (2–19), with frequencies of 48% (11), 69% (13), and 45% (17) in three of these.

Heart defects are a common associated malformation. For example, 25% of affected neonates in Boston (8) and 17.8% in Philadelphia (20) had heart defects. Atrial and ventricular septal defects, conotruncal defects, and left ventricular outflow tract obstructive defects, such as hypoplastic left heart syndrome, are most common heart defects (21). The infants with an associated heart defect were 2.9 times less likely to survive than the infants with congenital diaphragmatic hernia and no associated heart defect (20).

All children with congenital diaphragmatic hernia have some degree of pulmonary hypoplasia, which is characterized by a decreased number of airways, alveoli, and vascular generations (22–24). Both lungs and bronchi are usually hypoplastic, although the lung and

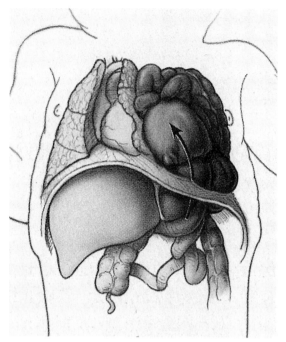

FIGURE 8.1   Shows in left-sided diaphragmatic defect the herniation of stomach and bowel into left side of thorax. (From Wenstrom KD: *N Engl J Med.* 2003;349:1888, 2003. Used with permission.).

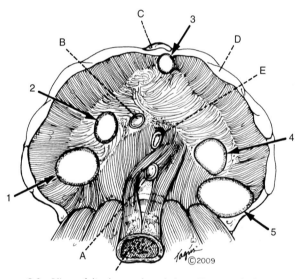

FIGURE 8.2   View of diaphragm from below, Showing the location of several types of defects: 1) Bochdalek hernia (rt) without loss of muscular rim; 2) Central hernia; 3) Morgagni hernia; 4) Bochdalek hernia (Lt) without loss of muscular rim; 5) Bochdalek hernia (Lt) with loss of muscular rim. Additional landmarks: A) aorta; B) inferior vena cava; C) sternum; D) rib; E) esophagus. Drawing adapted from Figure 1 in Am J Med Genet Part C Sem in Med Genet 2007; 145C:107, Figure 1 by K Ackerman, BR Pober. Used with permission.

tracheobronchial tree on the same side as the diaphragm defect are affected more severely. At bronchoscopy, in a series of 39 newborn infants in Japan (24), 18% and 38%, respectively, had anomalies of the tracheobronchial tree bronchi and bronchial hypoplasia on the affected side. The presence of these anomalies correlated with a worse prognosis.

An increased frequency of associated limb malformations has been reported, also, especially in infants with syndromic CDH (2, 6, 25, 26). In one study (2), 11% in a consecutive series of 146 infants with congenital diaphragmatic hernia had limb defects, such as monodactyly as a feature of the Cornelia de Lange Syndrome (MIM #122470). The limb deficiencies may be bilateral or unilateral. Among the unilateral cases, the affected limbs were equally likely to be ipsilateral or contralateral to the site of the diaphragmatic hernia (26).

In a case series of 117 stillborn infants with CDH and affected infants who died and had a postmortem examination (including infants with chromosome abnormalities), the most common skeletal abnormalities were anomalies of the ribs, including both absent and an extra rib, extra lumbar vertebrae, and spina bifida. The frequencies of all skeletal malformations were 31.2% in infants with syndromes and 17.8% in those without a specific syndrome (25). 30% of the males with congenital diaphragmatic hernia in one series of 60 autopsies were cryptorchid (23). 27% of the infants had an abnormality of the urinary system, including renal agenesis, renal dysplasia, and hydronephrosis.

An increased frequency of congenital diaphragmatic hernia has been noted also in infants with anencephaly and iniencephaly (27). An association with myelomeningocele, postulated to be a schisis association (28), has also been described.

Developmental Defect

The diaphragm forms as a membranous sheet that arises from several interconnected components and is complete by the eighth week of gestation (29–31).

Studies in the developing rat embryo showed that muscle precursor cells migrate from the somites in the cervical region into the membranous diaphragm (32).

The knock-out of the *Slit3* gene in mice showed that the central part of the diaphragm develops from the septum transversum (33).

Rat pups exposed in utero to the herbicide nitrofen have shown that the pleuroperitoneal folds, triangular-shaped structures, were derived from the mesoderm that develops in the human embryo between weeks 4 and 12 (34).

The mouse knockout of the gene *Fgf10 (-/-)* with lung agenesis had a primordial diaphragm. This was interpreted to mean that the development of the diaphragm did not depend on signals from lung tissue (35).

The most common left-sided Bochdalek hernia occurs because the dorsal mesentery of the esophagus does not fuse by the 10th week of gestation with the septum transversum, postulated to be of the pleuroperitoneal membrane on the left side of the diaphragm. (It is interesting to note that Bochdalek apparently described the lumbocostal triangles (36), but not the gap in the diaphragm to which his name is now applied (37, 38).

The less common Morgagni defects occur in openings between the sternal and costal heads (36) (Figure 8.2). This gap is closed usually by muscle fibers from the xiphoid cartilage (pars sternalis) and neighboring fibers (pars costales) [37].

Prevalence

Several population-based studies (6, 7, 15, 17, 39) have shown that the prevalence rate is 1:2,000 to 1:3,000 births. Prenatal detection by sonography has improved identification at birth.

Race

No apparent racial/ethnic differences have been identified.

Birth Status

An increased frequency of stillbirth has been reported. As two examples, the frequencies were 3% in the Northern Health Region of the United Kingdom during 1991–2001 (15) and 5.4% in a consecutive series of 203 infants with Bochdalek hernia in Boston (1972–1974, 1979–2003) [19] [Table 8-1].

Sex Ratio

A slight excess of affected males, such as 1.4:1=M:F (19), has been noted.

Sidedness

80 to 90% of the congenital diaphragmatic hernias are Bochdalek hernias; 85% of these are on the left side of the diaphragm, 10% on the right and 5% are bilateral (1).

Parental Age

No increase or decrease in maternal or paternal age has been reported. In one report (19), advanced paternal age was observed.

Twins

In a series of 203 consecutive infants with Bochdalek hernia, 8 (3.9%) were twin pairs and all were discordant, including five monozygous twins (19). While many instances of concordant monozygous twins have been reported, the experience in consecutive series has been that most are discordant. Pober et al. (19) postulated that spontaneous, epigenetic events could be a cause of the single affected, i.e., discordant, monozygous twins.

TABLE 8-1 *Apparent etiology: congenital diaphragmatic hernia**

	Isolated	Multiple anomalies
I. Mendelian disorders		
1. split-hand/split-foot		1**
2. Fryn Syndrome		1 (ref. Vargas)***
3. persistent Müllerian duct syndrome		1
4. Smith-Lemli-Opitz Syndrome		1
II. Chromosome abnormalities		
1. trisomy 21		1
2. trisomy 18		2(1) SHSF with trisomy 18
3. trisomy 13		1
4. tetrasomy 12p		1
5. deletion 4p		1
6. 46,XY, der(4)t (4:20)pat (unbalanced Translocation)		1
7. Deletion 15 - 46, XX, del 15 (pter→q26)		1
III. Syndromes		
1. Congenital diaphragmatic hernia with limb deficiency****		1
IV. Environmental factors		
1. Infant of diabetic mother		2
V. Twinning		
1. DZ	0	
2. Monozygous		(1***)
VI. Unknown etiology	14	16
	14	31/45 total (1 in 4,583)

Legends: * These affected infants were identified among 206, 244 liveborn and stillborn and elective terminations for fetal anomalies at Brigham and Women's Hospital in Boston (1972–1974, 1979–2000). Affected infants are not included whose mothers had planned to deliver at another hospital, prior to the detection of fetal anomalies.

** Infant had hereditary split-hand/split-foot syndrome and trisomy 18; one parent had SHSF Syndrome.

*** Monozygous twins with Fryns Syndrome, one with congenital diaphragmatic hernia:

Vargas J et al. Discordant phenotype in monozygotic twins with Fryns syndrome. *Am J Med Genet*. 2000;94:42–45.

**** Infant with left diaphragmatic hernia; absent right thumb; hemivertebrae T2, 3; 11 ribs n left.

( ) Infants listed under two apparent etiologies; counted only in one category.

Genetic Factors

Several types of genetic factors have been associated with the occurrence of congenital diaphragmatic hernia: several different chromosome abnormalities, specific chromosome deletions, spontaneous mutations, and autosomal recessive gene mutations (Table 8-1).

In three studies, 11.6% (6), 12% (40), and 9.5% (41), respectively, of affected fetuses and infants had a chromosome abnormality. Trisomy 18, 13, and 45, X have been the most frequently associated aneuploidies. The possibility of an associated chromosome abnormality is greatest in dysmorphic infants with multiple anomalies. In such infants, special testing of chromosome 12p by fluorescent in situ hybridization (FISH) in amniocytes or skin fibroblasts must be carried out to identify tetrasomy 12p (Pallister-Killian Syndrome: MIM #601803), which is always present in a mosaic pattern and is rarely identified in peripheral blood (42). The frequencies of tetrasomy 12p in two case series were 1% (17) and 1.5% (19). However, these are probably underestimates since the additional testing needed was not carried out routinely in all infants with CDH and associated anomalies.

Deletions, duplications, inversions, and translocations have been identified in almost all chromosomes in studies of infants with CDH and other anomalies. These deletions will be important in the search for the genes associated with CDH. The most common deletions identified have included: 1q41-q42, 3q22, 4p16, 8p23, and 15q26. Of these deletions, the 15q26 deletion is the most common (45). Common duplications have been 11q23.3-qter and 22pter-q11 (1, 31, 40, 43-45).

Infants with multiple malformations, including congenital diaphragmatic hernia, but no specific diagnosis and no chromosome deletion or duplication, may also be affected as the result of a spontaneous mutation. One example was a *de novo* mutation in FOG2 identified by Ackerman et al (46). Other candidate genes in the FOG2 pathway are: GATA4, GATA5, GATA6, and COUP-TF11, which are also part of the retinoic acid pathway (47). *SLIT2* and *SLIT3* are candidate genes that are migration molecules. The genes *RGMA* and *IGFR1* are in or near the 15q26 deletion (40). Systematic searches for de novo mutations in several candidate genes for causing congenital diaphragmatic hernia have not been published yet. No commercial testing is available yet for clinical use.

At least 10% of the infants with congenital diaphragmatic hernia and other anomalies have a specific syndrome (1, 7, 31, 48). These disorders include:

Fryns Syndrome (MIM %229850): coarse facial features, hypoplasia of fingernails, heart defects, genitourinary anomalies, and delayed development;

Simpson-Golabi-Behmel Syndrome (MIM #312870): overgrowth, coarse facial features, brachydactyly, polydactyly, heart defects, and renal anomalies; associated mutations in the gene encoding glypican-3 (GPC3) [300037], which maps to chromosome Xq26 (49);

Cornelia de Lange Syndrome (MIM #122470): growth restriction, distinctive facial features, absence of digits, hirsutism, and mental retardation; associated mutations in Nipped-B-Like (NPL) gene (50);

Donnai-Barrow Syndrome (MIM #222448): hypertelorism, high myopia, hearing loss, developmental delay,

proteinuria, associated mutations in LRP2, which encodes the multiligand receptor megalin (51);

Denys-Drash Syndrome (MIM #194080): ambiguous genitalia and male pseudohermephroditism; mutation in WT1-gene (52);

Matthew-Wood Syndrome (MIM 601186): pulmonary hypoplasia, anophthalmia/microphthalmia, heart defects; mutations in STRA6, a large group of "*st*imulated by *retinoic acid*" (STRA) genes (53);

Meacham Syndrome (MIM #608978): male pseudohermaphroditism with internal female genitals and complex heart defects; mutations in the C-terminal zink finger domains of WT1, a gene that plays a central role in the development of the diaphragm (54).

Environmental Factors

In a questionnaire-based interview with the mothers of 63 infants born with CDH in the Netherlands in the years 2000 to 2004, there was a significant association with excessive alcohol use around the time of conception (55).

Experimental studies and clinical observations suggest an association with vitamin A and retinoid metabolism (56, 57). First, in 1949 Anderson (58) reported the observation that vitamin A deficiency in pregnant rodents was associated with an increased rate of occurrence of CDH. The exposure to the herbicide nitrofen, which causes CDH in rat pups, can be reversed by vitamin A supplementation during pregnancy (59). Other compounds that induce congenital diaphragmatic hernia in rodent pups inhibit retinol dehydrogenase-2 (60).In a clinical study of 11 newborn infants with CDH, the plasma levels of retinol and retinol-binding protein were 50% less than in matched controls (p<0.0002 and <0.006, respectively) [61].

Combining the environmental and genetic factors in the development of the diaphragm, it has been noted that vitamin A and retinol are megalin ligands. The LRP2 mutation identified in the Donnai-Barrow Syndrome, which includes diaphragmatic hernia as a common feature of the phenotype, encodes megalin (51). Further studies will clarify the relationship between vitamin A, retinol, polymorphisms in LRP2, and the occurrence of "isolated" CDH.

Treatment and Prognosis

Associated factors that improve or worsen the prognosis of an infant with congenital diaphragmatic hernia have been identified in several clinical studies. A factor that improves the prognosis is the presence of a membranous sac around the hernia.

Factors associated with a worse prognosis include: an associated heart defect (20), location of the hernia on the right side, the presence of the stomach in the hernia, the presence of polyhydramnios during pregnancy, and a low lung-to-head-size ratio (1, 4, 8, 16–18).

Several treatments have been used in the newborn period that have improved the infants' chances of survival, including better treatments of respiratory insufficiency with inhaled nitric oxide, the use of exogenous surfactant, extracorporeal membrane oxygenation (ECMO), and more attention to clinical management of congestive heart failure. However, the novel treatment with fetal endoscopic tracheal occlusion has been shown to make no significant difference in survival to 90 days of life with this treatment (73%) in comparison to standard care (77%) [62].

The "hidden morbidity" of the infant with a repaired diaphragmatic hernia is pulmonary problems, including both obstructive and restrictive abnormalities. These clinical symptoms have been common in children who had been treated on ECMO as well as those whose diaphragm defect was closed with a patch. The factors include abnormalities of the chest wall, hypoplasia of the lung, bronchopulmonary dysplasia, and obstructive airway disease (63–65).

Genetic Counseling

The dramatic progress over recent years has impacted significantly the evaluation of the infant with CDH and other anomalies. The clinician's task is to determine whether or not the affected infant has the phenotype of a specific spectrum syndrome associated with CDH, as outlined above. For example, does the infant with CDH have the broad, anteverted nose and nail hypoplasia of the Fryns Syndrome (MIM #229850) or the pseudohermaphroditism and glomerulopathy of the Denys-Drash Syndrome (MIM #194080)?

Experience has shown that diagnostic testing is essential before accepting a clinical diagnosis of a specific syndrome. First, mosaicism for tetrasomy 12p should be looked for either in amniocytes or skin fibroblasts, as this abnormality is usually not identified in lymphocytes in blood samples (42). The second diagnostic testing is microarray CGH (comparative genomic hybridization) to identify either chromosome deletions or duplications. The importance of this testing has been illustrated by the delineation of deletions in either chromosome 15q26.2 or chromosome 8p 23.1 in patients considered clinically to have the Fryns Syndrome (43, 44).

If the affected infant has multiple anomalies and no visible chromosome deletions or duplications, the next step is mutation analysis of several candidate genes, when that becomes available commercially.

For the affected males, the possibility of X-linked inheritance should be considered (66). Associated malformations have included omphalocele, cleft palate, and cystic hygroma. No distinctive features have been identified in males with X-linked CDH in comparison to affected males without an X-linked mutation. Likewise, the "carrier" female has not been reported to have any abnormal physical features.

If the affected infant has no associated anomalies, no chromosome deletions/duplications or mutations, the parents can be counseled of a very low (1%) empiric recurrence risk (3, 17, 19).

Infants with CDH are being identified more and more frequently by prenatal screening by ultrasound. Once detected, chromosome analysis and microarray studies are indicated. The accuracy of the predicted phenotype is being established.

REFERENCES

1. Pober BR. Genetic aspects of human congenital diaphragmatic hernia. *Clin Genet.* 2008;74:1–15.
2. Weiner ES. Congenital posterolateral diaphragmatic hernia: new dimensions in management. *Surgery.* 1982;92:670–681.
3. Czeizel A, Kovacs M. A family study of congenital diaphragmatic defects. *Am J Med Genet.* 1985;21:105–115.
4. Adzick NS, Vacanti JP, Lillehi CW, O'Rourke PP, Crone RK, Wilson JM Fetal. diaphragmatic hernia: ultrasound diagnosis and clinical outcome in 38 cases. *J Pediatr Surg.* 1989;24:654–658.
5. Cunniff C, Jones KL, Jones MC. Patterns of malformation in children with congenital diaphragmatic defects. *J Pediatr.* 1990; 116:258–261.
6. Philip N, Gambarelli D, Guys JM, Camboulives J, Ayme S. Epidemiological study of congenital diaphragmatic defects with special reference to aetiology. *Eur J Pediatr.* 1991;150:726–729.
7. Torfs CP, Curry CJR, Bateson TF, Hondré LH. A population-based study of congenital diaphragmatic hernia. *Teratology.* 1992;46:555–564.
8. Fauza DO, Wilson JM. Congenital diaphragmatic hernia and associated anomalies: their incidence, identification and impact on prognosis. *J Pediatr Surg.* 1994;29:1113–1117.
9. Cannon C, Dildy GA, Ward R. A population-based study of congenital diaphragmatic hernia in Utah: 1988–1994. *Obst Gynecol.* 1996;86:959–963.
10. Tibboel D, Gang AVD. Etiologic and genetic factors in congenital diaphragmatic hernia. *Clini Perinatol.* 1996;23:689–699.
11. Martinez-Frias M-L, Prieto L, Urioste M, Bermejo E. Clinical/epidemiological analysis of congenital anomalies associated with diaphragmatic hernia. *Amer J Med Genet.* 1996;62:71–76.
12. Zhu J, Wang Y, Miao L. Epidemiological studies on 321 children with congenital diaphragmatic hernia in China. *Chung Hua Yu Fang/Hsueh Chih.* 1997;31:266–268.
13. Enns GM, Cox VA, Goldstein RB, Gibbs DL, Harrison MR, Golabi M. Congenital diaphragmatic defects and associated syndromes, malformations, and chromosome anomalies: a retrospective study of 60 patients and literature review. *Amer J Med Genet.* 1998;79:215–225.
14. Suda K, Bigras J-L, Bohn D, Hornberger LK, McCrindle BW. Echocardiographic predictors of outcomes in newborns with congenital diaphragmatic hernia. *Pediatrics.* 2000;105:1106–1109.
15. Stege G, Fenton A, Jaffray B. Nihilison in the 1990's: the true mortality of congenital diaphragmatic hernia. *Pediatrics.* 2003;112:532–535.
16. Downward CD, Jaksic T, Garza JJ, Dzakovic P, Nemes L, Jennings RW, Wilson JM. Analysis of an improved survival risk for congenital diaphragmatic hernia. *J Pediatr Surg.* 2003;38:729–732.
17. Tonks A, Wyldes M, Somerset DA, Dent K, Abhyankar A, Bagchi I, Lander A, Roberts E, Kilby MD. Congenital malformations of

the diaphragm: findings of the West Midlands Congenital Anomaly Register 1995 to 2000. *Prenat Diagn.* 2004;24:596–604.

18. VanDooren M, Tibboel D, Torfs C. The co-occurrence of congenital diaphragmatic hernia, esophageal atresia/tracheoesophageal fistula, and lung hypoplasia. *Birth Def Res (Part A): Clin Mol Teratol.* 2005;73:53–57.

19. Pober BR, Lin A, Russell MR, Ackerman KG, Chakravorty S, Strauss B, Westgate M-N, Wilson J, Donahoe PK, Holmes LB. Infants with Bochdalek diaphragmatic hernia: sibling precurrence and monozygotic twin discordance in a hospital-based malformation surveillance program. *Am J Med Genet.* 2005; 138A:81–88.

20. Cohen MS, Rychik J, Bush DM, Tian Z-Y, Howell LJ, Adzick NS, Flake AW, Johnson MP, Spray TL, Crombleholme TM. Influence of congenital heart disease on survival in children with congenital diaphragmatic hernia. *J Pediatr.* 2002;141:25–30.

21. Lin AE, Pober BR, Adatia I. Congenital diaphragmatic hernia and associated cardiovascular malformations: type, frequency, and impact on management. *Am J Med Gen Part C (Seminars in Medical Genetics).* 2007;145C:201–216.

22. Geggel RL, Murphy JD, Langleben D, Crone RK, Vacanti JP, Reid LM. Congenital diaphragmatic hernia: arterial structural changes and persistent pulmonary hypertension after surgical repair. *J Pediatr.* 1985;107:457–464.

23. Benjamin DR, Juul S, Siebert JR. Congenital posterolateral diaphragmatic hernia: associated malformations. *J Pediat Surg.* 1988;23:899–903.

24. Nose K, Kamata S, Sawai T, Tazuke Y, Usui N, Kawahara H, Okada A. Airway anomalies in patients with congenital diaphragmatic hernia. *J Pediatr Surg.* 2000;35:1562–1565.

25. VanDooren MF, Brooks AS, Tibboel D, Torfs CP. Association of congenital diaphragmatic hernia with limb-reduction defects. *Birth Def Res (Part A): Clin Mol Teratol.* 2003;67:578–584.

26. Evans JA. Diaphragmatic defects and limb deficiencies—taking sides. *Am J Med Genet Part A.* 2007;143A:2106–2112.

27. David TJ, Nixon A. Congenital malformations associated with anencephaly and iniencephaly. *J. Med Genet.* 1976;13: 263–265.

28. Dolk H, DeWals P, Gillerot Y, Lechat MF, Ayme S, Cornel M et al. Heterogeneity of neural tube defects in Europe: the significance of site of defect and presence of other major anomalies in relation to geographic differences in prevalence. *Teratology.* 1991;44:547–559.

29. O'Rahilly R, Müller F. *Human Embryology and Teratology.* New York: Wiley-Liss; 2001: 276–284.

30. Moore KL, Persaud TVN. *The Developing Human: Clinically Oriented Embryology.* 7th ed. Philadelphia: W. B. Saunders Company: 195–200.

31. Holder AM, Klaassens M, Tibboel D, de Klein A, Lee B, Scott DA. Genetics of congenital diaphragmatic hernia. *Am J Hum Gen.* 2007;80:825–845.

32. Babiuk RP, Zhang W, Clugston R, Allan DW, Greer JJ. Embryological origins and development of the rat diaphragm. *J Compar Neurol.* 2003;455:477–487.

33. Yuan W, Rao Y, Babiuk RP, Greer J, Wu JY, Ornitz DM. A genetic model for a central (septum transversum) congenital diaphragmatic hernia in mice lacking Slit3. *Proc Nat Acad Sci.* 2003;100:5217–5222.

34. Greer JJ, Cote D, Allan DW, Zhang W, Babiuk RP, Ly L, Lemke RP, Bagnall K. Structure of the primordial diaphragm and defects associated with nitrofen-induced CDH. *J Appl Physiol.* 2000; 89:2123–2129.

35. Babiuk RP, Greer JJ. Diaphragm defects occur in a CDH hernia model independently of myogenesis and lung formation. *Am J Physiol Lung Cell Mol Physiol.* 2002;283:L1310–L1314.

36. White JJ, Suzuki H. Hernia through the foramen of Bochdalek: a misnomer. *J Pediat Surg.* 1972;7:60–61.

37. Wells LJ. Development of the Human Diaphragm and Pleural Sacs Contributions to Embryology. 1957; no. 236, 35:108–134.

38. Kalousek DK, Fitch N, Paradice BA. *Pathology of the Human Embryo and Previable Fetus: Am Atlas.* New York: Springer-Verlag; 1990: 108–110.

39. Robert E, Kallen B, Harris J. The epidemiology of diaphragmatic hernia. *Eur J Epidemiol.* 1997;13:665–673.

40. Klaassens M, van Dooren M, Eussen HJ, Douben H, den Dekker AT, Lee C et al. Congenital diaphragmatic hernia of a candidate region by use of fluorescent in situ hybridization and array-based comparative genomic hybridization. *Am J Hum Genet.* 2005; 76:877–882.

41. Witters I, Legius E, Moerman P, Timmerman D, Van Assche FA, Fryns JP. Associated malformations and chromosomal anomalies in 42 cases of prenatally diagnosed diaphragmatic hernia. *Am J Med Genet.* 2001;103:278–282.

42. Bergoffen J, Punnett H, Campbell TJ, Ross AJ III, Ruchelli E, Zackai EH. Diaphragmatic hernia in tetrasomy 12p mosaicism. *J Pediatr.* 1993;122:603–606.

43. Kantarci S, Casavant D, Prada C, Russell M, Byrne J, Haug LW et al. Findings from aCGH in patients with congenital diaphragmatic hernia (CDH): a possible locus for Fryns Syndrome. *Am J Med Genet.* 2006;140A:17–23.

44. Slavotinek A, Lee SS, Davis K, Shrit A, Leppig KA, Rhim J et al. Fryns syndrome phenotype caused by chromosome microdeletions at 15q26.2 and 8p23.1. *J Med Genet.* 2005;42:730–736.

45. Klaassens M, Galjaard RJH, Scott DA, Brüggenwirth HT, van Opstal D, Fox MV et al. Prenatal detection and outcome of congenital diaphragmatic hernia (CDH) associated with deletion of chromosome 15q26: two patients and review of the literature. *Am J Med Genet Part A.* 2007;143A:2204–2212.

46. Ackerman KG, Herron BJ, Vargas SO, Huang H, Tevosian SG, Kochilas L et al. FOG2 is required for normal diaphragm and lung development in mice and humans. *PloS Genet.* 2005;1:58–65.

47. Kimura Y, Suzuki T, Kaneko C, Darnel AD, Moriya T, Suzuki S et al. Retinoid receptors in the developing human lung. *Clin Sci (Lond).* 2002;103:613–621.

48. Slavotinek AM. The genetics of congenital diaphragmatic hernia. *Semin in Perinatol.* 2005;29:77–85.

49. Li M, Shuman C, Fei YL, Cutiongco E, Bender HA, Stevens C et al. GPC3 mutation analysis in a spectrum of patients with overgrowth expands the phenotype of Simpson-Golabi-Behmel syndrome. *Am J Med Genet.* 2001;102:161–168.

50. Gillis LA, McCallum J, Kaur M, DeScipio C, Yaeger D, Mariani A et al. NIPBL mutational analysis in 120 individuals with Cornelia de Lange syndrome and evaluation of genotype-phenotype correlations. *Am J Hum Genet.* 2004;75:610–623.

51. Kantarci S, Al-Gazali L, Hill RS, Donnai D, Black GC, Bieth E et al. Mutations in LRP2, which encodes the multiligand receptor megalin, cause Donnai-Barrow and facio-oculo-acoustico-renal syndromes. *Nat Genet.* 2007;39:957–959.

52. Antonius T, van Bon B, Eggink A, van der Burgt I, Noordam K, van Heijst A. Denys-Drash syndrome and congenital diaphragmatic hernia: another case with the 1097G > A(Arg366His) mutation. *Am J Med Genet Part A.* 2008;146A:496–499.

53. Pasutto F, Sticht H, Hammersen G, Gillessen-Kaesbach G, Fitzpatrick DR, Nürnberg G et al. Mutations in STRA6 cause a broad spectrum of malformations including anophthalmia, congenital heart defects, diaphragmatic hernia, alveolar capillary dysplasia, lung hypoplasia, and mental retardation. *Am J Hum Genet.* 2007;80:550–560.

54. Suri M, Kelehan P, O'Neill D, Vadeyar S, Grant J, Ahmed SF et al. WT1 mutations in Meacham syndrome suggest a coelomic mesothelial origin of the cardiac and diaphragmatic malformations. *Am J Med Genet Part A.* 2007;143A:2312–2320.

55. Felix JF, van Dooren MF, Klaassens M, Hop WCJ, Torfs CP, Tibboel D. Environmental factors in the etiology of esophageal

atresia and congenital diaphragmatic hernia: results of a case-control study. *Birth Def Res (Part A): Clin Mol Teratol.* 2008; 82:98–105.

56. Greer JJ, Babiuk RP, Theband B. Etiology of congenital diaphragmatic hernia: the retinoid hypothesis. *Pediatric Res.* 2003; 53:1–6.

57. Gallot D, Marceau G, Coste K, Hadden H, Robert-Gnansia E, Laurichesse H et al. Congenital diaphragmatic hernia: a retinoid-signaling pathway disruption during lung development? *Birth Def Res (Part A): Clin Mol Teratol.* 2005;73:523–531.

58. Anderson DH. Effect of diet during pregnancy upon the incidence of congenital hereditary diaphragmatic hernia in the rat. *Am J Pathol.* 1949;25:163–185.

59. Babiuk RP, Thebaud B, Greer JJ. Reductions in the incidence of nitrofen-induced diaphragmatic hernia by vitamin A and retinoic acid. *Am J Physiol Lung Cell Mol Physiol.* 2004; 286:L973.

60. Mey J, Babiuk RP, Clugston R, Zhang W, Greer JJ. Retinal dehydrogenase-2 is inhibited by compounds that induce congenital diaphragmatic hernia in rodents. *Am J Pathol.* 2003;162: 673–679.

61. Major D, Cadenas M, Fournier L, Lederc S, Leclerc M, Cloutier R. Retinol status of newborn infants with congenital diaphragmatic hernia. *Pediatric Surg Int.* 1998;13:547–549.

62. Harrison MR, Keller RL, Hawgood SB, Kitterman JA, Sandberg PL, Farmer DL, Lee H, Filly RA, Farrell JA, Albanese CT. A randomized trial of fetal endoscopic tracheal occlusion for severe fetal congenital diaphragmatic hernia. *N Engl J Med.* 2003; 349:1916–1924.

63. Lund DP, Mitchell J, Kharasch V, Quigley S, Kuehn M, Wilson JM. Congenital diaphragmatic hernia: the hidden morbidity. *J Pediatr Surg.* 1994;29:258–264.

64. Muratore CS, Kharasch V, Lund DP, Shiels C, Friedman S, Brown C, Utter S, Jaksci T, Wilson JM. Pulmonary morbidity in 100 survivors of congenital diaphragmatic hernia monitored in a multidisciplinary clinic. *J Pediatr Surg.* 2001;36:133–140.

65. Trachsel D, Selvadurai H, Bohn D, Langer JC, Coates AL. Long-term pulmonary morbidity in survivors of congenital diaphragmatic hernia. *Pediatr Pulmonol.* 2005;39:433–439.

66. Carmi R, Meizner I, Katz M. Familial congenital diaphragmatic defect and associated midline anomalies: further evidence of an X-linked midline gene. *Am J Med Genet.* 1990;36:313–315.

Chapter 9

Cryptorchidism

Definition

One or both testicles cannot be palpated in the scrotum. A more specific definition, proposed by Scorer (1): the testis is undescended if it cannot be drawn down and held without tension at a distance of 4 cm below the symphysis pubis in the term male infant or 2.5 cm in the prematurely born male newborn. The word cryptorchidism, in Greek, means "hidden testis."

ICD-9:	752.5	(undescended testicle)
	752.500	(undescended testicle, unilateral unpalpable)
	752.514	(undescended testicles, bilateral)
	752.530	(ectopic testes, unilateral or bilateral)
ICD-10:	Q53.0	(ectopic testis)
	Q53.1	(undescended testicle, unilateral)
	Q53.2	(undescended testicle, bilateral)
	Q53.9	(undescended testicle, unspecified)
Mendelian Inheritance in Man:	#219050	Cryptorchidism (undescended testes)

Appearance

The scrotum appears unoccupied on one side (Figure 9-1) or both sides (Figure 9-2). The location of the undescended testicle can be intra-abdominal, in the inguinal canal, at the top of the scrotum, or in an ectopic location (2). At surgery in 108 consecutive boys (3), the locations were: 17% intra-abdominal, 16% at internal ring of inguinal canal, 53% at mid-canal, 10% at external ring, and 5% are absent.

By prenatal ultrasonography, it has been shown that there is no descent of testes before 23 weeks gestation and that descent occurs in 98% of male fetuses after 32 weeks (4).

The intra-abdominal testes of newborn infants have a normal number of germ cells. Spontaneous descent occurs rarely after one year of age. If the undescended testicle is not moved surgically or medically to the scrotum, germ cell development is impaired. The higher the location of the testis, the more severe the impairment of infertility with unilateral and bilateral cryptorchidism (50% in one study of males with unilateral cryptorchidism and 75% with bilateral [6]).

Associated Malformations

The frequency of undescended testes is higher among males born prematurely, in low birth weight infants, and in twins (1).

The most common associated abnormality is an inguinal hernia, as the processus vaginalis persists until the testis has reached its point of full descent. The persisting processus becomes the route of the inguinal hernia.

Another common association is with other genitourinary anomalies, such as hypospadias, hypoplasia of the penis, and bifid scrotum (7, 8).

Cryptorchidism has also been shown to be associated with malformations of the kidney and ureter on the same side of the body and anomalies of vertebrae T10 to S5 (9).

The cryptorchid male has a very significant risk of malignancy in the undescended testis (10). Spontaneous descent does not occur after one year of age, which makes treatment to move the scrotum to the testis essential. While the frequency of cancer of the testicle

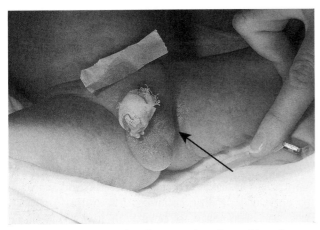

FIGURE 9.1 Penis covered with gauze after circumcision. Scrotum shows absence of left testicle. (arrow)

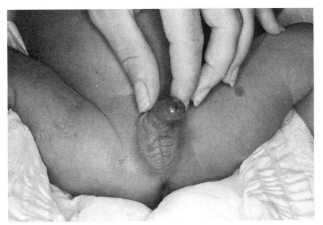

FIGURE 9.2 Shows scrotum with neither testicle present.

may not be reduced by this treatment, its detection is improved (11, 12).

Developmental Defect

Descent of the testicles is essential for the development of normal external genitals and the production of mature spermatozoa. These are development processes that are regulated by an intricate genetic network with many molecular interactions. The gene expression profiles are restricted in time and body segment and show a coordinated regulation. In the human, the differentiation of an indifferent genital anlage toward male or female genitals is initiated at around seven weeks of gestation. This process is dependent on the action of both androgens and estrogens. Research in humans, pigs, rats, mice, and other species has shown species-specific variations in the critical phases of testis development. In the human, the genital ridge forms at 49 days, the testis forms at 56 days, the intra-abdominal phase begins at 70 days, the inguinoscrotal phase begins at 182 days, and the testis is usually in the scrotum by 245 days (13).

The testis develops as a retroperitoneal organ, but appears to descend as an intraperitoneal organ (14).

The outgrowth of the gubernaculum (a gelatinous cylinder of undifferentiated mesenchyme that develops in the embryonic period and is attached to the region of the inguinal canal [14]) and the regression of the cranial suspensory ligament are the developmental processes that are essential to the descent of the testis into the scrotum (16, 17).

One theory focuses on the role of the gubernaculum, which is unique to the male fetus and is attached to the lower pole of the testis (18). The gubernaculum attains its greatest development between 16 and 24 weeks of gestation, just before the testis descends. There is debate as to whether the testis is "pulled" into the scrotum or is guided by the gubernaculum to the inguinal ring. The testis, epididymis, and gubernaculum move as a single entity through the inguinal canal (1). The testis reaches the scrotum, while the gubernaculum is regressing.

Another theory of the process of normal descent is that the gubernaculum is attached to the epididymis, not the testis, and that the epididymis precedes the testis down the inguinal canal into the scrotum (19). As a corollary of this hypothesis, 63% of 197 consecutive boys operated upon to correct cryptorchidism had "unfurled epididymides" (20).

Cryptorchidism is also considered to reflect abnormalities in the pituitary-hypothalamus-testis axis (9). After 16 weeks of gestation, the gubernaculum regresses in the female and increases in the male fetus, suggesting a sex difference in the endocrinologic aspects of this process. Fetal or placental gonadotropins induce the synthesis of androgens by the testis, which may stimulate the growth of the gubernaculum or the vas deferens, epididymis, and scrotum (13). Müllerian Inhibiting Substance (MIS) is also postulated to be involved in the swelling of the gubernaculum during the first phase of migration (12).

The role of sensitivity to androgens and androgen receptors is suggested by the fact that in humans with testicular feminization, the gubernaculum is abnormal and descent of the testes through the inguinal canal does not occur (21). Androgens have been postulated to control the inguinoscrotal phase of migration (12).

A deficiency of LH (lutenizing hormone) and a secondary deficiency of testosterone have also been reported in cryptorchid infants and children (22), suggesting that the pituitary-gonad axis is abnormal. Treatment with LH-RH nasal spray followed by human chorionic gonadotropin injected intramuscularly has been associated with success in the majority of the affected infants (23). However, the best treatment and its effectiveness remains an active debate (12).

Endocrine changes in the mothers of affected boys have also been implicated. The hypothesis is that a delay in the age of onset of her menses reflects a degree of hypogonadism in her that is a risk factor for her son's cryptorchidism (24).

Prevalence

The prevalence rates vary by several factors, including the infant's gestational age, or his postnatal age, birth weight, and the method for establishing the position of each testis. In general, the frequency at birth is 3 to 4% at birth and about 1% at three months of age (1, 12). By comparison, 30% of premature infants were cryptorchid in the 1960s (1). Since the third stage of testicular migration occurs between the 28th and the 35th week of gestation, male infants born before the 28th week will all be expected to be cryptorchid.

Significant, but unexplained, increases in the prevalence rates of cryptorchidism have been observed between the 1960s and 1980s in England (1, 8) and during the periods 1959–1961 and 1997–2001 in Demark (25). In spite of close collaboration among the investigators, significant differences in prevalence rates in infant boys in Denmark (9%) and Finland (2.4%) [25]) could not be explained.

Race

There is too little information available to determine whether or not there are differences between racial and ethnic groups. The prevalence rate among 1,002 consecutive Malaysian male newborns was 4.8%, with associations with low birth weight, prematurity, and other genital anomalies as observed in other populations (26).

Birth Status

The higher rate in premature infants has been established in many studies, reflecting the timing of the process of testis descent.

Sidedness

Small differences have been observed, but no consistent pattern.

Twins

The prevalence of cryptorchidism is higher among twins than singletons, but those observations are confounded by the fact that prematurity and low birth weight are more common among twins.

The concordance rates were much higher among monozygous than dizygous twins in one small number of twin pairs (24).

Genetic Factors

Chromosome abnormalities were identified in 5% of 110 boys with cryptorchidism with or without hypospadias in one study (27).

Family studies (24, 28) have shown that cryptorchidism is a familial disorder. In two studies the frequency among the fathers was 1.5% (24) and 3.9% (28), respectively, and higher among brothers: 6.2% (24) and 6.5% (28). The recurrence rate in brothers was higher when the index case had bilateral undescended testes.

Sufficient androgen receptor (AR) function is crucial for normal male differentiation. Mutations in the AR gene are uncommon in boys with hypospadias and cryptorchidism, the two most common malformations in male infants. The AR is highly polymorphic due to a glutamine repeat (aCAG segment), and a glycine repeat (aCGN segment). In gene sequencing of 232 cryptorchid men, 151 with hypospadias and 81 controls, the medial GGN lengths, but no increased CAG lengths, were higher in association with both cryptorchidism and hypospadias (29).

The single nucleotide polymorphism 12 (rs 6932902) in the estrogen receptor α gene (ESR1) was associated with the severity of the cryptorchidism, defined as the highest testicular position, in a study of 152 affected boys and 160 unrelated controls in Delaware (30).

Mice homozygous for the targeted deletion of the Insl3 locus have bilateral cryptorchidism with free moving testes and failure of development of the gubernaculum (16). The Insl3 gene has also been shown to be a factor in diethylstilbestrol-induced cryptorchidism in mice (31). Insl3 gene and its receptor Lgr8/great are candidate genes for cryptorchidism. Mutations in the Insl3 gene or its receptor were identified in 8 of 81 men with a history of cryptorchidism in one study (32), but at a lower rate in other studies (33). Mutations in the Insl3 receptor gene (RXFP2) were identified in 5 (0.8%) of 600 boys with cryptorchidism; and additional 8 (1.3%) of the 600 had Klinefelter Syndrome (47,XXY). These genetic abnormalities were more common in infants with bilateral and persistent cryptorchidism (34).

Genetic susceptibility to estrogenic endocrine disruptors is another theoretical cause of cryptorchidism. In a study of 63 cryptorchid males and 47 controls, the estrogen receptor alpha ESR1, which medicates the estrogenic effect of endocrine disruptors, was sequenced. The distribution of 15 SNPs (single nucleotide polymorphisms) was analyzed. Homozygosity for the AGATA haplotype occurred in 10 of 16 cryptorchid males and in none of the 47 controls (35).

Environmental Factors

Exposure to pesticides, which have anti-androgenic and/or estrogenic effects, has been implicated as a cause of the increased frequency of cryptorchidism in several rural populations (36–39). In one study in Germany (38) the concentrations of heptachloroepoxide and hexachlorobenzene in fat tissue collected at surgery in boys with cryptorchidism were higher than in fat from control children.

In the Ragusa district in Sicily (1998–2002), the cities in a "high pesticide impact" area, reflecting use in agriculture, had a significant association with newborns with hypospadias and cryptorchidism in comparison to the "low pesticide impact" areas (39).

A human "testicular dysgenesis syndrome" has been postulated as a potential effect of exposure to dibutyl phthalates in recent studies in humans (40, 41).

The male fetus exposed to diethylstilbestrol had at birth an increased frequency (8%) of cryptorchidism in comparison to 1% in controls (42).

An epidemiologic analysis showed an increased frequency of cryptorchidism in association with obesity in the mother, older age of the mother, maternal diabetes, and hypertension (43). In another study of 2,395 boys with cryptorchidism (44), there were additional correlations with other malformations (especially gastrointestinal and genitourinary) and breech presentation.

Treatment and Prognosis

The evaluation of cryptorchid boys with ultrasonography has been opposed as not necessary and as rarely finding the nonpalpable testis (45). The use of laparoscopy has been proposed as a better approach in the search for the testis not palpated than open exploration (46). Recently, magnetic resonance angiography has been recommended (47) as the most effective method to identify the undescended testis.

Genetic Counseling

The initial physical examination will establish whether or not the infant has other physical abnormalities. If the undescended testis is an isolated finding, close follow-up is needed during the first year. The current recommendation is to bring the testis down into the scrotum by either surgical or medical methods in the first year (11).

The parents of one affected son have an increased risk that a subsequent son will also be cryptorchid. The adult male, who had had treatment for unilateral cryptorchid in childhood, has been shown to have no evidence of infertility in comparison to controls (48). However, cryptorchid boys have very significant risks of developing testicular cancer in comparison to controls (49, 50).

REFERENCES

1. Scorer CG. The descent of the testis. *Arch Dis Child.* 1964;39: 605–609.
2. Hack WWM, Meijer RW, Bos SD, Haasnoot K. A new clinical classification for undescended testis. *Scand J Urol Nephrol.* 2003; 37:43–47.
3. Redman JF. Impalpable testes: observations based on 208 consecutive operations for undescended testes. *J Urol.* 1980;124: 379–381.
4. Rotondi M, Valenzano F, Bilancioni E, Spano G, Rotondi M, Giorlandino C. Prenatal measurement of testicular diameter by ultrasonography: development of fetal male gender and evaluation of testicular descent. *Prenat Diagn.* 2001;21:112–115.
5. Haziselimovic F, Herzog B, Buser M. Development of cryptorchid testes. *Eur J Pediatr.* 1987;146 (Suppl 2):S8–S12.
6. Kogan SJ. Fertility in cryptorchidism. An overview in 1987. *Eur J Pediatr.* 1987; 146(Suppl 2):S21–24.
7. Svensson J. Male hypospadias, 625 cases, associated malformations and possible etiological factors. *Acta Paediatr Scand.* 1979; 68:587–592.
8. John Radcliffe Hospital Cryptorchidism Study Group. Cryptorchidism: A prospective study of 7,500 consecutive male births, 1984–8. *Arch Dis Child.* 1992;67:892–899.
9. Cortes D, Thorup JM, Beck BL, Visfeldt J. Cryptorchidism as a caudal developmental field defect. A new description of cryptorchidism associated with malformations and dysplasias of the kidneys, the ureters and the spine from T10 to S5. *APMIS.* 1998; 106:953–958.
10. Reuter VE. Origins and molecular biology of testicular germ cell tumors. *Mod Pathol.* 2005;18(2):551–560.
11. American Academy of Pediatrics. Timing of elective surgery on the genitalia of male children with particular reference to the risks, benefits, and psychologic effects of surgery and anesthesia. *Pediatrics.* 1996;97:590–594.
12. Brucker-Davis F, Pointis G, Chevallier D, Fenichel P. Update on cryptorchidism: endocrine, environmental and therapeutic aspects. *J Endocrin Invest.* 2003;26:575–587.
13. Klonisck T, Fowler PA, Hombach-Klonish S. Molecular and genetic regulation of testis descent and external genitalia development. *Develop Biol.* 2004;270:1–18.
14. Pham SBT, Hong M K-H, Teague JA, Hutson JM. Is the testis intraperitoneal? *Pediatr Surg Int.* 2005;21:231–239.
15. O'Rahilly R, Müller F. *Human Embryology and Teratology.* 3rd ed. New York: Wiley-Liss, New York; 2001: 334–336.
16. Zimmermann S, Steding G, Emmen JMA, Brin K, Mann AO, Nayernia K, Holstein AF, Engel W, Adharn IM. Targeted disruption of the Insl3 gene causes bilateral cryptorchidism. *Mol Endocrinol.* 1999;13:681–691.
17. Pringle KC. Testicular proximity can induce gubernaculum formation after delivery. *J Pediatr Surg.* 2001;36:1708–1709.
18. Wensing CJ. The embryology of testicular descent. *Horm Res.* 1988;30:144–152.
19. Hadziselimovic F, Kruslin E. The role of the epididymis in descensus testis and the topographical relationship between the testis and epididymis from the sixth month of pregnancy until immediately after birth. *Anat Embryol (Berl).* 1979;155:191–186.
20. Mininberg DT. The epididymis and testicular descent. *Eur J Pediatr.* 1987;146:S28–S30.
21. Hutson JM, Donahoe PK. The hormonal control of testicular descent. *Endo Rev.* 1986;7:270–283.
22. Job JC, Toublanc JE, Chaussain JL, Gendrel D, Roger M, Canlorbe P. The pituitary-gonadal axis in cryptorchid infants and children. *Eur J Pediatr.* 1987;146(Suppl 2):S2–S4.
23. Waldschmidt J, Doede T, Vygen I. The results of 9 years of experience with a combined treatment with LH-RH and HCG for cryptorchidism. *Eur J Pediatr.* 1993;152(2):S34–36.

24. Czeizel A, Erödi E, Tóth J. Genetics of undescended testis. *J Urol.* 1981;126:528–529.

25. Boisen KA, Kaleva M, Main KM, Virtanen HE, Haavisto AM, Schmidt IM, et al. Difference in prevalence of congenital cryptorchidism in infants between two Nordic countries. *Lancet.* 2004;363:1264–1269.

26. Thong M-K, Lim C-T, Fatimah H. Undescended testes: incidence in 1,002 consecutive male infants and outcomes at 1 year of age. *Pediatr Surg Int.* 1998;13:37–41.

27. Yamaguchi T, Kitada S, Osada Y. Chromosomal anomalies in cryptorchidism and hypospadias. *Urol Int.* 1991;47:60–63.

28. Bjoro KJR, Dybvik T. Congenital abnormalities and growth patterns among cryptorchids boys. *Ann Chir Gynaecol.* 1983;72: 342–346.

29. Aschim EL, Nordenskjöld A, Giwercman A, landing KB, Rahayel Y, Jaugen TB, Grotmol T, Giwercman YL. Linkage between cryptorchidism, hypospadias, and GGN repeat length in the androgen receptor gene. *J Clin Endocrinol Metab.* 2004;89: 5105–5109.

30. Wang Y, Barthold J, Figueroa E, González R, Noh PH, Wang M, Manson J. Analysis of five single nucleotide polymorphisms in ESR1 gene in cryptorchidism. *Birth Def Res (Part A): Clin Mol Teratol.* 2008;82:482–485.

31. Emmen JMA, McLuskey A, Adham IM, et al. Involvement of insulin-like factor 3 (Insl3) in diethylstilbestrol-induced cryptorchidism. *Endocrinology.* 2000;141:846–849.

32. Ferlin A, Simonato M, Bartoloni L, Rizzo G, Bettella A, Dottorini T, Dallapicola B, Foresta C. The INSL3-LGR8/GREAT ligand-receptor pair in human cryptorchidism. *J Clin Endocrinol Metab.* 2003;88:4273–4279.

33. Bogatcheva NV, Agoulnik AI. Symposium: genetic aspects of male (in)fertility INSL3/LGR8 role in testicular descent and cryptorchidism. *Repro Bio Med Online.* 2004;10:49–54.

34. Ferlin A, Zuccarello D, Zuccarello B, Chirico MR, Zanon GR, Foresta C. Genetic alterations associated with cryptorchidism. *JAMA.* 2008;300:2271–2276.

35. Yoshida R, Fakami M, Sagagawa I, Hasegawa T, Kamatani N, Ogata T. Association of cryptorchidism with a specific haplotype of the estrogen receptor and gene: implication for the susceptibility to estrogenic environmental endocrine disruptors. *J Clin Endocrinol Metal.* 2005;90:4716–4721.

36. Garry VF, Schreinemachers D, Harkins ME, Griffith J. Pesticide appliers, biocides, and birth defects in rural Minnesota. *Environ Health Perspect.* 1996;104:394–399.

37. Weidner IS, Møller H, Jensen TK, Skakkebaek NE. Cryptorchidism and hypospadias in sons of gardeners and farmers. *Environ Health Perspect.* 1998;106:793–796.

38. Hosie S, Loff S, Witt K, Niessen K, Waag KL. Is there a correlation between organochlorine compounds and undescended testes? *Eur J Pediatr Surg.* 2000;10:304–309.

39. Carbone P, Giordano F, Nori F, Mantovani A, Taruscio D, Lauria L, Figà-Talamanca I. Cryptorchidism and hypospadias in the Sicilian district of Ragusa and the use of pesticides. *Reprod Toxicol.* 2006;22:8–12.

40. Fisher JS, MacPherson S, Marchetti N, Sharpe RM. Human "testicular dysgenesis syndrome": a possible model using *in-utero* exposure of the rate to dibutyl phthalate. *Human Repro.* 2003; 18:1383–1394.

41. Swan SH, Main KM, Lia F, Stewart SL, Kruse RL, Calafat AM, Mae CS, Redmon JB, Ternand CL, Sullivan S, Teague JL. Decrease in anogenital distance among male infants with prenatal phthalate exposure. *Environ Health Persp.* 2005;113:1056–1061.

42. Gill WB. Effects on human males of in *utero* exprosue to exogenous sex hormones. In: Mori T, Nagasawa H, eds. *Toxicity of Hormones in Perinatal Life.* Boca Raton, FL: CRC Press, Inc.; 1988: 161–177.

43. Berkowitz GS, Lapinski RH, Godbold JH, Dolgin SE, Holzman IR. Maternal and neonatal risk factors for cryptorchidism. *Epidemiology.* 1995;6:127–131.

44. Biggs ML, Baer A, Critchlow CW. Maternal, delivery, and perinatal characteristics associated with cryptorchidism: a population-based case-control study among births in Washington State. *Epidemiology.* 2002;13:197–204.

45. Elder JS. Ultrasonography is unnecessary in evaluating boys with a nonpalpable testis. *Pediatrics.* 2002;110:748–751.

46. Barqawi AZ, Blyth B, Jorden GH, Ehrlich RM, Koyle MA. Role of laparoscopy in patients with previous negative exploration for impalpable testis. *Urology.* 2003;61:1234–1237.

47. Eggener SE, Lotan Y, Cheng EY. Magnetic resonance angiography for the nonpalpable testis: a cost and cancer risk analysis. *J Urol.* 2005;173:1745–1750.

48. Miller KD, Coughlin MT, Lee PA. Fertility after unilateral cryptorchidism. *Horm Res.* 2001;55:249–253.

49. Swerdlow AJ, Higgins CD, Pike MC. Risk of testicular cancer in cohort of boys with cryptorchidism. *BMJ.* 1997;314:1507–1519.

50. Pettersson A, Richiardi L, Nordenskjold A, Kaijser M, Akre O. Age at surgery for undescended testis and risk of testicular cancer. *N Engl J Med.* 2007;356:1835–1841.

Chapter 10

Gastroschisis

Definition

A lateral abdominal wall defect, which occurs to the right of the umbilical cord and has no covering sac.

ICD-9:   756.710   (gastroschisis)

ICD-10:   Q79.3   (gastroschisis)

Mendelian Inheritance   230750   (gastroschisis)
in Man:

Appearance

The defect is usually less than 4 cm in diameter. Typically, the intestine protrudes, and occasionally other abdominal viscera as well (1–3). There is a fibrous coating over the protruding viscera, but not a covering sac. The umbilical cord is located in its normal position, and is not part of the gastroschisis defect (Figure 10-1 and 10-2).

Associated Malformations

The findings in many case series and population-based surveys have been published (4–23), as well as an international survey of 24 population-based malformations surveillance registries that identified 3,322 infants with gastroschisis (24) (Table 10-1). Most affected infants have no other malformations. There are two common related malformations: atresia or stenosis of the small intestine (25) and the amniotic band-related limb body wall complex (26). Each of these associated malformations is attributed to the process of vascular disruption.

An increased frequency of heart (12%) and genitourinary (7%) malformations was noted in a series of 121 cases evaluated in the period 1982–1999 at a referral medical center in Florida (21).

In a series of 621 infants with gastroschisis in California (1992–1997), 4% had significant heart defects, especially "right heart" lesions (27). Heart defects were not identified prenatally in a series of 26 fetuses with gastroschisis (28), although four of 21 survivors had significant heart problems, including supraventricular tachycardia and persistent pulmonary hypertension of the newborn.

Other associated abnormalities have been the amyoplasia type of arthrogryposis (17, 29) and cryptorchidism (30). In a series of 64 infants with gastroschisis,

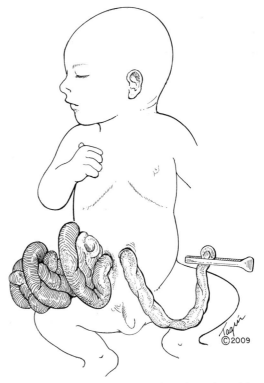

FIGURE 10.1 Diagram of gastroschisis, located on right side of umbilical cord.

two (3.1%) had amyoplasia (16). In a series of 225 individuals with amyoplasia, 12 (5.3%) had gastroschisis and 6 (2.7%) had bowel atresia (29).

In the international survey of 3,322 affected fetuses and infants (24), 86% of the infants had "isolated "gastroschisis. Among the infants with multiple anomalies, 1.2% had chromosomal abnormalities and 15% had specific syndromes. Among the other infants with multiple anomalies most had only one associated malformation, primarily a heart defect or a genitourinary anomaly. Two patterns of multiple anomalies were identified: Pattern A: gastroschisis, anencephaly/encephalocele, limb reduction defects, and/or cleft lip and palate; Pattern B: gastroschisis, indeterminate sex, anorectal atresia, spina bifida, and/or genitourinary anomalies.

Fetal imaging during pregnancy has documented the prenatal closure of the abdominal defect of gastroschisis in association with low segment atresia of the midintestine (31, 32). The infants with gastroschisis associated with bowel atresia have had a significantly higher frequency of growth restriction, amniotic fluid staining, and abnormalities in fetal activity (33).

Shortening of a limb and absence of a long bone have been observed in a few infants with gastroschisis (22).

Developmental Defect

Several theories have been proposed: 1) abnormal persistence of the umbilical vein that leads to failure of the skin to develop at that site (24); 2) early interruption of the right omphalomesenteric artery, which has been identified in an eight-week human embryo (35); 3) a body wall closure defect, which has its origin during the 3rd to 5th week postfertilization (36); 4) a rupture in utero of the membrane covering a hernia of the umbilical cord (37).

In general, it has been postulated that gastroschisis is present by eight weeks of gestation. This is illustrated by the case report of an embryo with gastroschisis and multiple anomalies who was estimated to be 51 days postfertilization age (38).

Gastroschisis developing later in gestation has also been documented (39). In these pregnancies the infant had a normal appearance initially by prenatal ultrasound. Later, at 14 to 16 weeks gestation the mother had an elevated level of maternal serum alpha-fetoprotein. Subsequently, gastroschisis was identified by ultrasound.

Animal models of gastroschisis have been developed in fetal rats (40), rabbits (41), and mice (42). These models have made it possible to study the role of and best treatments for the effects of meconium, interleukin-8 specifically, and the acute inflammatory exudates in the amniotic fluid on the intestine exposed in

TABLE 10-1 *Frequency of unrelated major malformations in infants with gastroschisis, from international survey (24)*

	n	%
Central nervous system (CNS) anomalies		
anencephaly	42	1.3
spina bifida	32	1.0
encephalocele	10	0.3
hydrocephalus	42	1.3
total CNS anomalies	147	1.4
Eye anomalies	10	0.3
Ear anomalies	1	0.0
All heart defects	83	2.5
VSD	37	1.1
ASD	10	0.3
other		
Cleft palate	9	0.3
Cleft lip with/without cleft palate	37	1.1
Esophageal atresia	2	0.1
Anorectal atresia	34	1.0
Cloacal exstrophy	4	0.1
Hypospadias	10	0.3
Indeterminate sex	34	1.0
Renal agenesis	15	0.5
Cystic kidneys	4	0.1
Other urinary tract	32	1.0
Exstrophy of bladder	10	0.3
Polydactyly	15	0.5
Syndactyly	6	0.2
Limb reduction defects	51	1.6
Other limb anomalies	84	2.6
Total limbs	154	4.9
Rib and sternum defects	11	0.3
Diaphragm defects	15	0.5
Arthrogryposis	17	0.5
Hydrops	8	0.2
Other defects	3.3	0.1
Total defects	615	

*From an international survey of 24 malformations surveillance registries (24); 86% of the 3,322 affected infants had isolated gastroschisis; 20% had either a chromosome abnormality or a specific syndrome; 404 infants had 615 associated non-syndromic major malformations (listed above).

gastroschisis (20). It has been suggested that the exposure of the gastrointestinal tract to amniotic fluid in utero could cause the dysmotility, e.g., hypoperistalsis, a common postoperative complication of gastroschisis (43).

Prevalence

To determine the prevalence of gastroschisis in population-based surveys, it is essential to exclude other abdominal wall defects: omphalocele, limb-body-wall defects and Cantrell Pentalogy. In addition, affected fetuses in pregnancies terminated electively should be included. Population-based studies in 1980–1990, with these qualifications, showed in Europe (9) that prevalence rate was 0.09 per 1,000.

An increase in the prevalence rate over the past 20 to 30 years has been documented in several populations: in Western Australia, the prevalence rate was 0.1/1,000 from 1980–1990 and 0.55/1,000 in 1997–1998 (16); in Norway, from 0.13/1,000 in 1967–1989 to 0.32/1,000 in 1998 (17); in southeast Georgia, from 0.08/1,000 from 1968–1975 to 0.23/1,000 from 1976–2000 (22); the prevalence rate in Japan increased from 0.13/1,000 in 1975–1980 to 0.25/1,000 in 1996–1997 (13).

Race/Ethnicity

Only limited information is available on ethnic differences in prevalence. Pacific Islanders in Hawaii (1986–1997) [12] appeared to have a much higher prevalence rate (0.33/1,000) than Caucasians in Europe (0.09/1,000) [9] and Japanese infants (0.05/1,000) in Japan (13). In Atlanta (23), the prevalence rate among mothers less than 24 years old was higher in white mothers in comparison to young black mothers. In a study in Texas (1996–2002) [44] the highest rate of occurrence was among Hispanics, then Caucasians, and least frequent in African Americans.

Birth Status

An increased frequency of stillbirths (8% [11]) and intrauterine fetal demise (10–15% [9–12], has been observed. Intrauterine growth restriction and small for gestational age births (22% in one study [17]) have also been more common in comparison to unaffected infants.

Sex Ratio

An excess of males to females, e.g., 1.7:1 (5) and 1.3:1 (11), was observed in some studies and an excess of females M:F:1:2.1 in others (22).

Sidedness

The defect is almost always to the right of the umbilical cord (Figures 10-1 and 10-2).

Parental Age

Both isolated gastroschisis and omphalocele have been more common among younger mothers (7, 11, 23, 27). This is true especially for gastroschisis. For the period 1984–1989 in Italy (7), the mean age of mothers of infants with isolated gastroschisis (n=32) was 23.7 ±

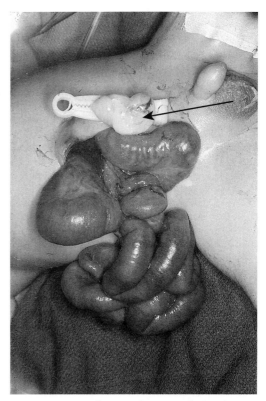

FIGURE 10.2 Newborn with gastroschisis, showing intestines protruding to the right of the white umbilical cord (arrow). (Courtesy of W. Hardy Hendren, M.D., Massachusetts General Hospital, Boston, MA).

3.8 years, isolated omphalocele (n=70) 28.3 ± 4.9, and control mothers 28.1 ± 5.1. In the period 1992–2000 in Philadelphia (27), the mean maternal age in the gastroschisis group (η=24) was 24.0 ± 5.4 years in comparison to 29.7 ± 7.2 years in the omphalocele group (η=22); p<0.01.

In Norway (19) the increased risk for gastroschisis correlated with the younger age of both the mother and the father.

In the international survey of 3,322 infants with gastroschisis (24), the mean maternal age was 21.9 years for infants with isolated gastroschisis, 27.05 years for malformation syndromes with gastroschisis (including chromosome trisomies), and 24.07 years for infants with nonsyndromic multiple anomalies, including gastroschisis.

Twinning

An increased frequency of twinning has been observed among the affected infants (21).

In three of four monozygous twin pairs and one of three dizygous twin pairs, both twins had gastroschisis (45).

Genetic Factors

Siblings with gastroschisis have been reported in several families (46–48). In a series of 127 families, the empiric recurrence risk was 4.7% (46). An affected mother and son (49) and affected sibs with an affected maternal grandfather and great-grandfather (50) have been reported.

Even though they are different types of anterior wall defects, gastroschisis and omphalocele have been observed in siblings (2, 51). In one family (51) a mother had one child with omphalocele, and, with a second husband, had one stillborn female with atresia of the colon and another daughter with gastroschisis.

The analysis of the familial aggregation of birth defects among 81 infants with gastroschisis showed an autosomal recessive pattern of inheritance for the infants with "isolated defects," but not among infants with gastroschisis and multiple defects (52).

In an analysis of 288 affected infants and 576 normal controls in 10 South American countries (1982–2005), the risk for having a child with gastroschisis correlated with a short cohabitation time between pregnancies, independent of maternal age (53). One interpretation was that, in those pregnancies, there was a higher likelihood of a "risky lifestyle," which could include exposure to drugs, alcohol, smoking, and poor nutrition.

The frequency of chromosome abnormalities was 2.7% in one population-based study in Hawaii (12). In the international survey of 24 registries (24), 1.2% of the infants had chromosome abnormalities: 15 of the 41 abnormalities were trisomy 18, 14 were trisomy 13, 4 sex chromosome anomalies, and 2 with trisomy 21.

Functional disruption of the bone morphogenetic protein-1 (BMP-1) in mice produced malformations similar to gastroschisis. However, mutation analysis with direct sequencing of exons 2 to 15 in the human BMP-1 gene showed no mutations in 11 children with gastroschisis (54).

In a case-control study (55) using DNA from 57 infants with gastroschisis and 506 controls, the presence in the infant of several gene polymorphisms involved in angiogenesis and blood vessel integrity was associated with an increased risk of gastroschisis. These polymorphisms included NPPA (atrial natriuretic peptide), ADD1 (alpha adducin1), ICAM 7 (intracellular adhesion molecule 7), and NOS3 (endothelial nitric oxide synthase). The risk was higher when the infant was homozygous for these polymorphisms. The risk for gastroschisis was 5 to 6 times greater if the mother smoked in the first trimester and the fetus had one or two of these polymorphisms in comparison to infants whose mothers did not smoke.

Environmental Factors

Exposure in pregnancy to several vasoactive compounds, including cocaine, cigarette smoking, salicylates, pseudoephedrine, and phenylpropanolamine, has been identified as a significant risk factors in several studies (56–59). In an analysis using human fetal livers, it was shown that genetic variation in SULT1A 3/4 (sulfotransferases) was a risk factor in the development of gastroschisis in the offspring of mothers who have taken acetaminophen (60).

In a population-based case-control study in California (61) of gastroschisis and lifestyle risk factors, the young, socially disadvantaged woman with a history of substance abuse had the highest risk for having a child with gastroschisis. Maternal hair analysis during the periconceptional period and pregnancy showed evidence of recreational drug use in 18% of 22 mothers of infants with gastroschisis in comparison to 8% for 25 controls (62).

In a case-control study of 55 infants with gastroschisis and 94 age-matched controls (63), the mothers of infants with gastroschisis had a significantly higher likelihood of smoking cigarettes or marijuana and eating a diet low in protein and in zinc than controls.

In an experimental study in CD-1 (hybrid) mice, a maternal diet of protein-zinc deficiencies and exposure to carbon monoxide produced gastroschisis (64).

Treatment and Prognosis

Clinically, infants with gastroschisis have been divided into two major groups, the simple group with 100% survival and no associated problems and the "complex cases" with associated atresia, perforation, infarction, and short bowel syndrome. The "complex cases" had a 28% mortality rate in one review (20).

The prognosis for the infant with gastroschisis is determined primarily by the condition of the exteriorized bowel. The examination of fetuses with gastroschisis showed that the development of the fibrous coating and edema of the loops of bowel occurred after the 30th week of gestation (65). The inflammatory response has been attributed to the bowel being exposed to amniotic fluid, and meconium in particular (66). The fetuses found prenatally to have severe perivisceritis and meconium-stained amniotic fluid had been more likely to be born prematurely (65). The presence of intestinal dilatation was predictive of the presence of bowel atresia (43). In turn, the presence of bowel atresia with gastroschisis has been a predictor of a higher frequency of perinatal morbidity and mortality (25).

Delivery by cesarean section (and avoidance of labor) has not been shown to improve the clinical outcome (67). Several techniques have been proposed to improve postoperative survival: amino-infusion (68), staged stretching of the abdominal cavity (69), the staged silo technique for gradual closure (70), a "gentle touch" method in which there is no manipulation of the bowel (71), and monitoring bladder pressure to decrease the complication of ischemia of the intestine and kidney (72). The staged closure approach has been associated with a longer length of stay and more days of mechanical ventilation, but lower frequency of infection and mechanical complications and a lower risk of long-term bowel dysfunction and reoperation (73).

Because recovery of function of the intestine after the repair of gastroschisis has been prolonged, an attempt was made to improve internal feeding with a prokinetic agent, such as erythromycin. However, a systematic, randomized study of treatment did not show improvement in the recovery time (74). Difficulty with oral feeding can be a prolonged, difficult problem for some children.

A comparison of survival rates of all infants born in New York State in the period 1983–1999 showed a lower survival rate among the black infants (75). Low birth weight and severe prematurity are also more common among the infants born to very young mothers (76).

An increased frequency of large placentas was reported in one case series (77). No systematic study of the placenta of infants with gastroschisis has been reported. The presence of numerous lipid droplets has been demonstrated by light and electron microscopy in the amniotic epithelium in association with gastroschisis (78).

Genetic Counseling

When diagnosed during pregnancy, cautious optimism is warranted. The pregnancy should be monitored by ultrasound to monitor for spontaneous closure of the abdominal wall defect, as this can be a serious or fatal complication. There is also an increased risk for stillbirth or intrauterine fetal demise. Chromosome analysis is warranted by CVS or amniocentesis, especially for the fetus with gastroschisis and other anomalies.

The examination of the affected infant at birth will confirm whether or not other structural abnormalities are present. The surgeon will have several options in the timing and the type of closure, as well as the monitoring of potential complications during the surgery.

In a future pregnancy, there is an empiric risk of recurrence of about 5%. The parents should be advised of the option of prenatal monitoring by ultrasound.

REFERENCES

1. Tibboel D, Verney-Keers C, Kluck P, Gaillard JLJ, Koppenberg J, Molenaar JC. The natural history of gastroschisis during fetal life: development of the fibrous coating on the bowel loops. *Teratology*. 1986;33:267–373.
2. Torfs C, Curry C, Roeper P. Gastroschisis. *J Pediatr*. 1990;116: 1–6.
3. Hunter A, Soothill P. Gastroschisis—an overview. *Prenatal Diag*. 2002;22:869–873.
4. Luck SR, Sherman JO, Raffensperger JG, Goldstein IR. Gastroschisis in 106 consecutive newborn infants. *Surgery*. 1985;98:677–683.
5. Roeper PJ, Harris J, Lee G, Neutra R. Secular rates and correlates for gastroschisis in California (1968–1977). *Teratology*. 1987;35:203–210.
6. Morrow RJ, Whittle MJ, McNay MB, Raine PAM, Gibson AAM, Crossley J. Prenatal diagnosis and management of anterior abdominal wall defects in the west of Scotland. *Prenat Diagn*. 1993;13:115–?.
7. Calzolari E, Volpato S, Bianchi F, Cianciulli D, Tenconi R, Clementi M, Calabro A, Lungarotti S, Mastroiacovo PP, Botto L, Spagnolo A, Milan M. Omphalocele and gastroschisis: a collaborative study of five Italian congenital malformation registries. *Teratology*. 1993;47:47–55.
8. Torfs CP, Velie EM, Oechsli FW, Bateson TF, Curry CJR. A population-based study of gastroschisis: demographic, pregnancy, and lifestyle risk factors. *Teratology*. 1994;50:44–53.
9. Calzolari E, Bianchi F, Dolk H, Milan M. Omphalocele and gastroschisis in Europe: a survey of three million births 1980–1990. EUROCAT Working Group. *Am J Med Genet*. 1995;58: 187–194.
10. Tan KH, Kilby MD, Whittle MJ, Beattie BR, Booth IW, Botting BJ. Congenital anterior abdominal wall defects in England and Wales 1987–93: retrospective analysis of OPCS data. *Brit Med J*. 1996;313:903–906.
11. Byron-Scott R, Haan E, Chan A, Bower C, Scott H, Clark K. A population-based study of abdominal wall defects in South Australia and Western Australia. *Paediatr Perinat Epidemiol*. 1998;12:136–151.
12. Forrester MB, Merz RD. Epidemiology of abdominal wall defects, Hawaii, 1986–1997. *Teratology*. 1999;60:117–123.
13. Suita S, Okamatsu T, Yamamoto T, Handa N, Nirasawa Y, Watanabe Y, Yanagihara J, Nishijima E, Hirobe S, Nio M, Gomi A, Horisawa M. Changing profile of abdominal wall defects in Japan: results of a national survey. *J Pediatr Surg*. 2000;35:66–72.
14. Di Tanna GL, Rosano A, Mastroiancovo P. Prevalence of gastroschisis at birth: retrospective study. *BMJ*. 2002;325:1389–1390.
15. Kidd JN Jr, Jackson RJ, Smith SD, Wagner CW. Evolution of staged versus primary closure of gastroschisis. *Ann Surg*. 2003;237:759–765.
16. Reid KP, Dickinson JE, Doherty DA. The epidemiologic incidence of congenital gastroschisis in Western Australia. *Am J Obstet Gynecol*. 2003;189:764–768.
17. Brantberg A, Blaas H-G K, Salvesen KA, Haugen SE, Eik-nes SH. Surveillance and outcome of fetuses with gastroschisis. *Ultrasound Obstet Gynecol*. 2004;23:4–13.
18. Arnold M. Is the incidence of gastroschisis rising in South Africa in accordance with international trends? *SAJS*. 2004;42:86–88.
19. Kazaura MR, Lie RT, Irgens LM, Didriksen A, Kapstad M, Egenaes J, Bjerkedal T. Increasing risks of gastroschisis in Norway: an age-period-cohort analysis. *Am J Epidem*. 2004;159: 358–363.
20. Wilson RD, Johnson MP. Congenital abdominal wall defects: an update. *Fetal Diagn Ther*. 2004;19:385–398.
21. Hwang P-J, Kousseff BG. Omphalocele and gastroschisis: an 18-year review study. *Genet Med*. 2004;6:232–236.
22. Goldkrand JW, Causey TN, Hull EE. The changing face of gastroschisis and omphalocele in southeast Georgia. *J Mat-Fetal Neonat Med*. 2004;15:331–335.
23. Williams LJ, Kucik JE, Alverson CJ, Olney RS, Correa A. Epidemiology of gastroschisis in Metropolitan Atlanta, 1968 through 2000. *Birth Defects Research (Part A): Clin Mol Teratology*. 2005;73:177–183.
24. Mastroiacovo P, Lisi A, Castilla EE, Martínez-Frias, Bermego E, Marengo L et al. Gastroschisis and associated defects: an international study. *Am J Med Genet Part A*. 2007;143A:660–671.
25. Cusick E, Spicer RD, Beck JM. Small-bowel continuity: a crucial factor in determining survival in gastroschisis. *Pedia Surg Int*. 1997;12:34–37.

26. Moerman P, Fryns J-P, Vandenberghe K, Lauweryns JM. Constructive amniotic bands, amniotic adhesions and limb body wall complex: discrete disruptive sequences with pathogenetic overlap. *Am J Med Genet.* 1992;42:470–479.

27. Kunz LH, Gilbert WM, Towner DR. Increased incidence of cardiac anomalies in pregnancies complicated by gastroschisis. *Am J Obst Gynecol.* 2005;193:1248–1252.

28. Gibbin C, Touch S, Broth RE, Berghella V. Abdominal wall defects and congenital heart disease. *Ultrasound Obstet Gynecol.* 2003;21:334–337.

29. Reid COMV, Hall JG, Anderson C, Bocian M, Carey J, Costa T, Curry C, Greenberg F, Horton W, et al. Association of amyoplasia with gastroschisis, bowel atresia, and defects of the muscular layer of the trunk. *Am J Med Genet.* 1986;24:701–710.

30. Lawson A, de la Hunt MN. Gastroschisis and undescended testis. *J Pediatr Surg.* 2001;36:366–367.

31. Bromley B, Shamberger RC, Benacerraf B. An unusual outcome for fetus with gastroschisis. *J Ultrasound Med.* 1995;14:69–72.

32. Tawil A, Comstock CH, Chang C-H. Prenatal closure of abdominal defect in gastroschisis: case report and review of the literature. *Pediat Develop Path.* 2001;4:580–584.

33. Dixon JC, Penman DM, Soothill DW. The influence of bowel atresia in gastroschisis on fetal growth, cardiotocograph abnormalities and amniotic fluid staining. *Brit J Obstet Gynaecol.* 2000;107:472–475.

34. de Vries PA. The pathogenesis of gastroschisis and omphalocele. *J Pediatr Surg.* 1980;15:245–251.

35. Hoyme HE, Jones MC, Jones KL. Gastroschisis: abdominal wall disruption secondary to early gestational interruption of the omphalomesenteric artery. *Semin Perinatal.* 1983;7:194–298.

36. Sadler TW, Carey JC, Feldcamp M. Gastroschisis: a schism for sure? *Proc Greenwood Center.* 2006;25:76–77.

37. Shaw A. The myth of gastroschisis. *J Pediatr Surg.* 1975;10:235–244.

38. Byrne J LB, Feldkamp ML. Seven-week embryo with gastroschisis, multiple anomalies, and physiologic hernia suggests early onset of gastroschisis. *Birth Def Res (Part A): Clin Mol Teratol.* 2008;82:236–238.

39. Torfs, Claudine. Personal communication. June 30, 2000.

40. Midrio P, Faussone-Pellegrini MS, Vannucchi MG, Flake AW. Gastroschisis in the rate model is associated with a delayed maturation of intestinal pacemaker cells and smooth muscle cells. *J Pediatri Surg.* 2004;39:1541–1547.

41. Oyachi N, Lakshmanan J, Ross MG, Atkinson JB. Fetal gastrointestinal mobility in a rabbit model of gastroschisis. *J Pediatr Surg.* 2004;39:366–370.

42. Brewer S, Williams T. Finally, a sense of closure? Animal models of human ventral body wall defects. *Bio Essays.* 2004;26:1307–1321.

43. Morrison JJ, Klein N, Chitty LS, Kocjan G, Walshe D, Goulding M, Geary MP, Pierro A, Rodeck CH. Intra-amniotic inflammation in human gastroschisis: possible aetiology of postnatal bowel dysfunction. *Br J Obstet Gynaecol.* 1998;105:1200–1204.

44. Husain T, Langlois PH, Sever LE, Gambello MJ. Descriptive epidemiologic features shared by birth defects thought to be related to vascular disruption in Texas, 1996–2002. *Birth Def Res (Part A): Clin Mol Teratol.* 2008;82:435–440.

45. Bugge M, Petersen MB, Christensen MF. Monozygotic twins discordant for gastroschisis: case report and review of the literature of twins and familial occurrence of gastroschisis. *Am J Med Genet.* 1994;52:223–226.

46. Torfs C, Curry CR. Familial cases of gastroschisis in a populations-based registry. *Am J Med Genet.* 1993;45:465–467.

47. Reece A, Thornton J, Stringer MD. Genetic factors in the aetiology of gastroschisis: a case report. *Eur J Ob Gyn Reprod Biol.* 1997;73:127–128.

48. Snelling CMH, Davies GAL. Isolated gastroschisis in successive siblings: a case report and review of the literature. *J Obstet Gynaeco Ca.* 2004;26:591–593.

49. Nelson TC, Toyama WM. Familial gastroschisis: a case of mother-and-son occurrence. *J Pediat Surg.* 1995;30:1706–1708.

50. Ventruto V, Stabile M, Lonardo F. Gastroschisis in two sibs with abdominal hernia in maternal grandfather and great-grandfather. *Am J Med Genet.* 1985;21:405–407.

51. Hershey DW, Marr CC, Adkins JC. Familial abdominal wall defects. *Am J Hum Genet.* 1988;43 (Suppl):A55.

52. Yang P, Beaty TH, Bkhoury MJ, Chee E, Stewart W, Gordis L. Genetic-epidemiology study of omphalocele and gastroschisis: evidence for heterogeneity. *Am J Med Genet.* 1992;44:668–675.

53. Rittler M, Castilla EE, Chambers C, Lopez-Camelo JS. Risk for gastroschisis in primigravidity, length of sexual cohabitation, and change in paternity. *Birth Def Res (Part A): Clin Mol Teratol.* 2007;79:483–487.

54. Komuro H, Mori M, Hayashi Y, Fukagawa M, Makino S-I, Takahara K, Greenspan DS, Momoi MY. Mutation analysis of the BMP-1 gene in patients with gastroschisis. *J Pediatr Surg.* 2001;36:885–887.

55. Torfs CP, Christianson RE, Iovannisa DM, Cheng S, Shaw GM, Lammer EJ. Selected gene polymorphisms, and their interaction with maternal smoking, as risk factors for gastroschisis. *Birth Def Res (Part A): Clin Mol Teratology.* 2006;76:723–730.

56. Haddow JE, Palomak GE, Holman MS. Young maternal age and smoking during pregnancy as risk factors for gastroschisis. *Teratology.* 1993;47:225–228.

57. Torfs CP, Katz EA, Bateson TF, Lam PK, Curry CJR. Maternal medications and environmental exposures as risk factors for gastroschisis. *Teratology.* 1996;54:84–92.

58. Martinez-Frias ML, Rodriquez-Pinilla E, Prieto L. Prenatal exposure to salicylates and gastroschisis: a case-control study. *Teratology.* 1997;56:241–243.

59. Werler MM, Sheehan JE, Mitchell AA. Association of vasoconstrictive exposures with risk of gastroschisis and small intestinal atresia. *Epidemiology.* 2003;14:349–354.

60. Adjei AA, Gaedigk A, Simon SD, Weinshilboum RM, Leeder JS. Interindividual variability in acetaminophen sulfation by human fetal liver: implications for pharmacogenetic investigations of drug-induced birth defects. *Birth Def Res (Part A): Clin Mol Teratol.* 2008;82:155–165.

61. Torfs CP, Velie EM, Oechsli FW, Bateson TF, Curry CJR. A population-based study of gastroschisis: demographic, pregnancy, and lifestyle risk factors. *Teratology.* 1994;50:44–53.

62. Morrison JJ, Chitty LS, Peebles D, Rodeck CH. Recreational drugs and fetal gastroschisis: maternal hair analysis in the periconceptional period and during pregnancy. *BJOG.* 2005;112:1022–1025.

63. Lam PK, Torfs CP. Interaction between smoking and malnutrition in infants with gastroschisis. *Birth Def Res (Part A): Clin Mol Teratology.* 2006;76:182–186.

64. Singh J. Gastroschisis is caused by the combination of carbon monoxide and protein-zinc deficiencies in mice. *Birth Def Res (Part B): Reprod Toxicol.* 2003;68:355–362.

65. Luton D, DeLagausie P, Guibourdenche J, Owry JF, Vuillard E, Sibony O, Farnoux C, Aigrain Y, Blot P. Prognostic factors of prenatally diagnosed gastroschisis. *Fetal Diagnosis & Therapy.* 1997;12:7–14.

66. Nichol PF, Hayman A, Pryde PG, Go LL, Lund DP. Meconium staining of amniotic fluid correlates with intestinal peel formation in gastroschisis. *Pediatr Surg Int.* 2004;20:211–214.

67. Salihu HM, Emusu D, Aliya ZY, Pierre-Lewis BJ, Druschel CM, Kirby RS. Mode of delivery and neonatal survival of infants with isolated gastroschisis. *Obstet Gynecol.* 2004;104:678–683.

68. Volumenic J-L, deLagausie P, Guibourdenche J, Quory J-F, Vuillard E, Saizou C, Luton D. Improvement of mesenteric

superior artery Doppler velocimetry by amnio-infusion in fetal gastroschisis. *Prenat Diag.* 2001;21:1171–1174.

69. Fishcer JD, Chun K, Moores DC, Andrews HG. Gastroschisis: a simple technique for staged silo closure. *J Pediat Sug.* 1995; 30:1169–1171.

70. Jona JZ. The "gentle touch" technique in the treatment of gastroschisis. *J Pediatr Surg.* 2003;38:1036–1038.

71. Patkowski D, Dzernik J, Baglaj SM. Active enlargement of the abdominal cavity—a new method for earlier closure of giant omphalocele and gastroschisis. *Eur J Pediatr Surg.* 2005;15: 22–25.

72. Tibboel D, Vermey-Keers C, Klück P, Gaillard JLJ, Koppenberg J, Molenaar JC. The natural history of gastroschisis during bowel loops. *Teratology.* 1986;33:267–272.

73. Kidd JW, Jackson RJ, Smith SD, Wagner CW. Evolution of staged versus primary closure of gastroschisis. *Am Surg.* 2003;237: 759–765.

74. Curry JI, Lander AD, Stringer M.D. A multicenter, randomized, double-blind, placebo-controlled trial of the prokinetic agent erythromycin in the postoperative recovery of infants with gastroschisis. *J Pediatr Surg.* 2004;39:565–569.

75. Salihu HM, Aliya ZY, Pierre-Louis BJ, Obuseh FA, Druschel CM, Kirby RS. Omphalocele and gastroschisis: black-white disparity in infant survival. *Birth Def Ref (Part A): Clin Mol Teratology.* 2004;70:586–591.

76. Emusu D, Salihu HM, Aliya ZY, Pierre-Louis BJ, Druschel CM, Kirby RS. Gastroschisis, low maternal age, and fetal morbidity outcomes. *Birth Defects Research (Part A): Clin Mol Teratology.* 2005;73:649–654.

77. Toriello HV. Gastroschisis: review of 80 patients. Proc Greenwood Genetics Center 2007 (in press).

78. Graefe MR, Benirschke K. Ultrasound study of the amniotic epithelium in a case of gastroschisis. *Pediatric Pathology.* 1990; 10:95–101.

Chapter 11

Heart Defects

Definition

A structural abnormality of the heart and great vessels (aorta and pulmonary arteries).

ICD-9:
(selected list)

745.000	(persistent truncus arteriosus; absent septum between aorta and pulmonary artery)
745.120	(corrected transposition of great vessels, L-transposition, ventricle inversion)
745.200	(tetralogy of Fallot)
745.490	(VSD [ventricular septal defect] not otherwise specified)
745.510	atrial septal defect; (ostium [septum] secundum defect)
745.100	(tricuspid atresia, stenosis, hypoplasia)
746.300	(congenital stenosis of aortic valve)
746.480	(other specified anomalies of the aortic valves; includes: aortic valve atresia)
746.505	(absence, atresia, or hypoplasia of mitral valve)
746.700	(hypoplastic left heart syndrome)
746.800	(dextrocardia *without* situs inversus [situs solitus])

747.000	(patent ductus arteriosus [PDA])
747.100	(preductal [proximal] coarctation of aorta)
747.200	(atresia of aorta)
747.300	(pulmonary artery atresia, absence, or agenesis)

ICD-10:

Q20.0	(common arterial trunk, persistent truncus arteriosus)
Q20.5	(discordant atrioventricular connection, includes corrected transposition)
Q21.0	(ventricular septal defect)
Q21.1	(atrial septal defect)
Q21.3	(tetralogy of Fallot)
Q22.4	(congenital tricuspid stenosis)
Q23.0	(congenital stenosis of aortic valve, includes congenital aortic atresia)
Q23.2	(congenital mitral stenosis and atresia)
Q23.4	(hypoplastic left heart syndrome)
Q24.0	(dextrocardia)
Q25.0	(patent ductus arteriosus)
Q25.1	(coarctation of aorta)
Q25.2	(atresia of aorta)
Q25.5	(atresia of pulmonary artery)

Mendelian Inheritance in Man:

#108900	(atrial septal defect with atrioventricular conduction defects)	
#120000	(coarctation of aorta)	
#140500	(malformation of heart)	
#217095	(conotruncal heart malformations; cthm)	
#241550	(hypoplastic left heart syndrome)	
#306955	(heterotaxy, visceral, X-linked)	
#603612	(atrial septal defect, secundum, with various cardiac and noncardiac defects)	
#606215	(atrioventricular septal defect; AVSD1)	
#605618	(tetralogy of Fallot syndrome, autosomal recessive)	

Historical Note

Charlotte Ferencz and colleagues (1) have suggested that the discipline of cardiology for children and adults was established by the heart clinics. The first such clinic for children was established at the Massachusetts General Hospital in Boston in 1910. The initial focus was to study acute endocarditis in children with rheumatic heart disease. In 1930, Dr. Edwards A. Park established the Cardiac Clinic at Harriet Home for Invalid Children and, significantly, chose Helen Taussig, M.D., as its director. This clinic became the site for innovations in the surgical repair of heart defects. Dr. Taussig wrote the book *Congenital Malformations of the Heart* in 1947, in which she described her experience with each abnormality.

Fellows training with Dr. Taussig, and later with Alexander Nadas, M.D., at Boston Children's Hospital, extended this clinical expertise all over the world.

Other leaders in the development of the expertise in clinical cardiology were Dr. Maude Abbott at McGill University in Montreal (6), Dr. John Keith, and later Dr. Richard Rowe at the Hospital for Sick Children in Toronto and Dr. Maurice Campbell in London. Each of these individuals recruited colleagues and fellows and carried out many different studies to characterize specific anatomic phenotypes, prevalence rates and plans for management. Several textbooks and atlases of heart defects were developed.

The progress in the surgical repair of heart defects developed in parallel with the expertise in clinical diagnosis and management. In 1938, Dr. Robert Gross at Boston Children's Hospital ligated a patent ductus arteriosus, the first surgical intervention. In 1945, the Blalock-Taussig operation was carried out to create a shunt to treat the symptoms of tetralogy of Fallot (7).

The advent of cardiac catherization improved significantly the determination of the specific abnormalities of heart defects (8).

In the 1980s, it began to be possible to use ultrasound to characterize the anatomy of the heart in the developing fetus (9). The four-chamber view in the routine "fetal survey" at 18 to 20 weeks of gestation led to the detection of 25% of the heart defects by the 1990s, although there was significant variation from medical center to medical center (10).

The early detection of the hypoplastic left heart by prenatal ultrasound suggested that the obstruction by the atretic aortic or mitral valves, if removed, could retain a functioning four-chamber heart. Trials of surgical repair, during pregnancy, are underway to test this important possibility (11).

Environmental factors that can cause heart defects began to be identified. During the national rubella epidemic in the 1960s, heart defects were established as a major component of the fetal effects. In the 1990s and 2000s insulin-dependent diabetes mellitus in the mother was recognized as another major cause of heart defects (12).

As chromosome abnormalities, such as trisomies 21, 18, and 13, were delineated in the 1960s, heart defects were found to be common in the affected infants. When it became possible to identify chromosome deletions, heart defects were found to be a frequent effect of common deletions, like the 22q11.2 deletion.

The advent of molecular studies began the process of identifying specific gene mutations associated with specific heart defects. Mutations were also identified that caused genetic syndromes, in which heart defects were a central feature, such as the Holt-Oram Syndrome (13). The advent of the microarray or array CGH (comparative genomic hybridization) has continued the process of unraveling mysteries with this technology.

During the 1990s, the possibility of preventing the occurrence of malformations, such as spina bifida and anencephaly, was tested with periconceptional supplementation with multivitamins and folic acid, in particular. In the analyses of the populations of women supplemented since 1998 in the United States, there has been more evidence that the frequencies of some heart defects in infants in those pregnancies have decreased, as well (14).

Appearance

The spectrum of heart defects identifiable in clinical evaluations and imaging studies includes internal defects in the atrial and ventricular septums, defective valves and extremely visible abnormalities of the aorta, pulmonary artery and, the venous connections to the heart. (Figures 11-1–11-4).

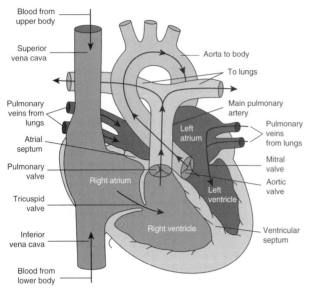

FIGURE 11.1 Normal heart and blood flow. (From Pediatric Cardiology Teaching Materials, Version 1.3, 2003, Pritchett & Hull Associates, Atlanta, GA)

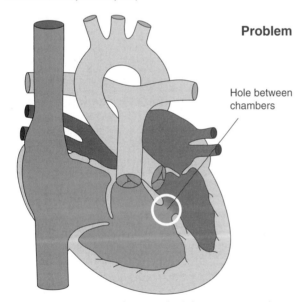

FIGURE 11.2 Ventricular septal defect. (From Pediatric Cardiology Teaching Materials, Version 1.3, 2003, Pritchett & Hull Associates, Atlanta, GA)

Visual aids, which made it easier for clinicians and parents to visualize the structural abnormalities, became available throughout atlases (4, 5) and websites, such as www.fetalecho.com.

Associated Malformations

Heart defects are the most common structural abnormality identified during pregnancy and in newborn infants. There is also a significant probability that the infant with a heart defect will have either associated heart defects or other non-heart malformations. For example, 20% of the infants with a ventricular septal

defect (after excluding conotruncal abnormalities and atrioventricular defects) had one other heart defect, such as infundibular pulmonary stenosis and aortic valve prolapse (15).

The high frequency of associated non-heart malformations has been established in many case series and population-based studies. An early example was the study by Greenwood et al (16) in 1975 of infants with heart defects who had been referred to Boston Children's Hospital. They reported that 25% had extracardiac anomalies. Later, the frequency of non-heart malformations was established in an unselected population of newborns with a congenital cardiovascular malformations in comparison to infants with no heart defect

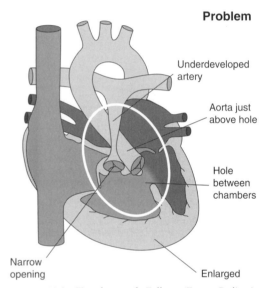

FIGURE 11.3 Tetralogy of Fallot. (From Pediatric Cardiology Teaching Materials, Version 1.3, 2003, Pritchett & Hull Associates, Atlanta, GA)

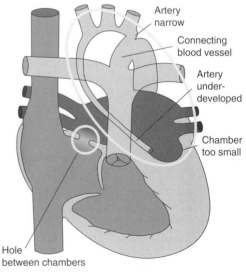

FIGURE 11.4 Hypoplastic left heart syndrome. (From Pediatric Cardiology Teaching Materials, Version 1.3, 2003, Pritchett & Hull Associates, Atlanta, GA)

in the population-based case-control study in the Baltimore-Washington area in the period 1981–1984 (1, 17). 1,090 (73%) of the 1,494 affected infants had an isolated cardiovascular malformation. Among the 404 (27%) with non-heart defects, the recognized etiologies included chromosome abnormalities in 187 (46%), syndromes and hereditary disorders in 74 (18.3%), possible syndromes in 17 (4.2%), and nonsyndromic malformations in 176 (31.2%).

As more sophisticated technologies have been developed, additional associated abnormalities have and will be detected in some infants with heart defects. Recently imaging by magnetic resonance imaging (MRI) and diffusion tensor imaging (DTI) has been used to evaluate infants with two major malformations, transposition of the great arteries and single ventricle, before surgery (18). The imaging showed widespread brain abnormalities before surgery, which suggested that these abnormalities had developed in utero. These changes could not be attributed to problems with blood flow during the surgical procedure.

Developmental Factors

The development of the heart is a very complex process. So, heart defects can be caused by abnormalities in several different developmental events.

Initially, mesodermal cells migrate to the midline, fuse at the primitive streak, and form a tube that beats spontaneously at days 21–23 (19, 20). Looping starts at day 23 and is complete by day 28. The four chambers of the heart develop from this tube. The heart normally forms a right-sided loop and creates a left-right asymmetry. The neural crest cells migrate from the neural folds into the outflow tract of the heart and the arteries of the aortic arch (21). Models of cell lineage analysis have suggested three different heart fields—one contributing primarily to the left ventricle, one to the right ventricle and atria, and one to the venous pole (20).

Edward Clark and his colleagues (22) showed in a series of experiments in the developing chick embryo that there are several processes underway during heart development that can produce structural abnormalities of the heart: 1) disordered intracardiac blood flow; 2) disordered cell migration; 3) altered patterns of cell death; 4) abnormal proliferation of extracellular matrix. Heart defects were subdivided into groups reflecting the affects of these four primary mechanisms of abnormal development. Heart defects were classified based on the apparent underlying type of developmental abnormality.

Family studies suggested that gene abnormalities could cause a clustering of related types of developmental abnormalities in close relatives (23–25). The comparison of close relatives with heart defects has shown, for example, that tetralogy of Fallot, transposition of the great arteries, and ventricular septal defect are more likely to occur in close relatives, suggesting that the affected relatives share a susceptibility to conotruncal defects. This clustering of heart defects has been confirmed in breeding studies of heart defects in Keeshond dogs (26). It is consistent also with the concept of the "segmental approach" to understanding heart defects, as postulated by Richard and Stella Van Praagh (27).

These family studies suggested that specific genes could affect certain aspects of heart development. Subsequently, molecular analyses have identified several of the genes associated with left and right outflow tracts. These genes include *HOX1.5*, *RXRA*, *SOX4*, and *NF1* in the neural crest cells, *jagged 1* in the right outflow tract, and *TFAPZB* in the ductus arteriosus (19).

This molecular technology made it possible, also, to identify polymorphisms in genes involved in relevant biologic processes, such as coagulation, cell-cell interaction, the inflammatory response, blood pressure regulation, and homocysteine metabolism, that are more subtle risk factors for the occurrence of heart defects. For example, the occurrence of 32 single nucleotide polymorphisms (SNPs) was determined in 155 infants with conotruncal heart defects compared to 437 infants without heart defects. Four SNPs showed significant associations: 1) prothrombin G20210A; 2) F7 promoter; 3) platelet glycoprotein IIIa; 4) atrial natriuretic precursor peptide (NPPA T2238C) [28]. Consistent with the model of multifactorial inheritance, additional associations with polymorphisms are expected to be identified.

Diseases that mothers have are another developmental factor in the occurrence of heart defects. Ferencz and her associates (29) identified in the Baltimore-Washington Infant Study several infants with heart defects whose mothers had had a hematologic disorder, such as von Willebrand Disease and a hemolytic anemia. One hypothesis developed was that the faulty synthesis of coagulation factors could lead to abnormalities of the blood of the embryo and could affect endothelial cell function. In another population-based study of the offspring of 1,239 mothers with hereditary hematologic disorders, there were 14 infants with a cardiovascular malformation, which was much greater number than the expected number 7.74 (p=0.027) [29].

Prevalence

The examination of spontaneous abortions (31–33) and stillborn (34) infants has shown that the incidence in these settings is higher than among liveborn infants at birth. In a consecutive series of 412 examinable specimens (8 to 28 weeks gestational age) collected between 1976 and 1983 in New York City (32), 277 fetuses had a normal chromosome karyotype. The spectrum of the heart defects identified (3 in 277 or 11/1,000) was considered similar to those seen in liveborn infants. Among 500 spontaneous abortions examined in a referral center for fetuses in Seattle (33), 289 were normal on external exam; 21 (7.3%) of these fetuses had a heart defect for a much higher prevalence rate (73/1,000) than in the consecutive sample in which chromosome analysis was performed. Ventricular septal defect (VSD) was the most common heart defect in both studies. In the New York Study (29), the VSD's were all the perimembraneous type.

Among stillborn infants in whom the heart was examined, 10% of 166 had heart defects (34). The most common cardiovascular abnormalities were ventricular septal defect (35%), atrial septal defect (10%), coarctation of the aorta (9.4%), and transposition of great arteries (9.1%).

Several factors influence the detection of heart defects and, thereby, the prevalence rate: the skill of the examiner, whether prenatal screening by ultrasound or echocardiography suggested the presence of a structural abnormality, the use of echocardiography in the evaluation of the infant of concern, and whether the evaluation of the child is only at birth or extends through the first year of life (1, 34, 35). The overall effect of these improvements has been an increase in the prevalence rates. For example, the Baltimore-Washington Infant Study (1981–1989) detected more heart defects (3.7/1,000) than the New England Regional Infant Cardiac Program (1969–1977) [2.03/1,000], which had a similar study design (36, 37).

An "epidemic" in the occurrence of ventricular septal defect (VSD) was reported in the years 1970–1977 (38). This observation and analyses of other populations (39) identified seasonal variation in the births of infants with VSD and led, initially, to the suggestion that an environmental exposure could be responsible for these changes. However, it was most likely that the increase was caused entirely by the increased detection of small defects in the muscular part of the interventricular septum after the use of echocardiography became a standard part of clinical evaluations (40).

The dramatic impact of imaging technology on the detection of VSDs was shown in studies in Israel (April to September, 1994) [41]. 1,053 consecutive newborn infants were examined with color Doppler echocardiography. When examined between 6 and 170 hours of age (mean 37 hours), 56 infants (53.2/1,000) were found to have a muscular VSD. All of the infants examined were asymptomatic. Only 6 of the 56 had a systolic heart murmur. Over the subsequent 10 months, 89% of these VSDs closed spontaneously. These findings raised the question as to whether a muscular VSD should be considered part of a normal developmental process and not a structural abnormality.

In view of these observations, what is the prevalence rate of the cardiovascular malformations in newborn infants? Very few studies have reported the prevalence rate at birth, Lin et al (42) reported a rate of 3.3/1,000 over a 15-year period in Boston (1972–1974, 1979–1990) in a consecutive sample, monitored at birth, which included liveborn and stillborn infants as well as elective terminations, because of fetal anomalies detected in prenatal studies. This rate is much lower than rates established after intensive follow-up evaluations. For example, a cohort of 19,044 liveborn were identified in the Kaiser Foundation Health Plan in 1959 to 1967 in California. In addition, there were 458 stillborn infants. Intensive follow-up of the liveborn infants over five years showed that the prevalence rate was 8.8/1,000 (34), a rate that is 2.7 times higher than the prevalence rate established at birth in the Boston study of Lin et al (42).

Race/Ethnicity

Prevalence rates have not been developed in major racial groups for the most common heart defects and related groups, using uniform methods of diagnosis.

Birth Status

The more severe heart defects are more likely to affect fetal growth and to be associated with stillbirth.

Sex Ratio

A predominance of affected males was noted for all diagnoses, and was significant statistically for transposition of the great arteries with intact ventricular septum, in the Baltimore-Washington Infant Study (1).

Parental Age

Some population-based studies, such as the Baltimore-Washington Infant Study (1), have evaluated possible correlations of specific heart defects with advanced or young maternal and paternal ages. No significant correlations have been established.

Twinning

The frequency of cardiovascular abnormalities is higher in monozygous (43) twins than in singletons. The excess of heart defects has been present in twin pairs that did not have the twin-twin transfusion syndrome (44).

The likelihood that each twin in an identical twin pair will be affected was 46% and 6.8% in two early case series in 1967 (45) and 1977 (46). In those two case series the likelihood that both of nonidentical twins were affected was 4.2% and 2.3% respectively. In a more recent case series of 1,743 infants with heart defects in South Italy (1999–2002), the concordance rate in 66 dizygous twin pairs was 13.6%, with both twins having a congenital heart defect (47). In this more recent study, echocardiography was used to identify cardiovascular malformations.

Genetic Factors

The delineation of the genetic factors in the causation of heart defects has paralleled the dramatic increase, over the past 40 years, in the delineation of the genetic factors that can cause all types of malformations. In the 1960s, the association of heart defects, as one of several anomalies, was recognized in the trisomies of chromosomes 21, 18, and 13. With the advent of banding techniques in the 1970s, more trisomies, more subtle deletions, and unbalanced translocations were recognized, primarily in infants with a heart defect as one of several heart and noncardiac malformations. In the 1980s, the technique of fluorescent in situ hybridization (FISH) made it easier to identify the common deletions associated with heart defects, such as 22q11.2 deletion (Di George Syndrome) and 7q11.23 deletion (Williams Syndrome).

Gene linkage studies in single families with many affected individuals made it possible to identify a gene region associated with a specific heart defect. For example, with this approach the *NKX2.5* gene was shown to be associated with the occurrence of an atrial septal defect (48). Since 2000, the association of tetralogy of Fallot, atrial septal defect, atrio-ventricular defect (AVSD), and X-linked heterotaxy with mutations in several different genes, have been identified primarily in studies of multiple affected related and unrelated individuals (Table 11-1).

Family studies and molecular techniques also led to the identification of specific mutations associated with hereditary syndromes that include heart defects, such as the Holt-Oram Syndrome (13). To date, several

malformation syndromes, which include heart defects, have been shown to be associated with specific mutations and to exhibit Mendelian inheritance (Table 11-2).

TABLE 11-2 *Mutations in genetic syndromes which include cardiovascular malformations*

	Gene	Syndrome	Mendelian Inheritance In Man
1.	TBX5 (58)	Holt-Oram Syndrome	(MIM #142900)
2.	KRAS PTPN1I SOS1 (59)	Noonan Syndrome	(MIM #163950)
3.	MKKS	McKusick-Kaufman Syndrome	(MIM #236700)
4.	DHCR7	Smith-Lemli-Opitz Syndrome	(MIM #270400)
5.	JAG1	Alagille Syndrome	(MIM #118450)
6.	CHD7	CHARGE Association	(MIM #214800)
7.	N1PBL	Cornelia de Lange Syndrome	(MIM #122470)

As these mutations have been delineated, clinicians have been challenged to delineate the entire phenotype carefully, as the pattern of the abnormalities can focus the diagnostic testing. Consider for example, the infant with absence or hypoplasia of the thumb and radius, which can occur in many malformation syndromes, including Holt-Oram (MIM #142900), Okihiro Syndrome (MIM #607323), lacrimo-auriculo-digital (LADD) syndrome (MIM #149730), Fanconi anemia (MIM #227650) and thrombocytopenia-radial-aplasia (TAR) [MIM %274000]. The associated physical features enable the clinician to be more selective in the testing.

Family studies had established the "familial" nature of "isolated," non-syndromic heart defects, before the

TABLE 11-1 *Mutations associated with cardiovascular malformations*

	Gene		Clinical Features	Reference
1.	*CFC1*	member of EGF-CFC gene family	transposition of great arteries (TGA) and double outlet right ventricle (DORV)	(49, 50)
2.	*CRDLD1*	novel cell adhesion molecule	sporadic atrio-ventricular septal defects (AVSD)	(51)
3.	*FOG2*	encodes zinc finger protein expressed in early heart development	tetralogy of Fallot	(52)
4.	*GATA4*	transcription factor essential for heart formation	atrial septal defects	(53)
5.	*JAG1*	a Notch ligand expressed in developing right side of heart	tetralogy of Fallot	(54)
6.	*α-myosin heavy chain 6 (MHC6)*	structural protein expressed at high levels in developing atria	atrial septal defect	(55)
7.	*NKx2.5*	homeodomain containing transcription factor crucial in heart development	tetralogy of Fallot	(56)
8.	*ZIC3*	zinc finger transcription factor	X-linked heterotaxy	(57)

specific gene mutations have been delineated. The findings in families with two affected relatives have suggested that there were related heart defects which were more likely to occur in affected siblings (23, 24).

The families of infants with the hypoplastic left heart syndrome (HLHS) illustrate the fact that a spectrum of mild to severe related abnormalities can occur among the first degree relatives, that is siblings and parents. The heritability of HLHS has been estimated to be 99%, which suggests that its occurrence is determined primarily by genetic factors. For example, among 193 family members of 38 affected infants studied in Cincinnati (60), screening by echocardiography showed that 22% of siblings had a cardiovascular malformation (CVM) and 18% of 126 first degree relatives had a range of CVM, including bicuspid aortic valve in 10% and HLHS in 4 (2%). Studies of a few affected individuals have identified a few gene mutations, including *Connexin 43*, *NKX2.5* and *NOTCH-1* (61). However, it seems likely that most of the gene mutations which cause HLHS remain to be identified.

The examination of the parents and brothers and sisters of children with heart defects have established empiric risks of recurrence, which confirm that the risk of occurrence is much higher than the prevalence rate of cardiovascular anomalies in the general population. For example, the study of the subsequent pregnancies after the birth of the first infant with a heart defect in 1,743 families (1999-2002) showed that the overall rate of recurrence of heart defects was 3.8%. In another echocardiographic study of 6,640 consecutive pregnancies (1990-1999), the recurrence rate of congenital heart defects was 2.7% (62).

Older studies, using physical examination and not echocardiography, established the recurrence risk of heart defects in the siblings (Table 11-3) and offspring (Table 11-4) of children with congenital heart defects. It will be very helpful for pediatricians, cardiologists, clinical geneticists and genetic counselors to have these studies repeated using echocardiography. It would also be essential that the index cases be evaluated to identify those with a genetic syndrome, more of which are known now.

Environmental Factors

In the early years of pediatric cardiology, the leading clinicians, like Maude Abbott (6), apparently assumed that heart defects were caused primarily by environmental factors. The recognized environmental factors now include maternal conditions, intrauterine infections, and medications (Table 11-5). Unfortunately, most of the exposures during pregnancy have not been evaluated in a large enough number of pregnancies to establish the risk more specifically, including the rate of occurrence and which defects are more common.

Maternal diabetes is one exception, as several studies have evaluated the frequency of specific defects. For example, in the National Birth Defects Prevention Study (69), 91 of 3,519 infants with heart defects were born to women with pregestational diabetes mellitus. This analysis showed that heart defects were 5 times (OR 4.64; 2.87–7.71) more common among the infants of diabetic mothers. 11 of 16 isolated heart defects were significantly more common. One notable example was tetralogy of Fallot (OR 4.89; 2.18–10.95).

Twenty-eight (14%) of 204 infants born to women with phenylketonuria had heart defects, primarily tetralogy of Fallot, coarctation of the aorta, and hypoplastic left heart syndrome (70). There was a dose-response relationship between the maternal phenylalanine level and the occurrence of heart defects in the exposed fetuses.

For more general exposures like maternal obesity, there is a significant increase in cardiovascular anomalies (OR 1.3; 95CI 1.12-1.51), but no specific cardiovascular abnormalities have been identified (71).

Intrauterine infections are often considered a potential cause of a congenital heart malformation. However, very few large-scale studies of the frequency of heart defects have been conducted. One exception was congenital rubella, which was shown in severe epidemiologic studies to be associated with an increased frequency of heart defects, in general, and patent ductus arteriosus and stenosis of the pulmonary artery and its branches, in particular. These abnormalities correlated with rubella infections in the first 12 weeks of pregnancy, and not later, reflecting presumably noninflammatory damage to the endothelial cells lining blood vessels (72).

TABLE 11-3 *Recurrence risk in siblings of child with heart defect*

	Several Studies (63)		Sweden (64)
	(1966–1976)	(1976–1985)	(1981–1986)
aortic stenosis	2.1%	2.0%	
atrial septal defect	2.6%	2.9%	
ventricular septal defect	2.9%	4.3%	
septal defects			1.1% (95 CI*:0.1-4.0%)
pulmonary stenosis	2.1%	2.0%	
tetralogy of Fallot	2.5%	2.8%	
coarctation of aorta	1.9%	1.8%	0 (95 CI:0-14%)
truncus	1.2%		1.1
hypoplastic left heart syndrome	2.2%	2.3%	
endocardial cushion defect	2.9%		

Legend: *95 CI = 95% confidence interval

TABLE 11-4 *Recurrence risk in children of one parent with heart defect.*

	Affected Father (65)	Affected Mother (65)	Affected Mother (66)	Affected Mother (67)	Affected Father (67)	Affected Mother (68)	Affected Father (68)
aortic stenosis	2.8%	6.4%	26.1%	17%	8.2%		
atrial septal defect	2.6%	5.7%	10.9%	13.7%	7.1%		
ventricular septal defect	2.5%	7.6%	21.8%				
pulmonary stenosis	2.%	3.9%	19.4%				
patent ductus arteriosus			10.8%				
tetralogy of Fallot	2.2%	4.9%				4.5%	1.6%
coarctation of aorta	2.4%	3.6%		6.5%	8.5%		

TABLE 11-5 *Environmental factors associated with heart defects*

	Reference
Maternal conditions	
insulin-dependent diabetes	(69)
maternal phenylketonuria	(70)
obesity	(71)
cigarette smoking	
alcoholism	
Intrauterine infections	(72)
rubella	
cytomegalovirus	
Medications	
thalidomide	(73)
13 cis-retinoic acid	(74)
valproate	(75)
phenobarbital	(76)
Monozygotic twins with and without twin-twin transfusion	(43)

Exposure to isotretinoin (13-cis-retinoic acid) is much less common, but more teratogenic than any other potential exposure in pregnancy. In the first case series of 154 isotretinoin-exposed pregnancies, the high rate of occurrence of conotruncal heart defects was established (74).

Exposures to anticonvulsant drugs occur in about 0.4% of pregnant women. The most teratogenic exposures are valproate and phenobarbital as monotherapy or polytherapy. Heart defects have been identified (75, 76), but the sample sizes have not been large enough to identify specific heart defects associated with these exposures.

Prevention

A case-control study of the fetal effects of periconceptional multivitamin use by pregnant women in Atlanta (1968–1980) showed a reduced risk for nonsyndromic heart defects in their infants (odds ratio 0.76; 95% confidence interval 0.60, 0.97) [77]. The reduced risks were strongest for outflow tract defects and ventricular septal defects. Subsequent studies have shown that elevated levels of homocysteine in the pregnant woman is a risk factor for the occurrence of heart defects in their infants (78). However, the presence of polymorphisms C677T and A1298C in the enzyme 5, 10-methylenetetrahydrofolate reductase (MTHFR) in the mothers and infants has not been associated with the occurrence of heart defects.

Treatment and Prognosis

The evaluations at birth lead to the decisions about medical treatment, further diagnostic studies, and the option of surgical repair. The timing and choices in surgery are based on the specific findings in each infant (79).

One promising new development is an aortic valvuloplasty late in the second trimester to promote growth and development of the left ventricle and to prevent the development of a hypoplastic left ventricle, as in hypoplastic left heart syndrome (80).

Genetic Counseling

As with each common malformation, the clinician's first question is to determine whether the congenital heart defect is an "isolated" abnormality or one of several malformations.

For the infant with multiple anomalies, there are features of a specific or recognizable syndrome. For those infants chromosome analysis has been the first diagnostic test to be carried out. The additional screening by fluorescent in situ hybridization (FISH) will be needed to identify deletions, such as 22q11.2, 1p36, and 7q11.2, associated with heart defects. It seems likely that additional deletions will be identified as microarray analysis is carried out on infants with heart defects, especially those with multiple anomalies.

The review of the pregnancy history will identify potentially relevant exposures.

In developed countries in which prenatal screening by ultrasound is common, this discussion of the occurrence of a heart malformation occurs during pregnancy. Experience has shown the value of repeating the studies of the infant's heart postpartum to confirm and clarify the specific pattern of abnormalities (81).

After the health status of the affected infant has been stabilized, the discussion will shift to the rate of occurrence of the same heart defect in subsequent pregnancies. The overall rate was shown to be 2.7% (62) and 3.8% (47) in two studies. Clinical examinations of affected infants and their brothers, sisters and parents, many years ago (63–68), established the empiric risks of recurrence for specific heart defects (Tables 11-3 and 11-4).

In planning for the next pregnancy, the use, before conception, of a multi-vitamin supplement that contains folic acid should be recommended.

An option to discuss is whether the at-risk fetus should be evaluated by ultrasound in the fetal survey or by the more detailed fetal echocardiography. This technology has improved significantly over the 1980s and 1990s, and further improvements are expected. However, the experience of the sonologist remains essential to successful prenatal detection of a heart defect (81).

REFERENCES

I. Books/Reviews

1. Ferencz C, Loffredo CA, Correa-Villaseñor A, Wilson PD. *Genetics and Environmental Risk Factors of Major Cardiovascular Malformations: The Baltimore-Washington Infant Study: 1981–1989. Perspectives in Pediatric Cardiology.* Vol. 5. Amark, NY: Futura Publishing Company, Inc.; 1997.
2. Lin A, Pierpont ME, eds. Heart development and the genetic aspects of cardiovascular malformations. Seminars in medical genetics. *Amer J Med Genet.* 2001;97:235–325.
3. Pierpont ME, Basson CT, Benson DW Jr, Gelb BD, Giglia TM, Goldmuntz E, et al. Genetic basis for congenital heart defects: current knowledge. *Circulation.* 2007;115:1–24.
4. Mullins CE, Mayer DC. *Congenital Heart Disease: A Diagrammatic Atlas.* New York: Wiley-Liss; 1988.
5. *Pediatric Cardiology Teaching Materials.* Atlanta: Pritchett & Hull Associates, Inc.; 2003.

II. Websites

www.cincinnatichildrens.org/health/heart-encyclopedia/anomalies/htm
www.fetalecho.com
www.kumc.org
www.mayoclinic.com
www.nemours.org

III. Articles

6. Ferrencz C. Origin of congenital heart disease: reflections on Maude Abbott's work. *Can J Cardiol.* 1989;5:4–9.
7. Blalock A, Taussig HB. The surgical treatment of malformations of the heart in which there is pulmonary stenosis or pulmonary atresia. *JAMA.* 1945;251:2123–2138.
8. Mayberry JC, Scott WA, Goldberg SJ. Increased birth prevalence of cardiac defects in Yuma, Arizona. *J Am Coll Cardiol.* 1992;16:1696–1700.
9. Allan L. Prenatal diagnosis of structural cardiac defects. *Am J Med Genet Part C (Seminar in Medical Genetics).* 2007;145C:73–76.
10. Bull C. Current and potential impact of fetal diagnosis on prevalence and spectrum of serious congenital heart disease at term in UK British Paediatric Cardiac Association. *Lancet.* 1999;356:2142–2147.
11. Tworetsky W, Wilkins-Haug L, Jennings RW, Van der Velde ME, Marshall AC, Marx GR et al. Balloon dilation of severe aortic stenosis in the fetus. Potential for Prevention of Hypoplastic Left Heart Syndrome Candidate Selection, Technique, and results of Successful Intervention. *Circulation.* 2004;110:2125–2131.
12. Wren C, Birrell G, Hawthorne G. Cardiovascular malformations in infants of diabetic mothers. *Heat.* 2003;89:1217–1220.
13. Basson CT, Bachinsky DR, Lin RC, Levi T, Elkins JA Soults J et al. Mutations in human TBX5 cause limb and cardiac malformation in Holt-Oram Syndrome. *Nat Genet.* 1997;15:30–35.
14. Botto L, Mulinare J, Erickson JD. Occurrence of congenital heart defects in relation to maternal multivitamin use. *Am J Epiderm.* 2000;151:878–884.
15. Glen S, Burns J, Bloomfield P. Prevalence and development of additional cardiac abnormalities in 1498 patients with congenital ventricular septal defects. *Heart.* 2004;90:1321–1325.
16. Greenwood RD, Rosenthal A, Parisi L, Fyler DC, Nadas AS. Extra cardiac abnormalities in infants with congenital heart disease. *Pediatrics.* 1975;55:485–492.
17. Ferencz C, Rubin JD, McCarter RJ, Boughman JA, Wilson PD, Brenner JI et al. Cardiac and noncardiac malformations: observations in a populations-based study. *Teratology.* 1987;35:367–378.
18. Miller SP, McQuillen PS, Hamrick S, Xu D, Glidden DV, Charlton N et al. Abnormal brain development in newborns with congenital heart disease. *N Engl J Med.* 2007;357:1928–1938.
19. Towbin JA, Belmont J. Molecular determinants of left and right outflow tract obstruction. *Am J Med Genet (Semin Med Genet).* 2000;97:297–303.
20. Andelfinger G. Genetic factors in congenital heart malformation. *Clin Genet.* 2008;73:516–527.
21. Kirby ML, Waldo KL. Neural crest and cardiovascular patterning. *Circ Res.* 1995;77:211–215.
22. Clark EB, Hu N. Developmental hemodynamic changes in the chick embryo from stage 18 to 27. *Circ Res.* 1982;51:810–815.
23. Fraser FC, Hunter AD. Etiologic relations among categories of congenital heart malformations. *Am J Cardiol.* 1975;36:793–796.
24. Corone P, Bonaciti C, Feingold J, Fromont S, Berthet-Bondet D. Familial congenital heart disease: How are the various types related? *Am J Cardiol.* 1983;51:942–945.
25. Gill HK, Splitt M, Sharland GK, Simpson JM. Patterns of recurrence of congenital heart disease. *J Am Coll Cardiol.* 2003;42:923–929.
26. Van Mierop HS, Patterson DF, Schwam WR. Hereditary conotruncal septal defects in Keeshond dogs: embryologic studies. *Am J Cardiol.* 1977;40:936–949.
27. Van Praagh R, Van Praagh S. Embryoligic et anatomie: clés pour le compréhansion des cardiopathies congénitales comlexes. *Cœur.* 1982;13:285–291.
28. Shaw GM, Iovannisci DM, Yang W, Finnell RH, Carmichael SL, Cheng S, Lammer EJ. Risks of human conotruncal heart defects associated with 32 single nucleotide polymorphisms of selected cardiovascular disease-related genes. *Am J Med Genet.* 2005;138A:21–26.

29. Ferencz C. The etiology of congenital cardiovascular malformations: Observations on genetic risks with implications for further birth defects research. *J Medicine*. 1985;16:497–508.

30. Khoury MJ, Waters GD, Martin ML, Edmonds LD. Are offspring of women with hereditary disorders of increased risk of congenital cardiovascular malformations? *Genetic Epidemiol*. 1991;8:417–423.

31. Semba R. Cardiovascular malformations found in 1286 externally normal human embryos alive in utero. *Teratology*. 1976; 13:341–344.

32. Ursell PC, Byrne JM, Strobino BA. Significance of cardiac defects in the developing fetus: a study of spontaneous abortions. *Circulation*. 1985;72: 1232–1236.

33. Chinn A, Fitzsimmons J, Shepard TH, Fantel AG. Congenital heart disease among spontaneous abortions and stillborn fetuses: prevalence and associations. *Teratology*. 1989;40: 475–482.

34. Hoffman JIE, Christianson R. Congenital heart disease in a cohort of 19,502 births with long-term follow-up. *Am J Cardiol*. 1978;42: 641–647.

35. Mitchell SC, Korones SB, Berendes HW. Congenital heart disease in 56,109 births: incidence and natural history. *Circulation*. 1971; 43: 323–332.

36. Ferencz C, Rubin JD, McCarter RJ, Brennen JI, Neill CA, Perry LW, Hepner SI, Downing JW. Congenital heart disease: prevalence at livebirth. The Baltimore-Washington Infant Study. *Am J Epiderm*. 1985;14:31–36.

37. Ferencz C. On the birth prevalence of congenital heart disease. *J Am Coll Cardiol*. 1990;16:1701–1702.

38. Cook D, Izakawa T, Rowe RD. An epidemic of ventricular septal defects. *Lancet*. 1980;1:1297–1298.

39. Rothman KJ, Fyler DC. Seasonal occurrence of complex ventricular septal defect. *Lancet*. 1974;ii:194–197.

40. Meberg A, Otterstad E, Froland G, Sorland S, Nitter-Hauge S. Increasing incidence of ventricular septal defects caused by improved detection rate. *Acta Paediatc*. 1994;83:653–657.

41. Rojuin N, Du Z-D, Barak M, Nasser N, Hershkowirz S, Milgram E. High prevalence of muscular ventricular septal defect in neonates. *J Am Coll Cardiol*. 1995;26:1545–1548.

42. Lin AR, Herring AM, Amstatz KS, Westgate M-N, Lacro RV, AL-Jufan M, Ryan L, Holmes LB. Cardiovascular malformations: changes in prevalence and birth status, 1972–1990. *Am J Med Genet*. 1999;84:102–110.

43. Mastroiacovo P, Castilla EE, Arpino C, botting B, Cocchi G, Goujard J et al. Congenital malformations in twins: an international study. *Am J Med Genet*. 1999;83:117–124.

44. Bahtiyar MO, Dulay AT, Weeks BP, Friedman AH, Copel JA. Prevalence of congenital heart defects in monochorionic/diamniotic twin gestations: a systematic literature review. *J Ultrasound Med*. 2007;26:1491–1498.

45. Nora JJ, Gilliland JC, Sommerville RJ, McNamara DG. Congenital heart disease in twins. *N Engl J Med*. 1967;277: 568–571.

46. Anderson RC. Congenital cardiac malformations in 109 sets of twins and triplets. *Am J Cardiol*. 1977;39:1045–1050.

47. Caputo S, Russo MG, Capozzi G, Morelli C, Argiento P, Di Salvo G et al. Congenital heart disease in a population of dizygotic twins: an echocardiographic study. *Internat J Cardiol*. 2005;102:293–296.

48. Schott JJ, Benson DW, Basson CT, Pease W, Silberbach GM, Moak JP et al. Congenital heart disease caused by mutations in the transcription factor NKX2-5. *Science*. 1998;281:108–111.

49. Goldmuntz E, Bamford R, Karkera JD, de la Cruz J, Roessler, Muenke M. CFC1 mutations in patients with transposition of the great arteries and double-outlet-right ventricle. *Am J Hum Genet*. 2002;70:776–780.

50. Shen MM, Schier AF. The EGF-CFC gene family in vertebrate development. *Trends Genet*. 2000;16:303–309.

51. Robinson SW, Morris CD, Goldmuntz E, Reller MD, Jones MA, Steiner RD Maslen CL. Missense mutations in *CRELD1* are associated with cardiac atrioventricular septal defects. *Am J Hum Genet*. 2003;72:1047–1052.

52. Pizzuti A, Sarkozy A, Newton AL, Conti E, Flex E, Digilio MC et al. Mutations of ZFPM2/FOG2 gene in sporadic cases of tetralogy of Fallot. *Hum Mut*. 2003;22:372–377.

53. Garg V, Kathiriya IS, Barnes R, Schuterman MK, King IN, Butler CA et al. GATA4 mutations cause human congenital heart defects and reveal an interaction with TBX5. *Nature*. 2003;424: 443–447.

54. Eldadah ZA, Hamosh A, Biery NJ, Montgomery RA, Duke M, Elkins R, Dietz HC. Familial tetralogy of Fallot caused by mutation in the jagged1 gene. *Hum Mol Genet*. 2001;10: 163–169.

55. Ching Y-H, Ghosh TK, Cross SJ, Packham EA, Honeyman L, Loughna S et al. Mutation in myosin heavy chain 6 causes atrial septal defect. *Nature Genetics*. 2005;4:423–428.

56. Goldmuntz E, Geiger E, Benson DW. NKx2.5 mutations in patients with tetralogy of Fallot. *Circulation*. 2001;104: 2565–2568.

57. Ware SM, Peng J, Zhu L, Fernbach S, Colicos S, Casey B, Towbin, Belmont JW. Identification and functional analysis of ZIC3 mutations in heterotaxy and related congenital heart defects. *Am J Hum Genet*. 2004;74:93–105.

58. McDermott DA, Bressan MC, He J, Lee JS, Aftimos S, Brueckner M et al. TBX5 genetic testing validates strict clinical criteria for Holt-Oram Syndrome. *Pediatr Res*. 2005;58:981–986.

59. Sarkozy A, Obregon MG, Conti E, Esposito G, Mingarelli R, Pizzuti A et al. A novel PTPN11 gene mutation bridges Noonan syndrome, multiple lentigines/LEOPARD syndrome and Noonan-like/multiple giant cell lesion syndrome. *Eur J Hum Genet*. 2004; 12:1069–1072.

60. Hinton RB Jr, Martin LJ, Tabangin ME, Mazwi ML, Cripe LH, Benson DW. Hypoplastic left heart syndrome is heritable. *J Am Coll Cardiol*. 2007;50:1590–1595.

61. Grossfeld PD. Hypoplastic left heart syndrome. It is all in the genes. *J Am Coll Cardiol*. 2007;50:1596–1597.

62. Gill HK, Splitt M, Sharland GK, Simpson JM. Patterns of recurrence of congenital heart disease. *J Am Coll Cardiol*. 2003;42: 923–929.

63. Nora JJ, Nora AH. Update on counseling the family with a first degree relative with a congenital heart defect. *Am J Med Genet*. 1988;29:137–142.

64. Pradat P. Recurrence risk for major congenital heart defects in Sweden: a registry study. *Genetic Epidemiol*. 1994;11:131–140.

65. Nora JJ, Nora AH. Maternal transmission of congenital heart diseases: new recurrence risk figures and the questions of cytoplasmic inheritance and vulnerability to teratogens. *Am J Cardiol*. 1987;59:459–463.

66. Whittemore R, Hobbins JC, Eagle MA. Pregnancy and its outcome in women with and without surgical treatment of congenital heart disease. *Am J Cardiol*. 1983;50:641–651.

67. Rose V, Gold RJM, Lindsay G, Allen M. A possible increase in the incidence of congenital heart defects among the offspring of affected parents. *J Am Coll Cardiol*. 1985;6:376–382.

68. Burn J, Brennan P, Little J, Holloway S, Coffey R, Somerville J et al. Recurrence risks in offspring of adults with major heart defects: results from first cohort of British collaborative study. *Lancet*. 1998;351:311–316.

69. Correa A, Gilboa SM, Besser LM, Botto LD, Moore CA, Hobbs CA et al. Diabetes mellitus and birth defects. *Am J Obstet Gynecol*. 2008;199:237.e1–9.

70. Rouse B, Azen C, Koch R, Matalon R, Hanley W, de la Cruz F et al. Maternal Phenylketonuria Collaborative Study (MPKUCS) Offspring: facial anomalies, malformations, and early neurological sequelae. *Am J Med Genet*. 1997;69:89–95.

71. Stothard KJ, Tennant PWG, Bell R, Rankin J. Maternal over-weight and obesity and the risk of congenital anomalies. A systematic review and meta-analysis. *JAMA.* 2009;301:636–650.

72. Webster WS. Teratogen Update: congenital rubella. *Teratology.* 1998;58:13–23.

73. Newman CGH. Teratogen Update: Clinical aspects of thalidomide embryopathy – a continuing preoccupation. *Teratology.* 1985;32:133–144.

74. Lammer EJ, Chen DT, Hoar RM, Agnish ND, Benke PJ, Braun JT et al. Retinoic acid embryopathy. *N Engl J Med.* 1985; 313:837–841.

75. Wyszynski DF, Nambisan M, Surve T, Alsdorf RM, Smith CR, Holmes LB. Increased rate of major malformations in offspring exposed to valproate during pregnancy. *Neurology.* 2005;64: 961–965.

76. Holmes LB, Wyszynski DF, Lieberman E. The AED (antiepileptic drug) Pregnancy Registry: a 6-year experience. *Arch Neurol.* 2004;61:673–678.

77. Botto LD, Mulinare J, Erickson JD. Occurrence of congenital heart defects in relation to maternal multivitamin use. *Am J Epidem.* 2000;151:878–884.

78. Verkleij-Hagoort A, Bliek J, Sayed-Tabatabaci F, Ursem N, Steegers E, Steegers-Theunissen R. Hyperhomocysteinemia and MTHFR polymorphisms in association with orofacial cleafts and congenital heart defects: a meta-analysis. *Am J Med Genet Part A.* 2007;143A:952–960.

79. Jones RA, Di Nardo J, Laussen PC, Howe R, La Pierre R, Matte G. *Comprehensive Surgical Management of Congenital Heart Disease.* London: Arnold Publishing; 2004.

80. Selamet Tierney ES, Wald RM, McElhinney DB, Marshall AC, Benson CB, Colan SD, Marons EN, Marx GR, Levine JC, Wilkins-Haug, Lock JE, Tworetsky W. Changes in left heart hemodynamics after technically successful *in utero* aortic valvuloplasty. *Ultrasound Obstet Gynecol.* 2007;30:715–720.

81. Allan L. Prenatal diagnosis of structural cardiac defects. *Am J Med Genet Part C (Seminars in Medical Genetics).* 2007;145C: 73–76.

Chapter 12

Hip Dysplasia

Definition

An abnormal development of the hip, including the acetabulum, which may cause the hip to be dislocated or subluxated. (This diagnosis replaces the term "congenital dislocation of the hip.")

ICD-9:	754.300	(congenital dislocation of hip)
ICD-10:	Q65.0 (unilateral)	(congenital dislocation of hip, unilateral)
	Q65.1 (bilateral)	(congenital dislocation of hip, bilateral)
	Q65.2 (unspecified)	(congenital dislocation of hip, unspecified)
Mendelian Inheritance in Man:	%142700	(acetabular dysplasia; includes congenital dislocation of developmental dysplasia of the hip)

Appearance

Developmental dysplasia of the hip (DDH) usually occurs in an infant with no other medical problems. The dislocation of the hip may occur during pregnancy, at birth, or after birth (1). (Figure 12-1)

The signs of unilateral dislocation of the hip are asymmetry of thigh creases, leg lengths, and ranges of motion. The Ortolani and Barlow maneuvers are used to evaluate the stability of the hip in the newborn and to reproduce the dislocation or subluxation. Ortolani described the sound of the "clunk" when the head of the femur slides over the posterior rim of the acetabulum and into the socket; this is also called the "sign of entry." In the Barlow maneuver, the "sound of exit," the leg is adducted, and with gentle pressure the head of the

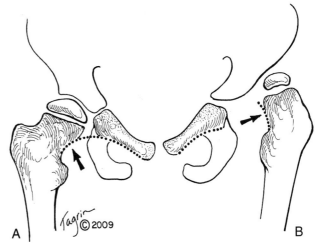

FIGURE 12.1 Shows normal hip on right (A) and dislocated hip on left (B).

femur slides over the posterior rim of the acetabulum out of the hip socket. The laxity of joint capsule decreases over the first weeks of life. As the laxity decreases, the "clunks" heard in either entry or exit from the hip socket disappear.

Since much of the head of the femur and the pelvis are cartilaginous at birth, it is difficult to determine the relationship between the head of the femur and the acetabulum in radiographs of newborn infants. In the older infant (6 to 12 months), with more ossification, the normal development of the acetabulum can be outlined or the presence of dislocation confirmed. (Figure 12-1)

Since the 1980s, ultrasound has been recommended and has been used to screen for dislocation or subluxation, by visualizing the Barlow and Ortolani maneuvers on the ultrasound screen. The sonography measures the thickening of the acetabular cartilage and the angle of the femur relative to the labium. Routine screening of all newborns has been recommended. While ultra-sound has been very helpful in confirming clinical diagnoses, the screening of newborns by ultrasound has produced a high frequency of false positive results and a higher rate of treatment of presumed congenital dislocation of the hips (3). Nevertheless, systematic comparisons have shown that ultrasound is a more sensitive indicator of an abnormality of the hip than radiography (4). The cost of a screening program is offset by a reduction in the money spent treating surgically affected infants diagnosed at an older age (5). The net effect of mass screening is that more children, many of whom are normal, require follow up until age 4 to 6 months when dysplasia of the acetabulum can be determined with radiographs (6). Unfortunately, even with newborn screening with ultrasound, dislo-cated hips continue to be diagnosed later in infancy.

Associated Malformations

Hip dysplasia or developmental dysplasia of the hip is associated with a higher frequency of torticollis and metatarsus adductus (1). In some studies (7, 8), the infants with torticollis and metatarsus adductus have had an increased frequency of congenital dislocation of the hip. However, in the evaluation of 349 children with idiopathic club feet followed an average of 8.4 years, the overall rate of hip dysplasia was less than 1% (9).

Developmental dysplasia of the hip is also a feature of the Legg-Perthes Disease (MIM: #150600), which is due to a vascular necrosis of the femoral head (10). This hip dysplasia becomes apparent in childhood; boys are affected more frequently than girls. This disorder is attributed to multifactorial inheritance, with a recur-rence risk of 2.6% in a sib of an affected infant (11).

An autosomal dominant familial hip dysplasia has also been identified (12).

Developmental dysplasia of the hip occurs also as a component of many skeletal dysplasias and monogenic disorders.

Developmental Defect

It has been postulated (11, 13) that dysplasia of the acetabulum and laxity of the joints are two abnormali-ties that lead to congenital dislocation of the hip. Carter and Wilkinson (13) postulated two genetic mechanisms were involved: a polygenic model of the hip dysplasia and autosomal dominant inheritance of laxity of the capsule around the hip joint. Wynne-Davies (14) in her own family studies confirmed this model.

The hip joint is first visible at eight weeks gestation, when a cleft is present between the acetabulum and the femoral head. The development has been considered complete by 11 weeks of gestation (15).

Anatomic studies have shown that the newborn infant is particularly vulnerable to dislocation of the hip. At birth, the acetabulum is more shallow than it is either earlier in fetal development (16) or later in child-hood (17, 18). Anatomic dissections have been carried out in affected newborn infants, who had died soon after birth, by two experienced individuals, Ignacio Ponseti in Iowa City, Iowa (18), and Peter Dunn in Bristol, England (19). Anatomic changes were identi-fied in the acetabular cartilage. The anatomic changes correlated with the clinical severity of the congenital hip dislocation.

Developmental orthopedic diseases, including develop-mental dysplasia of the hip, are common in several breeds of dogs (20). Factors identified in canine dyspla-sia have included joint laxity, abnormal pelvic muscles, and delayed ossification of the head of the femur (21).

Prevalence

It has been difficult to establish the prevalence of develop-mental dysplasia of the hip in specific populations because of variations in the methods and definitions used, as well as the training and experience of the examiners.

Race/Ethnicity

Among Caucasian infants in the United States the range of the prevalence rate has been 0.6 to 1.5 per 1,000 (22). Higher rates have been observed in Sweden [3.5/1,000] (23) and Israel [2.5/1,000] (24). In a recent study of 34,048 newborn infants evaluated clinically and sonographically (25), there were notable differences in prevalence rates: 5.5% of the Israeli population and 1.2% of Ethiopian Jews showed hip dysplasia by ultra-sound. The presence of congenital dislocation of the hip among Arabs and other Jews was 0.5% compared to 0.2% of Ethiopians.

The Bantus tribes in Africa (26) have a very low rate of occurrence of congenital dysplasia of the hip. Among the Cree-Ojibwa population the rate was 0.75/1,000 (27). However, these Native Americans also use the method of cradling newborn infants, which could increase the fre-quency of congenital dislocation of the hip.

Among the population in the United States and Canada, the prevalence rates among African Americans and Native Americans (28) is much lower than among Caucasians. Chinese also have a low prevalence rate (0.12/1,000) [29], whereas the rate among the Maori Polynesians is among the highest prevalence rates (2.55/1,000) [30].

Birth Status

"Isolated" developmental dysplasia of the hip has not been associated with an increased frequency of prema-turity or stillbirth.

Sex Ratio

Many more females than males are affected. In a series of 171 pedigrees derived from all affected individuals treated at a medical center in Italy (31), there were 499 individuals with developmental dysplasia of the hip (DDH). The sex ratio was F:M = 7.6:1.

Sidedness

The left hip is affected more frequently than the right. When DDH is bilateral, the left hip is more severely affected than the right (31). One explanation for the predilection for the left hip was the fact that the left leg was lying posteriorly in utero and that this leg was much more likely to be dislocated than the leg lying anteriorly (30).

Parental Age

A higher frequency among newborn infants of young mothers, ages 20 to 24, was noted in a study of 500 affected infants in Utah (32).

Twinning

In one study of 138 twin pairs the concordance rates were 3.4% among 29 monozygous twins and 2.8% among 109 sets of nonidentical fraternal twin pairs (33).

Genetic Factors

The familial nature of DDH has been established in several populations: females are affected more often than males; if a son is affected, the risk of recurrence in the next child is much higher than when a daughter is affected (Table 12-1).

If the index case has bilateral hip dysplasia, the risk of recurrence is higher than when the dysplasia is unilateral. These are characteristics of the process of multifactorial inheritance (13, 14, 34). However, complex segregation analysis has suggested a two-gene locus model in a sample of 171 pedigrees of families with affected individuals identified at a medical center in Italy (31), as well as in Utah (32).

Empiric recurrence risks have been established for first- and second-degree relatives (Table 12-1). Consistent with the model of multifactorial inheritance, the mothers of affected children and the fathers of affected boys (but not girls) had a more shallow acetabulum in radiographs than was found in controls.

Potential confounders in the evaluation of an affected infant are the co-incidence of either a hereditary hypermobility of the hip joint, or dysplasia of the acetabulum (35). In a study of 125 children with "ligamentous laxity" or joint hypermobility, 12% had had hip "clicks" at birth and 4% had congenital dislocatable hips. The features included some associated with the Ehlers-Danlos Syndrome and the Marfan Syndrome. Primary dysplasia of the acetabulum, not associated with dislocation of the hip, has been identified as a familial disorder (35).

Associated biomarkers, such as polymorphisms of type II collagen and vitamin D receptors (36), have not been identified yet in family studies of developmental hip dysplasia. However, the COL2A mutation in collagen has been associated with the Legg-Perthes Disease, a separate disorder associated with a vascular necrosis of the head of the femur (10).

Environmental Factors

The best-known nongenetic cause of developmental dysplasia of the hip is the breech presentation of the fetus in utero (37).

TABLE 12-1 *Empiric recurrence risk for Developmental dysplasia of the hip*

| | Index Cases | Rate of recurrence among first degree relatives | | | | |
		Total	Brothers	Sisters	Fathers	Mothers
A.	Utah (32): Females (n=236)	3.2%	1.8	6.3	0.8	2.5
	Males (n=54)	4.0%	6.3	5.7	0.0	1.9
B.	Edinburgh and Glasgow, Scotland (14): Females (n=147)	5.2%	2.3	25.6	0.0	1.4
	Males (n=45)	5.3%	5.6	20.0	0.0	2.2
C.	Budapest, Hungary (44): Females (n=1345)	4.7%	6.9	19.9	0.7	3.4
	Males (n=422)	6.1%	16.0	16.0	1.7	4.7
				Sibs		
D.	Oslo, Norway (34): Females (n=896)	3.3%		5.7	0.1	2.9
	Males (n=251)	4.4%		7.1	0.4	5.1

The susceptibility of the female fetus to maternal estrogens is a factor in the higher frequency of affected infant girls than boys. There is a higher frequency of DDH among firstborn infants than in subsequent births. Seasonality in the occurrence of DDH has also been noted (24).

Treatment and Prognosis

While screening for DDH by ultrasound in newborn infants has been recommended, it has also been noted that this screening has not decreased the frequency of congenital dysplasia of the hip (38). Furthermore, there are dangerous potential complications of the treatment, for example, the treatment of the DDH has been associated with avascular necrosis, which has been attributed to continuous compression of the cartilage between the femoral head and the acetabulum with the use of the Pavlik harness (39).

Based on the findings in the two randomized trials (40, 41), it was recommended that ultrasound screening focus on infants with clinical hip instability or with recognized risk factors, rather than universal screening (42).

The skill of the examiner is a crucial factor in early diagnosis. Even without screening by sonography in newborn infants, Hadlow and his associates showed over a 21-year period in New Zealand that the occurrence of congenital dislocation of the hip could be prevented in 90% of the affected infants with a careful, systematic approach (43).

Genetic Counseling

As with all other common malformations, the first step is to be certain that the affected infant has isolated developmental dysplasia of the hip and not an associated skeletal dysplasia or familial hypermobility.

The focus of the parents will be on the best treatment of the hip abnormality. Detailed follow-up is needed to ensure good treatment and to make certain avascular neurosis has not occurred. For subsequent discussions of genetic risk, empiric recurrence risk estimates are available, but only for Caucasians (Table 12-1) (14, 32, 34, 44).

Prenatal screening by ultrasonography has not shown to be useful or accurate. A careful evaluation at birth and subsequently of the newborn is essential to determining whether or not a newborn infant is affected.

REFERENCES

1. Aronsson DD, Goldberg MJ, Kling Jr TF, Roy DR. Developmental dysplasia of the hip. *Pediatrics.* 1994;94:201–208.
2. Soboleski DA, Babya P. Sonographic diagnosis of developmental dysplasia of the hip: importance of increased thickness of acetabular cartilage. *AJR.* 1993;161:839–842.
3. Yousefzadeh DH, Ramilo JL. Normal hip in children: correlation of US with anatomic and cryomicrotome sections. *Radiology.* 1987;165:647–655.
4. McEvoy A, Paton RW. Ultrasound compared with radiographic assessment in developmental dysplasia of the hip. *JR Coll Surg Edinb.* 1997;42:254–255.
5. Gray A, Elbouane D, Dezateux C, King A, Quinn A, Gardner F. Economic evaluation of ultrasonography in the diagnosis and management of developmental hip dysplasia in the United Kingdom and Ireland. *J Bone Jt Surg.* 2005;87-A:2472–2479.
6. O'Riordan C, Condon F, Conhyea D, Kaliszer M, O'Brien T. The role of ultrasound screening in hip dysplasia. *Irish Med J.* 2005; 98:147–149.
7. Iwahara T, Ikeda A. The ipsilateral involvement of congenital muscular torticollis and congenital dislocation of the hip. *JP Orthop Assoc.* 1962;35:1221.
8. Jacobs JE. Metatarsus varus and hip dysplasia. *Clin Orthop.* 1960;16:203–213.
9. Westberry DE, Davids JR, Pugh LI. Club foot and developmental dysplasia of the hip: value of screening hip radiographs in children with club foot. *J Pediatr Orthop.* 2003;23:503–507.
10. Miyamoto Y, Matsuda T, Kitoh H, Haga N, Obashi H, Nishimura G, Ikegawa S. A recurrent mutation in type II collagen gene causes Legg-Calve-Perthes disease in a Japanese family. *Hum Genet.* 2007;121:625–629.
11. Hall DJ. Genetic aspects of Perthes' disease: a critical review. *Clin Orthop.* 1986;209:100–114.
12. Cilliers HJ, Beighton P. Beukes familial hip dysplasia: an autosomal dominant entity. *Am J Med Genet.* 1990;36:386–390.
13. Carter CO, Wilkinson JA. Genetic and environmental factors in the aetiology of congenital dislocation of the hip. *Clin Orthop Rel Res.* 1964;33:119–128.
14. Wynne-Davies R. A family study of neonatal and late-diagnosis congenital dislocation of the hip. *J Med Genet.* 1970;315–333.
15. Watanabe RS. Embryology of the human hip. *Clin Orthop.* 1974;98:8–26.
16. Morville P. On the anatomy and pathology of the hip joint. *Acta Orthop Scand.* 1936;7:107–144.
17. Ralis Z, McKibbin B. Changes in the shape of the human hip joint during its development and their relation to its stability. *J Bon Jt Surg Br.* 1973;55:780–785.
18. Ponseti, IV. Morphology of the acetabulum in congenital dislocation of the hip. *J Bone Jt Surg.* 1978;60A:586–599.
19. Dunn PM. The anatomy and pathology of congenital dislocation of the hip. *Clin Orthopaedics.* 1976;119:23–27.
20. LaFond E, Breur GJ, Austin CC. Breed susceptibility for developmental orthopedic diseases in dogs. *J Am Anim Hosp Assoc.* 2002;38:467–477.
21. Morich K, Ohlerth S, reist M, Lang J, Riitano M, Schawalder P, Spreng D. Correlation of urinary nitric oxide concentrations with the development of hip dysplasia in Labrador retrievers. *The Veterinary Record.* 2003;153:423–427.
22. Harris LE, Stayura LA, Ramirez-Talavera PF, Annegers JF. Congenital and acquired abnormalities observed in live-born and stillborn neonates. *Mayo Clin Proc.* 1975;50:85–90.
23. Beckman L, Lemperg R. Normstrom: Congenital dislocation of the hip joint in Northern Sweden. *Clin Genet.* 1977;11: 151–153.
24. Chen R, Weissman, SL, Salama R, Klingberg MA. Congenital dislocation of the hip (CDH) and seasonality: the gestational age of vulnerability to some seasonal factor. *Amer J Epidem.* 1970; 92:287–293.
25. Eidelman M, Chezar A, Bialik V. Developmental dysplasia of the hip: incidence in Ethiopian Jews revisited: 7-year prospective study. *J Pediatr Orthop B.* 2002;11:290–292.
26. Roper A. Hip dysplasia in the African Bantu. *J. Bone Jt Surg.* 1997;58-B:155–158.

27. Walker JM. Congenital hip disease in a Cree-Ojibwa population: a retrospective study. *CMA Journal.* 1997;116:501–504.

28. Niswander JD, Barrow MV, Bingle GJ. Congenital malformations in the American Indian. *Social Biology.* 1975;22:203–215.

29. Emanuel I, Huang SW, Gutman LT, Yu FC, Lin CC. The incidence of congenital malformations in a Chinese population: the Taipei collaborative study. *Teratology.* 1972;5:159–170.

30. Howie RN, Phillips LI. Congenital malformations in the newborn: a survey of the National Women's Hospital 1964–1967. *NZ Med J.* 1970;71:65–71.

31. Sollazzo V, Bertolani G, Calzolari E, Atti G, Scapoli C. A two-locus model for non-syndromic congenital dysplasia of the hip (CDH). *An Hum Genet.* 2000;64:51–59.

32. Woolf CM, Koehn JG, Coleman SS. Congenital hip disease in Utah: The influence of genetic and non-genetic factors. *Amer J Hum Genet.* 1968;20:430–439.

33. Idelberger K. *Die Erbpathologie der sogenannten angeborenen Hüftverrenkung.* Munich and Berlin: Urban an Schwarzenberg; 1951.

34. Bjerkreim I, van der Hagen CB. Congenital dislocation of the hip joint in Norway. *Clin Genet.* 1974;5:433–448.

35. Beals RK. Familial primary acetabular dysplasia and dislocation of the hip. *Clin Orthop Relat Res.* 2003;406:109–115.

36. Granchi D, Stea S, Sudanese A, Toni A, Baldini N, Giuntia A. Association of two gene polymorphisms with osteoarthritis secondary to hip dysplasia. *Clini Orthop Relat Res.* 2002;403:108–117.

37. Dunn PM. Perinatal observations on the etiology of congenital dislocation of the hip. *Clin Orthopaedics.* 1976;119:11–22.

38. Morrisy RT, Cowie GH. Congenital dislocation of the hip. Early detection and prevention of the late complications. *Clin Orthop.* 1987;222:79–84.

39. Suzaki S, Yamamuro T. Avascular necrosis in patients treated with the Pavlik harness for congenital dislocation of the hip. *J Bone Jt Surg.* 1990;72-A:1048–1055.

40. Rosendahl K, Markestad T, Lie RT. Ultrasound screening for developmental dysplasia of the hip in the neonak: the effect on treatment rate and prevalence of late cases of late cases. *Pediatrics.* 1994;94:47–52.

41. Holen KJ, Tegnander A, Bredland T, Johansen OJ, Saether OD, Eik-Ness SH. Universal or selective screening of the neonatal hip using ultrasound? A prospective, randomised trial of 15,529 newborn infants. *J Bone Joint Surg.* 2002;84:886–890.

42. Elbourne D, Dezateux C. Hip dysplasia and ultrasound imaging of whole populations: the precautionary principle revisited. *Arch Dis Child Fetal Neonatal Ed.* 2005;90:F2–F3.

43. Hadlow V. Neonatal screening for congenital dislocation of the hip. *J Bone Jt Surg.* 1988;70–B:740–743.

44. Czeizel A, Tusnádn G, Vaczó G, Vizkelety T. The mechanism of senetic predisposition in congenital dislocation of the hip . *J Med Genet.* 1975;12:121–130.

Chapter 13

Holoprosencephaly

Definition

Holoprosencephaly is the term used for a spectrum of disorders, which reflect defective cleavage of the forebrain. The spectrum extends from the subtle arhinencephaly (absence of olfactory bulbs) and congenital pyriform aperture stenosis to absence of cleavage of the brain into two hemispheres in association with dramatic facial abnormalities, such as a single nostril (cebocephaly) or two fused eyeballs with a proboscis above the eyes.

ICD-9:	742.260	(holoprosencephaly not otherwise specified)
	742.261	(holoprosencephaly, semilobar)
	742.262	(holoprosencephaly, alobar)
	742.263	(arhinencephaly)
ICD-10:	Q04.1	(arhinencephaly)
	Q04.2	(holoprosencephaly)
	Q87.0	(cyclopia)
Mendelian Inheritance in Man:	%236100:	(familial alobar holoprosencephaly; holoprosencephaly 1; HPE 1; includes cyclopia);
	#157127:	(midline cleft syndrome; holoprosencephaly 2; HPE2);
	#142945:	(holoprosencephaly 3; HPE3)
	#142946:	(holoprosencephaly 4; HPE4)
	#609637:	(holoprosencephaly 5; HPE5)
	%605934:	(holoprosencephaly 6; HPE6)
	%609408:	(holoprosencephaly 8; HPE8)
	%202650:	(holoprosencephaly - agnathia)
	306990:	(holoprosencephaly with fetal akinesia/hypokinesia)
	147250:	(single median maxillary central incisor)

Appearance

The spectrum of the physical features of individuals with holoprosencephaly includes variations in the abnormalities of the brain and the facial features (1–10) [Figures 13-1–13-6].

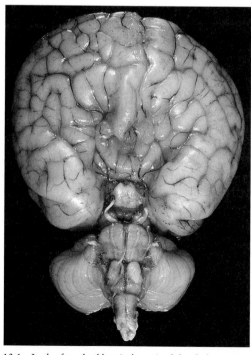

FIGURE 13.1   Lack of cerebral hemispheres in alobar holoprosencephaly.

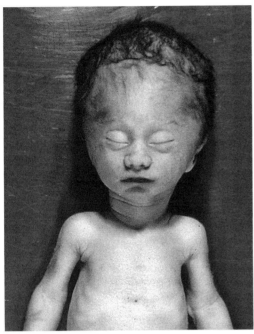

FIGURE 13.2 Normal facial features and enlarged head in an infant with holoprosencephaly.

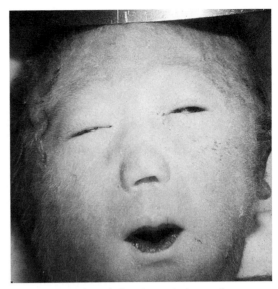

FIGURE 13.4 Cebocephaly—shows single nostril.

The three major groups of brain malformations are alobar (Figure 13-1), semilobar, and lobar holoprosencephaly. Within the alobar group, there are subdivisions in brain shape: pancake, cup, and ball types (3). A fourth and mildest type of brain malformation is the middle interhemispheric variant, in which the posterior frontal and parietal lobes have not separated in the midline, but the anterior and posterior portions of the cerebral hemisphere have separated (10).

The spectrum of the physical features of fetuses and infants which holoprosencephaly is defined by the abnormalities of the brain and face (Table 13-1, Figures 13-2–13-6).

DeMyer (1) suggested that "the face predicts the brain." While this is often true, many exceptions have been observed. In general (3, 7), the more severe the abnormality of the face, the more severe the associated brain abnormalities. A case series (8) of 50 affected fetuses diagnosed by prenatal studies showed that the alobar type occurred in 44%, semilobar in 33%, and lobar in 22%. A similar distribution was identified in other prenatal case series (11) and in population-based malformations registries and population-based malformations surveillance programs (12).

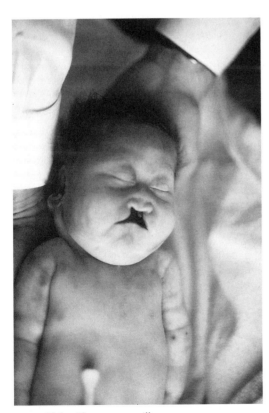

FIGURE 13.3 Absent premaxilla.

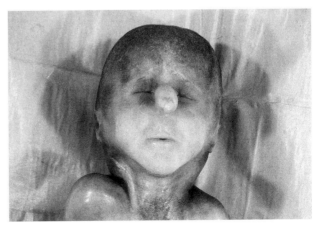

FIGURE 13.5 Ethmocephaly. (Courtesy of Mason Barr, M.D., University of Michigan, Ann Arbor, MI).

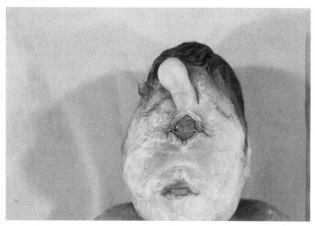

FIGURE 13.6   Cyclopia in infant with trisomy 13. (Courtesy of Mason Barr, M.D., University of Michigan, Ann Arbor, MI).

TABLE 13-1 *Correlation of facial features with associated holoprosencephaly phenotypes*

Phenotype	Face	Brain
Cyclopia (Figure 13-6)	Single eyeball; presence of proboscis; premaxilla abnormal	Absence of cleavage into two hemispheres; alobar holoprosencephaly (Figure 13-1)
Synophthalmia	Two fused eyeballs	Alobar holoprosencephaly
Ethmocephaly (Figure 13-5)	Severe hypotelorism with or without proboscis; nasal bones and maxilla absent fused	Alobar holoprosencephaly
Cebocephaly (Figure 13-4)	Hypotelorism; narrow anterior cranial fossa; single nostril; smooth upper lip without philtrum.	Alobar or less severe semi-lobar holoprosencephaly.
Median cleft lip (Figure 13-3)	Hypotelorism; flat nose; absence of premaxilla.	Alobar or less severe semi-lobar holoprosencephaly.
Single, central tooth incisor; or pyriform aperture stenosis	Hypotelorism	Varied from arhinencephaly to semi-lobar holoprosencephaly

There are several common associated findings that are part of the primary developmental abnormality. The olfactory bulbs and tracts are not present (4), which means that the affected infants have no sense of smell (5). The pituitary is often hypoplastic or deformed, which means that signs and symptoms of pituitary deficiencies are common clinical problems (5). Absence of the corpus collosum is especially common in alobar holoprosencephaly, as well as macrocephaly, hydrocephalus, and trigonocephaly (3). Two subtle, but consistent, findings in the mouth and upper lip are: absence of the superior labial frenulum between the upper lip and gum (13) and absence of the normal philtrum in the upper lip (14). (Figures 13.2, 13.4, 13.5 and 13.6)

Associated Malformations

In the review of all 63 infants with holoprosencephaly and arhinencephaly identified among 734,000 births (15), 55% of those with nonsyndromic holoprosencephaly had malformations not attributed to the brain defect. In other large population-based surveys (7,16), there was an increased frequency of neural tube defects, cleft lip, branchial arch anomalies, and polydactyly. These associated malformations were more common among stillborn infants and spontaneous abortions with holoprosencephaly than in liveborn infants with holoprosencephaly (7, 17).

In one series of 59 affected infants diagnosed prenatally (11), there were associated malformations (other than CNS and facial anomalies) in 86% of the infants with chromosome abnormalities, but in only 16% of the infants with no detected chromosome abnormality.

Developmental Defect

The early brain consists of prosencephalon, mesencephalon, and rhombencephalon. From the prosencephalon, the telencephalon (cerebral hemispheres) and diencephalon (thalamus and hypothalamus) develop. Interference with normal gastrulation in the third week of pregnancy has been postulated (18) to lead to the failure of the prosencephalon to "diverticulate" into two cerebral hemispheres. The analysis of serial sections of affected human embryos has been interpreted to show that the primary defect occurred at or before four weeks post-fertilization (19). In association with a failure to form two hemispheres in alobar prosencephaly, the thalamis and the corpora striata are undivided. There is also absence of the olfactory tracts and bulbs and the corpus callosum (3).

In semilobar holoprosencephaly, rudimentary cerebral lobes are present (3). The division into two cerebral hemispheres is never complete. In some infants, the olfactory bulbs and tracts are present; in others, they are hypoplastic. The corpus callosum is not a distinct bundle; some commissural fibers cross the midline.

In lobar holoprosencephaly, the cerebral hemispheres are well formed and are normal size (3). The olfactory bulbs and tracts and corpus callosum may be absent, hypoplastic, or normal.

The sonic hedgehog (SHH) signaling is central to the development process, as it is expressed in the mesoderm underlying the neural plate. The signal from the prechordal plate mesoderm induces ventral forebrain formation (22). Disrupting the ventralizing effect of SHH appears to lead to the occurrence of the classic forms of holoprosencephaly (9). For the milder phenotypes, such as the midline interhemispheric variant, disruption of the dorsalizing effect of bone morphogenetic protein may be the central change in signaling (9). A cascade of molecular processes, involving several developmental factors, has been identified in the development of the forebrain (20–26). These include the role of cholesterol synthesis (26), sonic hedgehog signaling (24), and the interrelationship with transcription factors Z1C2 (20) and SiX3 (25) and TGiF (23). Mutations in several of these developmental processes have been identified in a minority of the individuals with holoprosencephaly (see Genetics section below). Some affected individuals are heterozygous for one mutation. Others have two different mutations and reflect the effect of digenic inheritance (22). Unidentified modifier genes are postulated to explain the differences in the phenotypes of individuals with the same mutations.

Experimental studies, using cyclopamine-treated avian embryos, suggested that the specific phenotypes in the spectrum of craniofacial malformations, which included hypotelorism and facial clefts, were caused by reprogramming of the organizing center of the outgrowth and patterning of the mid and upper face (27).

Prevalence

Holoprosencephaly is the most common congenital malformation of the brain that is identified among embryos, but only about 5% of the affected embryos survive to the completion of pregnancy (7). In Japan, among 44,000 abortions, most of which were elective, there were 200 fetuses with holoprosencephaly, with an estimated prevalence rate of 1:250 (7). There have been several population-based studies of affected liveborn and stillborn infants and elective terminations for fetal anomalies (12, 15, 28–31). The prevalence rates of all types of holoprosencephaly were: in the North of England (1965–1998; 531,686 births) 0.12/1,000 (30); in Atlanta (1968–1992; 734,000 births) 0.1/1,000 (15); in the west of Scotland (1975–1994; 694,950 births) 0.07/1,000 [12] and in Hawaii (1986–1997) 0.11/1,000 (31).

In metropolitan Atlanta series (15), there were 53 cases of holoprosencephaly and 10 of arhinencephaly. The frequencies of the specific brain abnormalities in 71 infants with no identified chromosome abnormalities were: alobar (44%), semilobar (21%), lobar (7%), and unknown (21%). The face phenotypes identified in this series of 71 infants were: cyclopia (13%), ethmocephaly (1%), cebocephaly (18%), absence of premaxilla with median cleft lip (30%), and other less severe or unknown (38%) (28).

In a survey of 10.1 million births through eight population-based malformations registries (16), the prevalence of cyclopia associated with holoprosencephaly was 1:100,000 or 0.01/1,000 births. Infants with an identified chromosome abnormality were excluded, but chromosome analysis was not carried out on most of the affected infants.

Race/Ethnicity

No significant differences in the frequencies among major racial and ethnic groups have been reported. In the series of 25 infants with holoprosencephaly in Hawaii (1986–1997), there appeared to be a higher frequency among infants with Far East Asian and Filipino ancestry (31).

Birth Status

All case series and population-based surveys have shown an increased frequency of stillbirth, prematurity and neonatal death among infants with holoprosencephaly.

Sex Ratio

An excess of females has been observed in several population-based surveys (12, 15, 28–31). Among families with familial holoprosencephaly, an unexplained excess of affected females has been observed in individuals with isolated single maxillary central incisor (32).

Parental Age

Advanced maternal age has been reported in some series (31). This has been attributed to the occurrence of infants with trisomy 13, which is more common among the fetuses of older mothers and is often associated with holoprosencephaly.

Twinning

A casual relationship between holoprosencephaly and the twinning process has been proposed (33, 34). The excess of twinning has been observed also specifically in infants with cyclopia (16).

Very few monozygous (MZ) twin pairs have been reported (33, 35–37). Marked differences in the severity of the brain abnormalities were observed in concordant male twins (32). In a set of apparently MZ female triplets, one had holoprosencephaly, one was normal, and the third triplet was a fetus papyraceous (33). In one presumed monozygous twin pair, one twin had otocephaly and holoprosencephaly (37).

Genetic Factors

Several types of genetic abnormalities have been identified: single gene mutations (autosomal dominant and recessive and X-linked), chromosome deletions, and trisomies. Twelve (12) different chromosome regions have been identified as containing genes involved in the pathogenesis of holoprosencephaly.

The molecular studies, to date, have focused on a systematic analysis of the components of the sonic hedgehog pathway. Sonic hedgehog (SHH), a member of the Hedgehog family of secreted proteins, is a morphogen in several developmental events in the brain (21). The first mutation identified was reported in 1996 (38) in the critical region 7q36. The genes in which mutations have been identified are: sonic hedgehog (SHH), ZiC2 at 13q32 [39], SiX3 at 2p21 [40], and TG-interacting factor (TGIF) at 18p11.3 [22]. Two other candidate genes are the membrane receptor Patched (PTC), which forms a complex with the activated form of SHH and the zinc finger transcription factors GLI1 and 2 (21-23, 41). An additional holoprosencephaly locus at 14q13 has been postulated (42).

Mutational analysis in one population-based malformations registry showed that mutations in the recognized holoprosencephaly genes were only detected in less than 5% of the sporadic, non-familial cases (43). In a later study (44) sequence mutations in one of the four main holoprosencephaly-causing genes, SHH, ZiC2, SiX3, and TGiF, were detected in 20% of 339 affected individuals. 37% of 27 families with autosomal dominant holoprosencephaly had mutations in SHH (45).

Holoprosencephaly occurs occasionally in other mendelian malformation syndromes, such as 5% of infants with Smith-Lemli-Opitz (MIM #270400) with an associated defect in cholesterol biosynthesis and an occasional infant with Pallister-Hall Syndrome (MIM #146510), which is associated with mutations in the GLi3 gene.

In several case series (13, 15, 34, 46) about half of the affected fetuses and infants had an associated chromosome abnormality. Abnormalities of almost all chromosomes have been reported in association with holoprosencephaly. Trisomy 13 is the most common associated trisomy; trisomy 18 and triploidy are two other common aneuploidies. Deletions of 7q36, 18p, 2p21, and 13q are of specific interest because of the location of genes in the deleted regions which, when mutant, can be associated with holoprosencephaly. Submicroscopic deletions were identified in the SHH, ZiC2, SiX3 or TGiF genes in 4.7% of 339 individuals with severe holoprosencephaly and no mutations or chromosome abnormalities by quantitative PCR and multicolor fluorescent *in situ* hybridization (FISH) [44]. No microdeletions were found in 85 individuals with mild signs of this spectrum, such as the presence of a single maxillary central incisor and facial clefting.

Ninety-seven cases of nonsyndromic holoprosencephaly with no visible chromosome abnormalities were analyzed in 79 families (34). Segregation analysis in these 79 nuclear families suggested autosomal abdominal inheritance. There was familial aggregation in 23 of the 79 families. Penetrance was 82% for the major brain abnormalities, e.g., alobar, semilobar, and lobar holoprosencephaly, and 88% when all phenotypes were included. The risk of recurrence after the birth of isolated cases was 13%. (It should be noted that these studies were carried out before sequence analysis and FISH for microdeletions were available.)

Environmental Factors

Insulin-dependent diabetes mellitus in the mother is the most common environmental factor known to cause holoprosencephaly (47).

Exposure to an excessive amount of alcohol is another postulated cause (48), although less well documented.

Pregnant sheep that eat the mountain cabbage veratrum californicum may have lambs with holoprosencephaly and cyclopia. The plant contains cyclopamine and jervine reduce levels of cholesterol, the postulated mechanism of the teratogenic effect (49). Several other experimental models of producing holoprosencephaly in different species have been reported (50). One dramatic and species specific example, is all-trans retinoic acid (7.5 mg/kg) given by lavage on day 7 of gestations to C57BL/6N mice, which produced holoprosencephaly in the exposed pups (51).

Treatment and Prognosis

While holoprosencephaly is often a lethal abnormality, some affected children have survived for many years (52, 53). The survival of the affected infant varies with the specific phenotype. Virtually all infants with cyclopia, ethmocephaly, and cebocephaly die within a week of birth. Half of the children with alobar holoprosencephaly and a more normal face, but absence of the premaxilla, or lateral cleft lip, die before age 4–5 months, 30% live for at least one year, and a few live several years (52). For children with associated chromosomal abnormalities, the prognosis is often determined by the other structural abnormalities present. The prognosis is impacted by the profound developmental delay, the irregularities of the breathing and heart rate, and the difficulties in feeding. Diabetes insipidus occurred in 70% of 117 individuals in one case series; anterior pituitary deficiencies, such as hypothyroidism (11%), hypocortidism (7%) and growth hormone deficiency (5%) were much less common (54). In general, one cannot predict accurately how long an infant will survive. Often, the cause of death is not established by an autopsy.

Genetic Counseling

Holoprosencephaly has been shown to be very heterogeneous both in the associated phenotypic features and in the underlying etiology. Physical examination, chromosome analysis, imaging studies, array CGH, mutation analysis, and/or a postmortem examination are essential in establishing the phenotype and apparent cause.

Routine chromosome analysis is the first diagnostic test, as about half of the affected individuals will have a visible abnormality. The affected individual with a normal karyotype should be screened for point mutations and submicroscopic deletions. The mutation analysis of the several candidate genes has also shown that digenic inheritance, with two mutations in different genes, occurs in some infants with holoprosencephaly.

The empiric risk after the birth of an affected infant with a normal karyotype was 6% in one study (59) and 13% in another (34). (These studies were carried out before mutation analysis and studies for microdeletions were available.)

The primary brain malformation can be identified by ultrasound in the first trimester of pregnancy (56, 57). At 11 to 14 weeks normally a cross-section view of the fetal brain shows both choroid plexuses, an appearance called the "butterfly" sign (57). The absence of this "butterfly" configuration has been a marker of fetuses holoprosencephaly.

In families with familial transmission, autosomal dominant inheritance has been postulated. However, the individual with the mutation may or may not have abnormal physical features, an impressive example of variable expressively (22, 45).

Preimplantation genetic diagnosis has been achieved for familial holoprosencephaly associated with a mutation in sonic hedgehog (58).

REFERENCES

1. Demyer W, Zeman W, Palmer CG. The face predicts the brain: diagnostic significance of median facial anomalies for holoprosencephaly (arhinencephaly). *Pediatrics.* 1964;34:256–263.
2. Cohen MM, Jr. Problems in the definition of holoprosencephaly. *Am J Med Genet.* 2001;103:183–187.
3. Cohen MM Jr, Sulik KK. Perspectives on holoprosencephaly: Part II. Central nervous system, craniofacial anatomy, syndrome commentary, diagnostic approach, and experimental studies. *J Craniofac Genet Dev Biol.* 1992;12:196–244.
4. Cohen MM Jr. Perspectives on holoprosencephaly: Part III. Spectra, distinctions, continuities, and discontinuities. *Am J Med Genet.* 1989;34:271–288.
5. Muenke M, Gurrieri F, Bay C, Yi DH, Collins AL, Johnson VP, Hennekam RC, Schaefer GB, Weik L, Lubinsky MS et al. Linkage of a human brain malformation, familial holoprosencephaly, to chromosome 7 and evidence for genetic heterogeneity. *Proc Natl Acad Sci USA.* 1994;91:8102–8106.
6. Ming JE, Muenke M. Holoprosencephaly: from Homer to hedgehog. *Clin Genet.* 1998;53:155–163.
7. Yamada S, Uwabe C, Fujii S, Shiota K. Phenotypic variability in human embryonic holoprosencephaly in the Kyoto Collection. *Birth Defects Res (Part A): Clin Mol Teratol.* 2004;70:495–508.
8. Joó GJ, Beke A, Papp C, Tóth-Pál E, Szigeti Z, Bán, Z, Papp Z.l. Prenatal diagnosis, phenotypic and obstetric characteristics of holoprosencephaly. *Fetal Diag Ther.* 2005;20:161–166.
9. Fernandes M, Hébert JM. The ups and downs of holoprosencephaly: dorsal versus ventral patterning forces. *Clin Genet.* 2008;73:413–423.
10. Levey E, Hahn JS. Middle to interhemispheric variant of holoprosencephaly. A distinct cliniconeuroradiologic subtype. *Neurology.* 2002;59:1860–1865.
11. Chen C-P, Chern S-R, Lin C-J, Lee G-G, Wang W, Tzen C-Y. A comparison of maternal age, sex ratio and associated anomalies among numerically aneuploid, structurally aneuploid and euploid holoprosencephaly. *Genetic Counseling.* 2005;16:49–57.
12. Whiteford ML, Tolmie JL. Holoprosencephaly in the west of Scotland 1975–1994. *J Med Genet.* 1996;33:578–584.
13. Martin RA, Jones KL. Absence of the superior labial frenulum in holoprosencephaly: a new diagnostic sign. *J. Pediatr.* 1998;133:151–153.
14. Martin RA, Jones K, Benirschke K. Absence of the lateral philtral ridges: a clue to the structural basis of the philtrum. *Am J Med Genet.* 1996;65:117–123.
15. Rasmussen SA, Moore CA, Khoury MJ, Cordero JF. Descriptive epidemiology of holoprosencephaly and arhinencephaly in Metropolitan Atlanta, 1968–1992. *Am J Med Genet.* 1996;66:320–333.
16. Källén B, Castilla EE, Lancaster PAL, Mutchinick O, Knudsen LB, Martinez-Frias ML, Mastroiacovo P, Robert E. The cyclops and the mermaid: an epidemiological study of two types of rare malformation. *J Med Genet.* 1992;29:30–35.
17. Matsunaga EI, Shiota K. Holoprosencephaly in human embryos: epidemologic studies of 150 cases. *Teratology.* 1977;16:261–272.
18. Webster WS, Lipson AH, Sulik KK. Interference with gastrulation during the third week of pregnancy as a cause of some facial abnormalities and CNS defects. *Am J Med Genet.* 1988;31:505–512.
19. Müller F, O'Rahilly R. Mediobasal prosencephalic defects, including holoprosencephaly and cyclopia, in relation to the development of the human forebrain. *Am J Anat.* 1989;185:391–414.
20. Brown LY, Odent S, David V, Blayan M, Dubourg C, Apacik C et al. Holoprosencephaly due to mutations in ZiC2: Alanine tract expansion mutations may be caused by parental somatic recombination. *Hum Mol Gen.* 2001;10:791–796.
21. Marti E, Bovolenta P. Sonic hedgehog in CNS development: one signal, multiple outputs. *Trends Neurosci.* 2002;25:89–96.
22. Shiota K, Yamada S, Komeda M, Ishibashi M. Embryogenesis of holoprosencephaly. *Am J Med Genet Part A.* 2007;143A:3079–3087.
23. Aguillella C, Dubourg C, Attia-Sobol J, Vigneron J, Blayan M, Pasquier L et al. Molecular screening of the TGiF gene in holoprosencephaly: identification of two novel mutations. *Human Genet.* 2003;112:131–134.
24. DuHehr U, Gross C, Diebold U, Wahl D, Bendt U, Heidemann P et al. Wide phenotypic variability in families with holoprosencephaly and a sonic hedgehog mutation. *Eur J Pediatr.* 2004;163:347–352.
25. Ribiero LA, El-Jaick KB, Muenke M, Richiere-Costa A. SiX3 mutations in holoprosencephaly. *Am J Med Genet Part A.* 2006;140A:2577–2583.
26. Haas D, Morgenthaler J, Lacbawan F, Long B, Runz H, Garbade SF et al. Abnormal sterol metabolism in holoprosencephaly: studies in cultured lymphoblasts. *J Med Genet.* 2007;44:298–305.
27. Cordero D, Marcuio R, Hu D, Gaffield W, Tapadia M, Helms JA. Temporal perturbations in sonic hedgehog signaling elicit the spectrum of holoprosencephaly phenotypes. *J Clin Invest.* 2004;114:485–494.
28. Croen LA, Shaw GM, Lammer EJ. Holoprosencephaly: epidemiologic and clinical characteristics of a California population. *Am J Med Genet.* 1996;64:465–472.
29. Olsen CL, Hughes JP, Youngblood LG, Sharpe-Stimac M. Epidemiology of holoprosencephaly and phenotypic characteristics

of affected children: New York State, 1984–1989. *Am J Med Genet.* 1997;73:217–226.

30. Bullen PJ, Rankin JM, Robson SC. Investigation of the epidemiology and prenatal diagnosis of holoprosencephaly in the North of England. *Am J Obst Gynecol.* 2001;184:1256–1262.

31. Forrester MB, Merz RD. Epidemiology of holoprosencephaly in Hawaii, 1986–97. *Paediatr Perin Epidem.* 2000;14:61–63.

32. Suthers G, Smith S, Springbett S. Skewed sex ratios in familial holoprosencephaly and in people with isolated single maxillary central incisor. *J Med Genet.* 2005;36:924–926.

33. Schinzel AAGL, Smith DW, Miller JR. Monozygotic twinning and structural defects. *J. Pediatri.* 1979;95:921–930.

34. Odent S, Le Marec B, Munnich A, Le Merrer M, Bonaïti-Pellié C. Segregation analysis in nonsyndromic holoprosencephaly. *Am J Med Genet.* 1998;77:139–143.

35. Burck U, Hayek HW, Zeidler U. Holoprosencephaly in monozygotic twins—clinical and computer tomographic findings. *Am J Med Genet.* 1981;9:13–17.

36. Suslak L, Mimms GM, Desposito F. Monozygosity and holoprosencephaly: cleavage disorders of the "midline field." *Am J Med Genet.* 1987;28:99–102.

37. Reinecke P, Figgs C, Majewski F, Borchard F. Otocephaly and holoprosencephaly in only one monozygotic twin. *Am J Med Genet.* 2003;119A:395–396.

38. Roessler E, Belloni E, Gaudenz K, Jay P, Berta P, Scherer SW, Tsui L-C, Muenke M. Mutations in the human sonic hedgehog gene cause holoprosencephaly. *Nature Genetics.* 1996;14:357–360.

39. Brown SA, Warburton D, Brown LY, Yu C-Y, Roeder ER, Stengel-Rutkowski S, Hennekam RCM, Muenke M. Holoprosencephaly due to mutations in ZIC2, a homologue of *Drosophila odd-paired. Nature Genetics.* 1998;20:180–183.

40. Wallis DE, Roessler E, Hehr A, Nanni L, Wiltshire T, Richieri-Costa A, Gillessen-Kaesbach G, Zackai EH, Rommens J, Muenke M. Mutations in the homeodomain of the human SIX3 gene cause holoprosencephaly. *Nature Genetics.* 1999;22:196–198.

41. Villavicencio EH, Waterhouse PO, Iannac-Cone PM. The sonic hedgehog-patched-gli pathway in human development and disease. *Am J Hum Genet.* 2000;67:1047–1054.

42. Kamnasarn D, Chen C-P, Devriendt K, Mehta L, Cox DW. Defining a holoprosencephaly locus on human chromosome 14q13 and characterization of potential candidate genes. *Genomics.* 2005;85:608–621.

43. Nanni L, Croen LA, Lammer EJ, Muenke M. Holoprosencephaly: molecular study of a California population. *Am J Med Genet.* 2000;90:315–319.

44. Bendavid C, Haddad BR, Griffin A, Huizing M, Dubourg C, Gicquel I et al. Multicolor FISH and quantitative PCR can detect submicroscopic deletions in holoprosencephaly patients with a normal karyotype. *J Med Genet.* 2006;43:496–500.

45. Nanni L, Ming JE, Bocian M, Steinhaus K, Bianchi DW, de Die-Smulders C, Giannoti A, Imaizumi K, Jones KL, Del Campo M, Martin RA, Meinecke P, Pierpont MEM, Robin NH, Young ID, Roessler E, Muenke M. The mutational spectrum of the Sonic Hedgehog gene in holoprosencephaly: SHH mutations cause a significant proportion of autosomal dominant holoprosencephaly. *Hum Mol Genet.* 1999;13:2479–2488.

46. Moog U, Die-Smulders CE, Schrander-Stumpel CTRM, Engelen JJM, Hamers AJH, Frints S, Fryns JP. Holoprosencephaly: the Maastricht Experience. *Genet Counseling.* 2001;12:287–298.

47. Barr M Jr. Holoprosencephaly in infants of diabetic mothers. *J. Pediatr.* 1983;102:565–568.

48. Bönnemann C, Meinecke P. Holoprosencephaly as a possible embryonic alcohol effect: another observation. *Am J Med Genet.* 1990;37:431–432.

49. Cooper MK, Porter JA, Young EK, Beachy PA. Teratogen-medicated inhibition of target tissue response to Shh signaling. *Science.* 1998;288:1603–1607.

50. Cohen MM Jr, Shiota K. Teratogenesis of holoprosencephaly. *Am J Med Genet.* 2002;109:1–15.

51. Sulik KK, Dehart DB, Rogers JM, Chernoff N. Teratogenicity of low doses of all-trans retinoic acid in presomite mouse embryos. *Teratology.* 1995;51:398–403.

52. Barr M Jr, Cohen MM Jr. Holoprosencephaly survival and performance. *Am J Med Genet.* 1999;89:116–120.

53. Hahn JS, Plawner LL. Evaluation and management of children with holoprosencephaly. *Pediatr Neurol.* 2004;31:79–88.

54. Hahn JS, Hahn SM, Kammann H, Barkovich AJ, Clegg NJ, Delgado MR, Levey E. Endocrine disorders associated with holoprosencephaly. *J Pediatr Endocr Metab.* 2005;18:935–941.

55. Brown SA, Warburton D, Brown LY, Yu C-Y, Roeder ER, Stengel-Rutkowski S, Hennekam RCM, Muenke M. Holoprosencephaly due to mutations in ZIC2, a homologue of *Drosophila odd-paired. Nature Genetics.* 1998;20:180–183.

56. Turner CD, Silva S, Jeanty P. Prenatal diagnosis of alobar holoprosencephaly at 10 weeks of gestation. *Ultrasound Obstet Gynecol.* 1999;13:360–362.

57. Sepulveda W, Dezerega V, Be C. First-trimester sonographic diagnosis of holoprosencephaly. Value of the "butterfly" sign. *J Ultrasound Med.* 2004;23:761–765.

58. Verlinsky Y, Rechitsky S, Verlinsky O, Ozen S, Sharapova T, Masciangelo C, Morris R, Kulier A. Preimplantation diagnosis for sonic hedgehog mutation causing familial holoprosencephaly. *N Eng J Med.* 2003;348:1449–1454. 30 families.

59. Roach E, De Myer W, Conneally PM, Palmer C, Merritt AD. Holoprosencephaly: birth date, genetic and demographic analyses of 30 families. *Birth Defects: Original Article Series.* 1975; XI:294–312.

Chapter 14

Hypospadias

Definition

An abnormal opening of the urethra on the underside (ventral surface) of the penis.

ICD-9:	752.605	(hypospadias, first degree [1°], glandular, coronal)
	752.606	(hypospadias, second degree [2°], penile)
	752.607	(hypospadias, third degree [3°], perineal, scrotal)
	752.620	(congenital chordee with hypospadias)
	752.621	(congenital chordee alone)
ICD-10:	Q54.0	(hypospadias, glandular)
	Q54.1	(hypospadias, penile)
	Q54.2	(hypospadias, penoscrotal)
	Q54.3	(hypospadias, perineal)
Mendelian Inheritance in Man:	#146450	(hypospadias)
	241750	(hypospadias)

Appearance

Glandular hypospadias: In this mildest type of hypospadias, there is a long, slit-like urethral orifice that extends to the ventral surface of the glans (1) [Figures 14-1 to 14-3]. Sometimes there is, at birth, a membrane over the anterior end of the slit.

Penile Hypospadias

Typically there is a small (1 to 2 mm) opening along the urethra in the midline and on the underside (ventral surface) of the penis (2) [Figures 14-1 and 14-4].

Penoscrotal hypospadias: The abnormal opening is at the base of the penis, which is at the level of the scrotum (Figure 14-1).

Perineal hypospadias: The lowest abnormal opening in the urethra, located below the scrotum and on the perineum (Figure 14-1).

Chordee: This term refers to a congenital curvature or chordee of the penis, which is associated with a shortened ventral raphe. Chordee is usually present with hypospadias, but can occur without hypospadias.

Foreskin: Boys with hypospadias typically have a redundancy or excess of prepuce on the top of the penis (dorsally) and a deficiency of foreskin on the ventral side of the foreskin. The morphology of the foreskin affects the usefulness of this tissue in the surgical repair of hypospadias. In the examination of 174 affected males, the most common types or shapes of the foreskin were classified as: "monk's hood or one humped" in 25%, "cobra eyes or 2 humped" in 46% and "flat" in 14% (3).

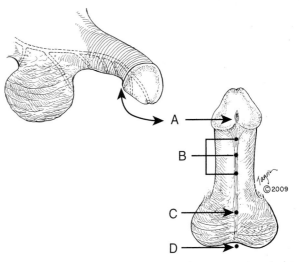

FIGURE 14.1 Diagram of location of ectopic opening of urethra in the different types of hypospadias: glandular (A), penile (B), penoscrotal (C) and perineal (D).

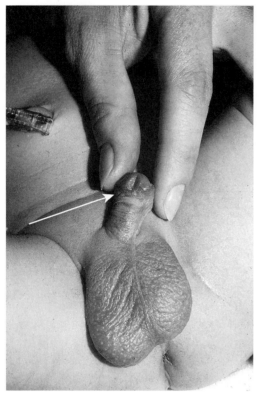

FIGURE 14.2   Shows ventral side of penis in newborn infant with glandular hypospadias (arrow) and defect in foreskin.

Associated Malformations

Hypospadias is an anomaly associated with deficient structure of the penis (2). There are two types of associated malformations, those in other genital structures, and those in nongenital structures.

In a review of 625 boys who had had surgical treatment for hypospadias (1952–1972), Svensson (4) identified the common associated genitourinary abnormalities: "hypoplasia" of the penis in 8%; cryptorchidism, 6%; and bifid scrotum, 4%. By using voiding cystourethrography, additional abnormalities were identified: vesicoureteral reflux in 6 (7%) of 84 studied obstructive and nonobstructive urethral folds in 32% and urethral recesses on the posterior wall in 13%. The frequency of other genitourinary anomalies was higher among children with more severe types of hypospadias in comparison to those with the milder forms (4).

The British Columbia Health Surveillance registry (5) identified among 295,656 male infants (1966–1981) additional anomalies in 20% of the affected boys: 60% had one other malformation, 18% had two, and 21% had three or more. In this registry, cryptorchidism and inguinal hernia were the most common other malformations (101/264: 38%). Heart defects (14%), gastrointestinal anomalies (9%), and club foot deformity (9%) were other common associated abnormalities.

In the analysis of 5,481 boys with hypospadias born in California (1983–1997), 70% had hypospadias as an "isolated" abnormality (6). 30% of the affected boys did have associated abnormalities. This analysis confirmed, also, the strong association of spina bifida with hypospadias. The observed/expected ratio (O/E) was 9.2 for the affected boys in California in comparisons to the O/E ratio of 18.3 in a similar study in Spain (7).

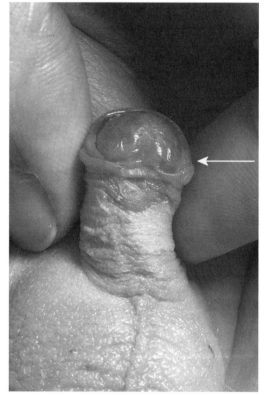

FIGURE 14.3   Shows ventral side of penis with glandular hypospadias (arrow) and foreskin defect.

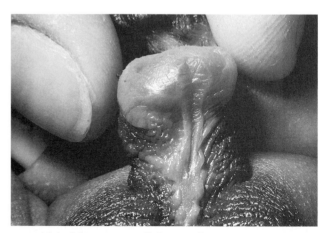

FIGURE 14.4   More severe penile hypospadias.

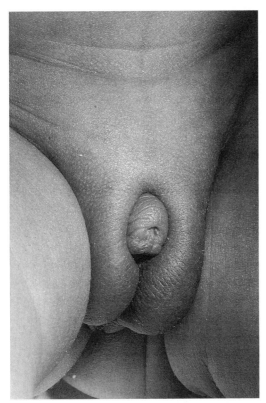

FIGURE 14.5 Penoscrotal hypospadias with small phallus and chordee in a prematurely born infant, diagnosed as having pseudovaginal perineoscrotal hypospadias.

Developmental Defects (8-10)

The urethral folds and groove are first visible in the sixth week (8). In the eighth week, in response to androgens, the genital tubercle in the male fetus elongates and forms the glans penis. The urogenital folds fuse, beginning proximally, to form the shaft of the penis by the 14th week. The curvature of the penis is most prominent in the 16th to 20th week, disappearing usually in the third trimester. The distal glandular urethra arises by ectodermal ingrowth and subsequently undergoes lamination, to produce the completed urethra in the fetus with 76 mm crown-rump length. The prepuce (foreskin) begins to develop after the formation of the glandular urethra. These developmental events are produced by a series of genes that lead to the expression of several hormones, including corticotrophin, gonadotropin and, later, thyrotropin (8, 9).

Significantly higher levels of plasma testosterone have been measured in male fetuses in comparison to female fetuses of 12 to 18 weeks gestation. The position of the urethral meatus, i.e., the degree of closure of the urethral groove, has been correlated with the level of testosterone (11).

The observed association of hypospadias with low birth weight or intrauterine growth restriction has led to hypotheses of the underlying cause. Akre and colleagues

(12) postulated that the occurrence of hypospadias is associated with early malfunction of the placenta, which causes decreased secretion of placental and fetal hormones and diminished fetal growth. A significant association with the mother having pre-eclampsia has also been observed (13). Another hypothesis is that hypospadias is more common when the levels of testosterone are low during pregnancy. Low levels of maternal testosterone at 6 to 14 weeks of gestation were identified in one study (14) in association with genital abnormalities and growth restriction in the male infants of these women. Studies in Denmark (15) showed that boys with hypospadias had, at age 3 months, elevated serum levels of the hormone FSH, but not elevated levels of either testosterone or LH. The higher levels of FSH were thought to reflect an increased gonadotropin drive of testicular function and a primary testicular dysfunction

Prevalence

The prevalence of hypospadias, including all degrees of severity, was 0.41% (1:250) in Minnesota (1940–1970) [16], 0.38% in Latin America (1967–1975) [17], and 0.41% in northern Italy (1978–1983) [18]. In these three studies the distribution of mild (glandular), moderate (penile), and more severe (perineoscrotal) types were: 77, 10, and 3%; 72, 18.5, and 9.5%; and 75, 21.4, and 3.6%, respectively.

Over the past 25 years, an increase in the frequency of hypospadias has been documented in many parts of the world, including Atlanta (19), Hungary (20), the Netherlands (21), and Singapore (13). One factor to consider in evaluating these increases is the impact of the sources of information. Many examining pediatricians do not record the specific location of the abnormality and simply record "mild" hypospadias. If this is glandular hypospadias, that is not considered a major malformation by some malformation surveillance programs. However, the term "mild" could also be used for an ectopic opening of the urethra just below the glans, which is technically "penile" hypospadias. Also, the precise location cannot be determined until the foreskin has been retracted, which may not occur until the infant is older and after the examinations are reviewed by a surveillance program. Another factor influencing prevalence rates is the higher frequency in low birth weight infants (12–14, 22, 23), which have been more likely to survive with improvements in care.

Race/Ethnicity

No significant differences between racial groups have been identified. In Singapore (13), the frequencies of hypospadias in Chinese, Malay, and Indian infants were very similar and did not differ from those in Caucasian infants (16–18).

Parental Age

In some (24), but not all (18, 25) studies, an increased frequency of hypospadias has occurred more often among the sons of older women. In another study (26), there was an increased risk for hypospadias among the extremes of maternal age: less than 20 years and over 40 years.

Birth Status

Infants with hypospadias are more likely to be small for gestational age (SGA) [defined as weight less than 10th centile] than unaffected controls (12, 18, 22). Likewise, hypospadias was ten times more common in SGA infants than in the general population with no correlation with the severity of the hypospadias (27). An increased frequency of hypospadias has been observed with decreasing birth weight, independent of gestational age (28).

Twinning

One study published in 1973 (29) showed that hypospadias was 8.5 times more common in monozygotic twins than in singletons.

With regard to concordance in twins, 9 twins were identified in the surveillance of 41,078 male births in northern Italy (18); three sets were monozygous, and in one set both twins were affected.

In an analysis of 18 pairs of twins, proven to be monozygous by microsatellite markers, 16 were discordant and the co-twin with the lowest birth weight had hypospadias (30).

Genetic Factors

Epidemiologic studies (17, 18, 25, 29, 31) have shown that the rates of occurrence of hypospadias among the brothers of an affected boy were 9.1% (18) and 9.7% (30). The heritabilities among first-degree relatives were 68% (17), 66.9% (18), 65% (25), and 74% (31) in the different studies.

The examination of 399 first-degree male relatives of 294 index cases showed that 4% also had hypospadias, a nine-fold increase in comparison to the general population (25). The more severe the hypospadias, the higher the rate of occurrence among the relatives (29, 30, 32).

The careful examinations by Farkas (1) of the 148 fathers and brothers of 122 boys with hypospadias showed that many (24.6%) had malformations of the external urethral meatus or prepuce, in comparison to 15.7% of 177 healthy men. Subfertility, due to lower motility of spermatozoa and a higher frequency of abnormal sperm morphology, is more common among the fathers of boys with hypospadias (25, 33).

Mutations in several genes have been associated with the occurrence of hypospadias (34):

1. Steroid 5-alpha reductase type 2 (SRD 4A2) [MIM #264600]: (These autosomal recessive mutations have been found in many 46,XY male pseudohermaphrodites, who have ambiguous external genitals, including varying degrees of hypospadias, a bifid scrotum, and blind vaginal pouch. At puberty they develop a male habitus with enlargement of the phallus and production of semen. This phenotype has been referred to as "pseudovaginal perineoscrotal hypospadias" [Figure 14-5].)

2. 17-beta hydroxysteroid dehydrogenase (HSD 17BB) [MIM #264300]: (The phenotype is similar to that produced by SRD5A2 deficiency: 46,XY individuals with undescended testes, normal epididymis, vas deferens, and seminal vesicles, but female external genitals. At puberty they develop gynecomastia and masculinize. Autosomal recessive.)

3. Androgen receptor gene (AR) [MIM *313700]: (The X-linked AR mutations identified in individuals with hypospadias have had other genitourinary malformations and signs of partial androgen insensitivity, not isolated hypospadias. Mutations in AR have been uncommon in boys and isolated, nonsyndromic hypospadias [35].)

4. Wilms tumor 1 gene (WT1): WT1 gene mutations are associated with the occurrence of two syndromes with genitourinary anomalies:
   a) Wilms tumor, aniridia, genitourinary anomalies, and mental retardation: MIM #194072;
   b) Denys-Drash Syndrome with nephropathy, Wilms tumor, and genital anomalies: MIM #194080.

However, heterozygous mutations in WT1 have been associated with mild effects on differentiation, including hypospadias and cryptorchidism (36).

In a systematic search for mutations in *SRDSA2*, *AR*, *WT1*, *SRY* and *SOX9* among 90 Chinese individuals with hypospadias, 16 different mutations were identified in 24 (27%) of these individuals (37). None had mutations in either *SRY* or *SOX9*.

Other potential genetic factors in the occurrence of "isolated" hypospadias are polymorphisms in these or related genes involved in development of the genital structures in male fetuses. The presence of these polymorphisms would be supportive of the concept that nonsyndromic "isolated" hypospadias occurs because of the multiple genetic and nongenetic interactions of multifactorial inheritance. Two examples of such polymorphisms are: polymorphisms in the *ESR1* and *ESR2* genes, which enclode the estrogen receptors *ER*α and *ER*β (38) and the V89L polymorphism in the 5-α-reductase gene (39). The presence of these two polymorphisms in males were associated with a reduced risk for developing hypospadias.

Studies of the mothers of affected boys have also identified genetic polymorphisms which decreased the risk. In Japan (40), the mothers with the CYP1A1 MSP1 variant had a decreased risk of having affected sons.

Families in which many men have had hypospadias have been reported (41, 42). Autosomal dominant (41) and autosomal recessive (42) inheritance have been postulated in different families. No molecular studies were carried out on the affected individuals.

Environmental Factors

Several exposures during pregnancy have been postulated to cause hypospadias: progesterone (43), phytoestrogens (44), diethylstilbestrol (45), and phthalates (46, 47). These hypotheses require confirmation by separate independent studies. For example, other analyses refute the association between exposure to progesterone and the occurrence of hypospadias (48).

An increased frequency of hypospadias has been noted, also, in some studies of the fetal effects of the anticonvulsant drugs, including carbamazepine (49) and valproate (50).

Male infants conceived by in vitro fertilization (51), especially with the intracytoplasmic sperm injection (ICSI) technique (52), have been shown to have an increased risk of developing hypospadias. This association with ICSI raises the question as to whether the sperm used in conception is conveying on the fetus genetic factors that had caused the father's reduced fertility.

Questions raised about the association of environmental exposures in pregnancy with the occurrence of hypospadias will be answered with more certainty with objective measurements. For example, measuring the blood level or urine level of the alleged teratogen in the mother provides objective confirmation of the exposure at the critical time in pregnancy. Careful study examinations of the physical features of the exposed fetus in infancy confirm the presence of the hypospadias and other features. This objectivity has been possible in some studies of phthalate exposure in pregnancy (47). The exposed boys had a reduced ano-genital distance and associated hypoplasia of the penis itself.

Treatment and Prognosis

Several surgical techniques have been used in the repair of hypospadias. Follow-up is recommended to identify physical abnormalities (53).

Genetic Counseling

As is true for all common malformations, the first question for the examining clinician to ask is whether it is an isolated anomaly or not.

TABLE 14-1 *Hypospadias: recognized etiologies and associations (excluding coronal hypospadias)**

	Isolated (n=91)	Multiple Anomalies (n=23)	Total (n=118)
Apparent etiologies			
1. Mendelian disorders			(8; 6.8%)
a. Opitz-Frias Syndrome		1	
b. Smith-Lemli-Opitz Syndrome		2	
c. Partial androgen resistance	2		
d. Pseudovaginal perineoscrotal hypospadias	1		
e. Alpha-thalassemia, homozygote; 45,X/46,XY		1	
f. Epidermolysis bullosa**	1		
2. Chromosome abnormalities			(5; 4.2%)
a. Trisomy 21 mosaic		1	
b. Chromosome 10p+ (de novo unbalanced translocation)		1	
c. Chromosome 4p-		1	
d. Chromosome 22q11.2 deletion		1	
e. Trisomy 13		1	
3. Syndromes			(1; 0.8%)
a. anencephaly with microphthalmia and split-hand deformity		1	
4. Twinning/multiple gestations			(6; 5.1%)
a. triplets	2***		
b. monozygous twins	1		
c. like-sex twins – unknown zygosity	1****		
d. dizygous twins◊	1	1	
5. Exposures in pregnancy			(7; 5.9%)
a. infants of diabetic mothers	5		
b. carbamazepine and lithium		1	
c. phenytoin	1		
6. Unknown etiology	78	13	(91; 77.1%)
	93	25	
	Total	118	(1:1,748)

Legends: * Infants with more severe hypospadias identified in the surveillance of 206,244 liveborn and stillborn infants and elective terminations at Brigham and Women's Hospital in Boston in 1972–1974, 1979–2000. Excludes infants with coronal or glandular hypospadias. Excludes infants whose mothers had planned to deliver at another hospital before the prenatal detection of fetal anomalies.

** Father and other relatives had also epidermolysis bullosa simplex, Werner-Cochrayne type, but not hypospadias.

*** Two sets of triplets only one affected. Zygosity not known.

**** Like-sex twin pair in which only one male had hypospadias.

◊ In dizygous twin pairs, only one infant had hypospadias.

The isolated type of hypospadias is to be expected. In the examination the common associated genital abnormalities, undescended testes and inguinal hernia should be looked for. Another option is to evaluate for abnormalities of the ureters and kidneys.

If the infant has ambiguous genitals, is dysmorphic, or has associated nongenital malformations, chromosome analysis, and chromosome microarray, should be considered routine tests. Additional testing options in the future may include analysis for mutations in genes associated with hypospadias, such as *WT1*, *SRD 4A2*, *HSD17BB* and *AR*.

In addition to the laboratory testing, the infant should have a diagnostic evaluation for having one of the many possible malformation syndromes associated with hypospadias (Table 14-1).

As part of the evaluation of the affected infant, the pregnancy history should be reviewed to identify potentially relevant exposures. Was the infant growth restricted? Did the affected infant's mother have preeclampsia or insulin-dependent diabetes mellitus? Does the father have hypospadias?

If there is no evidence of an environmental exposure or associated genetic abnormality, there should be a discussion of the empiric risk of recurrence in a subsequent pregnancy. The healthy parents with one affected son will have an approximate 10% risk that each subsequent son will have hypospadias. If the first affected son has more severe hypospadias, the risk appears to be greater.

REFERENCES

1. Farkas LG. Minor defects of the penis: microforms or stigmata of hypospadias and epispadias? *Plastic Reconstr Surg*. 1970;45: 480–486.
2. Van der Werff JF, Ultee J. Long-term follow-up of hypospadias repair. *Br J Plast Surg*. 2000;53:588–592.
3. Radojicic ZI, Perovic SV. Classification of prepuce in hypospadias according to morphological abnormalities and their impact on hypospadias repair. *J Urol*. 2004;172:301–304.
4. Svensson J. Male hypospadias, 625 cases, associated malformations and possible etiological factors. *Acta Paediatr Scand*. 1979; 68:587–592.
5. Leung TJ, Baird PA, McGillivray B. Hypospadias in British Columbia. *Am J Med Gen*. 1985;21:39–48.
6. Yang W, Carmichael SL, Shaw GM. Congenital malformations co-occurring with hypospadias in California, 1983–1997. *Am J Med Genet*. 2007; 143A:2627–2634.
7. Martinez-Frias ML. Spina bifida and hypospadias: a non-random association or an X-linked recessive condition? *Am J Med Genet*. 1994;52:5–8.
8. O'Rahilly R, Müller F. *Human Embryology & Teratology*. 3rd ed. New York: Wiley-Liss; 2001: 312–316.
9. Van der Werff JFA, Nievelstein RAJ, Brands e, Luijsterburg AJM, Vermeij-Keers C. Normal development of the male anterior urethra. *Teratology*. 2000;61:172–183.
10. Levitt SB, Freda EF. Hypospadias. *Pediatric Annals*. 1988;12: 48–57.
11. Abramovich DR. A possible cause of glandular hypospadias in man. *Arch Dis Childh*. 1974;49:66–67.
12. Akre O, Lipworth L, Cnattingius S, Sparén P, Ekbom A. Risk factor patterns for cryptorchidism and hypospadias. *Epidemiology*. 1999;10:364–369.
13. Chong JH, Wee CK, Kah S, Ho Y, Chan DK. Factors associated with hypospadias in Asian newborn babies. *J Perinat Med*. 2006; 34:497–500.
14. Key TJ, Bull D, Ansell P, Brett AR, Clark GM, Moore JW et al. A case-control study of cryptorchidism and maternal hormone concentrations in early pregnancy. *Br J Cancer*. 1996;73: 698–701.
15. Boisen KA, Chellakooty M, Schmidt IM, Kai CM, Damgaard IN, Suomi AM et al. Hypospadias in a cohort of 1072 Danish newborn boys: prevalence and relationship to placental weight, anthropometrical measurements at birth, and reproductive hormone levels at three months of age. *J Clin Endocrinol Metab*. 2005;90:4041–4046.
16. Sweet RA, Schrott HG, Kurland R, Culp OR. Study of the incidence of hypospadias in Rochester, Minnesota, 1940–1970, and a case-control comparison of possible etiologic factors. *Mayo Clin Proc*. 1974;49:52–57.
17. Monteleone Neto R, Castilla EE, Paz JE. Hypospadias: an epidemiological study in Latin America. *Am J Med Gen*. 1981; 10:5–19.
18. Calzolari E, Contiero MR, Roncarati E, Mattiuz PL, Volpato S. Aetiological factors in hypospadias. *J Med Gen*. 1986;23: 333–337.
19. Paulozzi LJ, Erickson JD, Jackson RJ. Hypospadias in two US surveillance systems. *Pediatrics*. 1997;100:831–834.
20. Czeizel A. Increasing trends in congenital malformations of male external genitalia. *Lancet*. 1985;ii: 462–463.
21. Pierik FH, Burdorf A, Nijman JM, de Muinck Keizer-Schrama SM, Juttmann RE, Weber RF. A high hypospadias rate in The Netherlands. *Human Reprod*. 2002;17:1112–1115.
22. Hussain N, Chagtai A, Herndon CDA, Herson VC, Rosenkrantz TS, McKenna PH. Hypospadias and early gestation growth restriction in infants. *Pediatrics*. 2002;109: 473–478.
23. Chambers CD, Castilla EE, Orioli I, Jones KL. Intrauterine growth restriction in like-sex twins discordant for structural defects. *Birth Def Res (Part A): Clin Mol Teratol*. 2006;76: 246–248.
24. Fisch H, Golden RJ, Libersen GL, Hyun GS, Madsen P, New MI, Hensle TW. Maternal age as a risk factor for hypospadias. *J Urol*. 2001;165: 934–936.
25. Czeizel A, Toth J, Erodi E. Aetiological studies of hypospadias in Hungary. *Hum Hered*. 1979;29: 166–171.
26. Bianca S, Ingegnosi C, Ettore G. Maternal and paternal risk actors for hypospadias. *Environ Health Perspectives*. 2005;113: A296.
27. Gatti JM, Kirsch AJ, Troyer WA, Perez-Brayfield MR, Smith EA, Scherz HC. Increased incidence of hypospadias in small-for-gestational age infants in a neonatal intensive-care unit. *BJU Internat*. 2001;87: 548–550.
28. Weidner IS, Moller H, Jensen TK, Shakkebaek NE. Risk factors for cryptorchidism and hypospadias. *J Urol*. 1999;161: 1606–1609.
29. Roberts CJ, Lloyd S. Observations on the epidemiology of simple hypospadias. *Brit Med J*. 1973;1:768–770.
30. Fredell L, Lichtenstein P, Pedersen NL, Svensson J, Nordenskjold A. Hypospadias is related to birth weight in discordant monozygotic twins. *J Urol*. 1998;160: 2197–2199.
31. Chen YC, Woolley PV Jr. Genetic studies on hypospadias in males. *J Med Genet*. 1971;8: 153–159.
32. Bauer SB, Retik AB, Colodny AH. Genetic aspects of hypospadias. *Urol Clin North Am*. 1981;8: 559–564.
33. Fritz C, Czeizel AE. Abnormal sperm morphology and function in the fathers of hypospadias. *J Reproduction and Fertility*. 1996;106: 63–66.

34. Manson JM, Carr MC. Molecular epidemiology of hypospadias: review of genetic and environmental risk factors. *Birth Def Res (Part A): Clin Mol Teratology*. 2003;67: 825–836.

35. Boehmer ALM, Nijman RJM, Lammers BAS, DeConinck SJF, Van Hemel JO, Themmen APN et al. Etiological studies of severe or familial hypospadias. *J Urol*. 2001;165: 1246–1254.

36. Pelletier J, Bruening WL, Li FP, Haber DA, Glaser T, Housman DE. WT1 mutations contribute to abnormal genital system development and hereditary Wilms' tumour. *Nature*. 1991;353:431–434.

37. Wang Y, Li Q, Xu J, Liu Q, Wang W, Lin Y et al. Mutation analysis of five candidate genes in Chinese patients with hypospadias. *Eur J Hum Gen*. 2004;12:706–712.

38. Ban S, Sata F, Kurahashi N, Kasa S, Moriya K, Kakizaki H et al. Genetic polymorphisms of *ESR1* and *ESR2* that may influence estrogen activity and the risk of hypospadias. *Hum Reprod*. 2008;23:1466–1471.

39. Thai HT, Kalbasi M, Lagerstedt K, Frisén L, Kockum I, Nordenskjöld A. The valine allele of the V89L polymorphism in the 5-alpha-reductase gene confers a reduced risk for hypospadias. *J Clin Endocrinol Metab*. 2005;90:6695–6698.

40. Kurahashi N, Sata F, Kasai S, Shibata T, Moriya K, Yamada H et al. Maternal genetic polymorphisms in CYP1A1, GSTM1 and GSTT1 and the risk of hypospadias. *Mol Hum Reprod*. 2005; 11:93–98.

41. Page LA. Inheritance of uncomplicated hypospadias. *Pediatrics*. 1979;63: 788–790.

42. Frydman M, Greiber C, Cohen HA. Uncomplicated familial hypospadias: evidence for autosomal recessive inheritance. *Am J Med Gen*. 1985;21: 51–55.

43. Carmichael SL, Shaw GA, Laurent C, Croughan M, Olney RS, Lammer EJ. Hypospadias and maternal intake of progestins and oral contraceptives. *Birth Def Res (Part A): Clin Mol Teratology*. 2004;70: 255.

44. North K, Golding J. A maternal vegetarian diet in pregnancy is associated with hypospadias. *BJU International*. 2000;85: 107–113.

45. Stillman RJ. In utero exposure to diethylstilbestrol: adverse effects on the reproductive tract and reproductive performance in male and female offspring. *Am J Obst Gynecol*. 1982;142: 905–921.

46. Skakkebaek NE, Rajpert-De Meyts E, Main KM. Testicular dysgenesis syndrome: an increasingly common developmental disorder with environmental aspects. *Human Reprod*. 2001;16: 972–978.

47. Swan SH, Main KM, Liu F, Stewart SL, Kruse RL, Calafat AM et al. Decrease in anogenital distance among male infants with prenatal phthalate exposure. *Environ Health Perspect*. 2005; 113:1056–1061.

48. Raman-Wilms L, Tseng AL, Wighardt S, Eimarson TR, Koren G. Fetal genital effects of first-trimester sex hormone exposure: a meta-analysis. *Obstet Gynecol*. 1995;85: 141–149.

49. Samrén EB, van Duijn CM, Christiaens GC, Hofman A, Lindhout D. Antiepileptic drug regimens and major congenital abnormalities in the offspring. *Ann Neurol*. 46:739–746, 1999.

50. Wyszynski DF, Nambisan M, Surve T, Alsdorf RM, Smith CR, Holmes LB. Increased rate of major malformations in offspring exposed to valproate during pregnancy. *Neurology*. 64:961–965, 2005.

51. Silver RI, Rodriguez R, Chang TSK, Gearhart JP. In vitro fertilization is associated with an increased risk of hypospadias. *J Urol*. 1999;161: 1954–1957.

52. Wennerholm U-B, Bergh C, Hamberger L, Lundin K, Nilsson L, Wikland M et al. Incidence of congenital malformations in children born after ICSI. *Human Reprod*. 2000;15: 944–948.

53. Van der Werff JF, Ultee J. Long-term follow-up of hypospadias repair. *Br J Plast Surg*. 2000;53:588–592.

Chapter 15

Limb Malformations

INTRODUCTION

Abnormalities of limb development are among the most common, most visible, and best known malformations. Accordingly, many studies have been conducted on systems of classification (1–4), apparent etiologies (5–6), prevalence rates (6–13) and, more recently, the cellular and molecular events during limb development (14–21).

Clinicians divide malformations into those that are "isolated," meaning no associated non-limb malformations, and "syndromic" or as part of multiple malformations. Declaring an abnormality "isolated" reflects the limited information available; imaging of viscera and inspection of the entire skeleton would be likely to identify additional structural abnormalities.

Many population-based (7–13) and large hospital-based consecutive case series (6) have reported the frequency of the common types of limb deficiencies: longitudinal deficiencies (includes both preaxial and postaxial deficiencies), terminal transverse limb defects (Table 15-1).

Each type of limb malformation, that is, polydactyly, syndactyly, terminal transverse limb defects, etc., has many etiologies. The apparent etiologies of the limb deficiencies have been evaluated in several studies (Table 15-2).

Many mutations with autosomal dominant or recessive inheritance have been identified in individuals with specific limb malformations (Table 15-3).

Fewer studies have been carried out on the association of limb defects with single nucleotide polymorphisms (22, 23).

A few limb malformations have been associated with exposures during pregnancy to drugs (24), including thalidomide, the anticoagulant Warfarin, the anticonvulsant drug phenytoin, and prostaglandin E_1 analogue misoprostol.

The classification of limb malformations will be improved when associated mutations can be identified readily and can be related to the normal cellular and molecular interactions during development (25). For now, we will be using a classification based on the pattern of the structural abnormalities. We present here these eleven types of limb malformations:

1. polydactyly
   a) postaxial
   b) preaxial
2. polysyndactyly
3. preaxial longitudinal deficiency
   a) absence of thumb/radius
   b) absence of first toe/tibia
4. postaxial longitudinal deficiency
   a) absence of fifth finger/ulna
   b) absence of fifth toe/fibula
5. split-hand/split foot
6. syndactyly
7. terminal transverse limb defects with nubbins
8. central digit hypoplasia

TABLE 15-1 *Frequency of limb malformations in newborn infants*

	terminal transverse limb defects	longitudinal		Intercalary defect	split-hand/ split-multiple foot	Unknown/Other
		preaxial	postaxial			
Italy (n = 173, 109) [11] (1978–1987)						
Upper limb						
unilateral	29	6	1	2	7	0
bilateral	2	3	0	0	2	1
Lower limb						
unilateral	5	0	2	4	0	0
bilateral	2	0	3	0	0	1
Both	7	0	0	2	1	2
TOTAL	45	9	6	8	10	4
	0.26/1,000	0.05/1,000	0.03/1,000	0.05/1,000	0.06/1,000	0.02/1,000
*Boston** (n = 161, 252) [340] (1972–1974, 79–94)						
upper	24	21	8	5	3	16
lower	6	0	4	3	4	2
Both	0	1	1	2	2	7
TOTAL	30	22	13	10	9	25
	0.19/1,000	0.14/1,000	0.08/1,000	0.06/1,000	0.06/1,000	0.15/1,000
France (n=118,265) [12] (1979-1987)						
TOTAL	57	15	10	11		36
	0.48/1,000	0.13/1,000	0.08/1,000	0.09/1,000		0.3/1,000
Hawaii (n=281, 866) [13] (1986–2000)						
TOTAL	70	34		9		12
	0.25/1,000	0.12/1,000		0.03/1,000		0.04/1,000

*McGuirk CK, Westgate M-N, Holmes LB. Limb deficiencies in newborn infants. Pediatrics 108:e64-71, 2001 (http://www.pediatrics.org/cgi/content/fall/108/4/e64)

TABLE 15-2 *Recognized etiologies of limb deficiencies**

Apparent etiology	Isolated (n=58)	Multiple anomalies (n=52)	Total (n=110)	Prevalence (n/1,000)
Mendelian Inheritance (e.g. Fanconi anemia)	10 (9%) 1+	7 (6%) 1+, 1*, 1	17 (15%)	0.11
Familial occurrence (e.g. uncle with split hand)	2 (2%)	2 (2%) 1*	4 (4%)	0.02
Chromosome abnormalities (e.g., tri 18, 4p-, 13q-)	0	7 (6%) 1+, 2*, 1++	7 (6%)	0.04
Known syndrome (excludes amniotic bands; Möebius syndrome; Poland's anomaly; and terminal forearm, hand, and foot defects with nubbins	0	6 (5%) 1+, 1*	6 (5%)	0.04
Teratogens Infants of diabetic mothers (IDM)	1 (0.9%) 1*	2 (2%)	3 (3%)	0.02
Misoprostol-exposed (27)	0	1 (0.9%)	1 (0.9%)	0.006
Presumed vascular disruption defects Amniotic band syndrome	7 (6%)	6 (5%) 2*	13 (12%)	0.08
Möebius syndrome	0	1 (0.9%)	1 (0.9%)	0.006
Poland's anomaly	0	3 (3%)	3 (3%)	0.02
Forearm defect with nubbins	4 (4%) 1*, 1++	0	4 (4%)	0.02
Absent hand with nubbins	4 (4%) 1*, 1++	0	4 (4%)	0.02
Foot defect with nubbins	1 (0.9)	0	1 (0.9%)	0.006
Other similar phenotypes	9 (8%)	2 (2%)	11 (10%)	0.07
Unknown cause	20 (18%)	15 (14%)	35 (32%)	0.22
Total	1*	3+, 3*		0.69/1,000

Excludes all maternal transfers with fetal abnormalities. 5 spontaneous abortions at <20 weeks, all infants with skeletal dysplasia, and 4 infants with brachydactyly. Based on findings in Active Malformations Surveillance Program (1972-74, 1979-1994) among 162,252 liveborn and stillborn infants and elective terminations at Brigham and Women's Hospital, Boston.

*Delivery by D and C
+Delivery by infusion.
++Children whose malformations have more than 1 cause.

*From: McGuirk CK, Westgate M-N, Holmes LB. Limb deficiencies in newborn infants. Pediatrics 108:e64-71, 2001 (http://www.pediatrics.org/cgi/content/fall/108/4/e64).

TABLE 15-3 *Mutations associated with limb malformations in humans**

Disorder	MIM**	Gene Location	Symbol	Protein affected
1. Acheiropody	200500	7q36	C7orf2	Homolog of limb region 1 in mouse
2. Al-Awadi/Raas-Rothschild/Schinzel	276820	3p25	WNT7A	Wingless-type MMTV integration site family 7A
3. Baller-Gerold syndrome	218600	8q24	RECQL4	RECQ protein-like 4
4. Campodactyly –arthro-pathy-coxa vara-pericarditis syndrome	208250	1q24-q25	PRG4	Proteolycan 4
5. CHARGE syndrome	21480	8q12.1	CHD7	Chromodomain helicase DNA-binding protein-7
6. Cornelia de Lange syndrome	122470	5p13.1	NIPB	Delangin
7. Cornelia de Lange syndrome	122470	Xp11	SMC1L1	SB1.8
8. Ectrodactyly, ectodermal dysplasia, and cleft lip/palate syndrome 3	604292	3q27	TP63	Tumor protein p63
9. Fanconi anemia, complementation	227650	16q24.3	FANCA	Fanconi anemia, complementation group A
10. Fanconi syndrome, group B	227650	Xp22.3	FANCB	Fanconi anemia, associated peptide 95 kb
11. Fanconi anemia, group C	227650	9q22.3	FANCC	FANCC peptide
12. Fanconi anemia, group D1	227650	13q12.3	BRCA2	BRCA2 peptide
13. Fanconi anemia, group D2	227650	3p25.3	FANCD2	FANCD2 peptide
14. Fanconi anemia, group E	227650	6p22	FANCE	FANCE peptide
15. Fanconi anemia, group F	227650	11p15	FANCF	FANCF peptide
16. Fanconi anemia, group G	227650	9p13	FANCG	FANCG peptide
17. Fanconi anemia, group J	227650	17q22	FANCJ	BRCA1 interacting protein
18. Fanconi anemia, group L	227650	2p16.1	FANCL	PHD finger protein 9
19. Fanconi anemia, group M	227650	14q21.3	FANCM	Fanconi anemia associated polypeptide
20. Fanconi anemia, group N	227650	16p12	PALB2	PALB2 protein
21. Fuhrmann syndrome	228930	3p25	WNT7A	Wingless-type MMTV integration site family 7°
22. Greig cephalopolysyndactyly syndrome	175700	7p13	GLI3	GLI-Kruppel family member GLI3
23. Hand-foot uterus syndrome	140000	7p15-p14.2	HOXA13	Homeobox-A13
24. Lacrimoauriculodentodigital syndrome (LADD)	149730	5p13	FGF10	Fibroblast growth factor 10
25. Lacrimoauriculodentodigital syndrome (LADD)	149730	10q26	FGFR2	Fibroblast growth factor 2
26. Okihiro syndrome	607323	20q13	SALL4	Sal-like 4
27. Pallister-Hall syndrome	146510	7p13	GLI3	GLI-Kruppel family member GLI3
28. Polydactyly, postaxial, types A1 and B	174200	7p13	GLI3	GLI-Kruppel family member
29. Polydactyly, preaxial, type IV	174700	7p13	GLI3	GLI-Kruppel family member GLI3
30. Polydactyly preaxial type 2	174500	7q36	LMBR1	Limb region 1, mouse homolog
31. Radioulnar synostosis with amegakaryocytic thrombo-cytopenia	605432	7p15-p14.2	HOXA11	Homeobox-A11
32. Split-hand/foot malformation, type 4	605289	3q27	TP63	Tumor protein p63
33. Split-hand/foot malformation type 3	600095	10q24		Dactylin
34. Syndactyly 5	186000	2q31-32	HOXD13	Homeobox-D-13
35. Tetra-amelia	273395	17q21	WNT3	Wingless homolog 3
36. Townes-Brocks syndrome	107480	16q21.1	SALL1	Sal-like 1
37. Ulnar-mammary syndrome	181450	12q24.1	TBX3	T-box 3
38. Weyer acrofacial oligodactyly	193530	4p16	EVC 1	EVC 1

Adapted from: Carey JC, Viskochil DH: Status of the Human Malformation Map: *Am J Med Genet* Part A 143A:2868–2885, 2007.

POLYDACTYLY, POSTAXIAL, TYPES A AND B (PEDUNCULATED POSTMINIMUS)

Definition

Type A postaxial polydactyly is an additional digit with a nail and interphalangeal joints that articulates with either the fifth metacarpal or fifth metatarsal. Type B pedunculated postminimus is an additional digit on the outer aspect of a hand or foot that consists of a pedicle at the end of which is a globular, skin-covered, cartilage-containing structure with a rudimentary nail.

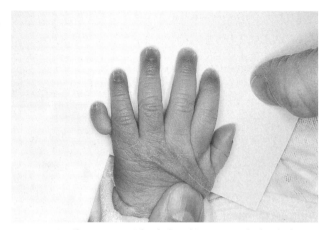

FIGURE 15.1 Shows postaxial polydactyly, type B at the level of proximal phalanx.

ICD-9:	755.005	(accessory fingers [postaxial polydactyly, type A])
	755.006	(skin tag [postaxial polydactyly, type B])
	755.020	(accessory toes [postaxial])
ICD-10:	Q69.0	(accessory finger [5]
	Q69.9	(polydactyly, unspecified)
Mendelian Inheritance in Man:	#174200	(polydactyly, postaxial, type A1)
	%602085	(polydactyly, postaxial, type A2)
	%607324	(polydactyly, postaxial, type A3)
	%608562	(polydactyly, postaxial, type A4)

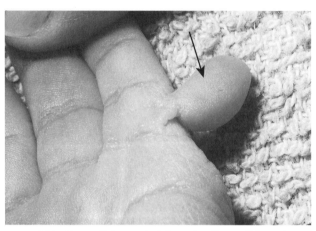

FIGURE 15.2 Extra digit attached by string-like pedicle to lateral aspect of fifth finger (arrow).

Historical Note

Temtamy and McKusick (27), based on the clinical observations, and the published literature, proposed that postaxial polydactyly be subdivided into two groups: Type A, meaning "fully developed extra digits"; Type B: "rudimentary extra digits or pedunculated postminimi." This classification has been accepted and is now standard terminology.

Appearance

In type A, the extra (sixth) finger or toe may deviate laterally and the interphalangeal joint may have little movement. (Figure 15-4 and 15-5) There may be a broad or bifid metacarpal or -tarsal or a sixth metacarpal or -tarsal.

In type B, the pedicle, usually 2 to 3 millimeters in diameter, is located most often on the lateral edge of the metacarpal-phalangeal joint or on the side of the proximal or middle phalanx of the fifth finger (Figures 15-1, 15-2) or toe. The pedunculated sixth toe is attached at the level of metatarsal-phalangeal joint or along the proximal phalanx of the fifth toe (27–31) (Figure 15-6).

A surgical classification of types I, II, and III has been developed (33). In Type I (the same as type B), a small neurovascular bundle is present within the skin pedicle or bridge. In Type II (also, type A) there is a bifid tip of the fifth metacarpal; the phalanges in the sixth finger are smaller than those in the fifth finger; there is clinodactyly of the sixth finger, and a hypoplastic fingernail. In Type III postaxial polydactyly, which is quite rare, there is a complete sixth metacarpal and phalanges of the most postaxial finger. There are subtle changes in the tendons, intrinsic muscles, and joint surfaces that may only become apparent in the teenage years (33).

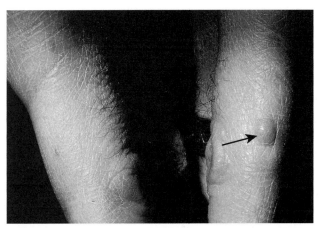

FIGURE 15.3   Scars on sides of fifth fingers of parent who was born with postaxial polydactyly, type B (arrow).

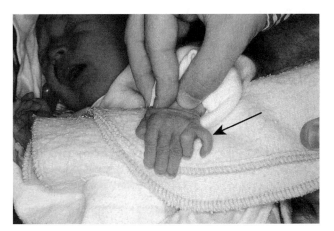

FIGURE 15.4   Shows postaxial polydactyly, type A (arrow) with the articulation at the level of the metacarpal-phalangeal joint.

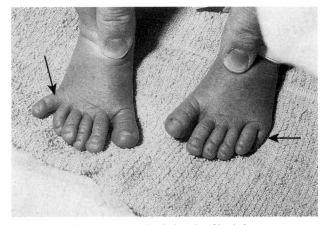

FIGURE 15.5   Type A postaxial polydactyly of both feet. (arrow)

Associated Malformations

Most, 88% of 4,756 affected individuals, in one study (34) had no associated malformations. Among the infants with associated malformations, there was a

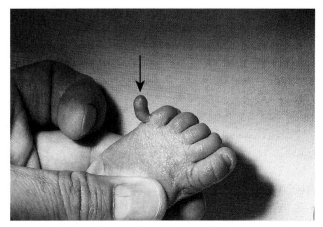

FIGURE 15.6   Type B postaxial polydactyly of left foot (arrow).

significantly increased occurrence of syndactyly, especially syndactyly of toes 2-3 and toes 4-5 (34). There is also a significant association with the occurrence of cleft lip, anophthalmia, polycystic kidneys, and cyclopia, each of which suggests recognizable phenotypes, such as trisomy 13 and Meckel-Gruber Syndrome (Mendelian Inheritance in Man #249000).

Over 100 different syndromes associated with polydactyly have been identified (35).

The variation in specific phenotypes makes it impossible to know for the infant with postaxial polydactyly, type B, and no affected relatives which associated molecular abnormality she/he has. This type of polydactyly can occur as the mildest expression of an autosomal dominant polysyndactyly mutation in GLI3 that is part of the spectrum of Greig cephalopolysyndactyly (36) or as an effect of a HOX 13 mutation that is part of the spectrum of preaxial polydactyly, Type IV (37). Mutation analyses of a large consecutive series of newborn infants are needed to determine the frequencies of the specific mutations (25).

Developmental Abnormality

The formation of an extra digit has been identified in the hands of Stage 16 human embryos (about 37 days postfertilization) and in the foot of Stage 17 (41 days postfertilization). Human embryos with an extension of the apical ectodermal ridge (AER) at the end of the developing limb in fetuses are predicted to be developing postaxial polydactyly (40). Theoretically, the presence of an ectopic specialized region of mesodermal cells, called the zone of polarizing activity (ZPA), on the posterior (lower) aspect of the developing limb controls anterior/posterior (A/P) patterning of the limb bud. Its presence could lead to the development of an extra, postaxial digit (polydactyly).

Mutations, which cause postaxial polydactyly with no other limb malformations, have been identified in mice. For example, the mutation toe-ulnar (tu) is associated with an extra digit with one or two phalanges in the forelimbs [28]. The mutation <u>Po</u> causes postaxial polydactyly in the forelimbs. An autosomal dominant gene with modifying genes is the postulated genetic mechanism.

Misexpression of the genes <u>sonic hedgehog</u> and <u>SOX9</u> have been shown to induce polydactyly in the mouse limb (39).

Prevalence/Race and Ethnicity

a) Spontaneous abortions

The frequency of polydactyly in Japan was much higher in embryos from spontaneous abortions than in liveborn infants (40). In the series of 36,380 embryos from induced abortions in Japan (38), the prevalence of all types of polydactyly was 0.35%. Among these 129 affected embryos only 29 had postaxial polydactyly: 12 affecting the hands and 17 affecting the feet. Preaxial polydactyly was much more common than postaxial polydactyly. Most had no other external anomalies.

In the Seattle case series of 1,924 elective terminations and 3,276 spontaneous abortions (41), 133 had limb defects and 20 had polydactyly. 67.9% of these 20 fetuses had postaxial polydactyly: 33% were bilateral: 30% had associated abnormalities.

b) Newborn infants

Africans in South Africa (43) and African Americans in the United States (31) show a frequency of about 1:100 (1%), which is 10 times more common than in Caucasians. The Japanese are the racial/ethnic group with the lowest frequency

Caucasians:	0.91: 1,000 isolated type B [31]
	0.25: 1,000 isolated type A
African Americans:	12.4: 1,000 isolated type B [31]
	0.16: 1,000 isolated type A
	0.12: 1,000 types A & B in same individual [31]
Africans (Nigeria):	19.9: 1,000 females [42]
	27.1: 1,000 males [42]
(South Africa)	10.4: 1,000 type not specified [43]
American Indian:	0.73: 1,000 type B only [44]
	1.07: 1,000 types A & B [44]
Japan:	0.08: 1,000 [48]

Sex Ratio

Males are more frequently affected than females; in one study 54 to 55% of infants with polydactyly of hands only, feet only, and hands and feet were males (34).

Sidedness

Bilateral polydactyly is much more common than unilateral polydactyly. However, when a unilateral malformation, the left hand or foot is affected more often. In one study (34), 77% of the 762 infants with unilateral polydactyly had an affected left hand, 56% of the infants with postaxial polydactyly of the foot had an affected left foot and 91% of the 11 infants with an affected hand and foot had polydactyly only on the left side.

Birth Status

A 1.6 to 1.8% frequency of perinatal death has been reported (46).

Twinning

The frequency of concordance in 47 sets of identical twins was 42.6%, although the report did not specify postaxial or preaxial location or type A or B (47).

Genetic Factors

Many family studies have been interpreted (31, 38) to show an autosomal dominant pattern of inheritance. In a consecutive series of births in Salt Lake City (31), autosomal dominant inheritance with reduced penetrance and variable expressivity was the interpretation of the findings.

In studies from the large consecutive series of affected newborn infants examined in Latin America (1967–1990), Orioli (48) reported that affected black fathers had a higher frequency of postaxial polydactyly in their offspring than either affected black mothers or affected nonblack mothers or fathers. She postulated that this effect in the children of affected black fathers reflected the effect of an X-linked recessive modifier gene on an autosomal dominant polydactyly gene. Subsequent segregation analyses from the same Latin American Collaborative Study of Congenital Malformations (ECLAMC) and a northeastern region of Brazil (49) suggested for affected black infants a multifactorial pattern of inheritance of postaxial polydactyly of the hands; no evidence of a major gene locus or a modifier gene was found. The authors concluded that the inheritance patterns of postaxial polydactyly of the hands differed from that of the feet.

In a separate analysis of the findings in the ECLAMC survey (46), significant differences were identified between the infant with postaxial polydactyly of the hand and the much less common postaxial polydactyly of the feet. It was postulated that the two phenotypes are separate entities.

In one early analysis by Sverdrup in 1922 (50), it was postulated that the parent with postaxial polydactyly type A could have children with either type A or type B;

the individual with type B could have infants with only type B, postaxial polydactyly (Figure 15-3). Subsequently, many families have been identified which disproved this hypothesis.

Molecular studies in several families with Greig Cephalopolysyndactyly have identified a mutation in the transcription regulator gene GLI3 on chromosome 7p13.6 [36, 51, 52]. Genotype-phenotype correlations have been made between the nature of the mutation and the presence of the more severe phenotypes of Pallister-Hall Syndrome and Greig Cephalopolysyndactyly. However, genotype-phenotype correlations have not been made with mutations in GL13 associated with only type A or type B postaxial polydactyly.

Linkage studies in large Turkish families with many affected individuals suggested a locus on 13q21-q32 (53) for type A postaxial polydactyly (MIM 602085) only. Separate loci on chromosome 19p13.1 were postulated in a Chinese family with type A or B (MIM 607324) [54] and on chromosome 7q21-q34 in a Dutch family with types A or B with or without associated syndactyly of toes 2-3 (MIM 608562) [55]. In the last of these families, one individual with type B only showed no evidence of linkage to the locus for individuals with type A, suggesting a separate genetic locus (or gene loci) for type B.

Environmental Factors

No teratogenic exposure during pregnancy has been shown to cause either type A or type B postaxial polydactyly.

Treatment and Prognosis

Often the type B polydactyly is removed by tying a suture tightly around the pedicle. The extra digit falls off after a few days, leaving a small bump at the site of the pedicle (29, 33). Surgical excision produces a better cosmetic result.

The surgical repair of postaxial polydactyly, type A of the hand is often done at age 2 to 3 years (33). If the extra digit is smaller than the normal digit it is always removed, but the hypothenar muscles and the ulnar collateral ligament are retained. For Type III postaxial polydactyly occasionally the most lateral digits is retained or portions of the fifth and sixth are retained.

In the repair of type A postaxial polydactyly of the foot, the strategy is usually to retain the more dominant of toes 5 and 6 (56).

Genetic Counseling

In the newborn infant with apparent "isolated" postaxial polydactyly, the surface examination will confirm the absence of dysmorphic features. However, more subtle anomalies may not be identified until the infant is older or has had studies, such as radiographs of the hands, feet, and vertebrae (57).

The empiric information available shows that "isolated" types A and B postaxial polydactyly are hereditary, but the mode of inheritance has been debated. Since varied expressivity and decreased penetrance have been observed, the affected parent should be counseled of an increased risk "up to 50%" for having an affected child.

If the affected parent has isolated polydactyly, type A or B, the risk is for having a child with an isolated form of polydactyly. The type of postaxial, i.e., type A or B, in the child is not always the same as in the affected parent.

If the affected infant has postaxial polydactyly as one of several malformations, the risk in subsequent children is that of the specific malformation syndrome.

POLYDACTYLY—PREAXIAL

Definition

An additional digit (thumb or first toe) or phalanx (triphalangism) on the medial or inner aspect of the hand or foot. The affected digit is usually the first, but is occasionally the second finger or toe.

ICD-9:	755.010	(accessory thumb)
	755.030	(accessory big toe)
ICD-10:	Q69.1	[accessory thumb(s)]
	Q69.2	[accessory toe(s); hallux]
Mendelian Inheritance in Man:	#174400	(polydactyly, preaxial I; thumb polydactyly; thenar anomaly; includes Fromont anomaly)
	#174500	(polydactyly, preaxial II; PPD2; polydactyly of triphalangeal thumb)
	%174600	(polydactyly, preaxial III; index finger polydactyly)
	#174700	(polydactyly, preaxial IV. A type of polysyndactyly).
	#603596	(polydactyly)
	601759	(preaxial hallucal, polydactyly)

Appearance

Hands. The additional finger or toe (Figure 15-9) is usually located on the medial aspect of the hand or foot (58–62). The appearance varies from a hypoplastic, small phalanx containing a nail that is dangling from the side of the thumb (Figure 15-7) or big toe to a hypoplastic digit that articulates with the first metacarpalphalangeal joint. Occasionally, there is a complete first digit with a separate metacarpal or metatarsal.

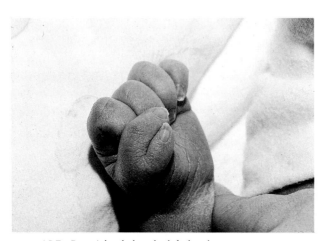

FIGURE 15.7   Preaxial polydactyly, left thumb.

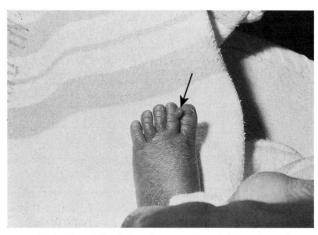

FIGURE 15.8   Preaxial polydactyly, second toe, left foot (arrow).

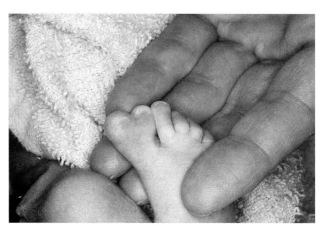

FIGURE 15.9   Preaxial polydactyly, first toe, right foot.

In triphalangism of the thumb, another type of preaxial polydactyly is an additional (third) phalanx. The triphalangeal thumb is in the normal position of the thumb.

Duplication of the index finger (or second toe) is a much less common type of preaxial polydactyly (Figure 15-8).

Wassel (63) proposed a classification of duplicated thumbs, with seven types.

I) bifid distal phalanx (accounts for 2 to 6% of thumb duplication[62])
II) duplicated distal phalanx (12 to 18% of thumb duplication [62])
III) bifid proximal phalanx (6 to 10% of thumb duplications [62])
IV) duplicated proximal and distal phalanx (43 to 52% of thumb duplications [62])
V) bifid metacarpal (4% to 14% of thumb duplications [62])
VI) duplicated metacarpal and thumb (3 to 6% of thumb duplications [62])
VII) triphalangism of the thumb, accompanied by a normal thumb (6 to 20% of thumb duplications [62])

However, these categories do not encompass all cases of thumb polydactyly. As was noted by Upton (64) in discussing an "unclassified" case, "the myriad of anatomic variations [on hand malformation] is almost endless."

Triphalangeal thumbs have also been subdivided into subgroups: opposable, non-opposable, and complicated preaxial polydactyly (65, 66). Anatomic dissections of resected polydactylous triphalangeal thumbs have shown that some do not have joints between the phalanges and metacarpals and others have only one interphalangeal joint, not two, between the three phalanges (67).

Population-based studies in several countries and large states in the United States (58–61) have shown that over 95% of the infants with preaxial polydactyly have an affected hand, with the affected foot very uncommon.

Feet. In the foot, Watanabe, Fujita, and Oka (32) identified four anatomic patterns of preaxial or medial-ray polydactyly in 36 feet of 22 patients: distal phalangeal type (22%), proximal phalangeal type (36%), metatarsal type (36%), and tarsal type (3%).

Studies of the vasculature of the different types of preaxial polydactyly of the thumb have shown that Wassel types I to VI thumbs had normal proximal vascular anatomy. For the additional digit, there were additional vessels from persistent medial arteries and the superficial palmar arch. However, the Wassel type VII triphalangeal thumb with a normal thumb had anomalous proximal feeding vessels (68).

Associated Malformations

Preaxial polydactyly occurs most often as an isolated abnormality, that is with no other associated malformations (58, 60). In malformation registries in Central-East France (1978–1993), Sweden (1973–1991), and California (1987–1992) [60], there were 1,694 infants with preaxial limb malformations: 31%, 6% and 24%, respectively, of infants with polydactyly of the thumbs had associated malformations or chromosome abnormalities. Among infants with polydactyly of the hallux (first toe), the frequency of those with associated malformations and chromosome abnormalities were: 27%, 13%, and 38%, respectively.

Preaxial polydactyly has been associated with many different syndromes (Table 15-4).

Well-described examples are the VACTERL Association (MIM# 174100), the Holt-Oram Syndrome (MIM# 142900), and the Townes-Brocks Syndrome (MIM# 107480).

In the analysis of 888 infants with thumb polydactyly in three populations surveyed (France, Sweden, and California [60]), 136 (15.3%) were considered to have a specific syndrome. The VACTERL Association was

the most common (51 of 888 or 5.7%). The Holt-Oram Syndrome was the most common syndrome attributed to a single mutant gene (17 of 888 or 1.9%).

Developmental Defect

The specific molecular events in humans with isolated preaxial polydactyly have not been determined.

The distribution of several genes, such as *A1x4, Gli3, C7orf2/Lmbr1* (69, 70), and ectopic location of other genes have all been shown to produce preaxial polydactyly in the mouse. For example, disruption of *A1x4* (*artistaless-related homeobox gene*) occurs in the semidominant mutations *Extra-toes (Xt)* and *Strong's Luxoid (Lst)* in the mouse (69, 71). The effect of disrupting *A1x4* is *Sonic hedgehog (Shh)* dependent.

In the heterozygote *(Xt/+)* *(extra toes)* mouse, there is preaxial polydactyly in the forelimb and the hindlimb. In *X-linked polydactyly (Xp1)* [71], there is preaxial polydactyly of the hindlimbs, sometimes in association with tibia hemimelia.

Sasquatch (Ssq) is another semidominant mutation in the mouse which affects the hindlimb (71). The Ssq mutation is postulated to interrupt the long-range cis-acting regulator of sonic hedgehog (Shh), which causes the preaxial polydactyly (72). Likewise in humans, disruption of Shh regulation is the most likely basis for preaxial polydactyly.

In several families with autosomal dominant triphalangeal thumbs this theory was confirmed, as mutations were identified in the long-range Shh enhancer (73).

In an experimental model of preaxial polydactyly produced in rat embryos exposed to 6-mercaptopurine riboside in utero, it was postulated that the drug-exposure delayed the onset of physiologic cell death (apoptosis) in the apical ectodermal ridge (74).

Another experimental model is misexpression of the basis helix loop-helix transcription factor dHAND on the anterior compartment of the limb bud, which induces ectopic expression of sonic hedgehog. This produced preaxial polydactyly in mouse limbs (75).

Prevalence

Population-based studies in France, Sweden, and California (60) and eleven countries in South America (59) showed these prevalence rates:

- Hands: preaxial polydactyly – isolated 0.07 to 0.19/1,000 (60) and 0.17/1,000 (59); with multiple anomalies 0.01 to 0.06/1,000 (60); triphalangism of thumbs – isolated 0.005 to 0.009/1,000 and 0.007/1,000 (59).
- Feet: preaxial polydactyly – isolated 0.02/1,000 (60) and triphalangism of the first toe with associated anomalies 0.0005/1,000 (60).

TABLE 15-4 *Preaxial polydactyly of hands and feet in Brigham and Women's Hospital, Boston (1972–1974, 1979–2000); 206, 224 livebirths, stillbirths and elective terminations for anomalies.*

Apparent Etiology	Left — Multiple	Left — Isolated Anomalies	Right — Multiple	Right — Isolated Anomalies	Both — Multiple	Both — Isolated Anomalies
I. Hands only, non-transfers:*						
1. Mendelian disorders						
Nager acrofacial dystosis				1		
Achondroplasia				1		
2. Chromosome abnormalities:						
Trisomy 18				1		1
3. Familial	1					
4. Syndromes						
VACTERL						1
5. Twinning						
DZ					1	
6. Unknown etiology	<u>18</u>	<u>1</u>	<u>22</u>	<u>3</u>	—	—
TOTAL	19	1	22	6	1	2/51
II. Feet only, non-transfers*						
1. Mendelian disorders						
Private syndrome						1
2. Chromosome abnormalities:						
Trisomy 13				1		
Triploidy						
(69,XXX)		1				
3. Unknown etiology	<u>1</u>	–	<u>5</u>	–	<u>2</u>	–
TOTAL	1	1	5	1	2	1

Legend: *No infants were identified who had preaxial polydactyly of both hands and feet.
Excludes infants whose mothers had planned to deliver at another hospital, but transferred care after the prenatal diagnosis of fetal anomalies.

Parental Ages

A significant increase in preaxial polydactyly of the thumb was identified among the infants of teenage mothers in Sweden and California (60).

Birth Status

In a survey in eleven South American countries (59), infants with thumb duplication had a lower mean birth weight and gestational age and their mothers had more frequent vaginal bleeding in the first trimester than their matched controls.

Race

Native Americans have a higher frequency of isolated preaxial polydactyly (0.25/1,000) [44] than occurs in Caucasians.

Case series in Japan (76) and China (77) showed that preaxial polydactyly was much more common than postaxial polydactyly. For example, in a review of 943 limb deformities treated in a clinic in Hokkaido, Japan (1968–1984), there were 155 with preaxial polydactyly of the arm and 8 with postaxial polydactyly (76).

Sex Ratio

There were significantly more males with preaxial polydactyly than females in California, Sweden, and eastern France: M:F = 409:318 (60). However, there was no difference in the sex ratio for infants with triphalangism of the thumb or preaxial polydactyly of the first toe.

Sidedness

Over 90% (674 of 722 infants in one study [60]) of the affected infants) have unilateral polydactyly. The right hand was much more often affected than the left (59, 60).

In contrast, triphalangism of the thumb was bilateral in half of the affected infants (60).

Twinning

There was a 3% frequency of twinning among 1,452 infants with preaxial limb malformations and 3.1% for polydactyly of the thumbs (60). This rate was considered higher than the expected population rate of 2%. However, no increase in the frequency of twinning was identified in the population-based studies in eleven countries in South America (59).

Several sets of monozygous twins have been discordant for preaxial polydactyly (78, 79). The rate of concordance in monozygous twins has not been established.

Genetic Factors

The likelihood of inheritance of the preaxial polydactyly varies with the anatomic type: highest frequency for thumb triphalangism and lowest for preaxial polydactyly of the first toe (59, 80–82).

The empiric risk of recurrence of preaxial polydactyly of the thumb has not been established for either the subsequent siblings of the affected child (with unaffected parents) or the offspring of the first affected member of the family. Families with two or more affected members with duplicated two-phalanx thumbs have been reported (80–82). A multifactorial pattern of inheritance has been considered more likely than monogenic inheritance (77).

Preaxial polydactyly, types II and III, with triphalangism of the thumb or index finger has been observed with apparent autosomal dominant inheritance in several families of several different ethnic/racial ancestries (80, 83, 84). Many, but not all, of the families have shown gene linkage to chromosome 7 q 36, which suggests genetic heterogeneity. The phenotype in one large family (84) varied from triphalangism of the thumb to preaxial polydactyly with either two or three phalanges to polysyndactyly. In some families absence or dysplasia of the radius or tibia has also occurred (83).

Environmental Factors

No human teratogens have been identified that causes isolated preaxial polydactyly of the thumbs or first toes. Preaxial polydactyly of the first toe occurs in infants of diabetic mothers, typically, as part of a phenotype of macrosomia and multiple anomalies (85).

Triphalangism of the thumb and preaxial polydactyly of the feet were features of the thalidomide embryopathy (86). Typically the polydactyly was one of multiple anomalies, not an isolated abnormality.

Treatment and Prognosis

The surgical repair is usually carried out by the end of the first year. Typically, the most hypoplastic, duplicated thumb is removed. The surgery includes removal of the extra thumb and reconstruction of the remaining thumb (87, 88). There is reconstruction of the collateral ligament, as well as correcting any deviation of the axis of the thumb. The remaining thumb does not have normal mobility. The inter-phalangeal joint becomes stiffer with age.

The repair of the triphalangeal thumb has special challenges and may require several procedures. All accessory parts, including the delta bone, must be removed, joint ligaments reconstructed, and deviations corrected (65, 66).

If not repaired in childhood, preaxial polydactyly is usually considered to have social consequences, with the affected individual hiding his/her hands. Surgical reconstruction in adults is usually very successful (89).

Genetic Counseling

Unilateral, preaxial polydactyly with two phalanges usually occurs in an infant with no other anomalies and no affected relatives. When evaluating an infant with preaxial polydactyly of the thumb, the examiner should examine the parents for hypoplasia of the thenar eminence, the Fromont anomaly. The polydactyly in the infant and hypoplasia of the thenar eminence in the parent could be different manifestations of an autosomal dominant condition (90). (Fig 15-10)

Two other patterns of varied physical findings have been observed in the parents of infants with preaxial polydactyly:

1) in infants with type I camptodactyly of the thumb or other fingers in one parent (91);
2) in infants with type II (triphalangism), some parents had a delta-shaped extra phalanx (92).

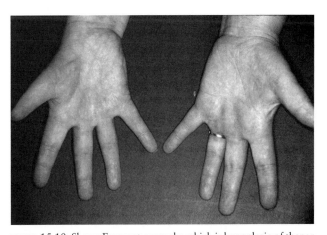

FIGURE 15.10 Shows Fromont anomaly, which is hypoplasia of thenar eminence of right hand of parent of an infant with preaxial polydactyly of one hand. (Courtesy of John M. Graham, Jr., M.D., Sc.D., Cedars-Sinai Medical Center, Los Angeles, CA.)

The empiric recurrence risk for unilateral, preaxial polydactyly with two phalanges in sibs and offspring of affected individuals has not been determined. The low frequency of reported families with two or more affected individuals and the low concordance in monozygous twins makes monogenic inheritance unlikely.

In contrast to isolated preaxial polydactyly with two phalanges, isolated preaxial polydactyly with triphalangism (with no associated malformations) is more likely to be due to an autosomal dominant gene. There is a high degree of penetrance of the mutation. The frequency of spontaneous mutations has not been determined. No commercial testing is available for this mutation.

Preaxial polydactyly is also a feature of many multiple anomaly syndromes.

Theoretically, preaxial polydactyly can be identified prenatally by ultrasound. The accuracy of this type of prenatal diagnosis has not been established.

POLYSYNDACTYLY

Definition

The presence of an extra digit (polydactyly) and a significant degree of webbing (syndactyly) between at least two fingers or toes on one hand or foot.

ICD-9:	755.005	(accessory fingers [postaxial polydactyly, type A]
	755.006	(skin tag [postaxial polydactyly, type B])
	755.010	(accessory thumbs [preaxial polydactyly])
	755.020	(accessory toes [postaxial])
	755.030	(accessory big toe [preaxial])
	755.100	(fused fingers)
	755.120	(fused toes)
ICD-10:	Q70.4	(polysyndactyly)
Mendelian Inheritance in Man:	%102510	(acropectorovertebral dysplasia; F-form of F Syndrome)
	#174500	(polydactyly, preaxial II; PPD2)
	#174700	(polydactyly, preaxial IV; includes crossed polydactyly, type I; CP1, included)
	%175690	(polysyndactyly, crossed)
	#186000	(synpolydactyly 1; SPD1)
	186200	(syndactyly, type IV; polysyndactyly, Haas type)
	^190605	(polydactyly, preaxial II;PPD2; includes triphalangeal thumb)
	#608180	(syndactyly 2; SPD2)
	%610234	(synpolydactyly 3)

Appearance

Polysyndactyly occurs in several relatively specific patterns of polydactyly and syndactyly. The first group identified was those attributed to autosomal dominant inheritance. The distinctive autosomal dominant phenotypes are:

1. Type II. Synpolydactyly: Vordingborg type (MIM: 186000) [93–98]
   polydactyly
   i) hands-partial or complete duplication of digit between fingers 3 and 4 (Figure 15-11)
   ii) feet-postaxial polydactyly, type B involving hands and postaxial polydactyly of feet (type A) with 5-6 syndactyly

syndactyly
   i) fingers 3-4
   ii) toes 4-5 and 5-6

Other features include camptodactyly of fingers and shortening of fifth fingers. In one family the males had hypospadias, possibly reflecting to the fact that HOXD is expressed in the urogenital folds during development (97).

Molecular basis: polyalanine expansion in HOXD13 gene (95).

2. Syndactyly 2; SPD2; fibulin-1 gene type (MIM#: # 608180) [99–103]
   polydactyly
   i) Hands – duplication of digit between fingers 3 and 4
   syndactyly
   ii) hands – partial syndactyly, fingers 3-4

Other distinctive features include fusion of metatarsals in feet and metacarpals in hands. The first affected family (99) was reported initially as having the Cenani-Lenz Syndrome. However, there were inconsistencies in the phenotype and molecular studies showed there was no expansion of polyalanines within the first exon of the HOXD13 gene, as occurs in Synpolydactyly, type II, Vordingborg type. Rather, decreased levels of fibulin 1-D were identified. This was caused by a reciprocal translocation t (12; 22) (p11.2; q13.3) with the breakpoint in chromosome 22 located in the intron between the last two exons of the fibulin 1-D. The translocation also interrupted the 5-prime untranslocated region of C12ORF2 on chromosome 12p (100).

3. Type II. Syndactyly, chromosome 14 type [105]; synpolydactyly 3 (MIM: %610234).
   polydactyly
   i) hands – bony element present between third and fourth metacarpals;
   ii) feet – postaxial polydactyly of feet with only five metatarsals;
   syndactyly
   i) hands – there is complete syndactyly between the third and fourth fingers with the third finger overriding the fourth;
   ii) feet – syndactyly between toes 4, 5 and 6.

Other features include hypoplastic distal phalanges of the thumbs, symphalangism of the first and second phalanges of the index fingers with camptodactyly of index fingers, osseous fusion of the third and fourth fingers at their tips, misshapen first and second phalanges of the first fingers. The carpal bones are hypoplastic and misaligned.

The feet showed hypoplasia of the distal phalanges of all toes. There is duplication of the distal phalanges of

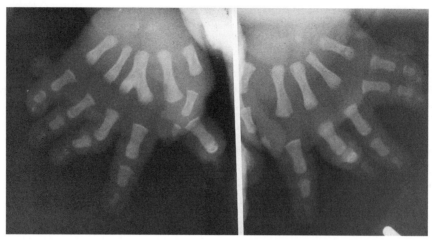

FIGURE 15.11   Extra third finger between fingers 3 and 4 in type II synpolydactyly; her affected son had only postaxial polydactyly.

the distal phalanges of the fifth toes. There is symphalangism of the first toes.

4. Preaxial polydactyly, type IV or crossed polysyndactyly: (MIM: #174700 and #175690) [105–108].
    <u>polydactyly</u>
    i) hands – postaxial, type B
    ii) feet – preaxial (duplication of first toe)
    <u>syndactyly</u>
    i) hands – fingers 3-4, most often (Figure 15-12), occasionally fingers 1-2
    ii) feet – toes 1-2-3 (Figure 15-13)

    Molecular basis: mutations in <u>GLI3</u> zinc-finger transcriptor factor gene.

5. Syndactyly type IV: Haas type: MIM: 186200 [109, 110]

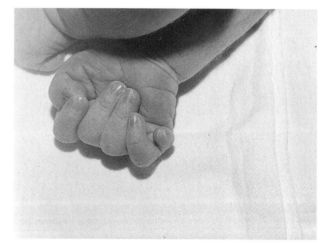

FIGURE 15.13   Syndactyly of fingers 3-4 and postaxial polydactyly of the right hand of the same infant shown in Figures 15.12 and 15.14.

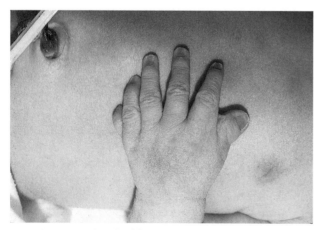

FIGURE 15.12   Syndactyly of fingers 1-2 (mild) and postaxial polydactyly, type B in infant with preaxial polydactyly, type IV (crossed polysyndactyly) in left hand.

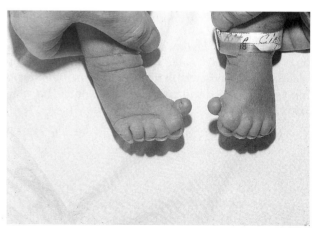

FIGURE 15.14   Duplication of first toe with syndactyly of toes 1, 2, and 3 in same infant with crossed polysyndactyly.

polydactyly

i) postaxial polydactyly of hands and feet with six metacarpals and metatarsals;

ii) hypoplastic triphalangism of thumb and hypoplasia of themar muscle;

Syndactyly:

i) complete syndactyly of some (fingers 3-5) or all fingers on both hands, but without bony fusion;

ii) toes: no syndactyly

iii) other features include absence of the tibia (110).

6. Triphalangeal thumbs-polysyndactyly (MIM: ^190 605) [ref. 111, 112]

polydactyly

i) hands – varies from thumb to an opposable thumb with a delta-shaped middle phalanx to triphalangeal index finger; can have two additional preaxial, but hypoplastic, digits lateral to the thumb; hypoplastic thenar eminence

ii) feet – pre-and postaxial polydactyly

syndactyly

i) hands – syndactyly between third, fourth and fifth fingers with synostosis of distal interphalangeal joints

7. F syndrome: Acropectorovertebral Dygenesis (MIM: %102510) [113]

polydactyly

i) hands- shortened thumb

ii) feet- duplication of first toe

syndactyly

i) hands- between thumb and index finger;

ii) feet- between duplicated first toe

Other features include stenoses of carpal and tarsal bones and dysgenesis of the first and second finger. Associated craniofacial abnormalities include brachycephaly, macrocephaly, dental dysplasia, and high and narrow palate. Pectus excavatum and spina bifida occultal are common.

The autosomal recessive phenotypes

These are more likely to be identified in inbred populations. They will be expected to have more severe abnormalities than the autosomal dominant disorders. One example was described in a large inbred Pakistani family (114):

polydactyly: central (insertional) or postaxial
              postaxial

syndactyly: fingers 3-4
              toes 4-5

Other features included: absence of middle phalanges of toes.

Associated Malformations

In general, none of these specific "isolated" polysyndactylies is associated with visceral malformations.

Developmental Defect

The molecular basis for the specific cellular events that lead to a specific pattern of polysyndactyly has only been described for a few phenotypes. One intriguing unanswered question is how the same gene mutation can produce different patterns in the hands and foot of the same individual, such as the preaxial polydactyly in the feet and postaxial polydactyly in the hands, which occurs in preaxial polydactyly, type IV or "crossed polysyndactyly."

Mutations have been identified in associations with three types of polysyndactyly in humans:

1) HOXD13 mutations in Type II synpolydactyly;

The mutation in Type II polysyndactyly, first reported by Muragki and associates in 1996 (94), is a polyalanine tract expansion in the HOXD13 gene. In general, there is a direct correlation between the length of the polyalanine repeat and the severity of the limb malformations (95, 97).

A 117-kb microdeletion, which removed HOXD9-HOXD13 and EVX2, has also produced this phenotype (102).

The most mildly affected, presumably heterozygous, individual had in each hand a single transverse crease, an accessory distal interphalangeal flexion crease presentation on the 3rd and 4th fingers and marked clinodactyly of the 5th fingers (37).

Homozygosity for this HOXD13 mutation is a much more severe abnormality (94) with associated oligodactyly and hypoplasia of the carpals, metacarpals, and phalanges.

2) GLI 3 mutations in type IV (or crossed) polysyndactyly.

Mutations in the GL13 zinc-finger transcription factor gene cause a wide spectrum of phenotypes: preaxial polydactyly type IV and postaxial polydactyly types A and B are the mild end of the severity spectrum, while Greig cephalopolysyndactyly and Pallister-Hall Syndromes are the more severe end. The genotype-phenotype correlations are being established, but have not been established for the isolated polysyndactyly (preaxial polydactyly type IV) yet.

3) Triphalangeal thumb – polysyndactyly has been shown, in Han Chinese families, to be associated with duplication of the ZPA regulatory sequence (SRS)

[115]. Point mutations have been identified in the long-range SHH enhancer in three other families with this phenotype (73).

Syndactyly type IV has been mapped to the same region 7q36 as triphalangeal thumb-polysyndactyly. The findings were interpreted to suggest that triphalangeal thumb-polysyndactyly and syndactyly, type IV are allelic with PPD2/PPD3.

A spontaneous mutation of HOXD13 with a poly-alanine expansion, as in human synpolydactyly, type II, has been identified in mice (116). There was a 21bp in-frame duplication within a polyalanine-encoding of the HOXD13 coding sequence. The duplication expands the number of alanine repeats from 15 to 22, as occurs in synpolydactyly, type II (spdh). The homozygotes (spdh/spdh) showed more severe malformations of forelimbs and hindlimbs, including polydactyly, syndactyly, and brachydactyly. The homozygotes lack preputial glands and the males do not breed.

The GLI3Δ699 mutant in the mouse carries a targeted mutation of the sequences encoding the DNA-binding domain at GLI3 locus (117). The Gli3 mutations are expressed in heterozygous in humans, but only in homozygotes ($GLI3^{\Delta699/\Delta699}$) in mice. The majority of the $GLI3^{\Delta699/\Delta699}$ embryos showed the polydactyly similar to that in Pallister-Hall syndrome, a central or insertional polydactyly (118).

Polysyndactyly has also been produced in transgenic mice. In one model (116) the chicken MSX2 promoter was used to target the expression of the Noggin gene. Noggin is an antagonist of several bone morphogenetic proteins (BMPs). The MSX2-noggin mutant mice showed syndactyly, postaxial polydactyly, and absence of ventral footpads and supernumerary ventral nails. The apical ectodermal ridge (AER) persisted longer than normal. The subectodermal mesoderm failed to undergo the normal pattern of apoptosis.

The mutation polysyndactyly (Ps) arose during neutron irradiation experiments and was characterized by Johnson (120) in 1969. Breeding studies showed that Ps was dominant and lethal in the homozygote (Ps/Ps). The extra digit was between digits III and IV; the first digit was broad and sometimes duplicated. Cell death was decreased in the interdigital areas of Ps/+ embryos.

The mouse knockout deficient in megf7/Lrp4, a lipoprotein receptor gene family, have growth restriction, polysyndactyly, and in some fetuses, abnormal development of teeth (121). In mouse limb bud cultures when the fibroblast growth factor 4 (fgf4) gain-of-function allele is activated, syndactyly between all digits and postaxial polysyndactyly are produced (130).

Rat fetuses exposed on days 9 and 10 of gestation to Triparanol, an inhibitor of 24 dehydrocholesterol reductase, develop preaxial syndactyly and postaxial polydactyly (123). This treatment modified sonic hedgehog signaling.

Prevalence

The prevalence rate of specific disorders has not been established in large population-based surveys.

In the Active Malformations Surveillance Program at Brigham and Women's Hospital in Boston (1972–1974, 1979–1994), 11 infants with specific polysyndactyly phenotypes (1:14,659) were identified among 166,252 livebirths, stillbirths, and elective terminations for anomalies. The most common was 6 infants (1:26,875) with preaxial polydactyly, type IV, or crossed polysyndactyly. In addition, five infants had one of these phenotypes:

1) Greig cephalopolysyndactyly (108);
2) Synpolydactyly, type II Vordingberg type; the affected mother had insertional polydactyly (Figure 15-11); her affected son had only postaxial polydactyly, type of each hand;
3) Acrocallosal syndrome;
4) Two private syndromes of multiple anomalies, each including polysyndactyly (125, 126).

Race/Ethnicity

No racial/ethnic differences have been established.

Birth Status

No increased frequency of miscarriage, stillbirth or premature births has been reported in association with any specific isolated polysyndactyly.

Sex Ratio

These phenotypes due to autosomal dominant and recessive mutations. No differences in sex ratio for any specific disorder has been described.

Sidedness

No asymmetry in the phenotypes has been established.

Parental Age

No alteration of the age of mothers or fathers of affected infants with any of these types of polysyndactyly has been reported.

Twinning

An increased frequency of twins has not been described for any of these phenotypes. No affected monozygous or dizygous twins have been reported.

Genetic Factors

The pattern of inheritance has been established in family studies for each of the specific types of polysyndactyly identified to date. Those highlighted above are almost all attributed to autosomal dominant inheritance. The likelihood of a spontaneous mutation for any of the 7 types described above has not been established for any, but appears to be low.

It seems likely that additional types of polysyndactyly will be identified in consanguineous families. These autosomal recessive phenotypes will be more severe, as a rule, than the autosomal dominant phenotypes.

Environmental Factors

No environmental exposure has been identified that causes a type of polysyndactyly.

Treatment and Prognosis

The repair is specific to the anatomic abnormalities.

Genetic Counseling

The first step is the physical examination to establish the phenotype. Since most of the specific types of polysyndactyly have been attributed to autosomal dominant genes and have a low rate of spontaneous mutation, it is likely that one parent will be affected, also. Sometimes the affected parent has had surgery in childhood for limb malformations, and is not aware of associated craniofacial features or genetic risk. These could have been considered "family resemblance," and not an "abnormality." This can be a sensitive issue to be explored carefully.

If it is possible to examine the affected parent, the pattern of changes in the hands and feet, and any other physical features, combined with those in the affected newborn, should make it possible to determine the type of polysyndactyly present.

Polysyndactyly is a feature of many multiple malformation syndromes. These should be considered in the infant who is dysmorphic or has associated malformations. Some examples are:

1. Sandrow Syndrome (127): dimelia of the fibula and ulna; severe limitation of flexion and pronation of both forearms; fixed bilateral talipes equinovarus; mirror hands with two digits fused; polysyndactyly of 10 rays on both feet.
2. Acrocallosal Syndrome (MIM: #200990): Duplication of first toe, postaxial polydactyly and absence of corpus callosum; mental retardation (128).
3. Bonneau Syndrome (MIM: 263630): Duplication of first toe, syndactyly of fingers 3-4 and heart defects (129).
4. Hirschsprung disease with heart defects, laryngeal anomalies, and preaxial polydactyly (MIM: 604211) [126].

The parents of a child with any type of polysyndactyly may ask to use prenatal ultrasound screening to rule out this diagnosis in the next pregnancy. Its accuracy has not been established.

LONGITUDINAL DEFICIENCY, PREAXIAL: ABSENCE/HYPOPLASIA OF THUMB AND/OR RADIUS

Definition

Absence or hypoplasia of the thumb, thenar eminence with or without hypoplasia, or absence of the radius.

ICD-9:	755.260	(preaxial longitudinal reduction defect of upper limb; absent radius (total or partial) and/or thumb with or without second finger (total or partial; includes isolated absent or hypoplastic thumb).
ICD-10:	Q71.4	(longitudinal reduction, defect of radius; radial club hand)
Mendelian Inheritance in Man:	312190	(radial aplasia, X-linked)

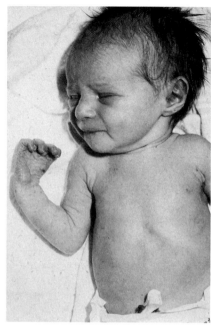

FIGURE 15.15　Absence of thumb and hypoplasia of radius.

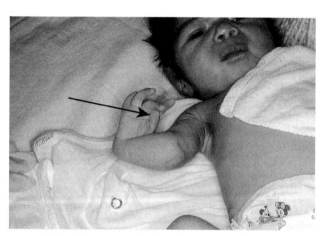

FIGURE 15.16　Hypoplasia of radius, but presence of thumb (arrow) in infant with thrombocytopenia and radial aplasia (TAR).

Appearance

The hypoplastic thumb can be in the normal location with a smaller than normal thenar eminence or more distally placed. The interphalangeal joint is often stiff.

Absence of the thumb usually occurs without a remnant or pedicle (Figures 15-15 and 15-17).

The thenar eminence is also hypoplastic (Figure 15-19).

When the hypoplastic thumb is "flail," (Figure 15-18), there is no articulation with the first metacarpal-phalangeal joint.

In the case of a "finger-like" thumb (Figure 15-20), the first finger is oriented parallel to the index finger, rather than in opposition, as is needed for the normal pincer grasp.

In one case series (141), the severity of the under-development of the thumb correlated with the degree of hypoplasia of the radius (Figure 15-15): the more severe the shortening of the radius, the greater the hypoplasia of the thumb.

In association with absence or hypoplasia of the thumb, there is often absence of the pulse from the radial artery in the wrist. This reflects absence of the radial artery, which anatomic (132) and surgical (133–136) dissections have shown to be a common association.

In children with hypoplastic thumbs, the first web space is often "tighter" than normal and may be more distally located. The intrinsic muscles, that is the abductor pollicis brevis and opponens brevis muscles, are either hypoplastic or absent. In more severe thumb hypoplasia, the flexor and extensor pollicis longus muscles may be absent. In association with hypoplasia of the radius, there are abnormal muscle attachments of both extensor and flexor muscles. When the forearm curves medially, because of absence of the radius, the brachialis muscle and median nerve form a "bowstring" across the elbow joint.

The muscles and neurovascular structures that arise from the lateral (preaxial) epicondyle are frequently absent (134). The muscles of the thenar eminence are deficient proportionate to the degree of hypoplasia of

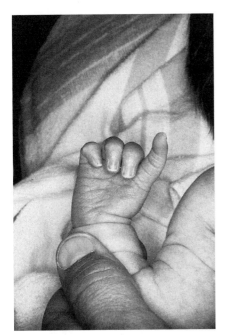

FIGURE 15.17   Absence of thumb with stiff index finger.

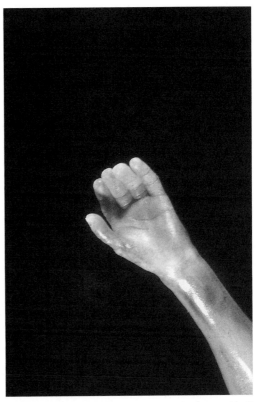

FIGURE 15.19   Hypoplastic thenar eminence in fetus with Fanconi Anemia.

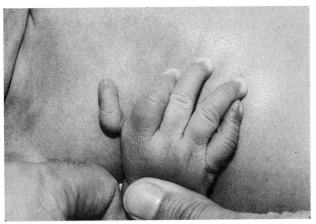

FIGURE 15.18   Dangling thumb.

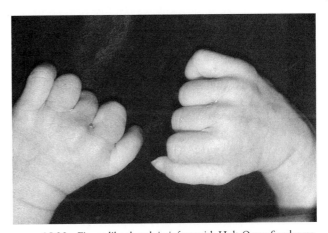

FIGURE 15.20   Finger-like thumb in infant with Holt-Oram Syndrome.

the thumb. There are often additional muscle abnormalities and deficiencies of the muscles throughout the arm with radial club hand, including those of the shoulder girdle and especially the forearm (132, 133).

The dissection of fetuses with absence of the radius showed three types of abnormal patterns of the arteries in the affected arm (137); 1) the arm was supplied by a single superficial axial artery; 2) absence of the radial artery with or without persistence of the median artery; the other vessels were present in their usual relationships; 3) the radial artery was present and had an unusual course. The first two of these vascular patterns were considered to represent the persistence of the embryonic arteries and a failure of the adult pattern

to develop. The third pattern was identified only in infants with thrombocytopenia-radial aplasia (TAR) syndrome, a genetic disorder in which there is absence of the radius, but the thumb is present (138).

Abnormalities of the carpal bones are common in individuals with absence or hypoplasia of the radius. Several patterns have been identified. For example, when the thumb was absent, the trapezium was also absent. The scaphoid was also absent or hypoplastic in association with absence or hypoplasia of the radius (135).

If the index finger is hypoplastic, the thumb is either absent or hypoplastic. Classifications have been proposed for thumb hypoplasia and hypoplasia or absence of the radius.

I. Thumb hypoplasia (131, 139, 140):
    Type I: minimal shortening and narrowing
    Type II: narrow thumb-index finger web space
        hypoplasia of intrinsic thenar muscles
        instability of metacarpophalangeal joint
    Type III:
        A: hypoplastic metacarpal; stable carpometacarpal
        B: partial aplasia of metacarpals; unstable carpometacarpal
    Type IV: floating thumb
    Type V: absent thumb
II. Absence or hypoplasia of radius (139, 141):
    Type I: short distal radius
        distal radial epiphysis decreased in growth; proximal epiphysis normal
        growth of thumb almost always hypoplastic
    Type II: hypoplastic radius
        both proximal and distal epiphyses have deficient growth
        growth of radius below normal
    Type III: partial absence or radius deficiency can be in proximal, middle, or distal portions
        absence of distal one or two thirds is most common
        ulna shortened, thickened and bowed
        hand is displaced radially
        wrist is unstable
    Type IV: total absence of radius
        hand deviated to marked degree
        wrist unstable
    Type V: absent proximal humerus, in addition to typical radial longitudinal deficiency in distal portion of radius

Associated Malformations

Absence or hypoplasia of the radius and thumb occurs as an "isolated" deformity with no other malformations, as well as in association with many malformation syndromes, mendelian disorders, and chromosome abnormalities.

In a case series (141) of 164 patients with abnormalities of the radius treated in a department of orthopedic surgery, most of the affected children had the more severe types of absence of radius (Types IV or V in the classification systems). The absent radius was an isolated finding in 33% of the affected individuals. Heart defects were identified in 32/104 (20%). Many children were considered to have a specific limb malformation

syndrome including: thrombocytopenia-radial aplasia (TAR) (MIM %274000) in 25/164 (15.2%), VACTERL Association (MIM 192350) in 22/164 (13.4%), Holt-Oram Syndrome (MIM #142900) in 7/164 (4.3%), and Fanconi Anemia (MIM #227650) in 1/164 (0.6%).

Developmental Defect

Limb development is a very complex process. The mesenchyme in the region of the future radius and ulna are identifiable by postfertilization week five or at 10 mm crown-rump length. Chondrification of the radius occurs between weeks 5 and 6 and ossification of the radius is present by week 7 (142).

Double mutant mice missing the homeobox containing genes MSX1 and MSX2 had shorter limbs that

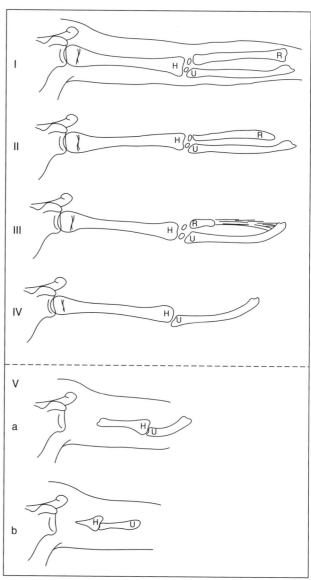

FIGURE 15.21   Classification of types I to V of absence/hypoplasia of radius.

lacked the anterior skeletal elements: radius/thumb and tibia/first toe (143). In the developing limb of these double mutant mice, there was no formation of the apical ectodermal ridge (AER) in the anterior portion of the ectoderm.

Developmental studies in which the tantalum foil barriers were inserted caudal to somite 4 prevented the caudal elongation of the mesonephros-produced limb reduction defects (144). No limb defects were seen when the foil barrier was placed into the intermediate mesoderm at the level of somite 21 or 25. These studies suggested that a signal from the mesonephros was necessary for normal limb development.

An interrelationship between the genes Tbx5 and SALL4 has been demonstrated in the developing mouse preaxial forelimbs and heart, where these genes interacted in regulating patterning and development (145). Mutations in TBX5 (146) and SALL4 (147) cause absence or hypoplasia of the thumb and/or radius, as common features of separate autosomal dominant disorders, the Holt-Oram Syndrome (MIM #142900) and the Okihiro Syndrome (MIM #607343), respectively. These disorders are distinguished by their associated features: Holt-Oram Syndrome with heart defects, a rounded shoulder with hypoplasia of the glenoid fossa, and an *os centrale* in the carpal bones (148); Okihiro Syndrome with hearing loss, Duane anomaly, and kidney malformations (149).

Prevalence

Among 1,575,904 births in Hungary (1975–1984), the birth prevalence rate for radius and tibial defects was 0.045/1,000 with 95% of these defects affecting the radius (150). Among 118,265 consecutive births in eastern France (1975–1987), 18 (0.15/1,000) had reduction deformities of the radius (12).

In the survey of the 4,024,000 residents of Denmark in 1943–1947, Birch-Jensen identified 625 with upper limb deformities 73 of whom had defects of the radius (1:55,123 or 0.02/1,000) [151].

Race/Ethnicity

No racial/ethnic differences have been described.

Birth Status

No increased frequency of prematurity or stillbirth has been established for infants with isolated aplasia or hypoplasia of the thumb or radius. However, these anomalies occur as a feature of many multiple anomaly syndromes some of which are associated with prematurity, stillbirth, small body size, and neonatal death.

Sex Ratio

In a case series of 64 patients with deficiency of the radius, there was an equal sex ratio:male:female=34:30 (139).

The 73 affected individuals with absence or hypoplasia of the radius identified in Denmark (1943–1947) included 44 males (60%) and 29 females (40%) [151].

In a case series of 139 individuals with congenital deficiencies of the radius and thumb in Northern California (131), there were 72 males (61%) and 47 females (39%).

Sidedness

In a case series of 64 individuals with hypoplasia or aplasia of the radius, 27 had a unilateral deformity (139).

In a case series of 164 affected individuals (141), 83 had a unilateral deformity: 36 affecting the right arm; 47, the left arm.

In the case series of 139 individuals in Northern California (131), 39% had unilateral deficiency of radius and thumb. In 70% of these, the right arm was affected.

Parental Age

Information on the average ages of the mothers and fathers of infants with a spinal preaxial deficiency in comparison to matched controls has not been reported.

Twinning

No increased frequency of twinning has been reported in individuals with anomalies of the thumb and radius.

Each of monozygous twins would be expected to be affected if one had a monogenic disorder, such as the Holt-Oram Syndrome.

Genetic Factors

Birch-Jensen (151) and Temtamy and McKusick (27) summarize many families in which there are a parent and child with absence or hypoplasia of the radius. In addition, many families have been identified with two affected children and unaffected parents. These families are postulated to represent autosomal dominant and autosomal recessive inheritance, respectively. However, these index cases were not evaluated for the associated genetic mutations or deletions in TBX5 (146) and SALL4 (147) or the microdeletion of 1q21.1 associated with the thrombocytopenia-absent-radius (TAR) syndrome (138) (Figure 15-16).

Environmental Factors

Absence or hypoplasia of the thumb and radius were common features of individuals with the thalidomide embryopathy. The spectrum of anomalies ranged from hypoplasia of the thenar eminence and thumb hypoplasia to triphalangism of the thumb to preaxial polydactyly (152). The affected infants usually had other anomalies, as well.

Currently, maternal diabetes is the environmental exposure that is most likely to be identified (153).

Treatment and Prognosis

The surgeon and the parents should discuss the severity of the abnormalities and their options soon after the affected infant's birth.

For the infant with hypoplasia of the thumb, there can be reassurance that the mild type I does not require surgery (154). (Figure 15-21) However, for the more severe deformities decisions must be made as to whether the thumb can be retained or whether it should be removed and the index finger pollicized. In general, it is recommended that the surgery be carried out between six and twelve months of age.

For the infant with absence of the radius, splinting of the soft tissues should begin early. The limb with this deficiency is typically limited by radial deviation of the forearm, the unstable wrist, impaired function of fingers, the shortened forearm and the small, weak thumb. Many treatments have been developed. One common approach is centralization of the ulna into the carpal bones, with straightening of the forearm. This procedure is often done at 6 to 12 months of age. If the thumb is hypoplastic, pollicization of the index finger (or conversion of the index finger to be an opposable first digit) is often carried out six months later.

Genetic Counseling

The first question for the clinician is whether the absence or hypoplasia of the thumb or radius is an "isolated" finding in an otherwise healthy infant or is one of several malformations.

If the infant appears to have no other anomalies, the clinician should look for subtle additional features illustrated by these specific phenotypes:

1. Holt-Oram Syndrome (MIM #142900). Usually affects both arms. Preaxial defects may include polydactyly or absence of thumb or finger-like thumb (Figure 15-20). The rounded shoulders may not be apparent in an affected newborn. As ossification continues during childhood, one can look for abnormalities of shoulder girdle and carpal bones in radiographs (146, 148). TBX5 mutations. Autosomal dominant.

2. Okihiro Syndrome (MIM #607323). Absence or hypoplasia of radius and thumbs, affecting both arms. Other features include Duane anomaly of cranial nerve function. Variety of kidney malformations. Associated hearing loss could be detected by newborn screening. SALL4 mutations (147, 149). Autosomal dominant.

3. Lacrimo-auriculo-dento-digital (LADD) Syndrome: MIM #149730). Abnormalities of nasolacrimal ducts and submandibular glands, hypoplasia, ear anomalies, hearing loss, and anomalies of thumb-duplicated triphalangism or hypoplasia. Other anomalies of hands and feet are less common. Mutations in fibroblast growth factor receptors 2 and 3 (155).

To identify these or any autosomal dominant disorders, it can be useful to examine each parent. Possibly one of them is more mildly affected than their affected infant and is not aware of the diagnosis.

4. Fanconi anemia (MIM #22760): Often affects both arms, primarily preaxial defects. A wide spectrum of other anomalies, including some in legs. Microcephaly, Café-au-lait spots. Pancytopenia develops. Identified initially by screening for sensitivity to diethylbutane (DEB). Mutation is one of 13 Fanconi Anemia complementation group genes. Autosomal recessive (156–158).

5. Thrombocytopenia radial aplasia (TAR) [MIM %274000]: Distinctive feature is presence of thumb in association with absence or hypoplasia of radius (Figure 15-16). Anomalies of legs are common. Very low platelet count present in newborn period. Familial, but not mendelian pattern of inheritance. Associated microdeletion of 1q21.1. Child inherits deletion from unaffected parent. An additional, yet unidentified, gene must be present to produce phenotype (138).

For the infant with apparent "isolated" absence or hypoplasia of the thumb or radius, these studies should be considered:

1. screening for mutations in TBX5
2. screening for mutations in SALL4
3. diethyebutane (DEB) stimulation tests
4. deletion studies, if thrombocytopenia – radial aplasia is a tentative clinical diagnosis
5. chromosome microarray (aCGH)

If the affected infant has negative results from the mutation screening, DEB stimulation test, and aCGH or karyotype, the possibility of autosomal dominant, autosomal recessive, or X-linked inheritance should be considered. Unfortunately no distinctive phenotype features have been identified for any of these presumed mendelian conditions. The positive family history has been the only means of suggesting a specific pattern of inheritance.

If the infant has multiple anomalies, including absence/hypoplasia of the radius or thumb and negative results from chromosome analysis and/or aCGH, the many multiple anomaly syndromes that include absence or hypoplasia of the thumb and radius should be considered. Some examples are:

1. X-linked radial ray deficiency (MIM *300378): absence of radius, hypoplasia of thumbs, heart defects, absent patella, contractures of hips and knees (159);
2. X-linked radial aplasia and anogenital anomalies (MIM 312190): an affected uncle and nephew with radial aplasia; variable hydrocephalus, hypospadias, and imperforate anus (160);

3. VACTERL Association with Hydrocephalus, X-linked (MIM #314390): affected males with the VACTERL spectrum of anomalies.

An infant with hypoplasia of the thumb and thenar eminence could have the Fromont Anomaly (90). This has been attributed to an autosomal dominant mutation. The affected individuals have had hypoplasia of the thenar eminence. Their affected relatives can have preaxial polydactyly.

There is no established empiric risk of recurrence after the birth of an infant with absence or hypoplasia of the thumb or radius. The risk could be affected by the findings in the recommended diagnostic studies.

LONGITUDINAL DEFICIENCY, PREAXIAL: ABSENCE/HYPOPLASIA OF TIBIA AND/OR FIRST TOE

Definition

Absence or hypoplasia of the first toe with or without hypoplasia or absence of the tibia.

ICD-9 code: 755.365 (preaxial longitudinal reduction defect of lower limb; absent tibia (total or partial) and/or great toe with or without second toe (total or partial))

ICD-10 code: Q72.5 (longitudinal reduction defect of tibia)

Mendelian Inheritance in Man: %188770 (tibia, hypoplasia of, with polydactyly)

275220 (tibia hemimelia)

Appearance

Absence or hypoplasia of the tibia occurs most often as an isolated, unilateral malformation with the fibula present. The first toe is often hypoplastic in association with absence of the distal tibia. (Figure 15-23). Most often there is a dramatic shortening of the tibia with a rigid club foot (equinovarus) deformity. The rigidity of the club foot reflects the effects of fusion of the bones in the ankle and foot (161–163).

A classification of the pattern of the absence and hypoplasia was developed in 1978 by Jones, Barnes, and Lloyd-Roberts (164), which is still used (163) [Figure 15-22]:

Type 1a: tibia not seen on radiograph; hypoplastic distal epiphysis of femur; fibula present;

1b: tibia not seen; normal epiphysis of distal femur; fibula present;

2: proximal tibia present; most of tibia is absent; fibula present;

3: proximal tibia is not seen, but distal portion of tibia is present; fibula present;

4: tibia is short; there is a spreading apart of the distal tibia and fibula.

The anatomic findings in several amputated affected lower legs have been described (165–171). The dissections showed that in the most severe deformities, the tibia was absent completely with no evidence of a fibrous or cartilaginous anlage of the tibia. There were synostoses of the calcaneus and talus, as well as other bones in the ankle and the tarsal bones (169). Anomalies

Type	Radiological Description	No. of limbs
1 a	• Tibia not seen • Hypoplastic lower femoral epiphysis	6
1 b	• Tibia not seen • Normal lower femoral epiphysis	12
2	• Distal tibia not seen	5
3	• Proximal tibia not seen	2
4	• Diastasis	4

FIGURE 15.22   Shows the spectrum of aplasia and hypoplasia of the tibia with an intact fibula (164).

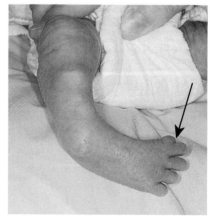

FIGURE 15.23   Hypoplasia of first toe (arrow) of right foot in association with absence of distal portion of tibia.

of the muscles were identified, such as absence or atrophy of the anterior tibial muscle. The patterns of the arteries were similar in several specimens: absence of the anterior tibial artery, a single major artery in the lower leg and a small secondary artery. The pattern of the arteries was a persistence of an immature network of vessels.

Associated Malformations

Many affected infants have adjacent defects that should be considered part of the primary developmental abnormality: preaxial polydactyly, shortening of the femur, coxa valga, congenital dislocation of the hip, and anomalies of a single vertebrae (162, 172).

The presence of distinctive associated malformations, such as split-hand or split-foot, suggests that the infant has a specific malformation syndrome, such as the tibia hemimelia-split-hand/split foot syndrome (173).

Many infants with absence or hypoplasia of the tibia will have multiple anomalies of unknown etiology (340).

Developmental Defect

The lower limbs are visible as limb buds at about 4 1/2 weeks postfertilization. The condensation of mesenchyme that will form the long bones is visible in the fifth week. Cartilage is present in these areas in the sixth week. Centers of ossification are visible in the diaphyses of bones in the 8th week and in all bones of the limbs by the 12th week. Development proceeds in a proximodistal sequence (142, 174).

The causes of absence or hypoplasia of the tibia are not known. Theoretically, there could be malfunction of the preaxial half of the apical ectoderm ridge (AER) after the formation of the femur in the proximal portion of the leg has begun.

Dominant hemimelia (Dh) is a dominant mutation in the mouse that arose spontaneously and is a model for absence of the tibia in humans. The Dh/+ mice are fertile. There is almost 100% penetrance of the Dh/+ phenotype on some genetic backgrounds. The absence of the tibia can be unilateral or bilateral and is always associated with absence of the spleen. If the tibia is hypoplastic, there is a deficiency of the distal portion. There is fusion of the ankle bones and variable deficiency or polydactyly of the preaxial digits (175). The limb deficiency is asymmetric, with more shortening of the left tibia than the right tibia (176). The shortening of the tibia in Dh/+ mice is associated with a decreased number of lumbar vertebrae. Whether absence/hypoplasia of the tibia in humans is associated with a decreased number of lumbar vertebrae has not been determined.

Prevalence

Some population-based surveys have reported the frequency of absence or hypoplasia of the tibia; 0.02/1,000 in British Columbia (1966–1984) [177] and 0.04/1,000 in eastern France (1979–1987) [256]. Unilateral defects are more common than bilateral and one of multiple anomalies is more common than an isolated defect (256).

Race/Ethnicity

The prevalence rates in different ethnic/racial groups have not been reported.

Birth Status

No data on infants with isolated absence of the tibia has been reported.

Sex Ratio

In one case series (172) of 13 individuals with tibia hemimelia, there were 7 males and 4 females.

Sidedness

In one case series (172), 9 of 11 involved the right tibia; in another series (8) of 18 affected individuals, 9 had an affected right leg and 9 had an affected left leg.

Parental Age

Abnormalities of maternal or paternal age have not been reported.

Twinning

In 1925, Ollerenshaw (165) described twin girls, who appeared to be identical, and each had absence of the tibia in the left leg. The operative specimen, when dissected, showed a bifid first toe and the presence of the proximal portion of the tibia, the diaphysis, and epiphysis.

Another set of identical twins had aplasia of the tibia, type Ia in one leg and type 4 in the other; the other twin had a normal right leg and a type II aplasia of the tibia in her left leg (178). Both twins had, also, a split hand deformity, which indicates that they had the tibia hemimelia-split-hand/split-foot syndrome (173).

Genetic Factors

Infants with absence of the tibia usually have an isolated, unilateral deformity and no affected relatives. A few families have been reported in which isolated tibia hemimelia was attributed to autosomal dominant (179, 162) or autosomal recessive (180, 181) inheritance.

Among the infants with absence or hypoplasia of the tibia with other associated malformations, many distinctive autosomal dominant (173, 182–185) and autosomal recessive (186–188) disorders have been described.

Environmental Factors

Absence of the tibia and preaxial polydactyly of the first toe is more common among infants of diabetic mothers (85). But, absence/hypoplasia of the tibia without preaxial polydactyly is not.

Absence of the tibia was also part of the spectrum of skeletal effects produced by exposure to thalidomide (190). The affected child would usually have other skeletal and visceral anomalies (86).

Treatment and Prognosis

The surgical treatment of absence of tibia has evolved. Initially, amputation at the knee was the usual treatment (161, 163, 166–168, 191). Infants with complete absence of the tibia (type I) had disarticulation of the knee.

More recently, leg lengthening procedures have been used successfully for infants with complete absence of the tibia (type Ia) or when the proximal tibia is present (type II) [191]. However, this type of reconstruction is difficult and takes a long-term commitment.

The presence of some proximal tibia and, therefore, some knee joint structure correlates with some function of the quadriceps. The proximal tibiofibular bifurcation synostosis was developed to stabilize the upper portion of the lower leg, with amputation at the below-the-knee level (192).

When an infant has absence of the tibia with shortening or malformations of the femur, the surgical management and options are much more complex (193).

Genetic Counseling

Absence of the tibia with no associated anomalies has shown, in some families, apparent autosomal dominant inheritance (162, 179) and, in others, autosomal recessive inheritance (180, 181), including MIM: 275220. Two families with affected brothers with only isolated absence of tibia and one family with affected individuals in three generations (grandfather, father, and daughter) were included in a case series of 57 affected individuals (162). However, no empiric risk of recurrence has been established for the next pregnancy of unaffected parents whose infant has absence/hypoplasia of the tibia with no other anomalies. In some inbred families with apparent autosomal inheritance of absence of tibia, there have been other anomalies.

There is limited information on the natural history of infants with isolated absence/hypoplasia of the tibia. They appear to have normal growth and development. No late onset deficits have been reported.

Experience has shown that there are several distinct hereditary phenotypes that include absence of the tibia. Several are autosomal dominant disorders:

1. absence of tibia, triphalangeal thumb and preaxial polydactyly (182); Mendelian Inheritance in Man #188770;
2. absence of tibia and split-hand, split-foot deformity (173);
3. absence of tibia with postaxial polysyndactyly (183);
4. tibia hemimelia-micromelia-trigonomacrocephaly (184);
5. tibia hemimelia diplopodia syndrome (185).

In addition, several distinct autosomal recessive phenotypes have been reported:

1. tibial hemimelia – cleft lip/palate (186);
2. tibial hemimelia-deafness syndrome (187);
3. absence/hypoplasia of tibia with polydactyly and retro-cerebellar arachnoid cyst (188); (Mendelian Inheritance in Man: 601027);
4. aplasia of tibia, bifurcation of femur and ectrodactyly (189), the Gollop-Wolfgang Complex (MIM %228250).

Unfortunately, molecular testing to confirm any of these specific phenotypes is not yet available.

As with any autosomal dominant disorder, variability of the physical features is to be expected. The family studies of individuals with absence of tibia and split-hand/split-foot deformity showed that some heterozygous individuals exhibited only hypoplasia of the first toe or postaxial polydactyly of both feet (173). The severe end of the spectrum can be monodactyly of all four limbs.

Prenatal screening by ultrasound may be used for reassurance for parents whose previous child had absence of the tibia. Unfortunately, the accuracy of the detection of absence or hypoplasia of the tibia has not been determined. The sensitivity of ultrasound in the detection of limb malformations, in general, has been poor.

LONGITUDINAL DEFICIENCY, POSTAXIAL: ABSENCE/HYPOPLASIA OF ULNA AND/OR FIFTH FINGER

Definition

Absence or hypoplasia of the fifth finger with or without hypoplasia or absence of the ulna.

ICD-9:   755.270 (postaxial longitudinal reduction of upper limb)

ICD-10:   Q71.5 (longitudinal reduction defect of ulna)

Mendelian Inheritance in Man: None

Appearance

Absence or hypoplasia of the ulna is much more likely to be a partial deficiency affecting only one arm (194–197). In one case series (194), 89% of the affected individuals had also absence of postaxial fingers. Syndactyly was present in 34%. With complete absence of the ulna there is often a marked flexion deformity of the elbow. The hand can be straight or angulated to the ulnar side of the wrist.

Often in association with absence of the ulna, there is bifurcation of the distal humerus and humeroradial synostosis and oligodactyly (196).

Classifications of the pattern of shortening of the ulna have been suggested by several individuals (194–196). Cole and Manske (195) added the characteristics of the thumb and first web space to the description of the appearance of the ulna (Figure 15-24):

Type I: hypoplasia of the ulna with the distal and proximal epiphyses of ulna present; normal first web space and thumb.

Type II: absence of the distal or middle one-third of the ulna; mild deficiency of thumb and first web space.

Type III: complete absence of ulna; moderate to severe deficiency of thumb and first web space; finger-like thumb; thumb index syndactyly; absence of extrinsic tendon function.

Type IV: fusion of radius to humerus; radio-humeral synostosis; forearm usually short; absence of thumb.

Type V: bifid humerus with absence of radius and ulna oligodactyly (196).

Type VI: proximal ulnar longitudinal dysplasia, associated with absence of radius and fingers and abnormalities of the shoulder (195).

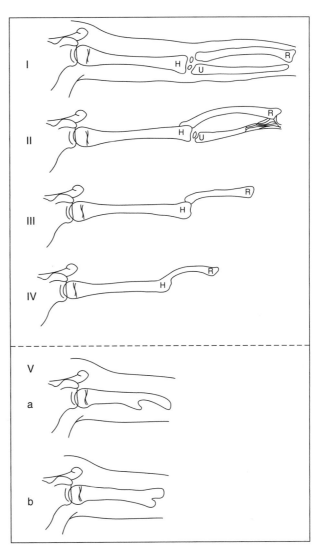

FIGURE 15.24 Classification of spectrum of deficiency of ulna. (Reprinted from Goldfarb CA et al: *J Bone Jt Surg.* 2005;87-A:2639–2648. Used with permission.)

Associated Malformations

Infants with unilateral absence of the ulna often have deformities of the other arm (194). In a case series (198) of 42 individuals with a unilateral deficiency, 22 (52.4%) had various anomalies of the other arm, including absence/hypoplasia of the radius and polydactyly, and 15 (35.7%) had anomalies of the legs, such as proximal focal femoral deficiency and fibula ray deficiency.

Two significant associations have been identified:

1. the unilateral absence or hypoplasia of the ulna, femur, and fibula (199); this association had been observed in 1949 by Birch-Jensen (151), who noted: "ulnar defects are fairly often attended by fibular defects."

2. the ulna-mammary syndrome in which there are deficiencies of the ulna, fibula and postaxial digits, hypogenitalism, and absence of one or both breasts, in association with mutations in the TBX3 gene (200, 201). Mutations in the TBX3 gene cause changes in the ulna and postaxial digits.

Developmental Defect

The mutation <u>ulnaless</u> in the mouse is an X-linked mutation, which disrupts the development of forelimbs and hindlimbs (202). The results are reductions of the forelimb, and less so, in the hindlimbs. <u>Ulnaless</u> altered the regulation of HOXD genes, specifically in the limbs, but not in the axial skeleton (203).

Gene knockouts of HOXA-11 and HDXD-11 in mice produced almost complete absence of both the radius and ulna as well as severe malformations of the kidneys (204).

Prevalence

Birch-Jensen (151) identified 19 individuals with absence of the ulna in his study of 4,024,000 Danes (1943–1947). The prevalence rate at birth was about 1:100,000 in the newborns surveyed and about 1:210,000 in the entire population.

In Sweden (8) [1965–1979], 855 infants with limb reduction defects were identified among 1,368,500 births. 38 (1:36,000) had ulnar hand reduction, 14 of which were unilateral, 3 were bilateral "isolated" malformations and the remainder (21;55%) were part of multiple malformations.

In eastern France (12), 123 of 118,265 consecutive births (1973–1981) had a limb deficiency (1:962); 10 (1:11,827) had absence of the ulna, 4 of which were "isolated." Among the 6 with multiple anomalies, the deficiency of the ulna was unilateral in 5 of the 6.

Regarding absence of the fifth finger only (Figure 15-25), complete or just the two distal phalanges, a survey of 161,252 liveborn and stillborn infants in Boston (1972–1974, 1979–1994) identified five with a unilateral deformity (3 left hand; 2 right hand) [340], for a frequency of 1:32,250 (0.003/1,000).

Race/Ethnicity

No prevalence rates have been established and compared among different ethnic or racial groups.

Birth Status

For isolated deficiency of the ulna, no increase in prematurity, stillbirth, or perinatal death has been reported.

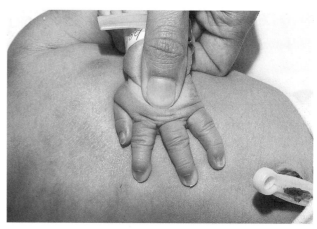

FIGURE 15.25 Absence of fifth finger and metacarpal, an isolated abnormality in a newborn infant.

Sex Ratio

The sex ratio was 19 males and 12 females in the survey in Denmark (151). Similarly, the male:female was 3:2 in one review (194).

Sidedness

No sidedness has been demonstrated in surveys of affected individuals (194).

Parental Age

No correlation with the ages of the mothers or fathers has been reported.

Twinning

The frequency of twinning has not been reported among infants with absence or hypoplasia of the ulna or fifth finger.

Genetic Factors

The molecular basis for absence of the ulna, unilateral or bilateral, has not been determined. However, the ulna-mammary syndrome (MIM #181450), in which these limb anomalies, genitourinary anomalies, and absence or hypoplasia of one or both breasts, is associated with mutations in TBX3. This is an autosomal dominant disorder.

Absence of the ulna and fibula are features of the phocomelia syndrome with anomalies of the kidney and intestine known as the Al-Awadi/Raas-Rothschild/Schinzel Phocomelia Syndrome (MIM #276820). Homozygous mutations in exon 4 and 3 have been identified in affected infants in two families (205, 206).

Environmental Factors

No teratogens in human pregnancies have been identified as a cause of absence or hypoplasia of the ulna.

Treatment and Prognosis

Treatment is individualized and less well-established than it is for isolated absence of the radius, tibia, or fibula. Some deformities are not amenable to surgical treatment (194). Release of the associated syndactyly and improvement in the thumb web space can improve the use of the hand.

Excision of the anlage of the ulna has been proposed as helpful in reducing the ulnar deviation of the arm in types II and IV (194).

Genetic Counseling

Isolated absence or hypoplasia of the ulna is usually unilateral. No etiology has been established. The parents of a child with either unilateral or bilateral absence/hypoplasia of the ulna have not been shown to have an increased risk of having a second affected infant.

In the families of the 19 affected individuals identified by Birch-Jensen in Denmark (151), none of the 61 siblings was affected. The 19 affected individuals had five unaffected children.

None of 65 individuals in a surgical case series (198) with deficiency of the ulna (42 unilateral; 23 bilateral) had an affected sib, parent, or other relative.

In one case series of 17 individuals with proximal ulnar longitudinal dysplasia, one affected infant had a sibling with bilateral amelia (196).

For the infant with absence of the ulna and other anomalies, several genetic syndromes should be considered:

1. Femur-fibula-ulna (FFU) syndrome, delineated by Lenz and Feldman in 1977 (MIM 228200), is usually sporadic. One family with two affected sibs has been reported.
2. The Al-Awadi/Raas-Rothschild/Schinzel Phocomelia Syndrome (MIM: #276820) is a more autosomal recessive syndrome of multiple anomalies which includes absence of the ulna, fibula, and tibia and curved or shortened radius, preaxial polydactyly, skull defects, and genitourinary anomalies (205, 206).
3. Proximal ulnar longitudinal dysplasia has been delineated among individuals with phocomelia (207). These individuals often have absence of radius and ulna and proximal femoral focal deficiency.
4. The ulna-mammary syndrome (MIM #181450) in which there are deficiencies of the ulna and postaxial fingers, absence of fibula, by pogenitalism absence of one or both breasts, in association with mutations in the TBX3 gene (200, 201).

LONGITUDINAL DEFICIENCY, POSTAXIAL: ABSENCE/HYPOPLASIA OF FIBULA AND/OR FIFTH TOE

Definition

Absence or hypoplasia of the fifth toe with or without absence or hypoplasia of the fibula.

ICD-9:   755.360 (longitudinal reduction defect of lower limb)

ICD-10:   Q72.6 (longitudinal reduction defect of fibula)

Mendelian   None
Inheritance
in Man:

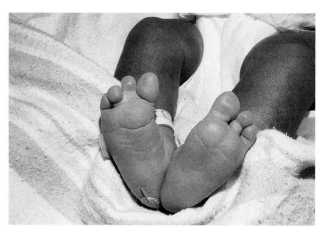

FIGURE 15.27 Shows feet of infant with absence of fifth toe in right foot and toes 4 and 5 in left foot.

Appearance

The absence or hypoplasia of the fibula is much more often unilateral than bilateral (208–213) (Figure 15-26). Usually the femur is shortened also. The shortened femur has an outward rotation, a lateral subluxation of the patella, and a shallow lateral condyle with a shallow sulcus. There may be a flattened eminence of the tibia with absence of the cruciate ligament. The tibia can be bowed or shortened with fusion of the bones in the ankle. Typically, the foot and ankle are in the talipes equinovalgus position (whereas with absence of the tibia, the foot and ankle are in the varus position).

There is a correlation of the severity of the postaxial deficiency in the foot with the severity of the hypoplasia of the fibula: the more tarsal and metatarsal bones that are absent, the greater the degree of shortening of the fibula (209). When there is absence of the lateral toes (Figure 15-27) and tarsal bones, there is a higher likelihood of fusion of the tarsal and ankle bones. Talocalcaneal fusion or coalition is the most common type of fusion. The valgus deformity is more severe and more rigid when talocalcaneal coalition is present.

A mild "fibular hemimelia syndrome" can be present even when the child has a fibula that appears normal in radiographs (214). These individuals can have limb shortening, absence of lateral toes, tarsal coalition, and a ball and socket ankle joint (215).

Three systems for classifying fibular hemimelia have been proposed by Coventry and Johnson in 1952 (208), Achterman and Kalamchi in 1979 (210), and Stanitski and Stanitski in 2003 (216):

Coventry and Johnson (208):

Type I: Shortening of the limb
     Partial unilateral absence of the fibula
     Little or no bowing of the tibia
     Little or no deformity of the foot
     No other anomalies
     Little disability
     Only treatment needed is a heel lift or arrest of epiphysis

Type II: Fibula completely or almost completely absent
     Unilateral deformity
     Anterior bowing of the tibia with a skin dimple
     Equinovalgus foot
     Absence or deformity of rays or tarsal bones
     Marked shortening of the extremity

Type III: Bilateral type I or II or type I or II in association with deformities elsewhere in the body, not including ipsilateral femoral shortening or delayed development of the capital femoral epiphysis and acetabulum.

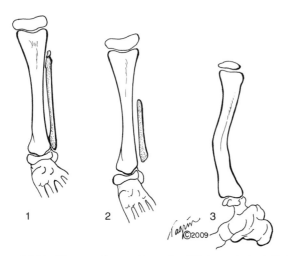

FIGURE 15.26 Diagram of normal lower leg (#1), hypoplasia of fibula (#2) and absence of fibula (#3). Adapted with permission from Achterman C, Kalamchi A: *J Bone Jt Surg.* 1979; 61B; 183.

Achterman and Kalamchi (210) subdivided type I:

Type IA: Proximal fibular epiphysis is distal to the level of the tibial growth plate and is often smaller than normal, whereas the distal fibular growth plate is proximal to the dome of the talus.

Type IB: Proximal fibula is absent for 30–50% of its length, whereas distally the fibula is present but does not support the ankle.

Stanitski and Stanitski (216) proposed this classification system:

Type I: Fibula is nearly normal
Type II: Small or miniature fibula, regardless of its position in the limb
Type III: Complete absence of the fibula.

Within each type of hypoplasia of the fibula, several variations may occur: the presence of coalition of the tarsal bones; reducing the number of foot rays from 1 to 5; the morphology of the tibiotalar and distal tibial epiphyses being horizontal, valgus or spherical (ball-and-socket).

The term "postaxial hypoplasia for the lower extremity" is more accurate. The term "fibular a/hypoplasia" understates the spectrum of anomalies that may be associated (217). Absence of the fifth toe is a rare anomaly. The infant with absence of the fifth toe should be evaluated for the spectrum of features of mild fibular a/hypoplasia.

Associated Malformations

Most infants with hypoplasia of the fibula have no associated anomalies.

Clubfoot was present in 16% of the 121 patients in a case series of fibular hemimelia (218). The presence of clubfoot is considered part of the developmental abnormality of absence or hypoplasia of the fibula.

Shortening of the femur and absence of the fifth finger and/or ulna are common associations (210, 212).

Several rare genetic disorders that include absence/hypoplasia of the fibula with other anomalies have been described (see Genetic Counseling, below).

Developmental Defect

The limb buds appear as elevations on the ventrolateral aspect of the body of the embryo toward the end of the fourth week (174). The cartilage of the early fibula is present in the sixth week. Ossification of all bones is visible by the 12th week.

Anatomic dissections of amputated lower limbs have confirmed the higher frequency of associated fusion of metatarsal, tarsal, and ankle bones (212, 219). In one series of five amputated lower limbs (219), there was dysplasia of the second or third metatarsal. This was a surprise finding, as the absent or abnormal metatarsals had been considered associated primarily with the fourth and fifth toes.

Prevalence

In a consecutive series of 161,252 liveborn and stillborn infants and elective terminations for malformations in Boston (340), two infants had absence of the fibula, one with five toes and the other with absence of the toes 4 and 5. The prevalence rate in this study was 1:80,626 or 0.012/1,000.

Race/Ethnicity

There is no information on the prevalence rates in different ethnic groups.

Birth Status

Isolated absence or hypoplasia of the fibula has not been associated with an increased frequency of prematurity, stillbirth, or perinatal death.

Sex Ratio

Some case series have had an excess of females (208) and others, an excess of males (210).

Sidedness

In a case series (208) of 81 affected individuals, those with the type I and type II deformities had an affected right leg more often than an affected left leg.

Parental Age

There is no information on the distribution of the ages of the mothers and fathers of affected infants.

Twinning

An association with an increased frequency of twinning has not been reported. In one set of monozygous twins, one infant had absence of the fibula and the other had split-hand deformity (220). These twins probably had the rare autosomal dominant syndrome of "fibular aplasia with ectrodactyly" (221). In another monozygous twin pair, one infant had absent fibula with split-hand deformity, while the other twin had no limb malformations (222).

Genetics Factors

Lewin and Opitz (211), in a review of both isolated and syndromic absence/hypoplasia of the fibula, noted that most affected infants have had no affected relatives.

Homozygous missense mutations in the dorsoventral patterning gene WNT7A have been identified in individuals with Fuhrmann Syndrome (MIM #228930) and Al-Awadi/Raas-Rothschild/Schinzel Phocomelia Syndrome (MIM #276820), a rare autosomal recessive disorder with hypoplasia of the fibula and ulna (249). WNT7A was noted to induce beta-catenin pathways, which control the formation of the apical ectodermal ridge (AER) in developing limb and dorsoventral polarity. The relationship between the two disorders has not been determined, although both are associated with mutations in WNT7A. Some phenotypic differences have also been identified.

Environmental Factors

No human teratogen has been shown to cause absence of fifth toe or absence/hypoplasia of fibula as either an isolated anomaly or as part of a multiple anomaly syndrome.

A few associations have been postulated. Graham (224) reported three individuals with absent/hypoplasia fibula among children born to two postulated teratogenic exposures: myomata of the mother's uterus and the early amnion rupture sequence. A cluster of infants with FFU (femur-fibula-ulna) dysostosis was reported in a malformations surveillance program in Lyon, France, in 1981 (224). No environmental cause was identified.

Infants of diabetic mothers with multiple anomalies have included some with absence of the fibula.

Treatment and Prognosis

For many years, the Syme's amputation was the recommended approach. This amputation is a modified ankle disarticulation (226). More recently (227), the Syme's amputation has been recommended for children with a leg length discrepancy between the two legs of over 7.5 cm or 15%, or when the foot was malformed.

The Ilizarov leg lengthening technique has also been used successfully for children with such severe limb shortening (213, 228). However, more hospitalizations and operations are needed with the leg-lengthening approach (229).

Orthopedists (230) have noted the challenge of developing a realistic treatment plan for the infant with significant leg length inequality. Many parents are reluctant to allow their child's foot to be amputated when the foot has a near normal appearance and the leg length discrepancy is not visually apparent.

For children with milder shortening of the tibia and fibula, the foot can be saved with the Gruca operation (231).

Genetic Counseling

Hypoplasia of the fibula can be missed in the newborn when the only apparent physical abnormality is the valgus foot deformity. So, confirming the absence or hypoplasia of the fibula is the essential first step.

The affected infant should be examined carefully for the presence of other malformations.

Isolated or nonsyndromic absence or hypoplasia of the fibula in one leg occurs most often without an affected parent or sibling. The empiric risk of recurrence in a subsequent pregnancy appears to be very low, but has not been established.

Several specific genetic syndromes have been identified in which absence or hypoplasia of the fibula is part of the phenotype.

1. Femur-fibula-ulna syndrome (FFU), delineated by Lenz and Feldman in 1977 (MIM 228200), is usually sporadic. Affected sibs were reported in one family (232).
2. Fibula aplasia with ectrodactyly (split-hand, split-foot) [MIM 113310] [221], a rare autosomal dominant disorder that is similar to the tibia aplasia-ectrodactyly syndrome.
3. Fuhrmann Syndrome (MIM #228930) with absence of fibula, bowed femurs, and poly-, syn- and oligodactyly (223) is a rare autosomal recessive phenotype.
4. Al-Awadi/Raas-Rothschild/Schinzel Phocomelia Syndrome (MIM #276820), a rare autosomal recessive phenotype that may include absence of the ulna, fibula and tibia, curved or shortened radius, preaxial polydactyly skull defects, and genitourinary anomalies (205, 233).
5. Volkmann dysostosis, a rare autosomal dominant phenotype, described by Lewin and Opitz (211): aplasia of fibula, hypoplasia of short thick tibia, abnormal ankle joints, and severe abduction of feet.

No commercial molecular testing is available yet to identify any malformation syndromes that include absence or hypoplasia of the fibula.

Absent/hypoplastic fibula is not a feature of any specific chromosome abnormality.

Prenatal screening by ultrasound is not very accurate in the detection of limb anomalies, in general (234). However, this screening will have higher accuracy and sensitivity in the subsequent pregnancy after the birth of the first affected infant in the family.

SPLIT HAND/SPLIT FOOT (SHSFM)

Definition

A median cleft of the hand or foot with absence or hypoplasia of the central elements and usually one or more digits on each side of a central cleft. The term ectrodactyly is sometimes used to refer to the split-hand/split-foot deformity; ectrodactyly means "aborted digit."

ICD-9:	755.250	(split-hand malformations; includes monodactyly and lobster-claw hand)
	755.350	(split-foot malformation; includes monodactyly and lobster-claw foot)
ICD-10:	Q71.6	(lobster-claw hand)
	Q72.7	(split foot)
Mendelian Inheritance in Man:	%183600	(SHSFM1; Type I): gene locus: 7q21-q22 (Ref. 235-238)
	%313350	(SHSFM2; X-linked): gene locus: Xq26 - q26.1 (239)
	%600095	(SHSFM3): gene locus: 10q24 (240-242)
	#605289	(SHSFM4): gene locus: 3q27 (243, 244)
	%606708	(SHFSM5): gene locus: 2q31 (245, 246)

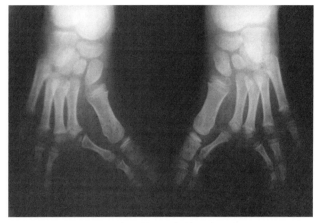

FIGURE 15.29   Radiographs of foot of affected mother.

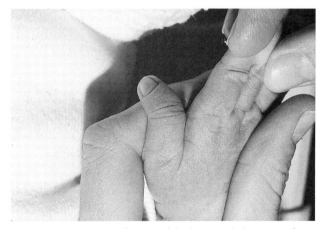

FIGURE 15.30   Minor deformity (delta-bone triphalangism) of one thumb of infant whose split-foot deformity is shown in Figure 15.28.

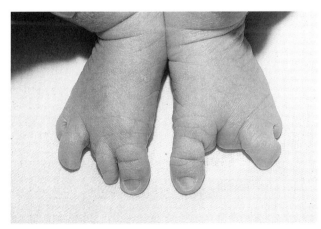

FIGURE 15.28   Split-foot deformity in the son of the affected mother in Figure 15.29.

Appearance

The affected hand in the split-hand/split-foot malformation (SHSFM) typically has a midline cleft that extends into the area of the third metacarpal or third metatarsal (Figures 15-28 and 15-29) with fingers(or toes) 1, 2, 4, and 5 present (151, 173, 249–259). The fingers or toes adjacent to the cleft may be normal or short with syndactyly and abnormal nails. Another common phenotype is a central deficiency with an in-curved, reduced first and fifth fingers. When the individual has a split foot deformity, the hands may show only a mild distal deficiency of one finger (Figure 15-31).

The typical deformity in the foot is a deficiency in the region of the second or third metatarsal (Figures 15-28 and 15-29). In the more severe expression, the cleft extends to the base of the metatarsals and only the first and fifth toes are present.

SHSFM occurs most often as an abnormality of one hand (151, 248, 256) [Table 15-5, Figure 15-32].

The hands are affected much more frequently than the feet. The term "atypical split hand" was used by Birch-Jensen (151) to refer to absence of the central ray with hypoplastic first and fifth fingers at each margin (Figure 15-32). He distinguished the "atypical" form from the "typical" by the fact that the "atypical" has more "reduction of the remaining rays."

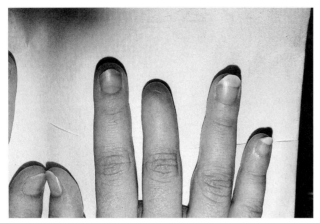

FIGURE 15.31 Deficiency of distal phalanx of third finger of the affected mother, whose foot deformity is shown in Figure 15.29.

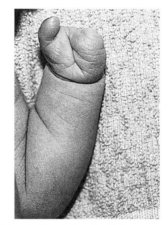

FIGURE 15.32 "Atypical" split hand of infant.

TABLE 15-5 *Split-hand/split-foot malformation*

	Hungary (15)	Boston (28)
Separate phenotypes		
I. Limbs only ("isolated")		
Hands only		
Bilateral	5	2
Unilateral	40	1
Feet only		
Bilateral	3	1
Unilateral	2	2 (1 Rt; 1 Lt)
Hands and Feet		
Bilateral	3	2
One hand, both feet	1	—
Subtotal	54	8
II. Multiple anomalies		
Hands and feet		
Bilateral	40	1[1]
Totals	94 in 1,566,666 or 1:16,666	9 in 161, 252 or 1:20,156[2]

Legend: (1) = An infant with autosomal dominant SHSFM, who also had trisomy 18.
(2) = prevalence among 161, 252 liveborn and stillborn infants and fetuses terminated because of anomalies identified prenatally in the years 1972–1974, 1979–1994 at Brigham and Women's Hospital in Boston (340); one infant's mother had planned to deliver at another hospital; if that infant is excluded, the prevalence rate was 8/161,252 or 1:20,156.

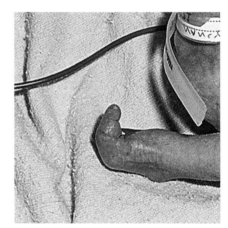

FIGURE 15.33 Monodactyly of one foot, an occasional manifestation of SHSFM.

Some distinctive limb malformations may also be caused by the SHSFM mutations.

1. Monodactyly (Figure 15-33), with only one finger or toe present can be an effect of several SHSFM mutations.
2. Hypoplasia of the distal tibia, syndactyly of two toes, and isolated cleft lip are other examples (238, 247).
3. Minor changes in the hands, such as deficiency of ends of one or more fingers (Figure 15.31) and medial deviation of the distal phalanx of the thumb (Figure 15-30) due to a "delta," an additional central phalanx.
4. Triphalangeal thumb, preaxial polydactyly, or absence of the first ray; the feet of these individuals do not show a distinctive preaxial change (257); this is associated with the SHSFM3 gene mutation.

The female carriers of the X-linked SHSFM may have mild limb abnormalities, such as hypoplasia of one or two fingers (250), but not the recognizable split-hand or split-foot abnormality.

In a consanguineous family with nine individuals with presumed autosomal recessive SHSFM, there was remarkable variability in the phenotype (258, 260). The hand malformations included syndactyly of various combinations of fingers (1-2, 2-3, 3-4, and 4-5), and toes (1-2, 3-4), as well as absence of toes 2, 3, and 4 and 3, 4, and 5. Some fingers and toes were broad. Some affected individuals had the more typical split-hand and split-foot malformations.

Associated Malformations

SHSFM types I, II, III, IV, and V are skeletal malformations; visceral anomalies are rare. One exception is an increased frequency of heart defects. In a retrospective review of 169 individuals with SHSFM types 1-5, the heart defects occurred in 10% of those with SHSFM1 and 47% with SHSFM5 (261).

There are many multiple malformation syndromes in which a split-hand or split-foot malformation occurs (258, 259, 262–264), such as the EEC syndrome (ectrodactyly, ectodermal dysplasia, and cleft lip/palate; MIM# 129900), and the limb-mammary syndrome (ectrodactyly, absence of breast tissue, cleft palate: MIM# 603543). Whenever a child with SHSFM has nonskeletal malformations, a separate and possibly distinctive, multiple anomaly syndrome would be a potential diagnosis.

Developmental Defect

The cause of the central cleft malformation has been postulated to be failure to maintain the apical ectodermal ridge (AER) in the central region of the upper or lower limb. This is suggested by the findings in the presumed analogous autosomal dominant mutation in the mouse: Dactylaplasia (Dac) [265]. The gene locus for Dac is syntenic with the chromosome 10q21 region in humans, a postulated locus of SHSFM3 (242). The developmental mechanism for the loss of central digits and metacarpals/metatarsals in Dac/+ embryos in dramatic cell death in the central portion of the AER. Breeding studies have suggested a two locus model, in which the dominant mutation leading to the split hand/foot malformation would be controlled by a second locus. Two molecular mechanisms have been identified that affect the synthesis of the *dactylin* gene, an insertion which produces a disrupting frameshift and an insertion that alters the amount or the integrity of the dactylin transcript (266).

Knockout mice with disruption of both the D1x5 and D1x6 genes, homologues of the *Distalless* gene in drosophila, have a progressive loss of median AER cells that are visible prior to embryonic day 11.5.

SHSFM4 and EEC syndrome are caused by mutations in p63, an ectoderm-specific p53-related transcription factor p63, and D1x proteins which co-localize in the nuclei of the cells in the AER (267).

A mouse mutant with absence of central digit rays, as in SHSFM, has been reported in which the primary genetic defect is in the cholesterol-modified form of Sonic hedgehog (SHH) [268]. This reduces the long-range signaling effects of SHH.

An alternative hypothesis, based on the findings in eight children with central clefts and six metacarpals, offered (269) that the primary defect is polydactyly of the middle finger and osseous syndactyly between the two middle finger metacarpals and the adjacent index and ring finger metacarpals.

Prevalence

The rates reported for all types of SHSFM have been: 1:71,857 (Birch-Jensen [151]), (combining typical and "atypical"); 1:16,666 (Hungary [248]); and 1:17,888 in Boston [340] (Table 15-5).

The anatomic distribution can be hands only, feet only, or affected hands and feet (Table 15-5).

Race/Ethnicity

Frequencies in separate race/ethnic groups have not been established.

Birth Status

No association with prematurity, stillbirth, or perinatal death has been reported.

Sex Ratio

In the large series in Hungary (248) the ratio of males:females in a series of individuals with isolated unilateral upper limb SHSFM was 27:13 (M:F).

In some family studies (241), an excess of affected males have been born to both affected males and females, a phenomenon referred to as segregation distortion (270).

Sidedness

In the series of 54 infants with isolated split-hand/split-foot identified in Hungary (1975–1984 [248]), there were 40 individuals with unilateral SHSFM with a predominance of the right side (25:15; right:left). In the 36 typical and 20 "atypical" cases identified in Denmark (151), 35 were unilateral with a predominance of affected right arms: 23:12 (Rt:Lt).

Parental Age

No significant changes in the distribution of the ages of the mothers and fathers of affected infants have been reported.

Twinning

No increase in the frequency of twinning has been reported.

Discordance for unilateral split-hand in monozygous twins has been reported (271, 326). In another monozygous twin pair (252), one twin had monodactyly of both arms, absence of the tibia and only two toes in each foot and a dysplastic ear and the co-twin had normal arms, but absence of the tibia in each leg. In another like-sex twin pair, one had bilateral split-foot, while the co-twin had a unilateral hypoplastic thumb (271).

Genetic Factors

Gene loci for at least five different SHSFM dominant mutations have been postulated. In addition, autosomal recessive inheritance has been postulated for the affected children of unaffected, consanguineous parents (260, 272). This pattern of inheritance has been questioned (273), suggesting instead the two locus model (one dominant and one recessive mutation) as observed in the mouse model *Dactylaplasia* (265).

The gene locus for SHSFM1 is postulated to be on chromosome 7q21 (235–238); SHSFM2 on an X chromosome (239); SHSFM3 on chromosome 10q24 (240–242); SHSFM 4 on chromosome 3q27 (243, 245), and SHSFM5 on chromosome 2q31 (245, 246).

In Type I the split-hand/split-foot malformation occurs in association with absence/hypoplasia of the tibia. Other malformations include distal bifurcation or hypoplasia of the femur, hypoplasia/aplasia of the ulna, aplasia of the patella, and hypoplasia of the first toes (274). An affected individual can have hypoplasia of one tibia and no SHSFM, while other relatives have SHSFM. The pattern of genetic transmission is often unusual, with the gene not penetrant in several individuals in a family, the phenomenon of premutation (275). Zlotogora (270) postulated that the pattern of transmission of Type II (SHSFM2) could be causally related to the expansion of a trinucleotide repeat sequence, which affects the expression of the mutant gene. Family studies (264) have shown that the gene for SHSFM, Type I is not linked to the mutation for SHSFM, Type II. Both affected fathers and affected mother have an excess of affected males, a phenomenon referred to as segregation distortion (241). The associated molecular changes have not been reported, nor whether this occurs in only Type I or Type II SHSFM families.

Submicroscopic tandem chromosome duplications affecting the SHSFM3 locus have been identified in individuals with either syndromic or nonsyndromic phenotypes of SHSFM (276, 277). Rapid diagnostic methods have been developed (276). These abnormalities were found to be more common than the p63 mutations identified only in SHSFM4.

In SHSFM4, there are median clefts of the hands and feet with absence or hypoplasia of the central digits and metacarpals/metatarsals. In studies of large families with many affected individuals, missense mutations were found within the DNA-binding domain of the p63 gene, which is a homologue of the p53 tumor suppressor gene (235, 244, 263, 274). The mode of inheritance is autosomal dominant with high penetrance (estimated 96%) [256]. Mutations in the p63 gene can produce four other autosomal dominant malformations with split-hand/split-foot malformations, in addition to SHSFM4, including EEC syndrome (Ectrodactyly, ectodermal dysplasia, and cleft lip (MIM# 129900); Limb-Mammary syndrome (MIM #603543); ADULT syndrome (Acro-dermato-ungal-lacrimal-tooth syndrome (MIM #103285); and ectrodactyly-cleft palate syndrome (MIM #129830). The fact that similar phenotypes are produced by mutations in the same gene suggests that the mutations involve functionally related molecular changes.

Autosomal recessive inheritance has been postulated in a few families in which affected sibs were born to unaffected parents who were related, i.e., consanguineous (260, 272). However, these patterns of transmission have also been attributed to the effect of a second gene on the SHSFM dominant mutation (273). Verma (272) described in one family with postulated autosomal inheritance atypical physical features, including radioulnar fusion and fusion of metacarpal and metatarsal bones.

SHSFM has been observed in association with several chromosome translocations and abnormalities, which has been very helpful in the search for the associated gene mutations. In addition, submicroscopic rearrangements have also been identified in individuals with SHSFM plus other non-limb malformations, such as hearing loss (278). SHSFM phenotypes can also occur in association with an interstitial deletion, which removes the SHSFM gene locus (246).

Environmental Factors

No exposure in pregnancy is known to cause the split-hand/split-foot malformations. No systematic case-control study of environmental exposures in individuals with SHSFM has been reported.

Treatment and Prognosis

Surgical repair can improve function and address some of the negative social reactions to the presence of a significant hand or foot deformity. One approach (279) to the repair noted three fundamentals for the surgical repair of a deep cleft deformity: 1) close the cleft with wide pedicled skin flaps that produce transverse scars; 2) the entire second finger ray should be moved adjacent to the third ray, after osteotomy at the metacarpal base; 3) excessive spread between the index and ring fingers should be prevented by reconstructing the interdigital ligament between them.

Genetic Counseling

In discussion with the parents, it will be helpful to decide upon the terms to be used, such as "split-hand" or "split-foot." The inappropriate terms, like "lobster-claw deformity" should be noted, as they could be included in some medical articles which they may read. The first question clinically is whether the affected infant has the nonsyndromic, "isolated" SHSF malformation or has a "syndromic" form with a wider spectrum of phenotypic features (258, 261). For infants with nonsyndromic SHSFM, confirmatory molecular testing can include mutation analysis of p63 and testing by microarray to identify genomic duplications or deletions.

For the infant with "atypical" split-hand deformity of one hand, more studies are needed, using new molecular diagnosis techniques, to determine whether or not this phenotype is different from bilateral SHSFM. Two family studies have suggested that "atypical" (unilateral) split-hand may be different. Birch-Jensen (151) identified 20 individuals with this phenotype who had 8 children, 51 sibs, and 33 nieces and nephews, none of whom had SHSFM. A family study by Widikund Lenz, the famous German geneticist who identified thalidomide as a teratogen, led him to conclude that this condition is "sporadic," that is not hereditary (326).

The associated physical features in syndromic SHSFM may include ectodermal changes, deafness, abnormal lacrimal ducts, cleft lip, and a variety of other limb malformations (261). The distinctive syndromes include EEC Syndrome, AEC Syndrome, limb-mammary syndrome, and ADULT Syndrome (279).

Chromosome analysis, and possibly microarrays, are appropriate in the evaluation of any infant with "syndromic" SHSFM.

The family history should be reviewed carefully to identify isolated limb defects, but not the split-hand or split-foot malformation, which could reflect the effect of the same mutation in close relatives.

Mutation analysis has improved significantly in recent years and more progress is expected. To date, some amazing differences in phenotypes have been associated with the same mutation. For example, ankyloblepharon-ectodermal defects and cleft lip and palate (AEC Syndrome: MIM# 106260) and the Rapp-Hodgkin Syndrome (RHS Syndrome; MIM# 129400), have been associated with the same mutation (c.1529C>T transition in exon 12 at position 510) [280]. In one family the mother had AEC Syndrome and her two affected daughters had RHS Syndrome (281).

Theoretically, prenatal screening by ultrasound could identify the fetus with the skeletal abnormalities of the SHSFM, as reported in the first trimester (282). However, the accuracy of this prenatal screening has not been established.

SYNDACTYLY

Definition

Persistence of webbing between two or more fingers or toes.

ICD-9:	755.100	(fused fingers)	
	755.110	(webbed fingers)	
	755.120	(fused toes)	
	755.130	(webbed toes)	
	755.190	(unspecified syndactyly)	
	755.191	(unspecified syndactyly, thumb and/or fingers, unilateral)	
	755.192	(unspecified syndactyly, thumb and/or fingers, bilateral)	
	755.193	(unspecified [webbed vs. fused] syndactyly thumb and/or fingers, not otherwise specified [NOS])	
	755.194	(unspecified syndactyly, toes unilateral)	
	755.195	(unspecified syndactyly, toes bilateral)	
	755.196	(unspecified syndactyly toes, NOS)	
	755.199	(unspecified syndactyly digits not known)	
ICD-10:	Q70.0	(fused fingers)	
	Q70.1	(webbed fingers)	
	Q70.2	(fused toes)	
	Q70.3	(webbed toes)	
	Q70.4	(polysyndactyly)	
	Q70.9	(syndactyly, unspecified)	
Mendelian Inheritance in Man:	%185900:	Syndactyly, Type I	
	#186000:	Syndactyly, Type II - a polysyndactyly; see page 154.	
	#186100:	Syndactyly, Type III	
	#186200:	Syndactyly, Type IV - a polysyndactyly; see page 155__	
	#186300:	Syndactyly, Type V	
	%212780:	Cenani-Lenz, Type VII	

Historical Note

Limb malformations, like syndactyly and polydactyly, are easy to identify and have been the focus of many studies. Clinicians (25, 105, 283–287) have offered several classifications for the many phenotypes of syndactyly. Unfortunately, some types labeled as "syndactyly" are, in fact, a "polysyndactyly." The earliest classifications were by Roblot in 1906 (283); by Julia Bell in 1953 (284); by Temtamy and McKusick in 1978 (285); Goldstein et al. in 1994 (105); and by Malik et al. in 2005 (287).

The most common types of syndactyly have been considered an "isolated" abnormality. Studies of mouse mutants, such as syndactylism (SM) [288], have shown that the genes mutated in a monogenic type of syndactyly are expressed in several tissues, which makes it reasonable that additional anomalies could be present. In the study of mouse mutants, associated skeletal anomalies were identified in fixed, cleared, stained skeletons (289, 28). However, skeletal imaging surveys have not been part of clinical studies in humans, making the designation "isolated" more tentative.

Hopefully, the identification of the mutations associated with specific phenotypes will delineate the critical steps that are interrupted and lead to a more developmental classification of the syndactylies (25).

To date, the associated mutations have been reported for only type III (290, 291) and type V (292), but systematic screening is not available commercially.

Appearance

In syndactyly, the skin between fingers or toes extends from the base of the affected digits out toward the tip. The skin in the "web" of syndactyly has the same appearance as the skin on the fingers. The extent of the syndactyly varies from "partial" to complete. The term "simple syndactyly" has been used when there is only persistence of skin between digits. The term "bridging syndactyly" refers to the presence of bony structures plus skin between fingers (293).

These are the specific types of syndactyly that have been described:

1. Type I (MIM %185900): Syndactyly between fingers 3 and 4 in association with syndactyly between toes 2 and 3 (Table 15-6 and 15-7; Figure 15-34).

Occasionally other digits are involved. Can be either bilateral or unilateral; can affect only the hands or only the feet (296).

A more severe, apparent homozygous expression of Type I syndactyly has also been described (286, 287). The phenotype included complete syndactyly, synostosis, and hypoplasia of phalanges. The gene map locus: 2q34-q36 (297, 298).

Syndactyly toes 2-3 without syndactyly of fingers 3 and 4 is the most common syndactyly (Figures 15-34 and 15-35). It has no medical significance and has been considered a minor anomaly (295). Future molecular

TABLE 15-6 *Syndactyly: Number of Cases Classified by Affected Interdigital Space*

	Isolated				Associated			
	South America (17) (η = 599,109)		Boston (η = 206,244)		South America (17) (η = 599,109)		Boston (η = 206,294)	
	Fingers	Toes	Fingers	Toes	Fingers	Toes	Fingers	Toes
Affected Digits								
1-2	1	4	1	2	3	2	1	3
2-3	1	70	*	*	2	11	*	*
3-4	18	7	6	2	2	4	6	2
4-5	1	13	-	8	1	5	4	6
1-3	0	1	0	2	0	0	0	0
2-4	1	2	0	1	0	0	3	1
3-5	1	0	1	0	1	0	1	1
1-2, 4-5	0	1	0	0	0	0	0	0
2-3, 4-5	0	0	0	0	1	0	0	0
1-4	0	2	0	0	0	0	0	0
2-5	2	0	2	1	1	0	0	0
1-5	0	0	0	0	2	1	3	0
Asymmetric	0	3	0	0	0	0	3	0
Total	25	103	9*	16*	13	23	21*	13*

Legends: Isolated = no other major malformations
Associated = other malformations present
South American (ref. 296) in 1967–1977
Boston (ref. 294–295) 1972–1974, 1979–2000
*data not recorded in Active Malformations Surveillance Program at Brigham and Women's Hospital in Boston, MA (15).

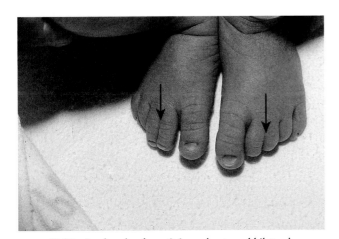

FIGURE 15.34 Syndactyly of toes 2-3, moderate and bilateral.

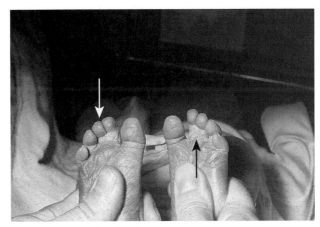

FIGURE 15.35 Syndactyly of toes 2-3.

studies will determine whether syndactyly of fingers 3-4 and toes 2-3 can be caused by the same mutation or if isolated syndactyly toes 2-3 can be caused by other mutations. Autosomal dominant.

2. Type II (MIM #186000): A polysyndactyly duplication of digit between fingers 3 and 4, postaxial polydactyly of hands or feet, syndactyly of fingers 3-4 and toes 4-5 (Figure 15-36). Autosomal dominant. Gene map locus: 2q31-q32.

3. Type III (MIM #186100): Syndactyly between fingers four and five. The fourth finger is flexed, i.e., camptodactyly. The fifth finger is shortened, with absence or hypoplasia of the middle phalanx (299). The syndactyly may involve fingers 3, 4 and 5. The toes are not affected. Autosomal dominant. Associated mutations have been identified in Connexin 43 (GJA1) [290, 291].

4. Type IV (MIM 186200): A polysyndactyly postaxial polydactyly of the hands and feet; syndactyly of all

TABLE 15-7 *Syndactyly: fingers 3-4*

Hand Affected	Non Transfers*		Transfers**	
	Isolated	Multiple Anomalies	Isolated	Multiple Anomalies
Left only	1	1		1[5]
		1[1]		1[6]
				1
				1[3]
Right only	2	1[2]		2[7]
		1		2[5]
				1[8]
				1
Side not known			1[5]	
			1[2]	
Bilateral	3	1[3]		7[5]
		1[4]		1[8]
		1[9]		1[10]
Totals	6	7	2	19

Recognized etiologies:
[1] = urethral atresia
[2] = triploidy with partial hydatidiform mole
[3] = amniotic band syndrome
[4] = triploidy mosaic (left 3-4; right hand 2-3)
[5] = triploidy
[6] = triploidy/no-molar
[7] = Down syndrome
[8] = triploid 18
[9] = unknown cause (right 3-4; left 4-5)
[10] = triploidy (left 3-4; right hand 2-3)

LEGEND: *Non-transfers = women who had always planned to deliver their infants at Brigham and Women's Hospital (BWH) in Boston. The total population was 206,224 liveborn and stillborn infants and elective terminations for fetal anomalies.

**Transfers = Women who had planned to deliver at another hospital, but transferred to deliver at BWH after the detection prenatally of a fetal abnormality.

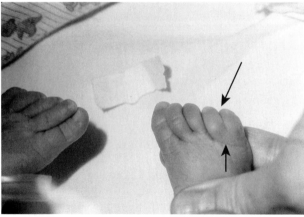

FIGURE 15.36   Syndactyly of toes 4-5.

fingers, but not toes. Autosomal dominant. Gene map locus: 7q36.

5. Type V (MIM #186300): Syndactyly (partial) of fingers 4 and 5, angulation and camptodactyly of fingers 4 and 5, fusion of metacarpals 4 and 5, shortening of some fingers and toes (300, 301). The mildest expression reported (299) was absence of distal phalangeal creases, enlargement of proximal interphalangeal joints, and partial fusion of metacarpals 4 and 5. In the feet there are various deformities of the metatarsals, valgus deviations of the toes, shortened fourth toes and shortened metatarsals 4 and 5. In one large Han Chinese family, a missense mutation was identified in the HOXD13 homeodomain 950A→G (292). Autosomal dominant.

6. Complete syndactyly: Fingers 2 to 5 or 1-4 and toes 2-5 or 1-4. A rare phenotype (296).

7. Syndactyly of toes 4-5 (Table 15-8) (Figure 15.36). This type of syndactyly was referred to as Type B in the classification of Julia Bell (284, 302). Autosomal dominant.

8. Cenani-Lenz syndactyly (303, 304): syndactyly of fingers with disorganization of phalanges, fusion of metacarpals, metatarsals and shortened long bones. Autosomal recessive.

9. Turkish family (286): syndactyly of toes; hypoplasia/absence of fingers 1, 2 and 5 and first toes; synostosis of metacarpals 3-4.

10. Pakistani family (287): syndactyly of toes 1-3; hypoplasia of phalanges in fingers and toes; synostosis of metacarpals 3-4.

TABLE 15-8 *Syndactyly: Toes 4-5*

Hand Affected	Non Transfers*		Transfers**	
	Isolated	Multiple Anomalies	Isolated	Multiple Anomalies
Left only	2			
Right only	4	1[1]		1[4]
		1[2]		
		2		
Bilateral	2	1[2]		2[2]
		1		1[5]
		1[3]		1[6]
				1[7]
				1[8]

Recognized etiologies:
[1] = Multiple anomalies: hereditary private syndrome ()
[2] = trisomy 21
[3] = trisomy 18 (4-5 left; 3-5 right)
[4] = amniotic band syndrome
[5] = trisomy 21 (4-5 left; 2-3 right)
[6] = acardia
[7] = anencephaly
[8] = trisomy 18

Legend: *Non-transfers = women who had always planned to deliver their infants at Brigham and Women's Hospital (BWH) in Boston. The total population was 206,224 liveborn and stillborn infants and elective terminations for fetal anomalies.

**Transfers = Women who had planned to deliver at another hospital, but transferred to deliver at BWH after the detection prenatally of a fetal abnormality.

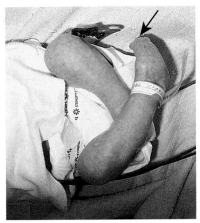

FIGURE 15.37   Syndactyly of toes 1-5.

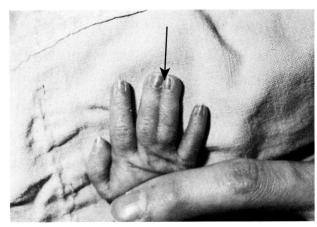

FIGURE 15.39   Syndactyly of fingers 3-4.

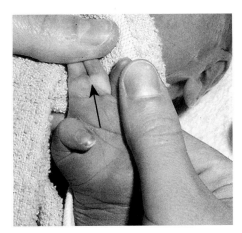

FIGURE 15.38   Syndactyly of fingers 2-3.

mice (28), including syndactylism (sm) [289], and fused toes (ft) [306], and in cattle, such as bovine syndactylism (sy) [307]. The anatomic studies of sm/+ in the gestational day 10–12 mouse embryos showed an increase in the thickness of the apical ectodermal ridge (AER), which was visible at gestational days 10–10.5. The ft mutation in the mouse is a novel dominant mutation that was produced by transgene insertion heterozygotes. The specific mechanism by which ft produces syndactyly has not been determined.

Studies of mouse embryos with syndactylism (sm) mutations (288) showed that the gene mutated in sm mice encodes the putative Notch ligand Serrate2. This suggests that Notch signaling is involved in early limb-bud patterning and AER formation.

Associated Malformations

Most infants with syndactyly have no other major malformations (Figures 15-34, 15-36, 15-37, 15-38 and 15-39). However, syndactyly is a feature of many malformation syndromes.

Among infants with syndactyly between fingers 3 and 4 in Boston (Table 15-7), none of the six infants with isolated syndactyly had an affected parent. Among those with multiple anomalies, the etiologies identified included triploidy (including mosaic and partial mole), trisomy 21, trisomy 18, amniotic band syndrome and urethral atresia (Table 15-7).

Developmental Defect

The formation of the fingers and toes is a complex process in which the normal pattern of five fingers and toes is produced with a minimal amount of skin between the digits at the base (305). Mutations that cause specific patterns of syndactyly have been identified in

Prevalence

"Isolated" syndactyly is the most common type of syndactyly. The most common locations in a study of 599,109 liveborn infants in Latin America (1967–1977) were syndactyly of toes 2-3, 0.12/1,000, for syndactyly of fingers 3-4, 0.03/1,000 and syndactyly of toes 4-5, 0.02/1,000 (296).

The prevalence rates in an Active Malformations Surveillance Program in Boston, which included liveborn and stillborn infants and elective terminations for fetal anomalies among 206,244 infant births were similar: "isolated" syndactyly 3-4 fingers 0.03/1,000 (Table 15-7), and "isolated" syndactyly toes 4-5 0.04/1,000 (Table 15-8).

Race/Ethnicity

A higher frequency of all syndactylies has been observed among Caucasians than in other ethnic groups in South America (296) and in the United States (308).

Birth Status

Among infants with isolated syndactyly, there is no evidence of an increased frequency of still-birth, miscarriage, or prematurity has not been reported. Among the many multiple anomaly syndromes in which syndactyly occurs, some have a high rate of miscarriages or still-birth, such as the chromosome abnormality triploidy, which is often associated with syndactyly of fingers 3 and 4 (Table 15-8).

Sex Ratio

A higher frequency of affected males was noted among Latin American infants with isolated syndactyly, including fingers 3-4 syndactyly, toes 2-3 syndactyly, and toes 4-5 syndactyly (296). Several authors of reports of cases of different syndactylies have also noted an excess of affected males. The question has been raised, but not settled, as to whether these pedigrees reflect Y-linked inheritance (285).

Sidedness

In South America among the individuals with syndactyly both the left and right limbs were affected similarly (296). In some groups bilateral involvement is more common than unilateral involvement. In the systematic examination of 7,157 newborn infants in Boston (Table 15-6) [295], there was no difference in frequency of syndactyly of toes 2-3 in the right and left foot.

Parental Age

No differences in the ages of mothers or fathers have been reported for any specific types of syndactyly.

Twinning

For isolated syndactyly attributed to autosomal dominant genes, such as types I, III, and V, concordance will be expected in monozygous twin pairs. Each of dizygous twins, like sibs, will have a 50% chance of being affected, if one parent is affected. No deviation from these expected patterns has been reported.

Genetic Factors

To date, most of the "isolated" syndactylies have exhibited autosomal dominant inheritance. The "new" Cenani-Lenz Syndrome (287, 304) has been attributed to autosomal recessive inheritance.

Ironically, polymorphisms in ft (fused toe) have been shown to account for a significant portion of childhood and adult obesity, prompting a change in the name of the gene from ft to FTO (fat mass and obesity associated) [309].

"Isolated" syndactyly has not been shown to have the characteristics of multifactorial inheritance.

Environmental Factors

Syndactyly can be a component of limb malformations attributed to the process of vascular disruption produced by the prostaglandin E_1 analogue misoprostol or as part of the "amniotic band limb deformity." However, syndactyly is not a specific distinctive component of any teratogen-induced phenotype.

Treatment and Prognosis

Regarding surgical repair, the most simple and complex syndactylies are corrected between 12 and 14 months of age (310). When a deformity involves both hands or feet, the procedure is performed on both at the same time, when the infants are younger, but not in the older child. The syndactylies affecting function more, such as thumb-index finger, are released earlier, between 6 to 12 months of age. However, the release or repair of simple syndactylies should not be repaired in newborns. In the surgery of syndactylies, fascial interconnections are always present and the release of this fascia is the most important step in the release. Digital nerves and arteries can have a wide variety of branching patterns within the web space. In general, more abnormal neurovascular configurations occur in the more complex malformations.

Genetic Counseling

Several of the many isolated syndactylies are hereditary, specifically Types I, III, and V, and are attributed to mutations with autosomal dominant transmission. Variable expressivity and non-penetrance occur in families with each of these mutations. (Types II and IV Syndactyly are also attributed to mutations with autosomal dominant inheritance, but are usually polysyndactylies and are presented in that section.)

The specific phenotype is established best after examination of several affected members of the family of the infant. As is typical of many genes with autosomal dominant inheritance, variation in the phenotype is common and the mildest expressions must be looked for carefully. An example of mild expression of Type III syndactyly was one affected woman who showed shortening of fingers, absence of the distal interphalangeal crease in an index finger, swollen interphalangeal joints, and partial fusion of the fourth and fifth metacarpals in contrast to the usual more severe deformities (292).

If an infant with "isolated" syndactyly has no affected relatives, molecular studies are needed to establish how often this infant is affected by a spontaneous mutation or another molecular mechanism, such as autosomal recessive or digenic inheritance. Unfortunately, commercial testing for the mutations postulated for each type of syndactyly is not yet available. One example of progress is in the identification of mutations in Connexin 43 (GJA1) in isolated Type III syndactyly (290, 291). Ultimately, as proposed by Winter and Tickle (25), a new classification is needed that reflects the underlying cellular and molecular abnormalities.

Prenatal diagnosis by ultrasonography will depend on the ability to identify more severe manifestations. Its accuracy has not been established.

TERMINAL TRANSVERSE LIMB DEFECTS (TTLD) WITH NUBBINS

Definition

An arm that ends at one of three levels, just above the elbow, the upper forearm, (Figure 15-42) or the wrist (Figures 15-40, 15-41), which has four or five tiny (5 mm) digit-like nubbins at the end. A similar leg deformity has been described at the level of the mid-foot and the toes. Only one arm or leg is affected.

ICD-9:   755.230   (absence of forearm and hand, includes infants with nubbin fingers attached to stump of forearm or elbow)
          755.330   (absence of lower leg or foot, includes infants with nubbin toes attached to stump of leg)

ICD-10:   Q71.2   (congenital absence of forearm and hand)
          Q71.3   (congenital absence of hand and finger(s))
          Q72.2   (congenital absence of both lower leg and foot)
          Q72.3   (congenital absence of foot and toe(s))

Mendelian   None
Inheritance
in Man:

Historical Note

No entry in Mendelian Inheritance in Man describes the specific phenotype of TTLD with nubbins. TTLD with nubbins affects only one arm or leg; all five fingers (or toes) are represented by tiny nubbins with tiny nails. "Unilateral adactylia" (MIM 102650) appears to be an

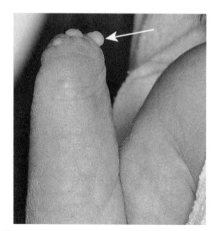

FIGURE 15.40   Shows terminal transverse limb defect (TTLD) at level of the wrist.

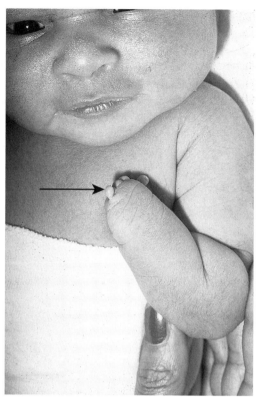

FIGURE 15.41   Another infant with TTLD with nubbins at the level of the wrist.

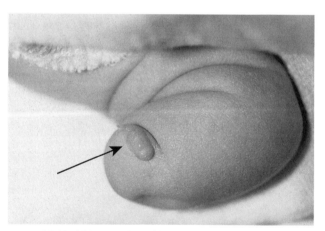

FIGURE 15.42   TTLD with nubbins at level of right proximal forearm.

autosomal dominant disorder; it also differs from the phenotype of TTLD with nubbins in that the nubbins are much larger and the thumb is present. "Congenital constricting bands" (MIM %217100) refers to the phenotype of the amniotic band syndrome that may affect more than one arm or leg; there is very little evidence that this condition is hereditary. The references cited within these two MIM entries include reports that describe TTLD with nubbins, such as Pauli et al. (311).

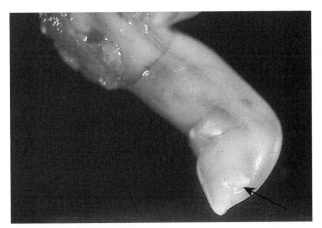

FIGURE 15.43 Shortened forearm of affected fetus (ref. 6) with arm bent at elbow. Nubbins visible near end of forearm (arrow).

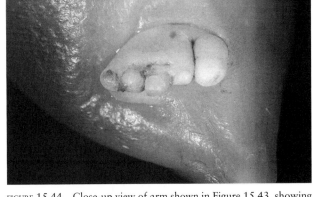

FIGURE 15.44 Close-up view of arm shown in Figure 15.43, showing the row of tiny digits on the edge of the stump of the forearm.

We present "TTLD with nubbins" as distinct from both unilateral adactylia and the amniotic band-limb deformity. All three phenotypes have been attributed, theoretically, to the process of vascular disruption.

Among hand surgeons, this phenotype of TTLD with nubbins has been referred to as the peromelic type of symbrachydactyly (312, 313).

Appearance

The arm is normal in appearance above the rounded end, which may be invaginated (314). The four or five digit-like nubbins are usually at the end of the "stump" or off-center (151, 315) [Figures 15-42, 15-43, 15-44].

These tiny (5 mm long) nubbins often have slit-like nails. Each nubbin may be separate (Figure 15-41), or a contiguous group (Figure 15-44). Histologic sections of the nubbins of one fetus (315) showed cartilage and bone. There were regularly spaced chondrocytes with coagulative necrosis, dystrophic calcification, and abundant osteoclastic activity (Figure 15-45).

In TTLD with nubbins at the level of the wrist, the nubbins are separate and distinct, usually with slit-like tiny nails (Figure 15-41).

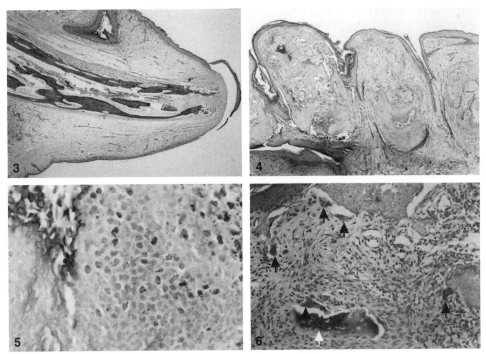

FIGURE 15.45 #3 shows that bone ends in distal portion of right arm; #4 cross section of three contiguous nubbins in Figure 15.44, each containing osteocartilaginous tissue; # 5 shows necrosis and calcification in the cartilage; #6 shows in nubbins well-formed bone (white arrow) and osteoclasts (black arrows). From article by Drapkin RI et al (315) [Figure 4, page 351]. Used with permission.

There are no midline clefts of the central metacarpals, no constriction rings, syndactyly, or crusted material at the ends of the "digits" and bands (strings) of tissue attached to the nubbins.

Associated Malformations

In general, most infants with terminal transverse limb defects with nubbins have no other major malformations. One infant with an affected forearm had an associated aneurysm of the left subclavian artery and dextrocardia (316).

Developmental Defect

Inferences as to the possible sequence of events have been made from several clinical observations. The major mechanisms postulated have been hypoperfusion with tissue loss and embolization. The observations include:

a) Vascular disruption is an occasional complication of the prenatal diagnosis procedure chorionic villus sampling [CVS] (317–320). In the initial report in 1991 of five early CVS-exposed infants with limb defects by Helen Firth and colleagues (317), one had TTLD with nubbins (Case 1). One theory as to the sequence of events is that the removal of villi causes blood loss, which in a few fetuses, leads to hypoperfusion, tissue hypoxia, endothelial cell damage, hemorrhage, and tissue loss (318). Los et al. (319) noted that the limb abnormalities that occur after CVS are located primarily in the upper part of the body. They postulated that CVS-induced abnormalities were caused by the abnormal transport of chemical substances, rather than hypovolemia and hypoxemia.

b) Embolization of material from the placenta to the brachial artery was postulated to be the cause of TTLD in three fetuses, based on the findings in anatomic dissections. One of the three infants had trisomy 21 and three nubbins at the end of the forearm stump (321).

c) Intense uterine contractions caused by the effect of the prostaglandin E_1 analogue misoprostol, as an abortifacient, administered at 6 to 8 weeks gestational age can produce vascular disruption attributed to hypoperfusion in the uterine artery followed by decreased blood flow in one limb, hypoxia, hemorrhage, and tissue loss (319, 322, 323); some misoprostol-exposed infants in one case series (323) had terminal transverse limb defects, but the presence of nubbins was not noted.

One theoretical basis for the presence of the tiny nubbins on the stump of the terminal limb deficiency is that these represent an attempt to regenerate the limb (324). The terminal limb deficiency would have been caused by a vascular "event," such as obstruction, which would destroy most, but not all, of the cells in the apical ectodermal ridge (AER). The AER produces the signals, specifically the fibroblast growth factor (FGF) family members, which are essential for the proximal-distal patterning of the limb (325). The remaining AER tissue has sufficient signaling capacity to produce the "regeneration" of distal limb structures, which are the tiny nubbins at the end of the shortened limb.

Prevalence Rate

Birch-Jensen (151) described all 625 individuals with upper limb defects identified among the 4,024,000 inhabitants of Denmark in the years 1943 to 1947. Many of the individuals with "amputations," described in the chapter entitled "Amputations and Symbrachydactylism," had TTLD with nubbins. Almost all of the photographs (Figures 572 to 609) show terminal transverse limb defects with nubbins. If we assume that all of these individuals had TTLD with nubbins, the prevalence rates by level were:

	Number	Prevalence Rate
Upper Arms:	9	1:270,000 (.004/1,000)
Forearm:	161	1:22,000 (.05/1,000)
Hand:	54	1:65,000 (.02/1,000)

A second source of information is the survey of 161,252 (liveborn and stillborn, and elective terminations) for anomalies in Boston (340). There were nine infants with TTLD with nubbins: forearm ($\eta = 4$) 1:40,000; hand ($\eta = 4$) 1:40,000; foot ($\eta = 1$) 1:161,252.

Race/Ethnicity

No data on the occurrence in different racial and ethnic groups has been reported.

Birth Status

There have been no reports that this phenotype as more common in stillborn infants and spontaneous abortions than in liveborn infants.

Sex Ratio

In the series in Denmark reported by Birch-Jensen (151), the sex ratio of individuals with affected forearms was: 69:92, M:F.

Sidedness

The TTLD with nubbins is always unilateral. For TTLD of the forearm, the left forearm was affected twice more often than the right (108:53) in the 161 affected Danes (151). In that population, the left hand was affected more frequentlyy than the right (34:20).

Parental Age

No associations have been reported.

Twinning

Three pairs of identical twins, discordant for terminal transverse limb defects at the levels of forearm or hand, were identified in an analysis of 872 infants with congenital limb reduction defects (1975–1984) in Hungary (326). There was no mention of nubbins being present, but these are visible in Figure 1 of the published report. (Table 15.9)

Genetic Factors

The most extensive information about the low rate of occurrence in close relatives was provided by Birch-Jensen in Denmark (151). Among the individuals with TTLD of the forearm, one of 585 sibs and one great-great maternal grandmother had amputation of one hand. None of the 82 children of affected individuals was affected.

Several families with two affected close relatives, including sibs, cousins, uncle/niece, or nephew, have been reported (311).

In the Boston series (340), one of the eight infants with an affected arm had a similarly affected aunt. Both the affected infant and her aunt had proximal forearm defects.

The potential effect of several associated genetic factors was suggested by the studies of 24 mother-infant

TABLE 15-9 *Prevalence of terminal transverse limb defects with nubbins:*

	Level of Defect	
	Denmark (2)*	Boston (12)**
A. Arms		
upper arm	9	0
upper forearm	161	4
wrist	54	4
B. Legs		
Distal foot at metatarsal		
Phalangeal joints	(not reported)	1

*Population: All 4,024,000 individuals in Denmark, 1943–1947 (see ref. 5).

**Population: 161,252 liveborn and stillborn infants and elective terminations for fetal anomalies in second trimester surveyed for limb deficiencies in 1972–74, 79–94 at Brigham and Women's Hospital, Boston (see ref. 12).

pairs with limb malformations, six (25%) of whom had TTLD with nubbins (22). The frequencies of protein S and C deficiency, methylenetetrahydrofolate reductase (C677 T variant) deficiency, prothrombin variant G20210A, and factor V Leiden and other risk factors were increased in several mothers and their affected infants.

Environmental Factors

The potential environmental causes include any substance, e.g., ergotamine, that would produce vasoconstriction of the main branchial artery.

Any cause of hypoperfusion in the first trimester of pregnancy, including the CVS procedure, the prostaglandin E_1 misoprostol, and placental trauma (327), with blood loss or intense uterine contractions, could theoretically produce this limb defect.

Treatment and Prognosis

There is no evidence that the child with terminal transverse limb defects with nubbins has an increased frequency of brain abnormalities. In a case series of 20 affected infants, none had other malformations and all had normal growth and development (328).

Genetic Counseling

In counseling, this phenotype should be considered a separate disorder and not the amniotic band-limb deformity. The limb deformities of the amniotic band syndrome include constriction rings, syndactyly, crusted ends of fingers with strands of amnion, and often involve more than one arm or leg. The spectrum of the amniotic band phenotypes can include some with associated brain abnormalities that would suggest a more negative prognosis.

Several phenotypes have some features similar to TTLD with nubbins, but notable differences:

a) Infants with unilateral adactylia (MIM 102650) have larger proximal phalangeal nubbins and the thumb is present, although hypoplastic (329, 330). It is attributed to autosomal dominant inheritance.

b) Adactylia occurs in several disorders (331, 332), but the affected digits are larger than the "nubbins" in this TTLD. Another distinct difference is the fact that the shortened digits are located at the metacarpal-phalangeal joint and affect both arms.

c) The limb deformities associated with homozygous alpha-thalassemia or Hemoglobin Barts can include nubbins at the level of the metacarpal-phalangeal joint (333–335). Usually more than one limb is affected. A terminal transverse limb defect that ends in the upper forearm or at the wrist, as occurs in TTLD with nubbins, has not been described in published descriptions of infants with Hemoglobin Barts.

d) Infants with the Adams-Oliver Syndrome (MIM: %100300) have terminal transverse limb defects with symmetrical and bilateral shortening or absence of the distal portions of fingers and toes. Scalp defects are also common (336). This disorder is attributed to autosomal dominant gene, but the mutation has not been identified.

The empiric recurrence risk in a subsequent sib, close relative or offspring of an affected individual appears to be very low. No specific risk has been established in recent family studies.

When absence of the hand or forearm is detected prenatally by ultrasonography, the identification of the tiny digit-like nubbins will confirm this diagnosis. This finding would provide the basis for a more positive prognosis.

CENTRAL DIGIT HYPOPLASIA

ICD-9:   None

ICD-10:   None

Mendelian Inheritance in   None
    Man:

Definition

Hypoplasia of the proximal portions of fingers 2, 3, and 4 and a normal or hypoplastic thumb and fifth finger.

Appearance

This is an isolated, typically unilateral upper limb defect (337, 151). Fingers 2,3 and 4 are affected primarily; some individuals have hypoplasia of fingers 2 to 5 or 3 to 5 (Figures 15-46–15-49).

The small fingers are usually located at the site of the normal proximal phalanx. A fingernail may be present or the shortened fingers are tapered and have no nail.

Sometimes the short "digits" are located on the inner aspects of the thumb or fifth finger (Figures 15-46, 15-48).

The thumb and fifth fingers are either normal in appearance or hypoplastic with shortening and stiff interphalangeal joints.

In some infants the metacarpal and carpal bones are shortened and hypoplastic.

We have identified a similar phenotype in the right foot of one infant (Figure 15-50). The first and fifth toes were hypoplastic, but larger than toes 2, 3, and 4, which were smaller and had small nails.

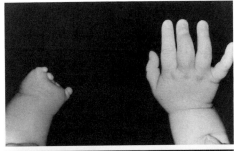
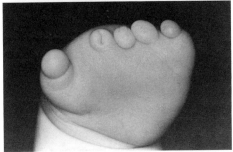

FIGURE 15.47 Left hand of affected infant with larger, but hypoplastic, thumb and fleshy knobs at metacarpal-phalangeal joints 2 to 5. Normal right hand. (From Graham JM et al:Pediatrics 78: 103–106, 1986. Used with permission.)

Associated Malformations

This is usually a unilateral deformity with no associated malformations.

More experience is needed to determine how often there are associated malformations or malformation syndromes.

Developmental Defect

The clamping of the uterine artery on day 15 to 16 of gestation in the rat was shown by Webster and his colleagues (339) to cause stasis of blood flow in the distal

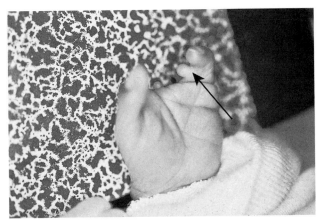

FIGURE 15.46 Palm view of the right hand of an affected infant. Shows the small digit-like structures (arrow) along inner aspect of fifth finger.

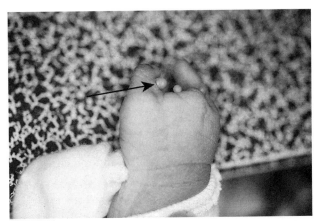

FIGURE 15.48 Dorsal view of the right hand of an affected infant. Shows the small digit-like structures along inner aspect of fifth finger (arrow).

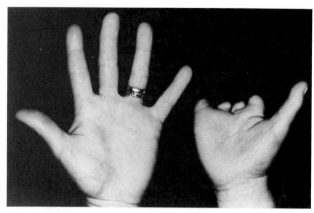

FIGURE 15.49   The right hand of the affected mother of the infant in Figure 15-47. She has a normal thumb, but hypoplasia of fingers 2 to 5. (From Graham JM Jr et al: Pediatrics 78:103-106, 1986. Used with permission.)

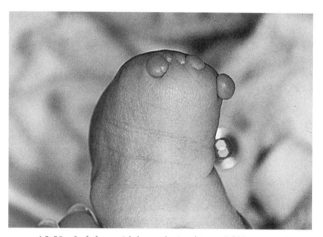

FIGURE 15.50   Left foot with hypoplasia of 1st and fifth toes and more severe underdevelopment of toes 2 to 4. Tiny nails visible in toes 3, 4, and 5.

part of the developing forelimb. Digits 2 to 4 were affected most often by hemorrhage and tissue loss. If the hemorrhage was severe, the digit primordia were destroyed and there was hypoplasia or complete loss of digits. With less extensive hemorrhage, there was constriction rings and syndactyly of the central digits. This is an experimental model of the process of vascular disruption.

Three affected women who were identical twins and the affected daughter of one were evaluated by Doppler flow studies (338). No vascular abnormalities were identified.

Prevalence

Four infants had an affected hand and a fifth had one affected foot in a survey in Boston of all limb malformations in 161,252 liveborn and stillborn infants and elective terminations of fetal anomalies in the second trimester of pregnancy. This was a prevalence rate of 0.02/1,000 or 1:40,313 for those with one affected arm and 1:161,252 for the infant with one affected leg.

Race/Ethnicity, Sex Ratio, and Parental Age

No information is available on a large number of affected individuals.

Birth Status

For the infant with an isolated deformity of one limb, an increased frequency of stillbirth or prematurity is not expected.

Twinning

Graham et al. (338) described affected identical twins, one of whom had a similarly affected daughter. One twin had an affected right hand and the other twin had an affected left hand. One twin had an affected daughter.

Genetic Factors

Individuals with this limb deformity have been reported in families in which there was an affected parent and child, suggesting autosomal dominant inheritance (338, 330).

Among the families with two affected relatives, there are families (337, 151, 330) in which one child has a terminal transverse limb defect that ends the proximal forearm and the affected cousin has central digit hypoplasia. The individuals through whom they are related had no limb malformations. The mechanism of the familial occurrence of these two types of limb malformationshas not been determined. However, it suggests that terminal transverse limb defects with nubbins and central digit hypoplasia are related abnormalities.

Environmental Factors

Infants exposed to the prenatal diagnosis procedure chorionic villus sampling (CVS) have been shown to have an increased frequency of a distinctive abnormality involving fingers 2, 3, and 4 (320). There can be a tapering and stiffness of these fingers and absence of the tip of the third finger. However, affected hands do not show the dramatic shortening of the central fingers as occurs in the phenotype being presented here. In addition, the infant affected after exposure to CVS may have additional associated abnormalities, such as infantile hemangiomas (340) or bowel atresia or club foot (341).

Treatment and Prognosis

The typical affected infant has one normal hand and no other malformations, which makes the prognosis excellent. When there is an adequate thumb, there will be a better prognosis for an adequate thumb to finger pinch, and a more limited disability.

Genetic Counseling

The initial examination will establish whether or not there are associated malformations.

The limited information available suggests that this "isolated" unilateral limb deformity is not associated with developmental delay or other malformations.

When an associated mutation has been identified in the familial cases, it can be determined whether the "sporadic" cases are caused by a similar spontaneous mutation.

An affected parent may have a 50% chance that each of her/his children will be affected, as well. The affected fetus could have a more severe limb deformity, such as terminal transverse limb defect with nubbins. Theoretically these unilateral limb deficiencies could be identified by prenatal screening by ultrasound. The accuracy of this type of prenatal detection has not been established.

For the clinician, two phenotypes are similar but can be distinguished:

1. The CVS-associated limb defect can cause hypoplasia, tapering and stiffness of the central fingers. However, the affected digits are longer than those in the phenotype presented here. In addition, the CVS-exposed infant with a limb defect may have other abnormalities, including hemangiomas, bowel atresia, or club foot (341–344).
2. The infant with an "atypical" split hand deformity may have a hypoplastic first and fifth finger on the affected hand. However, this phenotype does not include hypoplastic central digits. In the split hand deformity there may be evidence of a cleft, with either hypoplasia of only central metacarpals or a visible cleft in the center of the affected hand (151, 345).

REFERENCES

1. O'Rahilly R. Morphological patterns in limb deficiencies and duplications. *Amer J Anat.* 1951;89:135–193.
2. Hall CB, Brooks MB, Dennis JF. Congenital skeletal deficiencies of the extremities. Classification and fundamentals of extremities. Classification and fundamentals of treatment. *JAMA.* 1962; 181:590–599.
3. Swanson AB. A classification for congenital limb malformations. *J Hand Surg.* 1976;1:8–22.
4. Froster UG. Academicians are more likely to share each other's toothbrush than each other's nomenclature (Cohen, 1982). *Amer J Med Genet.* 1996;66:471–474.
5. Bod M, Czeizel A, Lenz W. Incidence at birth of different types of limb reduction abnormalities in Hungary 1975–1977. *Hum Genet.* 1983;65:27–33.
6. Czeizel A, Keller S, Bod M. An aetiological evaluation of increased occurrence of congenital limb reduction abnormalities in Hungary, 1975–1978. *Internat J Epidemiol.* 1983;12: 445–449.
7. Aro T, Heinonen OP, Saxen L. Incidence and secular trends of congenital limb defects in Finland. *Internat J Epidemiol.* 1982; 11:239–244.
8. Kallen B, Rahmani TMZ, Winberg J. Infants with congenital limb reduction registered in the Swedish register of congenital malformations. *Teratology.* 1984;29:73–85.
9. Froster-Iskenius UG, Baird PA. Limb reduction defects in over one million consecutive livebirths. *Teratology.* 1989;39: 127–135.
10. Bower C, Forbes R, Rudy E, Ryan A, Stanley F. *Report of the Birth Defects Registry of Western Australia 1980–2005.* Annual Report. King Edward Memorial Hospital for Women, western Australia, October, 2006.
11. Calzolari E, Manservigi D, Garani GP, Coechi G, Maguani C, Milan M. Limb reduction defects in Emilia Romagna, Italy: epidemiological and genetic study in 173,109 consecutive births. *J Med Genet.* 1990;27:353–357.
12. Stoll C, Alembik Y, Dott B, Roth MP. Risk factors in limb reduction defects. *Pediatric Perinat Epidemiol.* 1992;6: 323–338.
13. Forrester M, Merz RD. Descriptive epidemiology of limb reduction deformities in Hawaii, 1986–2000. *Hawaii Med J.* 2000;62: 242–247.
14. Zguricas J, Bakker WF, Heus H, Lindhout D, Heutink P, Hovias SER. Genetics of limb development and congenital malformations. *Plast Reconstr Surg.* 1998;101:1126–1135.
15. Grzeschik K-H. Human limb malformations: an approach to the molecular basis of development. *J Dev Biol.* 2002;46: 983–991.
16. Wilkie AOM. Why study human limb malformations? *J Anat.* 2003;202:27–35.
17. Bamshad M, Watkins WS, Dixon ME, Le T, Roeder AD, Kramer BE et al. Reconstructing the history of human limb development. Lessons from Birth. *Pediatric Research.* 1999;49: 291–299.
18. Zakany J, Duboule D. The role of Hox genes during vertebrate limb development. *Curr Opin Genet Dev.* 2007;17:359–366.
19. Scherz PJ, McGlinn E, Nissim S, Tabin CJ. Extended exposure to Sonic hedgehog is required for patterning the posterior digits of the vertebrate limb. *Dev Biol.* 2007;308:343–354.
20. Firulli BA, Redick BA, Conway SJ, Firulli AB. Mutations within helix 1 of twist1 result in distinct limb defects and variation of DNA-binding affinities. *J Biol Chem.* 2007;282: 27536–27546.
21. Barbosa AC, Funato N, Chapman S, McKee MD, Richardson JA, Olson EN, Yanagisawa H. Hand transcription factors cooperatively regulate development of the distal midline mesenchyme. *Dev Biol.* 2007;310:154–168.
22. Hunter AG. A pilot study of the possible role of familial defects in anticoagulation as a cause for terminal limb reduction malformations. *Clin Genet.* 2000;57:197–204.
23. Carmichael SL, Shaw GM, Iovannisci DM, Yang W, Finnell RH, Chang S et al. Risks of human limb deficiency anomalies associated with 29 SNPs of genes involved in homocysteine metabolism, coagulation cell-cell interactions, inflammatory response,

and blood pressure regulation. *Am J Med Genet Part A.* 2006; 140A:2433–2440.

24. Holmes LB. Teratogen-induced limb malformations. *Am J Med Genet.* 2002;112:297–303.

25. Winter RM, Trickle C. Syndactylies and polydactylies: embryological overview and suggested classification. *Eur J Hum Genet.* 1993;1:96–104.

26. Genest DR, Richardson A, Rosenblatt M, Holmes LB. Terminal transverse limb defects with tethering and omphalocele in a 17-week fetus following first trimester misoprostol exposure. *Clin Dysmorphol.* 1999;8:53–58.

27. Temtamy SA and McKusick VA. *The Genetics of Hand Malformations.* New York: Alan R Liss; 1978.

28. Johnson DR. *The Genetics of the Skeleton: Animal Models of Skeletal Development.* 1986, Oxford: Clarendon Press; 1986: 353.

29. Watson BT and Hennrikus WL. Postaxial type-B polydactyly. *J Bone Jt Surg.* 1997;79–A:65–68.

30. Woolf CM and Woolf RM. A genetic study of polydactyly in Utah. *Am J Hum Genet.* 1970;22:75–88.

31. Woolf CM and Myrianthopoulos NC. Polydactyly in American Negroes and Whites. *Am J Hum Genet.* 1973;25:397–404.

32. Watanabe H, Fujita S, Oka I. Polydactyly of the foot: an analysis of 265 cases and a morphological classification. *Plast Reconstr Surg.* 1992;89:856–877.

33. Mathes SJ, Hentz VR (Editors, Hand Surg Vol), *Plastic Surgery: The Hand Upper Limb, Part 2.* 2nd ed. Philadelphia: Saunders Elsevier, 2006: 246–249.

34. Castilla EE, Lugarinho R, da Graca Dutra M, Salgado LJ. Associated anomalies in individuals with polydactyly. *Am J Med Genet.* 1998;80:459–465.

35. Biesecker LG. Polydactyly: how many disorders and how many genes? *Am J Med Genet.* 2002;112:279–283.

36. Johnson JJ, Olivos-Glander I, Killoran C, Elson E, Turner J, Peters K et al. Molecular and clinical analysis of Greig cephalopolysyndactyly and Pallister Hall syndromes: robust phenotype prediction from the type and position of GLI3 mutations. *Am J Hum Genet.* 2005;76:609–622.

37. Kjaer KW, Hedeboe J, Bugge M, Hansen C, Friis-Henriksen K, Vestergaard MB. HOX D13 polyalanine tract expansion in classical synpolydactyly type Vordingborg. *Am J Med Genet.* 2002;110:116–121.

38. Shiota K, Matsunaga E. A Genetic and epidemiologic study of polydactyly in human embryos in Japan. *Jap J Hum Genet.* 1978;23:173–192.

39. Akiyama H, Stadler HS, Martin JF, Ishii TM, Beachy PA, Nakamura T, de Crombrugghe B. Misexpression of SOX9 in mouse limb bud mesenchyme induces polydactyly and rescues hypodactyly mice. *Matrix Biol.* 2007;26:224–233.

40. Nishimura H. Incidence of malformations in abortions. Congenital Malformations, Excepta Medica International Congress Series, eds FC Fraser, VA McKusick. Vol. 204, Amsterdam and New York: *Excerpta Medical*; 1970.

41. Stephens TD, Shepard TH. A review of limb defects in a large fetus collection. *Am J Hum Genet.* 1983;35:508–519.

42. Scott-Emuakpor AB and Madueke EDN. A study of genetic variation in Nigeria II. The genetics of polydactyly. *Hum Hered.* 1976;26:198–202.

43. Kromberg JGR and Jenkins T. Common birth defects in South African blacks. *So Afr Med J.* 1982;62:599–602.

44. Bingle, G.J. and J.D. Niswander. Polydactyly in the American Indian. *Am J Hum Genet.* 1975;27:91–99.

45. Neel JV. A study of major congenital defects in Japanese infants. *Am J Hum Genet.* 1958;10:398–445.

46. Castilla EE, da Graca Dutra M, Lugarinho da Fonseca R, Paz JE. Hand and foot postaxial polydactyly: two different traits. *Am J Med Genet.* 1997;73: 48–54.

47. Hay S, Wehrung DA. Congenital malformations in twins. *Am J Hum Genet.* 1970;22:662–678.

48. Orioli IM. Segregation/distortion in the offspring of Afro-American fathers with postaxial polydactyly. *Am J Hum Genet.* 1995;56:1207–1211.

49. Feitosa MF, Castilla E, da Graca Dutra M, Krieger H. Lack of evidence of a major gene acting on postaxial polydactyly in South America. *Am J Med Genet.* 1998;80:466–472.

50. Sverdrup A. Postaxial polydactylism in six generations of a Norwegian family. *J Genet.* 1922;12:214–240.

51. Radhakrishna U, Blouin J-L, Mehenni H, Patel UC, Patel MN, Solanki JV, Antonarakis SF. Mapping one form of autosomal dominant postaxial polydactyly type A to chromosome 7p15-q11.23 by linkage analysis. *Am J Hum Genet.* 1997;60: 597–604.

52. Radhakrishna UD, Bornholdt D, Scott HS. The phenotypic spectrum of GLI 3 morphopathies includes autosomal dominant preaxial polydactyly type IV and postaxial polydactyly type A/B; no phenotype prediction from the position of GLI3 mutations. *Am J Hum Genet.* 1999;65:645–655.

53. Akarsu AN, Ozbas F, Kostakogler N. Mapping of the second locus of postaxial polydactyly type A (PAP-A2) to chromosome 13q21-q32. *Am J Hum Genet.* 1997;61 (Suppl):A265.

54. Zhao H, Tian Y, Breedveld G. Postaxial polydactyly type A/B (PAP-A/B) is linked to chromosome 19p13.1-13.2 in a Chinese kindred. *Eur J Hum Genet.* 2002;10:162–166.

55. Galjaard RJ, Smits APT, Tuerlongs JHAM, Bais AG, Bertoli Avelia AM, Breedveld G et al. A new locus for postaxial polydactyly type A/B on chromosome 7q21-q34. *Eur J Hum Genet.* 2003;11: 409–415.

56. Morley SE, Smith PJ. Polydactyly of the feet in children: suggestions for surgical management. *Brit J Plast Surg.* 2001;54: 34–38.

57. Rogers JG, Levin S, Dorst JP, Temtamy SA. A postaxial polydactyly-dental-vertebral syndrome. *J Pediatr.* 1977;90: 230–235.

58. Castilla EE, Lugarinho da Fonseca r, da Grace Dutra M, Bermejo E, Cuevas L, Martinez-Frias M-L. Epidemiological analysis of rare polydactylies. *Am J Med Genet.* 1996;65:295–303.

59. Orioli IM, Castilla EE. Thumb/hallux duplication and preaxial polydactyly type I. *Am J Med Genet.* 1999;82:219–224.

60. Robert E, Harris J, Källén BAJ. The epidemiology of preaxial limb malformations. *Reprod Toxicol.* 1997;5:653–662.

61. Bellovits O. Genetical and epidemiological studies of polydactyly in Hungary. *Anthrop Anz.* 2003;61:413–419.

62. Cohen MS. Thumb duplication. *Hand Clinics.* 1998;12:17–27.

63. Wassel HD. The results of surgery for polydactyly of the thumbs: a review. *Clin Orthop.* 1969;64:175–193.

64. Upton J. Invited discussion: the true triplication of the thumb. A case of unclassified thumb polydactyly. *Ann Plastic Surg.* 2005; 55:324–326.

65. Wood VE. Polydactyly and the triphalangeal thumb. *J Hand Surg [Am].* 1978;3:435–444.

66. Miura T. Triphalangeal thumb. *Plast Reconstr Surg.* 1976;58: 587–594.

67. Islam S, Shinya F. Triphalangism in thumb polydactyly: an anatomic study on surgically resected thumbs. *Plast Reconstr Surg.* 1991;88:831–836.

68. Kitayama Y, Tsukada S. Patterns of arterial distribution in the duplicated thumb. *Plast Reconstr Surg.* 1983;72:535–541.

69. Panman L, Drenth T, Tewelscher P, Zuniga A, Zeller R. Genetic interactions of Gli3 and Alx4 during limb development. *Int J Devel Biol.* 2005;49:443–448.

70. Horikoshi T, Endo N, Shibta M, Heutink P, Hill RE, Noji S. Disruption of the C7orf2/Lmbr1 genetic region is associated with preaxial polydactyly in humans and mice. *J Bone Mineral Metab.* 2003;21:1–4.

71. Lyon MF, Searle AG. *Genetic Variants and Strains of the Laboratory Mouse.* 2nd ed. Oxford: Oxford University Press;1989:396–397.

72. Lettice LA, Horikoshi T, Heaney SJ, van Baren MJ, van der Linde HC, Breedveld GJ et al. Disruption of a long-range cis-acting regulator for Shh causes preaxial polydactyly. *Proc Nat'l Acad Sci.* 2002;99:7548–7553.

73. Gurnett CA, Bowcock AM, Dietz FL, Morcuende JA, Murray JC, Dobbs MB. Two novel point mutations in the long-range SHH enhancer in three families with triphalangeal thumb and preaxial polydactyly. *Am J Med Genet Part A.* 2007;143:27–32.

74. Scott WJ, Ritter EJ, Wilson JG. Ectodermal and mesodermal cell death patterns in 6-mercaptopurine riboside-induced digital deformities. *Teratology.* 1980;21:271–279.

75. McFadden DG, McAnally J, Richardson JA, Charité J, Olson EN. Misexpression of dHAND induces extra digits in the developing limb bud in the absence of direct DNA binding. *Development.* 2002;129:3077–3088.

76. Ogino T, Minami A, Fukada K, Kato H. Congenital anomalies of the upper limb among the Japanese in Sapporo. *J Hand Surg.* 1986;11-B:364–371.

77. Leung PC, Chan KM, Cheng JCY. Congenital anomalies of the upper limb among the Chinese population in Hong Kong. *J Hand Surg.* 1982;7:563–565.

78. Peterson SL, Rayan GM. Monozygotic twins discordant for thumb polydactyly. *Plast Reconstr Surg.* 2004;113:449–451.

79. Lajeunie E, Bonaventure J, El Ghouzzi V, Catalan M, Renier D. Monozygotic twins with Cronzon syndrome: concordance for craniosynostosis and discordance for thumb duplication. *Am J Med Genet.* 2000;91:159–160.

80. Woolf CM, Woolf RM. A genetic study of polydactyly in Utah. *Am J Hum Genet.* 1970;22:75–87.

81. De Smet L, Fabry G. Familial occurrence of unilateral biphalangeal duplication of the thumb. *Genet Couns.* 1992;3:31–34.

82. Nishikawa M, Bitoh N, Kikkawa F, Horil E, Mizutani S. Bilateral preaxial polydactyly: a possible dominant inheritant. *Arch Gynecol Obstet.* 2003;268:337–339.

83. Zguricas J, Heus H, Morales-Peralta E, Breedveld G, Kuyt B, Mumcu EF et al. Clinical and genetic studies on 12 preaxial polydactyly families and refinement of the localization of the gene responsible to a 1.9cM region on chromosome 7q36. *J Med Genet.* 1999;36:32–40.

84. Radhakrishna U, Blouin J-L, Solanki JV, Dhoriani GM, Antonarakis SE. An autosomal dominant triphalangeal thumb: polysyndactyly syndrome with variable expression in a large Indian family maps to 7q36. *Am J Med Genet.* 1996;66:209–215.

85. Martínez-Frías ML, Bermejo E, Cereijo A. Preaxial polydactyly of feet in infants of diabetic mothers: epidemiological test of a clinical hypothesis. *Am J Med Genet.* 1992;42:643–646.

86. Smithells RW. Defects and disabilities of thalidomide children. *Brit Med J.* 1973;1:269–272.

87. Kemnitz S, De SL. Preaxial polydactyly: Outcome of the surgical treatment. *J Ped Ortho.* 2002;11:79–84.

88. Tada K, Yonenobu KK, Tsuyuguchi Y, Kawai H, Egawa T. Duplication of the thumb. A retrospective review of 237 cases. *J Bone Jt Surg.* 1983;65A:584–588.

89. Cetik O, Uslu M, Cirpar M, Eksioglu F. Experience with the surgical treatment of radial polydactyly in adults. *Ann Plast Surg.* 2005;55:363–366.

90. Graham JM Jr, Brown FE, Hall BD. Thumb polydactyly as a part of the range of genetic expression for thenar hypoplasia. *Clin Pediatr.* 1987;26:142–148.

91. Falal F. Minor manifestations in preaxial polydactyly type I and Poland Syndrome. *Amer J Med Genet.* 1981;8:221–228.

92. Zguricas J, Snijders PJ, Hovius SE, Heutink P, Oostra BA, Lindhout D. Phenotypic analysis of triphalangeal thumb and associated hand malformations. *J Med Genet.* 1999;31:462–467.

93. Merlob P, Grunebaum M. Type II syndactyly or synpolydactyly. *J Med Genet.* 1986;23:237–241.

94. Muragaki Y, Mundlos S, Upton J, Olsen BR. Altered growth and branching patterns in synpolydactyly caused by mutations in HOXD13. *Science.* 1996;272:548–551.

95. Goodman FR, Mundlos S, Muragaki Y, Donnai D, Giovannucci-Uzielli ML, Lapi E et al. Synpolydactyly phenotypes correlate with size of expansions in HOXD13 polyalanine tract. *Proc Natl Acad Sci USA.* 1997;94:7458–7463.

96. Goodman FR, Majewski F, Collins AL, Scambler PH. A 117-kb microdeletion removing HOXD9-HOXD13 and EVX2 causes synpolydactyly. *Am J Hum Genet.* 2002;70:547–555.

97. Goodman FR. Limb malformations and the human Hox genes. *Am J Med Genet.* 2002;112:356–265.

98. Kuru I, Samli H, Yucel A, Bozan ME, Turkmen S, Solak M. Hypoplastic synpolydactyly as a new clinical subgroup of synpolydactyly. *J Hand Surg (Brit Europ Vol).* 2004;29B:6:614–620.

99. De Smet L, Debeer P, Fryns JP. Cenani-Lenz syndrome in father and daughter. *Genet Counsel.* 1996;7:153–157.

100. Debeer P, Schoenmakers EFPM, De Smet L, Van de Ven WJM. Co-segregation of an apparently balanced reciprocal t(12;22)(p11.2;q13.3) with a complex type of 3/3-prime/4 synpolydactyly associated with metacarpal, metatarsal and tarsal synostoses in three family members. *Clin Dysmorph.* 1998;7:225–228.

101. Debeer P, Schoenmakers EFPM, Thoelen R, Fryns J-P, Van de Ven WJM. Physical mapping of the t(12;22) translocation breakpoints in a family with a complex type of 3/3-prime/4 synpolydactyly. *Cytogenet Cell Genet.* 1998;81:229–234.

102. Debeer P, Schoenmakers EFPM, Thoelen R, Holvoet M, Kuittinen T, Fabry G, Fryns J-P, Goodman FR, Van de Ven WJM. Physical map of a 1.5 Mb region on 12p11.2 harbouring a synpolydactyly associated chromosomal breakpoint. *Europ J Hum Genet.* 2000;8:561–570.

103. Debeer P, Schoenmakers EFPM, Twal WO, Argraves WS, De Smet L, Fryns J-P, Van de Ven WJM. The fibulin-1 gene (FBLN1) is disrupted in a t(12;22) associated with a complex type of synpolydactyly. *J Med Genet.* 2002;39:98–104.

104. Malik S, Abbasi AA, Ansar M, Ahmad W, Koch MC, Grzeschik K-H. Genetic heterogeneity of synpolydactyly: a novel locus SPD3 maps to chromosome 14q11.2-q12. Clin Genet. 2006;69: 518–524.

105. Goldstein DJ, Kambouris M, Ward RE. Familial crossed polysyndactyly. *Amer J Med Genet.* 1994;50:215–223.

106. Reynolds JF, Sommer A, Kelly TE. Preaxial polydactyly type 4: variability in a large kindred. *Clin Genet.* 1981;25:267–272.

107. Radhakrishna U, Wild A, Grzeschik KH, Anonarakis SE. Mutation in GL13 in postaxial polydactyly type A. *Nature Genetics.* 1997;17:269–271.

108. Johnston JJ, Olives-Glander I, Killoran C, Elson E, Turner JT, Peters KF et al. Molecular and clinical analyses of Greig cephalopolysyndactyly and Pallister-Hall syndromes: robust phenotype predictor from the type and position of GLI3 mutations. *Am J Hum Genet.* 2005;76: 609–622.

109. Miura T, Nakamura MD, Horii E, Sano H. Three cases of syndactyly, polydactyly, and hypoplastic triphalangeal thumb: (Haas's malformation). *J Hand Surg.* 1990;15A: 445–449.

110. Rambaud-Cousson A, Dudin AA, Zuaiter AS, Thalji A. Syndactyly type IV/hexadactyly of feet associated with unilateral absence of the tibia. *Am J Med Genet.* 1991;40:144–145.

111. Balci S, Demirtas M, Civelek B, Pskin M, Sensoz D, Akarsu AN. Phenotypic variability of triphalangeal thumb-polysyndactyly syndrome linked to chromosome 7q36. *Am J Med Genet.* 1999;87:399–406.

112. Kantaputra PN, Chalidapong P. Are triphalangeal thumb-polysyndactyly syndrome (TPTPS) and tibia hemimelia-polysyndactyly-triphalangeal thumb syndrome (THPTTS) identical? A father with TPTPS and his daughter with THPTTS in a Thai family. *Am J Med Genet.* 2000;93:126–131.

113. Thiele H, McCann C, van't Padje S, Schwabe GC, Hennies HC, Camera G et al. Acropectorovertebral dysgenesis (F syndrome) maps to chromosome 2q36. *J Med Genet.* 2004;41:213–218.

114. Crow Y, Debeer P, Ali M, Malik S. A large Pakistani consanguineous family demonstrating a remarkable hand/foot syndrome comprising synpoly-and ectro-dactyly. *J Med Genet.* 2003;40 (Suppl1):S33.

115. Sun M, Ma F, Zeng X, Liu Q, Zhao X-L, Wn G-P et al. Triphalangeal thumb-polysyndactyly syndrome and syndactyly type IV are caused by genomic duplications involving the long range limb specific SHH enhancer. *J Med Genet.* 2007;45: 589–595.

116. Johnson KR, Sweet HO, Donahue LR, Ward-Bailey P, Bronson RT, Davisson MT. A new spontaneous mouse mutation of HOXD13 with a polyalanine expansion and phenotype similar to human synpolydactyly. *Hum Mol Gen.* 1998;7:1033–1038.

117. Hill P, Wang B, Rüther U. The molecular basis of Pallister-Hall associated polydactyly. *Hum Mol Gen.* 2007;16:2089–2096.

118. Biesecker LG, Graham JM Jr. Pallister-Hall Syndrome. *J Med Genet.* 1996;33:585–589.

119. Wang C-KL, Omi M, Ferrari D, Cheng H-C, Lizarraga G, Chin H-J, Upholt WB, Dealy CN, Kosher RA. Function of BMPs in the apical ectoderm of the developing mouse limb. *Devel Biol.* 2004;269:109–122.

120. Johnson DR. Polysyndactyly, a new mutant gene in the mouse. *J Embryol Exp Morph.* 1969;21:285–294.

121. Johnson EB, Hammer RE, Herz J. Abnormal development of the apical ectodermal ridge and polysyndactyly in Megf 7-deficient mice. *Hum Mol Genet.* 2005;14:3523–3538.

122. Lu P, Minowada G, Martin GR. Increasing Fgf4 expression in the mouse limb bud causes polysyndactyly and rescues the skeletal defects that result from loss of Fgf8 function. *Development.* 2006;133:33–42.

123. Gofflot F, Hars C, Illien F, Chevy F, Wolf C, Picard JJ, Roux C. Molecular mechanisms underlying limb anomalies associated with cholesterol deficiency during gestation: implications of Hedgehog signaling. *Hum Mol Gen.* 2003;12:1187–1198.

124. Nelson K, Holmes LB. Malformations due to presumed spontaneous mutations in newborn infants. *N Engl J Med.* 1989; 320:19023.

125. Holmes LB, Redline RW, Brown DL, Williams AJ, Collins T. absence/hypoplasia of the tibia, polydactyly, retro-cerebellar arachnoid cyst and other anomalies: an autosomal recessive disorder. *J Med Genet.* 1995;32:896–900.

126. Huang T, Elias ER, Mulliken JB, Kirse DJ, Holmes LB. A new syndrome: heart defects, laryngeal anomalies, preaxial polydactyly, and colonic aganglionosis in sibs. *Genet Med.* 1999;1:104–108.

127. Sandrow RE, Sullivan PD, Steel HH. Hereditary ulnar and fibular dimelia with peculiar facies. A case report. *J Bone Jt Surg (Am).* 1977;52:367–370.

128. Elson E, Perveen R, Donnai D, Wall S, Black GC. De novo GLI3 mutation in acrocallosal syndrome: broadening the phenotypic spectrum of GLI3 defects and overlap with murine models. *J Med Genet.* 2002;39:804–806.

129. Stoll C, Gasser B. Polysyndactyly, complex heart malformations, cardiopathy, and hepatic ductal plate anomalies: an autosomal recessive syndrome diagnosed antenatally. *Am J Med Genet.* 2003;119A:223–227.

130. James MA, McCarroll HR Jr, Manske PR. The spectrum of radial longitudinal deficiency: a modified classification. *J Hand Surg.* 1999;24A: 1145–1155.

131. James MA, Greene HD, McCarroll HR Jr, Manske PR. The association of radial deficiency with thumb hypoplasia. *J Bone Joint Surg Am.* 2004;86-A:2196–2125.

132. Stephens TD. Muscle abnormalities with radial aplasia. *Teratology.* 1983;27:1–6.

133. Lamb DW. Radial club hand: a continuing study of 68 patients with 117 club hands. *J Bone Jt Surg.* 1977;59:1–13.

134. Heikel HVA. Aplasia and hypoplasia of the radius. Studies on 64 cases and on epiphyseal transplantation in rabbits with the imitated defect. *Acta Orthop Scand Suppl.* 1959;39: 1–155.

135. Riordan CD. Congenital absence of the radius: 15-year follow-up. *J Bone Jt Surg.* 1955;37-A:1129–1140.

136. Lourie GM, Lins RE. Radial longitudinal deficiency. A review and update. *Hand Clinics.* 1998;14:85–99.

137. Van Allen MI, Hoyme HE, Jones KL. Vascular pathogenesis of limb defects. Radial artery anatomy in radial aplasia. *J Pediatr.* 1982;101:822–837.

138. Klopocki E, Schulze H, Strauss G, Ott CE, Hall J, Trotier F et al. Complex inheritance pattern resembling autosomal recessive inheritance involving a microdeletion in thrombocytopenia-absent radius syndrome. *Am J Hum Gen.* 2007 ;80:232–240.

139. Bayne LG, Klug MS. Long-term review of the surgical treatment of radial deficiencies. *J Hand Surg (AM).* 1987;12: 165–179.

140. Manske PR, McCarroll HR Jr, James M. Type III-A hypoplastic thumb. *J Hand Surg.* 1995;20A:246–253.

141. Goldfarb CA, Wall L, Manske PR. Radial longitudinal deficiency: the incidence of associated medical and musculoskeletal conditions. *J Hand Surg.* 2006;31A:1176–1182.

142. O'Rahilly R, Müller F. *Human Embryology & Teratology.* 3rd ed. New York: Wiley-Liss; 2001: 381–394.

143. Lallemand Y, Nicola MA, Ramos C, Bach A, Cloment CS, Robert B. Analysis of Msx1; Msx2 double mutant reveals multiple roles for Msx genes in limb development. *Development.* 2005;132:3003–3014.

144. Smith DW, Torres RD, Stephens TD. Mesonephros has a role in limb development and is related to thalidomide embryopathy. *Teratology.* 1996;54:126–134.

145. Koshiba-Takeuchi K, Takeuchi JK, Arruda EP, Kathiriya IS, Mo R, Hui C, Srivastava D, Bruneau BG. Cooperative and antagonistic interactions between Sall4 and Tbx5 pattern the mouse limb and heart. *Nat Genet.* 2006;38:175–183.

146. Borozdin W, Bravo Ferrer Acosta AM, Bamshad MJ, Botzenhart EM, Froster UG, Lemke J, Schinzel A et al. Expanding the spectrum of TBX5 mutations in Holt-Oram syndrome: detection of two intragenic deletions by quantitative real time PCR and report of eight novel point mutations. *Hum Mutat.* 2006;27: 975–976.

147. Kohlhase J, Schubert L, Liebers M, Rauch A, Becker K, Mohammed SN et al. Mutations at the SALL4 locus on chromosome 20 result in a range of clinically overlapping phenotypes, including Okihiro syndrome, Holt-Oram syndrome, acro-renal-ocular syndrome, and patients previously reported to represent thalidomide embryopathy. *J Med Genet.* 2003; 40:473–478.

148. Hurst JA, Hall CM, Baraister M. The Holt-Oram Syndrome. *J Med Genet.* 1991;28:406–410.

149. Okihiro MM, Tasaki T, Nakano KK, Bennett BK. Duane syndrome and congenital upper limb anomalies. A familial occurrence. *Arch Neurol.* 1997;34:174–179.

150. Evans JA, Vitez M, Czeizel A. Congenital abnormalities associated with limb deficiency defects: a population study based on cases from the Hungarian Congenital Malformation Registry (1975–1984). *Am J Med Gen.* 1994;49:52–66.

151. Birch-Jensen A. *Congenital Deformities of the Upper Extremities.* Commission: Andelsbogtrykkeriet i Odense and Det danske Forlag, 1949, pages 74–89.

152. Newman CGH. Teratogen update: clinical aspects of thalidomide embryopathy – a continuing preoccupation. *Teratology.* 1985;32:133–144.

153. Martínez-Frías ML. Epidemiological analysis of outcomes of pregnancy in diabetic mothers: identification of the most characteristics and most frequent congenital anomalies. *Am J Med Genet.* 1994;51:108–113.

154. Manske PR, McCarroll HR Jr. Reconstruction of the congenitally deficient thumb. *Hand Clinics.* 1992;8:177–196.

155. Rohmann E, Brunner HG, Kayserili H, Uyguner O, Nurnberg G, Lew ED et al. Mutations in different components of FGF signaling in LADD syndrome. *Nature Genet.* 2006;38:414–417.

156. Glanz A, Fraser FC. Spectrum of anomalies in Fanconi anemia. *J Med Genet.* 1982;19:412–416.

157. Auerbach AD, Rogatko O, Schroeder-Kurth TM. International Fanconi Anemia Registry: relation of clinical symptoms to diepoxybutane sensitivity. *Blood.* 1989;73:391–396.

158. Kutler DI, Singh B, Satagopan J, Batish SD, Berwick M, Giampietro PF et al. A 20-year perspective on the Inter-national Fanconi Anemia Registry (IFAR). *Blood.* 2003;101:1249–1256.

159. Galjaard R-JH, Kostakoglu N, Hoogeboom JJM, Breedveld GJ, van der Linde HC, Hovius SER et al. X-linked recessive inheritance of radial ray deficiencies in a family with four affected males. *Eur J Hum Genet.* 2001;9:653–658.

160. Gibson CC, Genest DR, Bieber FR, Holmes LB. X-linked phenotype of absent radius and anogenital anomalies. *Am J Med Genet.* 1993;45:743–744.

161. Kalamchi A, Dawe RV. Congenital deficiency of the tibia. *J Bone Jt Surg.* 1985;67-B:581–584.

162. Schoenecker PL, Capelli AM, Millar EA, Sheen MR, Haher T, Aiona MD, Meyer LC. Cogenital longitudinal deficiency of the tibia. *J Bone Jt Surg.* 1989;71-A:278–287.

163. Fixsen JA. Major lower limb congenital shortening: a mini review. *J Pediatr Orthopaed.* 2003;12:1–12.

164. Jones D, Barnes J, Lloyd-Roberts GC. Congenital aplasia and dysplasia of the tibia with intact fibula. Classification and management. *J Bone Jt Surg Br.* 1978;60B:31–39.

165. Ollerenshaw R. Congenital defects of the long bones of the lower limb. *J Bone Jt Surg.* 1925;7:528–552.

166. Evans EL, Smith NR. Congenital absence of tibia. *Arch Dis Child.* 1926;1:194–229.

167. Dankmeijer J. Congenital absence of the tibia. *Anat Rec.* 1935;62:179–194.

168. Gray JE. Congenital absence of the tibia. *The Anatomical Record.* 1948;101:265–273.

169. Diamond LS. Tarsal coalition in paraxial hemimelia of lower extremity. *Orthopaedic Review.* August 1979;VIII(8):91–99.

170. Williams L, Wientroub S, Getty CJM, Pincott JR, Gorden I, Fixsen JA. Tibia dysplasia. A study of the anatomy. *J Bone Jt Surg.* 1983;65-B:157–159.

171. Miller LS, Armstrong PF. The morbid anatomy of congenital deficiency of the tibia and its relevance to treatment. *Foot Ankle.* 1992;13:396–399.

172. Hudgins L, Jaffe K, Mosca V. Tibia hemimelia: report of 11 cases, review of the literature and proposed classification system. *Am J Hum Gen.* 1995;57 Suppl (4):94:A21.

173. Majewski F, Küster W, ter Haar B, Goecke T. Aplasia of tibia with split-hand/split-foot deformity. Report of six families with 35 cases and considerations about variability and penetrance. *Hum Genet.* 1985;70:136–147.

174. Moore KL, Persaud TVN. *The Developing Human: Clinically Oriented Embryology.* 7th ed. Philadelphia: Saunders;2003: 395–399 and 410–423.

175. Morin B, Owen M, Ramamurthy GV, Holmes LB. Pattern of skeletal malformations produced by Dominant hemimelia (Dh). *Teratology.* 1999;60:348–355.

176. Owen MH, Coull BA, Holmes LB. Asymmetry of skeletal effects of Dominant hemimelia. *Birth Defects Res (Part A): Clin Mol Teratol.* 2006;76:474–482.

177. Froster-Iskenius VG, Baird PA. Limb reduction defects in over one million consecutive livebirths. *Teratology.* 1989;39:127–135.

178. Dayer R, Kaelin AJ. Tibial hemimelia in monozygotic twins. *J Bone Jt Surg.* 2003;85-B (Suppl III):268.

179. Clark MW. Autosomal dominant inheritance of tibia miromelia. *J Bone Jt Surg.* 1975;57-A:262–264.

180. Emani-Ahari Z, Mahloudji M. Bilateral absence of the tibia in three siblings. *Birth Defects.* 1974;10(5):197–200.

181. McKay M, Clarren SK, Zoru R. Isolated tibia hemimelia in sibs: an autosomal-recessive disorder. *Am J Med Genet.* 1984;17: 603–607.

182. Pashayan H, Fraser FC, McIntyre JM, Dunbar JS. Bilateral aplasia of the tibia, polydactyly and absent thumb in father and daughter. *J Bone Jt Surg.* 1971;53B:495–499.

183. Rambaud-Cousson A, Dudin AA, Zuaiter AS, Thalji A. Syndactyly type IV/hexadactyly of feet associated with unilateral absence of the tibia. *Am J Med Gen.* 1991;40: 144–145.

184. Wiedemann HR, Opitz JM. Unilateral partial tibia defect with preaxial polydactyly, general micromelia and trigonmacrocephaly with a note on "developmental resistance." *Am J Med Genet.* 1983;14:467–472.

185. Narang IC, Mysorekar VR, Mathur BP. Diplopodia with double fibula and agenesis of tibia. *J Bone Jt Surg.* 1982;64B: 206–209.

186. Richieri-Costa A. Tibia hemimelia-cleft lip/palate in a Brazilian child born to consanguineous parents. *Am J Med Genet.* 1987; 28:325–329.

187. Carraro A. Assenz congenital delle tibia e sordomutismo nel Quattro fratelli. *Chic Organi Mov.* 1931;16:429–438.

188. Holmes LB, Redline RW, Brown DL, Williams AJ, Collins T. Absence/hypoplasia of tibia, polydactyly, retrocerebellar arachnoid cyst, and other anomalies: an autosomal recessive disorder. *J Med Genet.* 1995;32:896–900.

189. Kohn G, El Shawwa RE, Grunebaum M. Aplasia of the tibia with bifurcation of the femur and ectrodactyly: evidence for autosomal recessive inheritance. *Am J Med Genet.* 1989;33: 172–175.

190. McCredie J, Willert H-G. Longitudinal limb deficiencies and the sclerotomes. *J Bone Jt Surg (Br).* 1999;81-B:9–23.

191. Hosny GA. Treatment of tibia hemimelia without amputation: preliminary report. *J Pediatr Orthop.* 2005;14:250–255.

192. Davids JR, Meyer LC. Proximal tibiofibular bifurcation synostosis for the management of longitudinal deficiency of the tibia. *J Pediatr Orthop.* 1998;18:110–117.

193. Pappas AM. Congenital abnormalities of the femur and related lower extremity malformations: classification and treatment. *J Pediatr Orthop.* 1983;3:45–60.

194. Bayne L. Ulnar club hand. In: Greeen DP, ed. *Operative Hand Surgery.* 3rd ed. New York: Churchill Livingstone; 1993: 288–303.

195. Cole RJ, Manske PR. Classification of ulnar deficiency according to the thumb and first web. *J Hand Surg (Am).* 1997;22: 479–488.

196. Leroy JG, Speeckaert MT. Humeroradioulnar synostosis appearing as distal humeral bifurcation in a patient with distal phocomelia of the upper limbs and radial ectrodactyly. *Am J Med Genet.* 1984;18:365–368.

197. Swanson AB, Tada K, Yonenobu K. Ulnar ray deficiency: its various manifestations. *J Hand Surg.* 1984;9A:658–664.

198. Evans JA, Vitez M, Czeizel A. Congenital abnormalities associated with limb deficiency defects: a population study based on cases from the Hungarian Congenital Malformation Registry (1975–1984). *Am J Med Genet.* 1994;49:52–66.

199. Lenz W, Feldmann U. Unilateral and asymmetric limb defects in man: delineation of the femur-fibula-ulna complex. *Birth Defects: Orig Art Series.* 1977;13:269–285.

200. Schinzel A. Ulnar-mammary syndrome. *J Med Genet.* 1987; 24:778–781.

201. Bamshad M, Lin RC, Law DJ, Watkins WS, Krakowiak PA, Moore ME et al. Mutations in human TBX3 alter limb, apocrine and genital development in ulnar-mammary syndrome. *Nature Genet.* 1997;16:311–315.

202. Peichel CL, Prabhakaran B, Vogt TF. The mouse ulnaless mutation deregulates posterior HOXD gene expression and alters appendicular patterning. *Development.* 1997;124:3481–3492.

203. Herault Y, Fraudeau N, Zákány J, Duboule D. Ulnaless (Ul), a regulatory mutation inducing both loss-of-function and gain-of-function of posterior Hoxd genes. *Development.* 1997;124: 3493–3500.

204. Davis AP, Witte DP, Hsieh-Li HM, Potter SS, Capecchi MR. Absence of radius and ulna in mice lacking hoxa-11 and hoxd-11. *Nature.* 1995;375:791–795.

205. Woods CG, Stricker S, Seemann P, Stern R, Cox J, Sherridan E et al. Mutations in WNT7A cause a range of limb malformations, including Fuhrmann Syndrome and Al-Awadi/Raas-Rothschild/Schinzel Phocomelia Syndrome. *Am J Hum Genet.* 2006;79:402–408.

206. Lonardo F, Sabba G, Laquetti DV, Monica MD, Scareno G. Al-Awadi/Raas-Rothschild Syndrome: two new cases and review. *Am J Med Genet Part A.* 2007;143A:3169–3174.

207. Goldfarb CA, Manske PR, Busa R, Mills J, Carter P, Ezaki M. Upper-extremity phocomelia re-examined: a longitudinal dysplasia. *J Bone Jt Surg.* 2005;87-A:2639–2648.

208. Coventry MB, Johnson EW. Congenital absence of the fibula. *J Bone Jt Surg.* 1952;34A:941–955.

209. Hootnick D, Boyd NA, Fixsen A, Lloyd-Roberts GC. The natural history and management of congenital short tibia with dysplasia or absence of the fibula. *J Bone Jt Surg.* 1977; 59-B:267–271.

210. Achterman C, Kalamchi A. Congenital deficiency of the fibula. *J Bone Jt Surg Br.* 1979;61B:133–137.

211. Lewin SO, Opitz JM. Fibular a/hypoplasia: review and documentation of the fibular developmental field. *Am J Med Gen Suppl.* 1986;2:215–238; Developmental Field Concept: 425–448.

212. Grogan DP, Holt GR, Ogden JA. Talocalcaneal coalition in patients who have fibular hemimelia or proximal femoral focal deficiency. *J Bone Jt Surg.* 1994;76-A:1363–1369.

213. Gibbons PJ, Bradish CF. Fibular hemimelia: a preliminary report on management of a severe abnormality. *J Pediatr Orthop Part B.* 1996;5:20–26.

214. Searle CP, Hildebrand RK, Lester EL, Caskey PM. Findings of fibular hemimelia syndrome with radiographically normal fibulae. *J Pediatr Orthop.* 2004;13:184–188.

215. Pappas AM, Miller JT. Congenital ball-and-socket ankle joints and related lower-extremity malformations. *J Bone J Surg.* 1982;64-A:672–679.

216. Stanitski DF, Stanitski CL. Fibular hemimelia: a new classification system. *J Ped Orthopae.* 2003;23:30–34.

217. Stevens PM, Arms D. Postaxial hypoplasia of the lower extremity. *J Pediatr Orthop.* 2000;20:166–172.

218. Caskey PM, Lester EL. Association of fibular hemimelia and club foot. *J Pediatr Orthopaed.* 2002;22:522–525.

219. Hootnik DB, Levensohn EM, Packard DS Jr. Midline metatarsal dysplasia associated with absent fibula. *Clin Orthopaed Rel Res.* 1980;150:203–206.

220. Halal F. Monozygotic twins discordant for fibular aplasia. *Am J Med Genet.* 1991;41:434–437.

221. Evans JA, Reed MH, Greenberg CR. Fibular aplasia with ectrodactyly. *Am J Med Genet.* 2002;113:52–58.

222. Paes BA. Discordant fibular aplasia in twins. *Am J Med Genet.* 1995;55:225–228.

223. Lipson AH, Kozlowski K, Barylak A, Marsden W. Fuhrmann Syndrome of right-angle bowed femora, absence of fibulae and digital anomalies: two further cases. *Am J Med Genet.* 1991; 41:176–179.

224. Graham JM Jr. Limb anomalies as a consequence of spatially-restricting uterine environments. In: Fallon JF, Caplan AI, eds. *Limb Development and Regeneration, Part A.* New York: Alan R. Liss, Inc.; 1983: 413–422.

225. Robert JM, Griband P, Robert E. A local outbreak of femoral hypoplasia or aplasia and femoral-fibula-ulnar-complex. *J Génét Hum.* 1981;29:379–394.

226. Canale ST, Beaty JH. *Operative Pediatric Orthopaedics.* 7th ed. St. Louis: Mosby; 1995: 215–217.

227. Choi H, Humer SJ, Bowen JR. Amputation or limb-lengthening for partial or total absence of the fibula. *J Bone Jt Surg (Am).* 1990;72:1391–1399.

228. Catagni MA, Bolano L, Cattaneo R. Management of fibular hemimelia using the Ilizarov method. *Orthopedic Clin N Am.* 1991;22:715–722.

229. Naudie D, Hamdy RC, Fassier F, Morin B, Duhaime M. Management of fibular hemimelia: amputation or limb lengthening. *J Bone Jt Surg.* 1997;79-B:58–65.

230. Letts M, Vincent N. Congenital longitudinal deficiency of the fibula (fibular hemimelia). Parental refusal of amputation. *Clin Orthop Related Res.* 1993;287:160–166.

231. Thomas IH, Williams PF. The Gruca operation for congenital absence of the fibula. *J Bone Jt Surg.* 1987;69–13: 587–592.

232. Zlotogora J, Rosenmann E, Menashe M, Robin GC, Cohen T. The femur, fibula, ulna (FFU) complex in siblings. *Clin Genet.* 1983;24:449–452.

233. Olney RS, Hoyme HE, Roche F, Ferguson K, Hintz S, Madan A. limb/pelvis hypoplasia/aplasia with skull defect (Schinzel phocomelia): distinctive features and prenatal detection. *Am J Med Genet.* 2001;103:295–301.

234. Kevern L, Warwick D, Wellesley D, Senbaga R, Clarke NMP. Prenatal ultrasound: detection and diagnosis of limb abnormalities. *J Ped Orthop.* 2003;23:251–253.

235. Genuardi M, Pomponi MG, Sammito V, Bellussi A, Zollino M, Neri G. Split-hand/split-foot anomaly in a family segregating a balanced translocation with breakpoint on 7q22.1. *Am J Med Genet.* 1993;47:823–831.

236. Scherer SW, Poorkaj P, Allen T, Kim J, Geshuri D, Nunes M, Soder S, Stephens K, Pagon RA, Patton MA, Berg MA, Donlon T, Rivera H, Pfeiffer RA, Naritomi K, Hughes H, Genuardi M, Guerrieri F, Neri G, Lovrein E, Magenis E, Tsui LC, Evans JP. Fine mapping of the autosomal dominant split hand/split foot locus on chromosome 7, band q21.3-q22.1. *Am J Hum Genet.* 1994;55:12–20.

237. Crackower MA, Scherer SW, Rommens JM, Hui CC, Poorkag P, Soder S, Cobben JM (to be added). Characterization of the split hand/split foot malformation locus SHSFM1 at 7q21.3-q22.1 and analysis of a candidate gene for its expression during limb development. *Hum Mol Genet.* 1996;5:571–579.

238. Tackels-Horne D, Toburen A, Sangiorgi E, Gurrieri F, deMollerat X, Fischetto R, Causio F, Clarkson K, Stevenson RE, Schwartz CE. Split hand/split foot malformation with hearing loss: first report of families linked to the SHFM1 locus in 7q21. *Clinical Genetics.* 2001;59:28–36.

239. Faiyaz-ul-Hague M, Zaidi SHE, King lm, Haque S, Patel M, Ahmad M, Siddique T, Ahmad W, Tsui L-C, Cohn DH.

Fine mapping of the X-linked split-hand/split foot malformation (SHFM2) locus to a 5.1-Mb region on xq26.3 and analysis of candidate genes. *Clin Genet.* 2005;67:93–97.

240. Nunes ME, Schutt G, Kapur KP, Luthardt F, Kukolich M, Byers P, Evans JP. A second autosomal split hand/split foot locus maps to chromosome 10q24-q25. *Hum Mol Genet.* 1995;4: 2165–2170.

241. Duijf PHG, van Bokhoven H, Brunner HG. Pathogenesis of split-hand/split-foot malformation. *Hum Mol Genetics.* 2003; 12:R51–R60.

242. Roscioli T, Taylor PJ, Bohklen A, Donald JA, Masel J, Glass IA, Buckley MF. The 10q24 linked split hand/split foot syndrome (SHFM3): narrowing of the critical regions and confirmation of the clinical phenotype. *Am J Med Genet.* 2004;124A: 136–141.

243. Ozen RS, Baysal BE, Devlin B, Farr JE, Gorry M, Ehrlich GD, Richard CW. Fine mapping of the split-hand/split-foot locus (SHSFM 3) at 10q24: evidence for anticipation and segregation distortion. *Am J Hum Genet.* 1999;64:1646–1654.

244. Lanakiev P, Kilpatric MW, Toudjarska I, Basel D, Beighton P, Tsipouras P. Split-hand/split-foot malformation is caused by mutations in the p63 gene on 3q27. *Am J Hum Genet.* 2000;67: 59–66.

245. Goodman FR. Limb malformations and the human HOX genes. *Am J Med Genet.* 2002;112:256–265.

246. Bijlsma EK, Knegt AC, Bilardo CM, Goodman FR. Increased nuchal translucency and split hand/foot malformation in a fetus with an interstitial deletion of chromosome 2q that removes the SHFM5 locus. *Prenat Diagn.* 2005;25:39–44.

247. Hoyme HE, Jones KL, Nyhan WL, Pauli RM, Robinow M. Autosomal dominant ectrodactyly and absence of long bones of upper or lower limbs: further clinical delineation. *J Pediatr.* 1987;111:538–543.

248. Czeizel AE, Vitéz M, Kodaj I, Lenz W. An epidemiological study of isolated split-hand/foot in Hungary, 1975–1984. *J Med Genet.* 1993;30:595–596.

249. Graham JB, Badgley CE. Split-hand with unusual complications. *Am J Hum Genet.* 1995;7:44–50.

250. Rogala EJ, Wynne-Davies R, Littlejohn A, Gormley J. Congenital limb anomalies: frequency and aetiological factors. Data from the Edinburgh Register of the Newborn (1964–68). *J Med Genet.* 1974;11:221–233.

251. Temtamy SA, McKusick VA. *The Genetics of Hand Malformations.* New York: Wiley-Liss 1978: 53–71.

252. Bujdoso G, Lenz W. Monodactylous splithand-splitfoot. A malformation occurring in three distinct genetic types. *Eur J Pediatr.* 1980;133(3):207–15.

253. Viljoen DL, Beighton P. The split-hand and split-foot anomaly in a central African Negro population. *Am J Med Genet.* 1984;19(3):545–52.

254. Spranger M, Schapera J. Anomalous inheritance in a kindred with split hand, split foot malformation. *Eur J Pediatr.* 1988; 147:202–205.

255. Ahmad M, Abbas H, Haque S, Flatz G. X-chromosomally inherited split-hand/split-foot anomaly in a Pakistan kindred. *Hum Genet.* 1987;75:169–173.

256. Stoll C, Alembik Y, Dott B, Roth MP. Risk factors in limb reductions defects. *Paed Perinat Epidemiol.* 1992;6: 323–338.

257. Elliott AM, Reed MH, Roscioli T, Evans JA. Discrepancies in upper and lower limb patterning in split hand foot malformation. *Clin Genet.* 2005;68:408–423.

258. Elliott AM, Evans JA, Chudley AE. Split hand foot malformation (SHFM). *Clin Genet.* 2005;68:501–505.

259. Elliott AM, Reed MH, Chudley AE, Chodirker BN, Evans JA. Clinical and epidermiological findings in patients with central ray deficiency: split hand foot malformation (SHFM) in

Manitoba, Canada. *Amer J Med Genet (Part A).* 2006;140A: 1428–1439.

260. Gul D, Oktenli C. Evidence for autosomal recessive inheritance of split hand/split foot malformation: a report of nine cases. *Clin Dysmorph.* 2002;11:183–186.

261. Elliott AM, Evans JA. The association of split hand foot malformation (SHFM) and congenital heart defects. *Birth Def Res (Part A): Clin Mol Teratol.* 2008;82:425–434.

262. Celli J, Duijf P, Hamel BC, Bamshad M, Kramer B, Smits AP et al. Heterozygous germline mutations in the p53 homolog p63 are the cause of the EEC syndrome. *Cell.* 1999;99:143–153.

263. van Bokhoven H, Brunner HG. Splitting p63. *Am J Hum Genet.* 2002;71:1–13.

264. Rinne T, Hamel B, van Bokhoven H, Brunner HG. Pattern of p63 mutations and their phenotypes – update. *Am J Med Genet Part A.* 2006;140A:1396–1406.

265. Chay CK. Dactylaplasia in mice: A two-locus model for developmental anomalies. *J Hered.* 1981;72:234–237.

266. Kraus P, Lufkin T. Dlx homeobox gene control of mammalian limb and craniofacial development. *Am J Med Genet Part A.* 2006;140A:1366–1374.

267. Iacono NL, Mantero S, Chiarelli A, Garcia E, Mills AA, Morasso MI et al. Regulation of Dlx5 and Dlx6 gene expression by p63 is involved in EEC and SHFM congenital limb defects. *Development.* 2008;135:1377–1388.

268. Lewis PM, Dunn MP, McMahon JA, Logan M, Martin JF, St. Jacques B, McMahon AP. Cholesterol modification of sonic hedgehog is required for long-range signaling activity and effective modulation of signaling of Ptc 1. *Cell.* 2002;105:599–612.

269. Jones NF, Kono M. Cleft hands with six metacarpals. *J Hand Surgery.* 2004;29A:720–726.

270. Zlotogora J. On the inheritance of the split hand/split foot malformation. *Am J Med Gen.* 1994;53:29–32.

271. Schmidt A. Unilateral split hand in one of monozygotic twins. *Hum Genet.* 1983;64:301–302.

272. Verma IC, Joseph R, Bhargava S, Mehta S. Split-hand and split-foot deformity inherited as an autosomal recessive trait. *Clin Genet.* 1976;9:8–14.

273. Zlotogora J, Nubani N. Is there an autosomal recessive form of the split hand and split foot malformation? *J Med Gen.* 1989;26:138–140.

274. Palmer SE, Scherer SW, Kukolich M, Wijsman EM, Tsui L-C, Stephens K, Evans JP. Evidence for locus heterogeneity in human autosomal dominant split hand/split foot malformation. *Am J Med Genet.* 1994;50:21–26.

275. Witters IN, Van Bokhoven A, Goossens A, Van Assche F-A, Fryns J-P. Split-hand/split-foot malformation with paternal mutation in the p63 gene. *Prenatal Diagn.* 2001;21: 1119–1122.

276. Everman DB, Morgan CT, Lyle R, Laughridge ME, Bamshad MJ, Clarkson KB et al. Frequency of genomic rearrangements involving the SHFM3 locus at chromosome 10q24 in syndromic and non-syndromic split-hand/foot malformation. *Am J Med Genet Part A.* 2006;140A:1375–1383.

277. Lyle R, Radhakrishna U, Blouin JL, Gagos S, Everman DB, Gehrig C et al. Split-hand/split-foot malformation 3 (SHFM3) at 10q24, development of rapid diagnostic methods and gene expression from the region. *Am J Med Genet Part A.* 2006; 140A:1384–1395.

278. Everman DB, Morgan CT, Clarkson K, Guirieri F, McAuliffe F, Chitayat D, Steveson RE. Submicroscopic rearrangements involving the SHFM1 locus on chromosome 7q21-22 are associated with split hand/foot malformation and sensorioneural hearing loss. *J Med Genet.* 2005;42:292.

279. Ueba Y. "Cleft hand." In: Buck-Gramcko D, ed. *Congenital Malformations of the Hand and Forearm.* London: Church Livingstone; 1999: 199–209.

280. Bertola DR, Kiim CA, Albano LMJ, Scheffer H, Meijer R, von-Bokhoven H. Molecular evidence that AEC syndrome and Rapp-Hodgkin syndrome are variable expression of a single genetic disorder. *Clin Genet.* 2004;66:78–80.

281. Dianzani I, Garelli E, Gustavsson P, Carando A, Gustafsson B, Dahl N, Anneren G. Rapp-Hodgkin and AEC syndromes due to a new frameshift mutation in the TP63 gene. *J Med Genet.* 2003;40(12):e133.

282. Haak MC, Cobben JM, van Vagt JM. First trimester diagnosis of split-hand/foot by transvaginal ultrasound. *Fetal Diagn Ther.* 2001;16:146–149.

283. Roblot G. *La syndactylie congénitale.* Paris: Maulde. Doumencet Cie.; 1906.

284. Bell J. On syndactyly and its association with polydactyly. In: Penrose LS, ed. *Treasury of Human Inheritance.* London: Cambridge University Press; 1953.

285. Temtamy SA, McKusick VA. *The Genetics of Hand Malformations.* New York: Alan R. Liss; 1978: 303.

286. Percin BF, Percin S, Egilmez H, Sezgin I, Ozbas F, Akarsu AN. Mesoaxial complete syndactyly and synostosis with hypoplastic thumbs: an unusual combination or homozygous expression of syndactyly type I. *J Med Genet.* 1998;35:868–874.

287. Malik S, Ahmad W, Grzeschik K-H, Koch MC. A simple method for characterizing syndactyly in clinical practice. *Genetic Counseling.* 2005;16:229–238.

288. Sidow A, Bulotsky M, Kerrebrock AW, Bronson RT, Daly MJ, Reeve MP et al. Serrate2 is disrupted in the mouse limb-development mutant syndactylism. *Nature.* 1997;389: 722–725.

289. Gruneberg H. Genetical studies on the skeleton of the mouse. XVIII: Three genes for syndactylism. *J Genet.* 1956;54: 113–145.

290. Paznekas WA, Boyadjiev SA, Shapiro RE, Daniels O, Wollnik B, Keegan CE et al. Connexin 43 (GJA1) mutations cause the pleiotropic phenotype of oculodentodigital dysplasia. *Am J Hum Genet.* 2003;72:408–418.

291. Richardson R, Donnai D, Meire F, Dixon MJ. Expression of Gja1 correlates with the phenotype observed in oculodento-digital syndrome/type III syndactyly. *J Med Genet.* 2004;41: 60–67.

292. Zhao X, Sun M, Zhao J, Leyva JH, Zhu H, Yang W et al. Mutations in HOXD13 underlie Syndactyly Type V and a novel brachydactyly-syndactyly syndrome. *Am J Hum Genet.* 2007; 80:361–371.

293. Halal F. Dominant inheritance of syncamptodactyly of the second and third toes with foot and lower limb asymmetry and scoliosis. *Am J Med Genet.* 1985;22:149–156.

294. Nelson K, Holmes LB. Malformations due to presumed spontaneous mutations in newborn infants. *N Engl J Med.* 1989; 320:19–23.

295. Leppig KA, Werler MM, Cann CI, Cook CA, Holmes LB. Predictive value of minor anomalies: I. Association with major malformations. *J Pediatr.* 1987;110:531–537.

296. Castilla EE, Paz JE, Orioli-Parreiras IM. Syndactyly: frequency of specific types. *Am J Med Genet.* 1980;5:357–364.

297. Bosse K, Betz RC, Lee Y-A, Wienker TF, Reis A, Kleen H et al. Localization of a gene for syndactyly type I to chromosome 2q34-q36. *Am J Hum Genet.* 2000;67:492–497.

298. Ghadami M, Majidzadeh AK, Haerian BS, Damavandi E, Yamada K, Pasallar P et al. Confirmation of genetic homogeneity of syndactyly Type 1 in an Iranian family. *Am J Med Genet.* 2001;104:147–151.

299. Johnston O, Kirby W Jr. Syndactyly of the ring and little fingers. *Am J Hum Gen.* 1955;7:80–82.

300. Robinow M, Johnson GF, Broock GJ. Syndactyly Type V. *Am J Med Gen.* 1982;11:475–482.

301. Al-Qattan MM. Variable expression of isolated familial long-ring-little syndactyly. *J Hand Surg.* 2000;25B:400–402.

302. Nogami H. Polydactyly and polysyndactyly of the fifth toe. *Clin Orthopod Rel Res.* 1984;204:261–265.

303. Cenani A, Lenz W. Total syndactylia and total radioulnar synostosis in 2 brothers. A contribution on the genetics of syndactylia. *Z Kinderheilkd.* 1967;101:181–190.

304. Nezarati MM, McLeod DR. Cenani-Lenz syndrome: report of a new case and review of the literature. *Clin Dysmorph.* 2002;11:215–218.

305. Wang CK, Omi M, Ferrari D, Cheng HC, Lizarraga G, Chin HJ, Upholt WB, Dealy CN, Kosher RA. Function of BMPs in the apical ectoderm of the developing mouse limb. *Dev Bio.* 2004;269:109–122.

306. van der Hoeven F, Schimmang T, Volkmann A, Mattei MG, Kyewski B, Rüther U. Programmed cell death affected in the novel mouse mutant Fused toes (Ft). *Development.* 1994; 120:2601–2607.

307. Wöhlke A, Kuiper H, Distl O, Drögemüller C. The bovine aristaless-like homeobox 4 (ALX4) as a candidate gene for syndactyl. *Cytogenet Genome Res.* 2006;115:123–128.

308. Chung CS, Myrianthopolous NC. Racial and prenatal factors in major congenital malformations. *Am J Hum Gen.* 1968;20: 44–60.

309. Dina C, Meyre D, Gallina S, Durand E, Körner A, Jacobson P et al. Variation in FTO contributes to childhood obesity and severe adult obesity. *Nature Genetics.* 2007;39:724–726.

310. Upton J. III. Management disorders of Separation - Syndactyly. Mathes SJ (Editor), Henz VR (Editor, Hand Surgery Volumes). *Plastic Surgery.* 2nd ed. Vol. VIII, *The Hand and Upper Limb, Part 2* xxxxxx: Saunders Elsevier; 2006: chap. 204, pp. 139–150.

311. Pauli RM, Lebovitz RM, Meyer RD. Familial recurrence of terminal transverse defects of the arm. *Clin Genet.* 1985;27: 555–563.

312. Blauth W, Gekeler J. [Morphology and classification of symbrachydactylia]. *Handchirurgie.* 1971;3:123–128.

313. Buck-Gramcko D. Symbrachydactyly: a clinical entity. *Tech Hand Up Extrem Surg.* 1999; 3:242–258.

314. Kallemeier PM, Manske PR, Davis B, Goldfarb CA. An assessment of the relationship between congenital transverse deficiency of the forearm and symbrachydactyly. *J Hand Surg.* 2007;32A:1408–1412.

315. Drapkin RI, Genest DR, Holmes LB, Huang T, Vargas SO. Unilateral transverse arm defect with subterminal digit nubbins. *Ped Develop Path.* 2003;6:345–354.

316. Robinow M, Schatzman ER, Oberheu K. Peromelia, ipsilateral subclavian atresia, coarctation, and aneurysms of the aorta resulting from intrauterine vascular occlusion. *J Pediatr.* 1982; 101:84–87.

317. Firth HV, Boyd PA, Chamberlain P, MacKenzie IZ, Lindenbaum RH, Huson SM. Severe limb abnormalities after chorion villus sampling at 56–66 days' gestation. *Lancet.* 1991;337: 762–763.

318. Van Allen MI. Structural anomalies resulting from vascular disruption. *Pedi Clin N Amer.* 1992;39(2):255–277.

319. Los FJ, Brandenburg H, Niermeijer MF. Vascular disruptive syndromes after exposure to misoprostol or chorionic villus sampling. *Lancet.* 1999;353:843–844.

320. Golden CM, Ryan LM, Holmes LB. Chorionic villus sampling: a distinctive teratogenic effect on fingers? *Birth Def Res (Part A): Clin Mol Teratology.* 2003;67:557–562.

321. Hoyme HE, Jones KL, Van Allen MI, Saunders BS, Benirschke K. Vascular pathogenesis of transverse limb reduction defects. *J Pediatr.* 1982;101:839–843.

322. Gonzalez CH, Marques-Dias MJ, Kim CCAE. Congenital abnormalities in Brazilian children associated with misoprostol

misuse in the first trimester of pregnancy. *Lancet.* 1998; 351:1624–1627.

323. Vargas FR, Schuler-Faccini L, Brunoni D, Kim C, Meloni VFA, Sugayama SMM et al. Prenatal exposure to misoprostol and vascular disruption defects: a case-control study. *Am J Med Genet.* 2000;95:302–306.

324. Muneoka K, Han M, Gardiner DM. Regrowing limbs: can people regenerate body parts? *Scientific American.* 2008;298: 56–63.

325. Mariani FV, Ahn CP, Martin GR. Genetic evidence that FGFs have an instructive role in limb proximal-distal patterning. *Nature.* 2008;453:401–406.

326. Métneki J, Czeizel AE, Evans JA. Congenital limb reduction defects in twins. *Eur J Pediatr.* 1996;155:483–490.

327. Viljoen DL. Porencephaly and transverse limb defects following severe maternal trauma in early pregnancy. *Clin Dysmorph.* 1995;4:75–78.

328. Ghany JF, Holmes LB. Terminal transverse limb defects (TTLD) with nubbins. *Birth Def Res (Part A): Clin Mol Teratol.* 2008;82:359.

329. Graham JM Jr, Brown FE, Struckmeyer CL, Hallowell C. Dominantly inherited unilateral terminal transverse defects of the hand (adactylia) in twin sisters and one daughter. *Pediatrics.* 1986;78:103–106.

330. Neumann L, Pelz J, Kunze J. Unilateral terminal aphalangia in father and daughter – exogenous or genetic cause? *Am J Med Genet.* 1998;78:366–370.

331. Al-Sanna'a N, Adatia I, Teebi AS. Transverse limb defects associated with aorto-pulmonary vascular abnormalities: vascular disruption sequence or atypical presentation of Adams-Oliver syndrome? *Am J Med Genet.* 2000;94:400–404.

332. Johnson VP, Munson DP. A new syndrome of aphalangy, hemivertebrae and urogenital-intestinal dysgenesis. *Clin Genet.* 1991;39:311–312.

333. Chitayat D, Silver MM, O'Brien K, Wyatt P, Waye JS, Cliu DHK, Babul R, Thomas M. Limb defects in homozygous alpha-thalassemia: report of three cases. *Am J Med Gen.* 1997;68:162–167.

334. Harmon JV Jr, Osathanondh R, Holmes LB. Symmetrical terminal transverse limb defects: report of a twenty-week fetus. *Teratology.* 1995;51:237–242.

335. Abuelo DN, Forman EN, Rubin LP. Limb defects and congenital anomalies of the genitalia in an infant with homozygous α-thalassemia. *Am J Med Genet.* 1997;68:158–161.

336. Whitely CB, Gorlin RJ. Adams-Oliver syndrome revisited. *Am J Med Gen.* 1991;40:319–326.

337. Pauli RM, Lebovitz RM, Meyer RD. Familial recurrence of terminal transverse defects of the arm. *Clin Genet.* 1985;27: 555–563.

338. Graham JM Jr, Brown FE, Struckmeyer CL, Hallowell C. Dominantly inherited unilateral terminal transverse defects of the hand (adactylia) in twin sisters and one daughter. *Pediatrics.* 1986;78:103–106.

339. Webster WS, Lipson AH, Brown-Woodman PDC. Uterine trauma and limb defects. *Teratology.* 1987;35:253–260.

340. McGuirk CK, Westgate M-N, Holmes LB. Limb deficiencies in newborn infants. *Pediatrics.* 2001;108:e64–e71 (http://www.pediatrics.org/cgi/content/full/108/4/e64).

341. Burton BK, Schulz CJ, Angle B, Burd LI. An increased incidence of haemangiomas in infants born following chorionic villus sampling (CVS). *Prenat Diagn.* 1995;15:209–214.

342. Stoler JM, McGuirk CK, Lieberman E, Ryan L, Holmes LB. Malformations reported in chorionic villus sampling exposed children: a review and analytic synthesis of the literature. *Genet Med.* 1999;1:315–322.

343. Burton BK, Schulz CJ, Burd LI. Spectrum of limb disruption defects associated with chorionic villus sampling. *Obstet Gynecol.* 1992;79:726–730.

344. Firth H. Chorionic villus sampling and limb deficiency – cause or coincidence? *Prenat Diagn.* 1997;17:1313–1330.

345. Métneki J, Czeizel AE, Evans JA. Congenital limb reduction defects in twins. *Eur J Pediatr.* 1996;155:483–490.

Chapter 16

Microphthalmia/Anophthalmia

Definition

A very small eye (microphthalmia) or absence of the eye (anophthalmia) may be a unilateral or bilateral abnormality.

ICD–9:	743.000	(anophthalmos)
	743.100	(microphthalmos; small eyes)
ICD–10:	Q11.1	(anophthalmos)
	Q11.2	(microphthalmos)
Mendelian Inheritance in Man:	%251600	(microphthalmos, isolated I; MCOP1; microphthalmia, autosomal recessive)
	309700	(microphthalmia; includes X-linked microphthalmia and anophthalmia with mental retardation)
	#610093	(microphthalmia; isolated 2; MCOPS; autosomal recessive)
	#611038	(microphthalmia, isolated 3; MCOP3)
	#206900	

Appearance

In microphthalmia, the volume of the eye is reduced (Figures 16-1 & 16-2).

One definition of "simple" microphthalmia is an eye whose axial length is two standard deviations below the mean age-matched control measurements. In "simple" microphthalmia, the eye is normal, aside from the small size (1, 3). Microphthalmia can be associated with many different structural abnormalities of the eye, such as cataracts and coloboma of the iris (Figure 16-3).

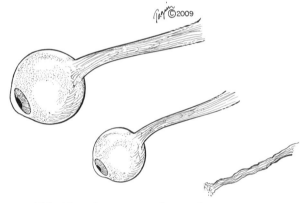

FIGURE 16.1   Normal eye compared to small or microphthalmia eye compared to anophthalmia (absence of eye).

Anophthalmia is a total absence of the tissues of the eye. The extreme form of microphthalmia can only be distinguished from apparent anophthalmia by dissection of tissues and histologic sections of tissues in the orbit.

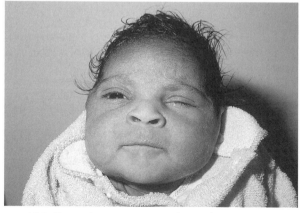

FIGURE 16.2   External appearance in newborn infant—microphthalmia of left eye.

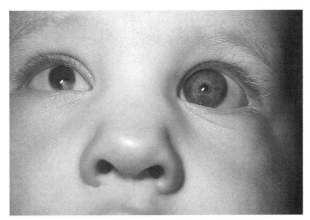

FIGURE 16.3 Microphthalmia of right eye with associated coloboma. (Courtesy of David S. Walton, M.D., Boston, MA)

In one study (4) of 17 individuals with clinical anophthalmia, the imaging by computerized tomography (CT) showed in each patient (100%) a vestigial globe (range 1-7 mm) and the presence of the optic nerve in the orbit. All individuals with small optic nerves in both eyes had evidence of abnormalities of the brain in neuroimaging. This population in Saudi Arabia was notable in having a very high rate (53%) of consanguinity, suggesting an underlying genetic basis with autosomal recessive inheritance for the clinical anophthalmia.

Individuals with microphthalmia/anophthalmia may have hypothalamic and pituitary deficiencies (5), which can be a major risk factor in anesthesia (6).

Associated Malformations

Several case series (2–6) and population-based surveys (7–16) have demonstrated the heterogeneity of the eye abnormalities, the associated malformations, and the apparent etiologies. Non-eye malformations were more common in infants with anophthalmia (63%), than in microphthalmia (30%) in Scotland [12].

Among the 45 infants with anophthalmia and 55 with bilateral microphthalmia identified among two million liveborn and stillborn infants in California (1989–1997), anomalies of the ears, brain, genitals, mouth (i.e., cleft lip/palate), and syndactyly were common associations (14).

The apparent etiologies for 60 infants with anophthalmia/microphthalmia identified in Alberta Province (1991–2001) were: 11/60 (18%) had other eye anomalies (coloboma, cataract, aniridia, etc); 16/60 (27%) had multiple anomalies; 20/60 (33%) had an associated chromosome abnormality and 13/60 (22%) had a specific syndrome, including Aicardi Syndrome (MIM #225750) and Walker-Warburg Syndrome (MIM #236670) [13].

In the population-based survey in Spain (1, 116, 212 live births and 8,442 stillbirths (1980–1995), the recognized associations among 240 infants with microphthalmia/anophthalmia were: 10% isolated, 58% multiple malformations, and 33% syndromes (11). Several significant and specific associations were identified:

Anophthalmia/microphthalmia with coloboma;
Microphthalmia with congenital cataract;
Anophthalmia/microphthalmia with holoprosencephaly.

Developmental Defect

The eyes develop from several sources: neural ectoderm, somatic ectoderm, neural crest, and mesoderm. Complex inductive processes and invaginations must occur. The retina develops as part of the wall of the brain. The components of the eye are derived from several sources: the optic vesicle is derived from the forebrain; the lens from the surface ectoderm; the optic cup by invagination of the optic vesicle; the optic nerve fibers arise in the retina and grow into the brain (17–20).

The identification of mutations associated with the occurrence of microphthalmia, and anophthalmia with and without other malformations began in recent years. Since anophthalmia and microphthalmia arise very early in development, the genes in which mutations are expected are those involved in early brain development (19, 20): PAX6 (paired box gene 6), SOX2 (sex determining region Y-box family of transcription factors), and OTX2 (orthodenticle protein homolog 2), which are considered to control each stage of eye development. PAX6 plays distinct roles in the development of the lens and retina. It is also expressed in the prosencephalon, telencephalon, diencephalons, and the olfactory bulbs. PAX6 has been postulated to be "master control gene" of eye development. SOX2 mediates gene regulation. The mutations in SOX2 have been associated with severe eye abnormalities (20, 21). OTX2 is expressed in early developing forebrain, midbrain, and retinal pigment epithelium and throughout the optic vesicle. The spectrum of eye abnormalities caused by mutations in OTX2 has been broader than those caused by SOX2 mutations. Mutations, signaling molecules, and transcription factors, which operate downstream to PAX6, SOX2, and OTX2, such as FOXC1, FOXE3, PLTX3 and MAF, are predicted to cause milder eye abnormalities (19–22).

Variation in expression can produce microphthalmia in one individual and a more severe abnormality in another. This has been shown to occur in mutations in SIX3 with some individuals having holoprosencephaly and others having microphthalmia and iris coloboma (23).

The mutations <u>microphthalmia</u> (mi) and <u>ocular</u> <u>retardation</u> (or) have been identified in the mouse (19). The mutated gene microphthalmia-associated transcription factor (Mitf) is a member of the basic-helix-loop-helix leucine zipper family of transcription factors (MIM *156845). The <u>or</u> phenotype is caused by a mutation in CHX10, a gene which encodes a homeobox transcription factor (24).

Mice with PAX2 mutations have malformations of the eye and kidney. The same mutation has been identified in two families with the renal-coloboma syndrome (25).

Prevalence

Prevalence rates of microphthalmia and anophthalmia in population-based surveys in several countries, including Italy (8), England (10), Spain (11), Canada (13), and Sweden (16)) have been 0.1-0.2/1,000.

Race/Ethnicity

In California (14) there were no significant differences in prevalence rates between whites, blacks, Asians, and foreign-born Hispanics.

Sex Ratio

No significant excess of males or females has been reported.

Birth Status

Among infants with isolated microphthalmia and anophthalmia, no changes in miscarriage and stillbirth rate, labor, delivery, or body size have been reported.

Twinning

In California (14), both microphthalmia and anophthalmia were twice as common in twins and other multiple births, as in singletons. However, in Sweden (16)

TABLE 16-1 *Etiologic heterogeneity of infants with microphthalmia and anophthalmia identified at Brigham and Women's Hospital, Boston**

	Microphthalmia		Anophthalmia	
	Isolated	Multiple Anomalies	Isolated	Multiple Anomalies
1. *Mendelian inheritance*	0		0	
X-linked syndrome of brain, eye and urogenital anomalies**		1		0
CHARGE Association		1		0
2. *Chromosome abnormalities*	0		0	
trisomy 13		5		3
trisomy 21		3		0
trisomy 9		2		0
trisomy 18		1		0
3. *Syndromes*	0		0	
arrhinencephaly with median cleft lip		1		0
holoprosencephaly with esophageal atresia and microtia		0		1
anencephaly with split-hand/split foot deformity		1		(1)***
anencephaly with absence of one eye and other anomalies		0		2
4. *Exposures*	0	0	0	0
5. *Twinning*	0	0	0	0
6. *Unknown etiology*	<u>4</u>	<u>4</u>	<u>2</u>	<u>0</u>
	4	18	2	6
Total		22****		8****

Legends: * The affected infants were identified in the Active Malformations Surveillance Program in the survey of 206,244 liveborn and stillborn infants and elective terminations for fetal anomalies in the years 1972–74, 79–2000. These infants were born to women who had always planned to deliver at this hospital and excludes infants whose mothers transferred for care after the prenatal detection of anomalies.

    ** Male infant with microphthalmia, corneal pannus, cataracts, uveal hypoplasia, retinal hypoplasia, optic nerve hypoplasia and blepharoptosis, in family with other affected males (ref. 35).

    *** Infant with anencephaly and split-hand/split-foot deformity of both hands; had microphthalmia of left eye and anophthalmia of right eye.

    **** Prevalence rate: microphthalmia: 22/206,244 = 0.11/1,000 or 1:9,375

    Prevalence rate: anophthalmia: 8/206,244 = 0.04/1,000 or 1:25,781.

there was no significant increase in the rate of twinning among infants with microphthalmia and anophthalmia.

In two sets of identical twins each twin was affected (26, 27). Neither family was consanguineous. There were no other affected relatives. In one family, each twin had microphthalmia of one eye and the other eye was either normal or had a chorioretinal coloboma.

Parental Age

In Sweden (16) in the period 1965–2001, there was a significant increase of infants with isolated anophthalmia/ microphthalmia among mothers over 40 years old.

No correlations with paternal age have been reported.

Genetic Factors

Several types of associated genetic abnormalities have been identified, including chromosome abnormalities, single mutant genes, and specific syndromes with no associated mutation identified yet. (Tables 16-1 and 16-2).

Chromosome abnormalities have been identified in 20 to 30% of affected infants, with trisomy 13 the most common association (11, 13).

Many families with parent-to-child transmission and a smaller number of X-linked inheritance (MIM %309800) have been reported. Family studies (12) support the hypothesis that there are several monogenic conditions that include microphthalmia or anophthalmia.

Mutations in SOX2 (28), OTX2 (29), SIX6 (30) and RAX (31) have been identified in individuals with anophthalmia or microphthalmia. The autosomal recessive mutations in CHX10 (32) have been identified in populations with a higher frequency of consanguinity. Systematic population-based studies (12) have identified few mutations in these candidate genes, suggesting that further research is needed to make molecular studies a practical option.

Environmental Factors

Theoretically, intrauterine infections with rubella, toxoplasmosis, and cytomegalovirus are potential causes

TABLE 16-2

A. Clinical diagnoses – no mutation analysis available

Mendelian Inheritance in Man (MIM)	Pattern of anomalies
206920	Waardenburg anophthalmia with limb anomalies (4 toes on foot and synostosis of metacarpals 4-5)
%251600	Microphthalmia with mental retardation (autosomal recessive)
%301590	X-linked microphthalmia with ankyloblepharon and mental retardation
%309800	X-linked Lenz microphthalmia with multiple anomalies
600776	Fryns anophthalmia syndrome with multiple anomalies
No MIM number	Holoprosencephaly, microphthalmia or anophthalmia and microtia [36]

B. Isolated microphthalmia/anophthalmia – molecular analysis available

Mendelian Inheritance in Man (MIM)	Gene	Pattern of anomalies
#610093	CHX10	Isolated anophthalmia/microphthalmia(autosomal recessive) [37]
#610092	CHX10	Isolated microphthalmia with coloboma 3; MCOPCB3
601881	RAX	Anophthalmia and microphthalmia with sclerocornea [31]

C. Multiple anomaly syndromes with molecular analysis available

Mendelian Inheritance in Man (MIM)	Gene	Pattern of anomalies
#206900 ^600992	SOX2	Anophthalmia and microphthalmia and developmental delay (21, 28)
#300166	BCL6 copressor gene	Microphthalmia, dental anomalies, heart defects and developmental delay (autosomal dominant)
#309801	HCCS	X-linked microphthalmia with linear skin defects
601186	STRA6	Matthew-Wood Syndrome with anophthalmia or microphthalmia, agenesis of lung, eventration of diaphragm and heart defects (autosomal recessive) [38]
607932	BMP4	Anophthalmia, short digits, genitourinary and brain malformations
#610125	OTX2	Microphthalmia, brain anomalies, joint laxity and developmental delay (29)

of anophthalmia and microphthalmia. However, the large malformation surveillance programs worldwide rarely report these associations.

Eye anomalies, including microphthalmia, have been reported in children with the fetal alcohol syndrome (33) and the thalidomide embryopathy (34).

Exposure to Benomyl, a fungicide, was postulated to cause anophthalmia but population-based studies (8) and clinical evaluations did not confirm this hypothesis.

Treatment and Prognosis

The facial appearance of the infant with anophthalmia and microphthalmia can be improved with the placement of protheses.

The habilitation of the affected infant is a significant challenge that is much more complex when there are associated anomalies of the brain and other structures, such as the heart or kidneys.

Genetic Counseling

The first step is the clinical evaluation to establish the clinical phenotype and diagnosis. Chromosome analysis and microarray analysis are essential components of this evaluation.

Many genetic syndromes are associated with the occurrence of microphthalmia and anophthalmia (Table 16-1 and 16-2).

The following are examples, subdivided by the presence of an identified mutation and the presence or absence of associated malformations:

Predicting the empiric recurrence risk after the birth of the first affected child born to healthy parents will be improved with more extensive family studies of affected infants who have had mutation analysis. Gonadal mosaicism has been the basis for the second affected infant of healthy parents with SOX2 (28) and OTX2 (29) mutations.

Microphthalmia can be a chance finding by prenatal ultrasound screening. Sometimes the small eyeball has been seen early in pregnancy; late development of microphthalmia has also been documented (39). The accuracy of prenatal detection of microphthalmia by ultrasound screening has not been established.

REFERENCES

1. Traboulsi EL, ed. *Genetic Diseases of the Eye.* Oxford Monographs on Medical Genetics No. 36. New York: Oxford University Press; 1998.
2. O'Keefe M, Webb M, Pashby RC, Wagman RD. Clinical anophthalmos. *Brit J Ophthalmol.* 1987;71:635–638.
3. Weiss A, Koussef B, Ross E, Longbottom J. Simple microphthalmos. *Arch Ophthalmol.* 1989;107:1625–1630.
4. Jacquemin C, Mullaney PB, Bosley TM. Ophthalmological and intracranial anomalies in patients with clinical Anophthalmos. *Eye.* 2000;14:82–87.
5. Brodsky MC, Frindik JP. Hypothalamic- hypophysial dysgenesis as a neuroimaging correlate of pituitary hormone deficiency in anophthalmia. *Am J Ophthalmol.* 1996;122:747–8.
6. Brodsky MC, Conte FA, Taylor D, Hyot CS, Mrak RE. Sudden death in septo-optic dysplasia: report of 5 cases. *Arch Ophthal Mol.* 1997;115:66–70.
7. Clementi M, Turolla L, Mammi I, Tenconi R. Clinical anophthalmia: an epidemiological study in Northeast Italy based on 368,256 consecutive births. *Teratology.* 1992;46:551–553.
8. Spagnolo A, Bianci F, Calabro A, Calzolari E, Clementi M, Mastroiacovo P et al. Anophtalmia and benomyl in Italy: a multi-center study based on 940,615 newborns. *Reprod Toxicol.* 1994;397–403.
9. Stoll C, Alembik Y, Dott B, Roth MP. Congenital eye malformations in 212,479 consecutive births. *Ann Genet.* 1997;40: 122–128.
10. Dolk H, Busby A, Armstrong BG, Walls PH. Geographical variation in anophthalmia and microphthalmia in England, 1988–1994. *Brit Med J.* 1998;317:909–910.
11. Bermejo E, Martinez-Frias M-L. Congenital eye malformations: clinical-epidemiological analysis of 1,124,654 consecutive births in Spain. *Am J Med Genet.* 1998;75:497–504.
12. Morrison D, Fitzpatrick D, Hanson I, Williamson K, van Heyringen V, Fleck B et al. National study of microphthalmia, anophthalmia, and coloboma (MAC) in Scotland: investigation of genetic aetiology. *J Med Genet.* 2002;39:16–22.
13. Lowry RB, Kohat R, Sibbald B, Rouleau J. Anophthalmia and microphthalmia in the Alberta Congenital Anomalies Surveillance System. *Can J Ophthalmol.* 2005;40:38–44.
14. Shaw GM, Carmichael SL, Yang W, Harris JA, Finnell RH, Lammer EJ. Epidemiologic characteristics of anophthalmia and bilateral microphthalmia among 2 million births in California, 1989–1997. *Am J Med Genet.* 2005;137A:36–40.
15. Chuka-Okosa CM, Magulike NO, Onyekouwa GC. Congenital eye anomalies in Enugs, South-eastern Nigeria. *West African J Med.* 2005;24:112–114.
16. Källen B, Tornqvist K. The epidemiology of anophthalmia and microphthalmia in Sweden. *Eur J Epidemiol.* 2005;20:345–350.
17. O'Rahilly R, Müller F. *Human Embryology & Teratology.* 3rd ed. New York: Wiley-Liss; 2001: 467–470.
18. Moore KL, Persaud TVN. *The Developing Human: Clinically Oriented Embryology.* 7th ed. Philadelphia: WB Saunders Co.; 2003: 466–483.
19. Graw J. The genetic and molecular basis of congenital eye defects. *Nature Reviews/Genetics.* 2003;4:876–888.
20. Hever AM, Williamson KA, van Heysingen V. Developmental malformations of the eye: the role of PAX6, SOX2 and OTX2. *Clin Genet.* 2006;69:459–470.
21. Fantes J, Ragge NK, Lynch S-A, McGill NI, Collin JRO, Howard-Peebles PN et al. Mutations in SOX2 cause anophthalmia. *Nature Genetics.* 2003;33:1–2.
22. Hagstrom SA, Pauer GJT, Reid J, Simpson E, Crowe S., Maumenee IH, Traboulsi EI. SOX2 mutation causes anophthalmia, hearing loss, and brain anomalies. *Am J Med Genet.* 2005;138A:95–98.
23. Wallis DE, Roessler E, Hehr U, Nanni L, Wiltshire T, Richieri-Costa A et al. Mutations in the homeodomain of the human SIX3 gene cause holoprosencephaly. *Nature Genet.* 1999;22: 196–198.
24. Burmeister M, Novak J, Liang MY, Basu S, Ploder L, Lawes NL et al. Ocular retardation mouse caused by Chx10 homeobox null allele: impaired retinal progenitor proliferation and bipolar cell differentiation. *Nat Genet.* 1996;12:376–384.
25. Schimmenti LA, Cunliffe HE, McNoe LA, Ward TA, French MC, Shim HH et al. Further delineation of renal-coloboma syndrome in patients with extreme variability of phenotype and identical PAX2 mutations. *Am J Hum Genet.* 1997;60: 869–878.

26. Rains DE, McCoy DA, Nelson EJ. Bilateral microphthalmos in monozygous twins. *Ann Ophthalmol.* 1972;4:646–652.

27. Leatherbarrow B, Kwartz J, Noble JL. Microphthalmos with cyst in monozygous twins. *J Pediatr Ophthalmol Strabismus.* 1990;27:294–298.

28. Ragge NK, Lorenz B, Schneider A, Bushby K, deSanctis L, deSanctis U et al. SOX2 anophthalmia syndrome. *Am J Med Genet.* 2005;135A:1–7.

29. Ragge NK, Brown AG, Poloschek CM, Lorenz B, Henderson RA, Clarke MP et al. Heterozygous mutations of OTX2 cause severe ocular malformations. *Am J Hum Genet.* 2005;76:1008–1022.

30. Gallardo ME, Rodríguez de Córdoba S, Schneider AS, Dwyer MA, Ayuso C, Bovolenta P. Analysis of the developomental Six6 homeobox gene in patients with anophthalmia/microphthalmia. *Am J Med Genet.* 2004;129A:92–94.

31. Voronina VA, Kozhemyakina EA, O'Kernick CM, Kahn ND, Wenger SL, Linberg JV, Schneider AC, Mathers PH. Mutations in the human RAX homeobox gene in a patient with anophthalmia and sclerocornea. *Hum Mol Genetics.* 2004;13:315–322.

32. Bar-Yosef U, Abuelaish I, Harel T, Hendler N, Ofir R, Birk OS. CHX10 mutations cause non-syndromic microphthalmia/anophthalmia in Arab and Jewish kindreds. *Hum Genet.* 2004; 115:302–309.

33. Strömland K. Ocular involvement in the Fetal Alcohol Syndrome. *Survey of Ophthalmology.* 1987;31:277–284.

34. Miller MT, Strömland K. Ocular motility in thalidomide embryopathy. *J Ped Ophthalmol Strab.* 1991;28:47–54.

35. Duker JS, Weiss JS, Siber M, Bieber FR, Albert DM. Ocular findings in a new heritable syndrome of brain, eye and urogenital abnormalities. *Am J Ophthalmol.* 1985;99:51–55.

36. Guion-Almeida ML, Richieri-Costa A, Zechi-Ceide RM. Holoprosencephaly spectrum, ano/microphthalmia, and first branch arch defects: evidence for a new disorder. *Clin Dysmorphol.* 2008;17:41–46.

37. Faiyaz-Ul-Haque M, Zaidi SH, Al-Mureikhi MS, Peltekova I, Tsui LC, Teebi AS. Mutations in the CHX10 gene in non-syndromic microphthalmia/anophthalmia patients from Qatar. *Clin Genet.* 2007;72:164–166.

38. Golzio C, Martinovic-Bouriel J, Thomas S, Mougou-Zrelli S, Grattagliano-Bessières B, Bonniè M et al. Matthew-Wood Syndrome is caused by truncating mutations in the retinol-binding protein receptor gene STRA6. *Am J Hum Genet.* 2007;80: 1179–1187.

39. Blazer S, Zimmer EZ, Mezer E, Bronshstein M. Early and late onset microphthalmia. *Am J Obst Gynecol.* 2006;194: 1354–1359.

Chapter 17

Microtia

Definitions

Microtia is a malformed and underdeveloped ear that is always smaller than the normal, unaffected external ear. The spectrum of severity is from a small ear to a rudimentary ear (1). Anotia is complete absence of the ear.

ICD-9: 744.010 (absence of ear)
        744.210 (microtia; hypoplastic pinna and absence or stricture of external auditory meatus)

ICD-10: Q16.0 (congenital absence of ear [auricle])
         Q16.1 (congenital absence, atresia and stricture of external auditory canal)

Mendelian %251800 (microtia with meatal
Inheritance   atresia and conductive
in Man: deafness)
          %600674 (microtia-anotia)
          %608814 (lateral semicircular canal malformation, familial, with external and middle ear abnormalities)

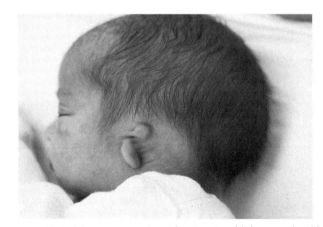

FIGURE 17.1   Monozygous twin with microtia of left ear and mild deformity of right ear (See Figure 17.2 below).

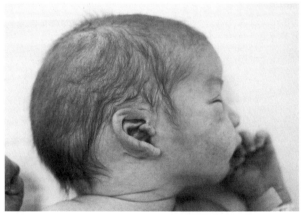

FIGURE 17.2

Appearance

A graded system of severity of microtia was suggested in 1926 by Marx (2):

Grade I: The ear is small, but the morphology of the pinna is normal.
Grade II: The ear is smaller, and its structure is partially maintained.

Grade III: Only a narrow remnant formed by a lobule and a small amount of cartilage is present (Figures 17-1–17-5).
Grade IV: Anotia, complete absence of the ear (Figure 17-6).

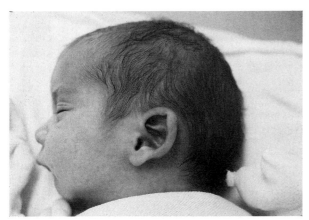

FIGURE 17.3 Monozygous twin of infant shown in Figures 17.1 and 17.2, with near normal left ear and microtia of right ear (figure 17.4).

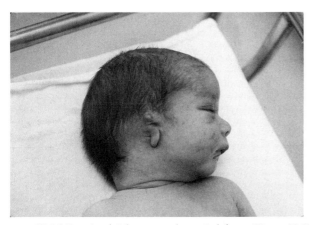

FIGURE 17.4 Microtia of right ear, as shown in left ear (Figure 17.1) of identical twin.

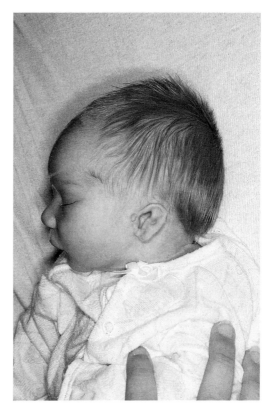

FIGURE 17.5 Infant with microtia of left ear and anotia of the right ear (See Figure 17.6 below).

With a moderate ear deformity, the external auditory canal can be normal or stenotic. With severe microtia, the meatus and external canal are absent, i.e., aural atresia (3). The more severe the ear deformity, the greater the probability that the middle ear ossicles will be either malformed or absent (4).

Fusion of the malleus and incus is common. If the cavum conchae was present, abnormalities of the ossicles were slight (4). Magnetic resonance imaging has shown that infants with grade II microtia do not have hypoplasia of the eustachian tube (5).

Microtia with only a rudimentary ear (Grade III) is associated with a conductive hearing loss of 50 to 70 dB and occasionally with sensorineural hearing loss (3) and hypoplasia of the eustachian tube cartilage (5).

The most common phenotype is unilateral microtia.

Infants with bilateral microtia usually have one less severely affected ear. Bilateral involvement occurs in about 50% of infants with syndromic microtia, but in only about 15% of the infants with isolated, non-syndromic microtia (6).

As the infant grows, the adjacent structures, such as the mandible, may show subnormal growth and

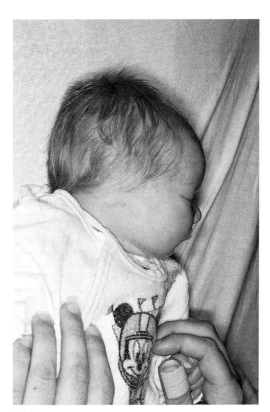

FIGURE 17.6

appear hypoplastic. The affected ear will never reach the size of the normal ear (7).

Associated Malformations

In children with isolated microtia, two studies (8, 9) have shown that there is no increased frequency of kidney malformations. Jaffe (8) carried out intravenous pyelograms on 45 children with unilateral microtia; none had any renal malformations. In another study (9) of 26 affected individuals, 2 were found to have only minor asymptomatic abnormalities of the ureters. However, screening for associated renal anomalies is recommended for children with many "syndromic" forms of microtia.

Unilateral, but not bilateral, nonsyndromic microtia was associated with a significant rate of occurrence of hypoplasia and abnormalities of cervical spine fusion in one study (11).

27% of the isolated cases of microtia in one case series (12) had either preauricular tags or sinuses.

In the large population surveys in California, Sweden, and France (13), two significant associations were identified:

1) microtia/anotia, holoprosencephaly and an/ microphthalmia.
2) microtia/anotia, neural tube defect and facial cleft.

678 infants with microtia or anotia were identified in the Texan Birth Defect Registry (14). The recognized etiologies included chromosome abnormalities in 10% and monogenic disorders in 5%. 52.5% of the infants had "isolated microtia/anotia." There were several notable associations with other malformations: acardia (1 infant), abnormal vertebrae (12.5%), heart defects (6.6%), reduction defects in upper (primarily radial ray defects) (6.1%) and lower limb (3.4%), cleft lip or cleft palate (11.7%), absence/hypoplasia of lung (2.2%), anophthalmia/microphthalmia (2.2%), and congenital diaphragmatic hernia (1.4%).

Developmental Defect

The ear develops from the first and second branchial arches. The otic placode is visible by days 21–22 post-fertilization (1). The anterior crus of the helix and the tragus are the components of the ear derived from the mandibular arch. The hyoid arch, from the maxillary arch, contributes the helix, antihelix, scapha, antitragus, and lobule. By the end of the sixth week, three hillocks are present at the caudal border of the first arch and three more on the cephalic border of the second arch. 13 cis-retinoic acid (isotretinion) or Accutane, when taken by mouth, can produce unusual ear malformations apparently by altering the development of the six hillocks (15, 16). The effect of retinoic acid on these hillocks has been postulated to be the basis for the microtia that occurs in some Accutane-exposed fetuses (16).

Days 20–22 post-fertilization were the period of greatest sensitivity during which exposure to thalidomide produced anotia; exposure to thalidomide in days 23–29 produced microtia (17).

Prevalence

In several case series and population-based studies (6–13, 18–24) microtia was much more common than anotia. The prevalence rate in California (13) of all cases of anotia was 3.3/1,000 and of isolated anotia was 1.1/1,000 in comparison to 35.2/1,000 for all cases of microtia and 18.3/1,000 for isolated microtia.

Race/Ethnicity

The highest rates of microtia and anotia groups have been observed in Hispanics, including both U.S.-born (1.9/10,000), and foreign-born Hispanic infants (2.1/10,000) in comparison to 0.9, 1.0, and 1.1 for white, black, and Asian infants, respectively (24).

Among newborn infants, isolated or nonsyndromic microtia was usually unilateral: 88% in Italy (6), 82% in Venezuela (22), 95% in California (24), and 91% in seven countries in South America (12) (Table 17-1).

A high prevalence rate of 1.74/1,000 was observed among 46,041 live births in two hospitals in Quito, Ecuador (12). There was a higher rate of more severe (grade III) microtia, in particular, in Quito.

Birth Status

An increased frequency of prematurity, low birth weight, reduced intrauterine growth, and neonatal mortality was observed among infants with microtia and anotia in the Italian Multicentre Birth Defects Registry (1983–1992; 1,173,794 births) [6].

Sex Ratio

A 60:40 ratio of affected males to females has been observed in several case series and population-based studies in New Mexico (9), Italy (6), California (13), Japan (21), and Mexico (23).

Sidedness

Many studies have shown that the unilateral microtia is more common on the right side: 58% in Japan (21), 57% in Italy (6), and 67% in New Mexico (9).

TABLE 17-1 *Microtia among infants born at Brigham and Women's Hospital, Boston (1972–1974, 1979–2000)*

	Non Transfers	
	Isolated	Multiple Anomalies
I. Mendelian Inheritance		
1. Nager's Acrofacial dysostosis (MIM: 154400)		2
2. Treacher Collins Syndrome (MIM: #154500)		1
3. Fanconi Anemia (MIM: #22760)		1
II. Chromosome Abnormalities		0
III. Specific Syndromes		
1. Hemifacial microsomia	1	6** (incl. 1 twin)
2. VACTERL Association		2** (incl. 1 twin)
3. Holoprosencephaly		1
IV. Maternal Conditions		0
V. Twinning		
Monozygous	2	
Dizygous		1 (2**)
VI. Unknown Etiology	9	5
Total	12***	19***

Legends: In each twin pregnancy, only one infant was affected.

* Affected infants were identified in the Active Malformations Surveillance Program among 206,244 liveborn and stillborn infants and elective terminations for fetal anomalies. Infants born to mothers who had planned to deliver at another hospital, before the prenatal detection of anomalies, are not included.

** Two of the three affected dizygous twins are listed under specific diagnoses; hemifacial macrosomia and VACTERL Association

*** The prevalence rates were: 1:17,187 for isolated microtia and 1:10,855 for microtia with other anomalies.

Parental Age

A maternal parity effect, that is a higher frequency among children born in the fourth or higher pregnancies, was observed in an analysis of births in France, Sweden, and California (1973–1991) [13] and later in California (1989–1997) [24]. This was observed also in Quito, Ecuador, an area of high prevalence (12).

Twinning

In a population of 1,173,794 births (6), there was one set of male twins among 172 infants with microtia; one of the twins had microtia and the co-twin did not.

13 monozygous and 22 dizygous twin pairs with isolated microtia, identified in three treatment centers, showed concordance rates of 38.5 % and 4.5 % respectively(25). In one set of reported monozygous twins, both twins had severe microtia of the right ear (26). In another set of identical twins, the most severe microtia affected the right ear in one infant and the left side in the other; the opposite ears were mildly affected. (Figures 17-1 to 17-4).

Among one set of fraternal triplets, one had microtia (3).

Genetic Factors

The empiric risk of recurrence appears to be low. Among 114 infants with non-syndromic microtia in Italy (6), one had affected relatives in three generations and another four affected infants had other affected relatives. In a Czech series of 100 affected individuals, 4% had an affected first-degree relative (20).

In the family studies of 70 affected Navajos, the occurrence rate among first-degree relatives was 5.7% (9).

Families in which there were several individuals with microtia have been reported. In one reported family with five affected members, there was no clear pattern of inheritance (27). In several families, autosomal dominant inheritance was postulated (28). In another family with possible autosomal dominant inheritance, the severity varied from mild microtia to bilateral microtia (29). In one family, the father had microtia of the left ear and his son had microtia of the right ear.

Several families have been reported in which unaffected parents have had two or more affected children with unilateral or bilateral isolated microtia, which has been interpreted as suggestive of autosomal recessive inheritance (30). No distinctive physical features have been identified that distinguish between the autosomal recessive "isolated microtia" phenotype and the presumed autosomal dominant phenotype.

Mutations in TCOF1 gene, which are present in most individuals with Treacher Collins Syndrome (MIM #154500), were not present in one father and son with non-syndromic unilateral microtia (31). In one family with SALL1 mutations, some affected members had only atretic ears and others had features of hemifacial microsomia, including epibulbar dermoid and asymmetry of the mandible (32).

Mutations in HOXA2 (33) and fibroblast growth factor 3 (FGF3) [34] have been identified in consanguineous families with phenotypes that include microtia and associated adjacent anomalies. The HOXA2 variant was in a highly conserved amino acid and not found in any controls. This was identified in a consanguineous family in Iran with bilateral microtia, mixed symmetrical severe to profound hearing loss, and partial cleft palate. Two homozygous mutations in FGF3 were found in four individuals from two unrelated families with the autosomal recessive syndromic deafness syndrome LAMM-complete labyrinthine aplasia, microtia and microdontia (MIM 610706).

In an on-going study of isolated microtia, the array-base technology has been used to assess whether copy number variants are an associated and significant finding (35).

Environmental Factors

Both microtia and anotia have been produced by exposure during pregnancy to isotretinoin (13-cis-retinoic acid) [36], thalidomide (17, 37) and mycophenolate mofetil (38). These ear deformities are part of the pattern of distinctive anomalies produced by each drug.

A higher rate of microtia and anotia occurs among infants of diabetic mothers (6).

Treatment and Prognosis

Surgical reconstruction can begin during infancy or before grade school (3). Cartilaginous ribs can be used to form the framework for a reconstructed ear. Chondrocytes obtained from the cartilage in the deformed ear can be used to generate tissue-engineered cartilage (39). A more normal looking ear can usually be formed. This surgical repair brings a significant amount of psychological relief to most affected children.

Genetic Counseling

Since microtia is a feature of many different malformation syndromes, the first step is to establish the phenotype. Since some clinicians have postulated that microtia is "a microform of hemifacial microsomia" (40), features of this phenotype, such as asymmetry of the mouth and mandible, facial nerve palsy and skeletal anomalies, should be looked for.

For isolated non-syndromic microtia, there is an empiric rate of recurrence in sibs of 3 to 8%; rates specific by race and sex of the index case have not been established.

The rare autosomal recessive forms of nonsyndromic microtia have not been shown to have phenotypic features that distinguish this type from the more common "sporadic," nonsyndromic microtia. The infant with isolated, nonsyndromic microtia does not need to have renal ultrasound, as systematic studies (8, 9) have not shown an increased frequency of significant malformations of the kidney. However, these studies are indicated if the child has syndromic microtia (10).

For microtia as part of a specific syndrome, the risk of recurrence is whatever is appropriate for that syndrome.

Specific syndromes to consider include:

1. Hemifacial microsomia (MIM: %154400); see page 288

2. Nager's acrofacial dysostosis (MIM: %154400)
3. Treacher Collins Syndrome (MIM: #154500)
4. Branchio-oto-renal syndrome (MIM: #113650)
5. CHARGE Association (MIM: #214800); see page 285

Prenatal diagnosis by ultrasound would only be realistic for severe microtia and anotia. The accuracy of detection by prenatal ultrasound screening has not been determined.

REFERENCES

1. Rogers BO. Microtic, lop, cup and protruding ears: four directly related inheritable deformities? *Plast. Reconstr. Surg.* 1968; 41:208–231.
2. Marx H. Die Missbildungen des Ohres. In: Henke F, Lubarsch O, eds. *Handbuch der Spez Path Aanat Hist.* Berlin: Springer; 1926;12:620–625.
3. Eavey RD. Ear malformations. *Pediatric Clinics of North America.* 1996;43:1233–1244.
4. Harada O, Ishii H. The condition of the auditory ossicles in microtia. *Plast Reconstr Surg.* 1972;50:48–53.
5. Imai Y, Matsuo K, Imai N. Resonance imaging of the Eustachian tube cartilage in microtia. *Cleft Palate-Craniofac J.* 1997;35:26–34.
6. Mastroiacovo P, Corchia C, Botto LD, Lanni R, Zampino G, Fusco D. Epidemiology and genetics of microtia-anotia: a registry-based study on over one million births. *J Med Genet.* 1995; 32:453–457.
7. Fukuda O. The microtic ear: survey of 180 cases in ten years. *Plast Reconstr Surg.* 1972;53:458–463.
8. Jaffe BF. The incidence of ear diseases in the Navajo Indians. *Largyngoscope.* 1969;79:21–26.
9. Aase JM, Tegtmeier RE. Microtia in New Mexico: evidence for multifactorial causation. *Birth Defects.* 1977; XIII:113–116.
10. Wang RY, Earl DL, Ruder RO, Graham JM Jr. Syndromic ear anomalies and renal ultrasounds. *Pediatrics.* 2000;108:e32–40 (http://www.pediatrics.org/egi/content/full/108/2/e32)
11. Kaye CI, Rollnick BR, Hauck WW, Martin AO, Richtsmeir JT, Nogatoshi K. Microtia and associated anomalies: statistical analysis. *Am J Med Genet.* 1989;34:574–578.
12. Castilla EE, Orioli IM. Prevalence rates of microtia in South America. *Internat J Epid.* 1986;15:364–368.
13. Harris J, Källén B, Robert E. The epidemiology of anotia and microtia. *J Med Genet.* 1996;33:809–813.
14. Seeley C, Scheuerle A. Population- based analysis of birth defects associated with anotia/microtia. Proc Greenwood Genetic Center 2007;26:61–62.
15. Hummler H, Korte R, Hendrickx AG. Induction of malformations in the cynomolgus monkey with 13-cis retinoic acid. *Teratology.* 1990;42:263–272.
16. Lammer EJ. Preliminary observations on isotretinoin-induced ear malformations and pattern formation of the external ear. *J Craniofac Genet Dev Biol.* 1991;11:292–295.
17. Miller MT, Strömland K. Ocular motility in thalidomide embryopathy. *J Ped Ophthalmol Strab.* 1991;28:47–54.
18. Melnick M, Myrianthopoulos N. *External Ear Malformations: Epidemiology, Genetics, and Natural History.* Birth Defects: Original Article Series Volume XV, No. 9, New York: A.R. Liss, Inc.; 1979.
19. Takahashi H, Maeda K. Survey of familial occurrence in 171 microtia cases. *Keisei Geka.* 1982;25:310–319.
20. Smahel Z, Horák I. Craniofacial changes in unilateral microtia. An anthropometric study. *J Craniofac Genet Develop Biol.* 1984; 4:7–16.

21. Okajima H, Takeichi Y, Umeda K, Baba S. Clinical analysis of 592 patients with microtia. *Acta Otolaryngol (Stockh).* 1996;Suppl 525:18–24.

22. Sánchez O, Méndez JR, Gomez Y, Dania Guerra E. Estudio clinico epidemiológico de la microtia. *Invest Clin.* 1997;38:203–217.

23. Llano-Rivas I, González-del Angel A, del Castillo V, Reyes R, Carnevale A. Microtia: a clinical and genetic study at the National Institute of Pediatrics in Mexico City. *Arch Med Res.* 1999;30:120–124.

24. Shaw GM, Carmichael SL, Kaidarova Z, Harris JA. Epidemiologic claracteristics of anotia and microtia in California, 1989–1997. *Birth Def Res (Part A):Clin Mol Terat.* 2004;70:472–475.

25. Artunduaga MA, Quintanilla-Dieck MDL, Greenway S, Betensky R, Nicolau Y, Hamdan U et al. A classic twin study of external ear malformations, including microtia. *N Engl J Med.* 2009;361: 1216–1217.

26. Hussain M, Ball EA, Moss AL. Ipsilateral microtia in monozygotic twins: an unusual concordant phenotype. *Plast Reconstr Surg.* 2004;113:1293–1294.

27. Zankl M, Zang KD. Inheritance of microtia and aural atresia in a family with five affected members. *Clin Genet.* 1979;16:331–334.

28. Orstavik KH, Medbo S, Mair IWS. Right-sided microtia and conductive hearing loss with variable expressivity in three generations. *Clin Genet.* 1990;38:117–120.

29. Balci S, Boduroglu K, Kaya S. Familial microtia in four generations with variable expressivity and incomplete penetrance in association with type ± syndactyly. *Turkish J. Pediatr.* 2001;43: 362–365.

30. Schmid M, Schroder M, Langenbeck U. Familial microtia and conductive deafness in three siblings. *Am J Med Genet.* 1985; 22:327–332.

31. Thiel CT, Rosanowski F, Kohlhasc J, Reis A, Rauch A. Exclusion of TCOF1 mutations in a case of bilateral Goldenhar syndrome and one familial case of microtia with meatal atresia. *Clin Dysmorphol.* 2005;14:67–71.

32. Kosaki R, Fujimaru R, Samejima H, Yamada H, Izumi K, Iijuma K, Kosaki K. Wide phenotype variations within a family with SALL1 mutations: isolated external ear abnormalities to Golenhar syndrome. *Am J Med Genet Part A.* 2007;143A: 1087–1090.

33. Alasti F, Sadeghi A, Sanati MH, Farhadi M, Stollar E, Somers T, Van Camp G. A mutation in HOXA2 is responsible for autosomal-recessive microtia in an Iranian family. *Am J Hum Gen.* 2008;82:982–991.

34. Tekin M, Oztürkmen AH, Fitoz S, Birnbaum S, Cengiz FB, Sennaroğlu L et al. Homozygous FGF3 mutations result in congenital deafness with inner ear agenesis, microtia and microdontia. *Clin Genet.* 2008;73:554–565.

35. Artunduaga MA, Quintanilla-Dieck ML, Greenway SC, Herman DS, DePalma SR, McDonough B et al. Rare de novo copy number variant identifies new locus in non-syndromic microtia/anotia. *Plast Reconstr Surg.* 2010;125(June 2010 Suppl):24.

36. Lammer EJ, Chen DT, Hoar RM, Agnish NO, Benke PJ, Braun JT et al. Retinoic acid embryopathy. *N Engl J Med.* 1985;33: 837–841.

37. D'Avignon M, Barr B. Ear abnormalities and cranial nerve palsies in thalidomide children. *Arch Otolaryngol.* 1964;80: 136–140.

38. Perez-Aytes A, Ledo A, Boso V, Saenz P, Roma E, Poveda JL, Vento M. In utero exposure to mycophenolate mofetil: a characteristic phenotype? *Am J Med Genet Part A* 2008;146A:1–7.

39. Kamil SH, Vacanti MP, Vacanti CA, Eavey RD. Microtia chondrocytes as a donor source for tissue-engineered cartilage. *Laryngoscope.* 2004;114:2187–2190.

40. Bennum RD, Mulliken JB, Kaban LB, Murray JE. Microtia: a microform of hemifacial microsomia. *Plast Reconstr Surg.* 1985;76:859–863.

Chapter 18

Neural Tube Defects

INTRODUCTION

Failure of the neural tube to close in the fourth week after fertilization results in a neural tube defect. Several clinical phenotypes have been identified (in order of frequency): anencephaly, myelomeningocele, encephalocele, lipomeningocele, meningocele, cloacal exstrophy, and the lateral meningocele (Table 18-1).

Clinical evaluations have shown that some affected infants have other anomalies and others appear to be an "isolated" neural tube defect. Several apparent etiologies have been identified. For example, a few of the affected infants have mendelian disorders, specific syndromes and associated chromosome abnormalities. Only a few environmental causes have been identified, with insulin-dependent diabetes mellitus the most common. Two anticonvulsant drugs, valproate and carbamazepine, taken in the early weeks of pregnancy are associated with a significant risk for an associated myelomeningocele. Further study is needed to determine whether other anticonvulsant drugs are associated with this risk and whether or not the risk includes other types of neural tube defects.

To date, it is notable that exposure to valproate is associated with a significant risk primarily for myelomeningocele, but not anencephaly. Presumably, that difference reflects a site-specific cellular and molecular effect of valproate.

The progress made in the study of dozens of mouse models with neural tube defects has shown that there are several cellular and molecular effects of specific mutations (1). One can only speculate at this time that several mutations will be identified in human embryos in association with the occurrence of the different neural tube defects. Will the genetic mechanisms be more likely minor general differences or subtle duplications, rather than major mutations?

A role for environmental factors, in addition to maternal diabetes and exposure to anticonvulsant drugs, has been postulated. The effect of folic acid and multivitamin supplementation has been documented in many studies. The hope is that other factors will be identified in the ongoing clinical research studies on these common malformations. One new addition to this list is the effect of maternal obesity, although the mechanism has not been determined (2).

The findings in the infants with neural tube defects born at the Boston Lying-In Hospital, and later the Brigham and Women's Hospital, illustrate the many different causes that can be identified (3). Some neural tube defects were so rare, that they are not listed in the table: iniencephaly (1 infant), cloacal exstrophy (2 infants), lateral meningocele (1 infant), and myelomeningocele associated with a molar pregnancy. However, for all types of neural tube defects there are many more causes to be identified. Most are of unknown etiology.

REFERENCES

Harris MJ, Juriloff DM. Mouse mutants with neural tube closure defects and their role in understanding human neural tube defects. *Birth Def Res (Part A): Clin Mol Teratol.* 2007;79: 187–210.

Anderson JL, Waller DK, Canfield MA, Shaw GM, Watkins ML, Werler MM. Maternal obesity, gestational diabetes, and central nervous system defects. *Epidemiology.* 2005;16:87–92.

Holmes LB, Driscoll S, Atkins L. Etiologic heterogeneity of neural tube defects. *N Engl J Med.* 1976;294:365–369.

TABLE 18-1 *Recognized etiologies of neural tube defects (NTD): Brigham and Woman's Hospital, Boston**

Etiology	Anencephaly (n=116)	Myelomeningocele (n=89)	Encephalocele (n=35)	Meningocele (n=10)	Lipomeningocele (n=5)
1. Mendelian disorders	0	0	5.7%	0	0
2. Syndromes	0	0	8.6%	0	0
3. Chromosome abnormalities	2.6%	10.1%	11.4%	10%	0
4. Teratogens					
a) IDM**	6.9%	4.5%	5.7%	10%	0
b) Drugs-meds	0	2.2%***	0	0	40%****
5. Twinning	6%	1.1%	0	0	0
6. Unknown etiology	84.5%	82.1%	68.6%	80%	60%
Prevalence rate:	1:1,778	1:2,317	1:5,893	1:20,624	1:41,249

Legend: * Data from Active Malformations surveillance Program at Brigham and Women's Hospital (Boston) in the years 1972–1974, 1979–2000. During that period 206,244 liveborn and stillborn infants and elective terminations for fetal anomalies are surveyed. The prevalence rate for all types of NTDs was 1:796.

** IDM = infants of diabetic mothers.

*** One infant exposed to valproate during pregnancy and another to carbamazepine.

**** One infant had been exposed to phenytoin during pregnancy and another to phenytoin and phenobarbital.

ANENCEPHALY

Definition

A severe, lethal malformation of the brain in which there is a lack of most of the cranial vault and absence of much of the brain. The word "an-encephaly' means technically "without brain."

ICD-9:	740.000	(absence of brain)
	740.010	(acrania)
	740.020	(anencephaly)
ICD-10:	Q00.0	(anencephaly includes acrania)
	Q00.1	(craniorachischisis)
Mendelian Inheritance in Man:	%206500	(anencephaly)
	301410	(anencephaly-spina bifida; neural tube defects, X-linked)

Appearance

Four phenotypes have been identified. The most common type, isolated anencephaly, has no cranium (Figures 18-1, 18-2 and 18-3).

The top of the head is a mass of tissue with no recognizable landmarks (1–6). There is absence of major segments of the brain, such as prosencephalon, mesencephalon, and part of the rhombencephalon (5). What remains appears to be a vascular structure and degenerated tissue above the brain stem structures. The eyes are prominent, and the bony forehead ends at the edge of the brain mass. The ears are thickened and often prominent. The neck is short. The term meracrania refers to anencephaly confined to the cranium.

The second phenotype is anencephaly with an open spine or rachischisis or craniorachischisis (Figure 18-4). The open abnormal brain extends down through the lower cranium, foramen magnum, and the cervical and upper thoracic vertebrae.

A third phenotype is anencephaly with retroflexion, a marked backward flexion of the neck. This is similar to, but to be distinguished from, iniencephaly.

A fourth phenotype is the occurrence of both anencephaly and spina bifida in the same infant (Figure 18-5).

The frequencies of these four phenotypes have been determined in population-based malformation surveys (7). For example, in the United Kingdom and Ireland, between 1980 and 1987, 68% of the affected infants had isolated anencephaly, 4% anencephaly with retroflexion, and 28% had anencephaly with either rachischisis or spina bifida. In the same time period in Europe

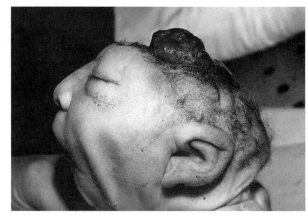

FIGURE 18.1   Side view that shows absence of skull over top of head, the protruding brain tissue, and the thickened, simple ear shape.

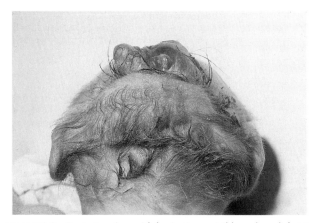

FIGURE 18.2   Posterior view with brain tissue visible and no defect in occipital region.

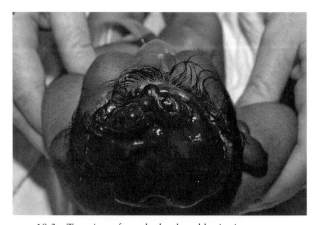

FIGURE 18.3   Top view of poorly developed brain tissue.

and Malta, the frequencies of these phenotypes were somewhat different: 93%, 1%, and 6% respectively.

Associated Malformations

Cleft palate and absence of the pituitary are common associated features and are considered part of the underlying abnormality, not separate defects. The adrenal cortex is thin because of the decreased stimulation by ACTH, reflecting the pituitary deficiency.

Among fetuses with anencephaly, the frequencies of associated malformations were 19% (8) and 38% (2) in two case series. Among liveborn and stillborn infants, the frequencies were 14.4% for liveborn and 11.6% for stillborn infants in British Columbia (9) and 24% in the United Kingdom (10). The frequencies of non-neural malformations were higher in infants with both anencephaly and spina bifida, 33.3% and 40%, respectively (9, 10).

The common associated non-neural malformations are cleft lip, diaphragmatic hernia, a wide spectrum of renal anomalies, cryptorchidism, and hypospadias (1, 2, 9, 10, 11, 12). The frequency of cleft lip and palate has been 10%; omphalocele and diaphragm defects, 5%. In one report (13) the diaphragm defect was primarily "central" or "high diaphragm" defects rather than the more common Bochdalek pleuroperitoneal defect.

Seller and Kalousek (8) noted that the pattern of associated non-neural malformations varied with the level of the defect. Cleft lip and palate, congenital heart defects, omphalocele, and congenital diaphragmatic hernia occurred in association with anencephaly, anencephaly with rachischisis, and upper spina bifida. By contrast, mid-level spina bifida was associated with defects in the abdominal region, such as accessory spleen, non-rotation of gut, and Meckel diverticulum. They considered cleft lip and palate a reflection of the failure of the anterior portion of the neural tube to close. They postulated that these non-neural malformations "are mechanically induced by the particular specific maldevelopment of the neural tube and its surrounding tissue during neurulation."

Developmental Defect

Anencephaly becomes visible in the fourth week postfertilization (5, 6). The neural tube should be closed completely rostrally by stage 12. One co-twin with anencephaly was considered to be at stage 13, which is 28–30 days gestation (14). When the neural tube remains open, the exposed brain will degenerate throughout the fetal period.

The primary defect appears to be failure of fusion of the cerebral portion of the neural folds (15). The alternative explanation of reopening the closed neural tube seems much less likely, based on the information available (2, 5, 6).

Marin-Padilla (16) developed another theory from the analysis of the disarticulated skulls and skeletons of twelve 7 to 8 month gestation age fetuses with anencephaly. He identified multiple vertebral anomalies and an altered shape of the base of the skull, facial, and cranial bones. He postulated that the structural

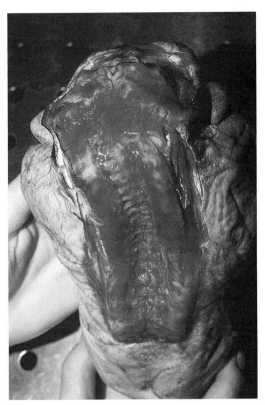

FIGURE 18.4 Shows cranioschisis, an extensive closure defect of brain that extends through occiput and into upper thoracic vertebrae.

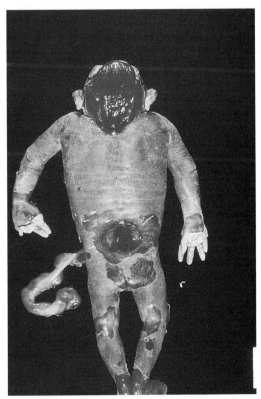

FIGURE 18.5 Posterior view of macerated fetus with anencephaly and lumbosacral spina bifida.

abnormality of the base of the skull, especially the sphenoid bone, was unable to fulfill its function, because of the primary abnormality of mesodermal tissue in anencephaly. Using radiography and cephalometric analyses (17), the findings by Marin-Padilla (16) were confirmed. Some, but not all, anencephalic fetuses had a malformed and much smaller posterior cranial fossa.

The analysis of total gangliosides in the cerebral remnant in 37 and 30 week gestational age infants, by mass spectrometry and high performance thin layer chromatography, showed that all gangliosides characteristic of brain tissue were present, but the relative proportions were markedly different from age-matched normal brains (18).

Exencephaly in mice looks like anencephaly in humans, except that brain tissue is present. The pattern of closure of the neural tube has been determined in developing mice (19). Correlations with human abnormalities have been postulated (20), such as defective closure of Zone 2 produces meracrania (anencephaly confined to cranium) and defective closure 2 for holocranium (anencephaly with open upper thoracic spine [rachischisis]). However, embryologists have reported that human embryos show a pattern of closure that is not the same as in mouse embryos (15, 21).

Over 190 different mouse mutants and strains of mice have neural tube defects, most of which are only exencephaly (19, 22). The studies of the cellular effects of the mutations suggest many mechanisms by which exencephaly can develop: abnormalities of cell number, gap, anchors, transcription, active regulation, and basal lamina. Studies of the embryos from the SELH/Bc strain have shown that all embryos exhibit a developmental error (failure to elevate: Zone B), but most recover and only 20% develop exencephaly (23). This could be a model of the process of multifactorial inheritance which leads to the development of anencephaly. Such details are not available from affected human embryos.

Prevalence

The prevalence rates have varied with the gestational age of the fetuses surveyed, race/ethnicity, geographic area, and socioeconomic and health status:

a) spontaneous abortions: A survey of 1,213 intact embryos in Japan (24), excluding twins and pregnancies terminated because of maternal illness, showed that 4 (0.34% or 1 in 300) of the 1,186 embryos had neural tube defects, two with anencephaly, and two with spina bifida. The prevalence rate of anencephaly was, therefore, 1 in 600 or 1.6/1000. Anencephaly was also a common neural tube defect in spontaneous abortions in London (25) and New York (26): 11 of 36 fetuses with CNS defects in London and 3 of 9 fetuses with neural tube defects in New York had anencephaly with or without rachischisis.

b) spontaneous abortions and livebirths: Surveys of spontaneous abortions in London (25) in 1971–1974 and New York City (26) in 1977–1981 showed significant differences in prevalence rates for neural tube defects (NTD) in those two cities, and in comparison to two high prevalence areas, Edinburgh, Scotland, and Belfast, Northern Ireland: New York (10.2/1,000 sp. ab.; 0.9/1,000 term births); London (36.2/1,000; 3.0/1,000); Edinburgh (41.2/1,000; 5.3/1,000); Belfast (55.6/1,000; 6.3/1,000). The rates of NTD among spontaneous abortions were ten-fold (10x) higher among spontaneous abortions than in liveborn infants in all four cities. Some of the affected embryos had associated chromosomal abnormalities, although not all were studied successfully: 10.6% of 94 specimens in London and 8.1% of 86 in New York.

c) severity of defect and prevalence rates: There has also been a correlation of the severity of the defect, such as the extent of the associated rachischisis, with higher prevalence rates (27, 28).

d) decreasing prevalence: The prevalence rates of all types of neural tube defects have decreased over the past 50 years, beginning long before the advent of periconceptional folic acid supplementation. A major factor in determining the prevalence rate in newborn infants, since 1980, has been the impact of prenatal detection of affected fetuses by ultrasound and the elective termination of these pregnancies (29–32). The Active Malformations Surveillance Program in Boston (31) in the years 1972–1990 showed that by 1990 fetuses with anencephaly were detected by either the fetal survey by ultrasound or maternal serum alpha-fetoprotein screening, and that the parents chose to terminate each of these pregnancies. In France, the prenatal detection rate (1979–1999) was 96%. 73% of those pregnancies with affected fetuses were terminated (32). Therefore, estimates of prevalence rate must consider the time period, the intrinsic differences between several major ethnic/racial groups, and the impact of prenatal diagnosis and elective termination of pregnancies in which the fetus has been found to have anencephaly.

Race

Population-based studies in the 1960s–1980s showed differences in the prevalence rates between racial/ethnic groups, unrelated to folic acid supplementation, prenatal diagnosis, or elective termination of an affected fetus (Tables 18-2 and 18-3).

A dramatic illustration of geographic differences was shown in Texas (1981–1986) when the rate in 1,000 births varied from 0.2-0.3/1,000 in West Texas and to more than 0.5/1,000 in East Texas and along the Rio Grande River (40).

TABLE 18-2 *Examples of prevalence rates in different populations and time periods.*

	Anencephaly (rate/1,000)	
Native American	1980–1988 (33)	0.13 to 0.36
California (30)	1983–1987 (30)	0.27
Hawaii	1988–1994 (34)	0.3
Australia:	1980–1989 (29)	0.6 to 0.73
East Ireland:	1980–1994 (35)	0.5 to 1.8
China		
Northern (rural):	1992–1993 (27)	0.9
Southern (rural):	1992–1993 (27)	0.4
Korea	1993–1994 (36)	0.3 to 0.4
India	2002–2003 (37)	2.5
(Uttar Pradesh; rural)		
Ghana	1991–1992 (38)	0.8
Venezuela	1993–1996 (39)	0.75

TABLE 18-3 *Prevalence rates within different racial and ethnic groups in three areas of the United States*

U. S. – Caucasian	Time Period	Rate/1,000
TEXAS (40)	1981–1986	
White males		0.3
White females		0.49
Hispanic males		0.39
Hispanic females		0.62
Black males		0.18
Black females		0.3
BROOKLYN (41)	1968–1976	
White		0.55
Black		0.4
Puerto Rican		0.73
LOS ANGELES (42)	1973–1977	
White		0.45
Hispanic		0.77
Black		0.32

Sex Ratio

An excess of affected females has been identified in many studies (43–46), but not all (30). Several interpretations have been made about this association. Knox (43) and James (44) suggested that the excess of females was greater in populations with the higher frequencies of occurrence of anencephaly. The analysis of 147 fetuses in London (45) with neural tube defects attributed to multifactorial inheritance, i.e., excluding infants with chromosome abnormalities and NTD as part of genetic syndromes, showed that there was an excess of females in fetuses with isolated anencephaly and anencephaly with rachischisis. However, there was an excess of males with lumbar and sacral spina bifida. By comparison, the analysis of 165 infants (live births and fetal deaths) with isolated anencephaly and 28 with nonisolated anencephaly in California (30) showed an equal number of males and females. There was an excess of males with "high" or "thoracic" spina bifida.

Parental Age

No consistent correlation of maternal or paternal age with the occurrence of anencephaly has been reported. There was no difference among the mothers of affected infants in California (1983–1987) [30] or British Columbia (1958–1985) [46], but there was an excess of young mothers in Eastern Ireland (1980–1994) [35].

Birth Status

An increased rate of prematurity, low birth weight, spontaneous abortion, and stillbirths among fetuses and infants with anencephaly has been reported (25, 26).

Twins

An increased frequency of twinning among infants with anencephaly has been demonstrated in several population-based studies. In the analysis of 1,560 infants with anencephaly, encephalocele, and myelomeningocele in New South Wales, Australia (1965–1973), 35 twin pairs (2.2%) were identified (29).

In a study of 3,584 infants and aborted fetuses with anencephaly in eight populations surveyed for malformations in the 1970s and 1980s (47), the rate of twinning was 2.3% to 6.4%. Among the different phenotypes with anencephaly, the rate of twinning was 5.6% in those with chromosome abnormalities, 5.4% with anencephaly and other malformations, and 3.9% among infants with isolated anencephaly.

In a prenatal diagnosis center in Israel (1997–2004), there were 26 infants with anencephaly among 300 consecutive pregnancies (48). 7 of 26 affected infants were twin pregnancies, all of which were dichorionic and discordant for anencephaly. 7 of the 26 twin pregnancies had been conceived by in vitro fertilization, using intracytoplasmic sperm injection (ICSI).

Monoamniotic (identical twins; MZ) are usually discordant for anencephaly, as was illustrated in a case series from the literatures of 11 twin pregnancies (49). The concordance rate for neural tube defects was 21.4% for monozygous (MZ) twins and 5.5% for dizygous (DZ) twins. In one set of female MZ twins, one had anencephaly and the other had myelomeningocele.

Monoamniotic (MZ) twin pairs in which both have a neural tube defect are quite rare. Examples reported include: both twins having anencephaly (50); one with anencephaly and the other with encephalocele (51); one with anencephaly and the other with spina bifida of cervical vertebrae and hemivertebrae in the upper thoracic spine (52); and one with anencephaly and the other with holoprosencephaly (53) have been reported. In such concordant MZ twins, autosomal recessive inheritance has been postulated (54).

Genetic Factors

Among the many studies of genetic markers associated with neural tube defects, some have included DNA samples from infants with anencephaly. No anencephaly-specific gene mutations have been identified.

Several infants with anencephaly have been born to parents who are related, which suggests that some rare autosomal recessive genes can cause anencephaly (54). The anatomic findings were not described, so it is not known if there are distinctive phenotypic characteristics in infants with autosomal recessive anencephaly.

A few families have had an apparent X-linked pattern of inheritance, with anencephaly in some relatives and myelomeningocele in others (55, 56). The observation that the mother's sisters' children are more likely to have infants with anencephaly than other relatives has been interpreted as support for X-linked inheritance for anencephaly in some families (57). The NAP1L2 gene, which maps to Xq12-q24, is one candidate gene for X-linked neural tube defects (58).

Chromosome abnormalities have been identified in 1 to 2% of fetuses with anencephaly (59–61). A higher rate (11%) was identified in a study of 9 infants with anencephaly and other major malformations (60). Several infants with abnormalities of chromosome 2 have had a neural tube defect, including instances of anencephaly (62, 63). Aside from that association, no specific chromosome abnormalities have been associated with anencephaly.

After the demonstration in several studies that supplementation with folic acid in the weeks just before and after conception appeared to decrease the occurrence of anencephaly, myelomeningocele, and several other malformations (64), research studies focused on identifying mutations and polymorphisms that predisposed to the occurrence of these malformations. The initial focus was on genetic differences in the metabolism of folic acid. Several genetic polymorphisms have been identified which when present in the pregnant woman are associated with an increased risk for all types of neural tube defects, including the C677T polymorphism in methylenetetrahydrofolate reductase (MTHFR) (21), and the R653Q polymorphism of the C1-synthase enzyme (65). The presence of the 19-bp deletion polymorphism in intron-1 of dihydrofolate reductase in the mother appeared to decrease her risk (66). No polymorphism or mutation associated only with the occurrence of anencephaly has been identified.

Genetic abnormalities have also been looked for in pathways not involved in folate metabolism. These include the PAX transcription factors (67) and the genes involved in planar cell polarity, such as VANGL1 (68). One fetus homozygous for a FOXN1 mutation had anencephaly as well as severe combined immune deficiency (69).

It is not possible, yet, to screen the fetus or infant with anencephaly or her/his mother to identify the genetic abnormalities that led to the occurrence of this malformation.

Environmental Factors

Brian MacMahon and Stella Yen (70) described dramatic epidemics of anencephaly and spina bifida in the 1930s in Providence and Boston. No explanation was ever established. Subsequently, several environmental factors have been postulated to cause anencephaly, in particular, and neural tube defects, in general: hyperthermia (71), blighted potatoes (72), insulin-dependent diabetes in the mother (73), and excessive obesity (74).

Exposure during the first weeks of pregnancy to the anticonvulsant drugs carbamazepine (75) and sodium valproate (76) are associated with an increased risk for neural tube defects, primarily myelomeningocele and rarely anencephaly (77).

Prevention

In 1991, the evidence that periconceptional supplements with folic acid could decrease the risk for anencephaly and other neural tube defects came from using these supplements to decrease the occurrence of the second affected child among couples with one affected child (78). Proof that these supplements would prevent the first occurrence of neural tube defects came in separate, systematic studies in 1992 and in 1999 in Hungary (79) and China (80), respectively.

In the United States, the Food and Drug Administration required, by January 1998, the fortification of U.S. enriched grain products with folic acid. This was done with the goal of reducing the occurrence of anencephaly and all other types of neural tube defects. Data from 21 population-based birth defects surveillance programs in the years 1995–2002 (81) showed that, following fortification, there were significant declines in the occurrence of anencephaly and spina bifida among births to Hispanic women and non-Hispanic white women. There was no significant decline in the birth of infants with either anencephaly or spina bifida among non-Hispanic black mothers.

While these and other studies (82, 83) have shown an unequivocal benefit from fortification of enriched grains among major racial/ethnic groups, it has been disappointing to see that many developed countries, such as European countries, have not mandated this fortification. As a result, prevention has relied on voluntary supplementation, which does not reach as many pregnant women and, as a result, more infants with folic acid–preventable anencephaly (and spina bifida) have been born (84).

Recent studies (85) suggest that a supplement of vitamin B12 should be added to the periconceptional folic acid tablet. The prevention of a greater number of infants with anencephaly or spina bifida would be prevented by using both vitamin B12 and folic acid.

Treatment and Prognosis

Anencephaly is a fatal condition. The affected fetuses may be stillborn or, if born alive, survive only a few hours or days. After detection by ultrasound during pregnancy, elective termination of the pregnancy is a common management choice.

Genetic Counseling

The infants with non-syndromic anencephaly are attributed to the additive effect of genetic "differences" and environmental factors (Table 18-4).

While genetic risk factors have been identified in research projects, the specific factors responsible for the birth of a single affected infant cannot be determined, yet, through genetic testing available in commercial laboratories.

Family studies have shown that if the first affected infant has anencephaly, the second affected infant is more likely to have anencephaly than any other type of neural tube defect (86). This was documented in a study in North America in the years 1975 to 1978 among 831 pregnancies. After the birth of a child with a neural tube defect, 87.2% of the subsequent affected fetuses had the same defect (86). For the 14 families whose previous child had anencephaly and a subsequent child had a NTD, 13 or the 14 recurrences were also anencephaly.

The empiric recurrence risks in different populations have varied by the baseline prevalence of NTDs: an area of higher prevalence has a higher rate of recurrence. For example, in Ireland and Wales, when the prevalence rate was 7-8/1,000 births, the recurrence risk of one affected child was 5% (87). Later in Ireland, when the prevalence rate of all neural tube defects was 3/1,000, the empiric recurrence risk was 3.3% (88).

TABLE 18-4 *Apparent etiologies in infants with anencephaly*

Etiologies	Multiple Isolated	Anomalies Phenotype	Unknown
I. Mendelian	0	0	0
II. Chromosome abnormalities*	0	3*	
III. Maternal conditions			
a) Infants of diabetic mothers	1	2	5
IV. Twinning**			
Identical twins	3		1
Non-identical twins	3		
V. Unknown etiology	30	19	49
	37	24	55/116***

* = the chromosome abnormalities were: unbalanced translocations (2) and 46,XX/47,XY+18 (1).

** = six sets of twins; both males were affected in one set presumed to be non-identical; three sets of twins were considered identical, based on placentation, and only one twin in each pair had anencephaly.

*** = these 116 affected infants were identified among 206,244 liveborn and stillborn infants and elective terminations for anomalies surveyed at Brigham and Women's Hospital in Boston in the years 1972–1974, 1979–2000. Infants born to women who had planned to deliver at another hospital before prenatal detection of the anencephaly have been excluded.

By comparison, in Italy, a country with a lower prevalence rate, the empiric recurrence risk was 1.8%. In British Columbia, when the prevalence rate was 1.6/1,000 the recurrence rate was 2.1% (89).

The question has been raised (90) as to whether parents with an increased risk for anencephaly and spina bifida, have also an increased risk for having an infant with "isolated" hydrocephalus (90). This association has not been confirmed in recent studies.

For the mother of an affected fetus or infant, daily periconceptional supplementation with multivitamins and 4 mg folic acid is recommended. While there is ample evidence in Hispanic and non-Hispanic white families that the risk of having a second affected infant is reduced by this supplementation, it does not *guarantee* that the next infant born to that couple will be unaffected.

Prenatal screening in high-risk pregnancies, such as the pregnant women with insulin-dependent diabetes mellitus, will be carried out to make certain the fetus does not have either anencephaly or other types of neural tube defects.

Experience has shown that anencephaly can be detected by prenatal ultrasound in the first trimester.

CLOACAL EXSTROPHY

Definition

This is a malformation syndrome of the lower abdomen, spine, and genitourinary tract that includes omphalocele, exstrophy of the bladder, divided genital structures, bowel anomalies, imperforate anus, and a lumbosacral skin-covered myelocystocele.

ICD-9:	759.824	(cloacal dysgenesis)
	741.98	(meningocystocele)
ICD-10:	Q64.1	(exstrophy of urinary bladder)
	Q42.3	(imperforate anus)
	Q42.9	(congenital absence, atresia and stenosis of large intestine)
	Q43.4	(duplication of intestine)
	Q43.7	(persistent cloaca)
Mendelian Inheritance in Man #:	258040:	OEIS complex (omphalocele-exstrophy-imperforate anus-spina defects)
	%600057:	exstrophy of bladder

Historical Note

This pattern of anomalies has been observed for many, many years, as was illustrated by the early report in 1709 (91). Several reports appeared in the 1960s and 1970s by Roberta Spencer (92), a pediatric surgeon, by Bruce Beckwith (93), a pediatric pathologist, and by Patricia Hayden (94), a pediatrician, and her colleagues.

John Carey (95), a clinical geneticist, brought this phenotype to wider attention in 1978 and suggested the acronym OEIS: omphalocele-exstrophy-imperforate anus–spinal defects.

Before 1960, this malformation syndrome was considered lethal (96). However, by the mid-1970s improvements by surgeons, anesthesiologists, and critical care physicians and nurses had increased survival to 50%. By the 1980s, survival had continued to improve (97).

John Lattimer, an experienced pediatric urologist, emphasized the need for a team approach to provide care for the multiple medical and surgical problems of infants with cloacal exstrophy (98).

In the 1980s the association with monozygotic twinning was noted. It was suggested that the abnormality was caused by the twinning process (99). Blighting of a conjoined twin was another postulated cause (100) that was suggested by the frequent observation of a "vanishing twin" earlier in the pregnancy.

The advent of magnetic resonance imaging (101) and ultrasound (102) have made it possible to improve the evaluation of affected infants for potential tethering of the cord and renal abnormalities that require early surgical treatment.

Recently questions have been raised about the common practice of converting surgically an affected male to be raised as a female because of the hypoplasia and division of the genital structures. However, these 46,XY "females," when older, have been found to retain interests and attitudes typical of males and some have declared themselves males (103).

Appearance and Associated Malformations

The affected infant appears normal above the abdomen, but has multiple, severe defects of the abdominal organs, genitourinary structures, spine, and sometimes deformities of the legs (92–95, 104–113).

The omphalocele is located lower on the abdomen than the more common "central," isolated omphalocele and often contains the liver and small intestines.

The bladder is exstrophied and has hemibladders on either side of the protruding cecum.

Often the ileum is prolapsed through a vesicointestinal fistula. The cecum and anus are absent. There may be duplications of the colon and appendix, and rotation of the intestine (Figures 18-8 and 18-9).

Many affected infants have persistence of the urogenital sinus. The genital tubercles are hypoplastic and are divided, with one on each side of the exstrophied bladder. Most males have undescended testes. Affected females have a short atretic vagina that is sometimes duplicated; likewise, the uterus may be absent or duplicated.

The symphysis pubis is separated. The pubic rami may be hypoplastic and sometimes are oriented anteriorly.

The skin-covered lumbar protrusion, which may be large, is an enormously dilated central canal of the spinal cord (Figures 18-7 and 18-10). This protrusion passes through a defect in the vertebrae within a meningocele and expands into a terminal cyst (Figure 18-6).

The meningocele is lined with arachnoid. The terminal cyst is lined with ependyma and is referred to as a myelocystocele. Some have associated lipomas and are referred to as lipomyelocystoceles. There is always tethering of the spinal cord. In the dissection of these lipomas, choristomas, containing intestine, stomach, and testes, have been identified (107).

Images from magnetic imaging (101), ultrasound (102), and radiography (114) can identify the spectrum of internal anomalies of the vertebrae and spinal cord that are present in all affected individuals. All have occult spinal dysraphism (114). Magnetic resonance imaging showed, in a study of 15 affected children (101), that each infant had a terminal cyst of the central canal of the spinal cord that was tethered and had herniated through the area of vertebrae defects. The imaging showed that 5 (33%) of the 15 had a Chiari I malformation. There was

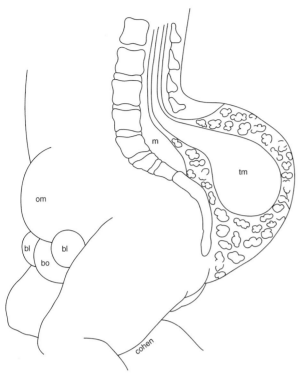

FIGURE 18.6 Sagittal view that shows large terminal cyst from the enlarged central canal of spinal cord. (From Cohen AR: *Neurosurgery.* 1991;28:834–843. Used with permission.)

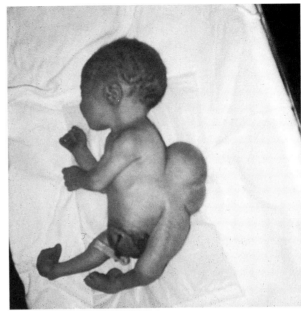

FIGURE 18.7 Side view of newborn with cloacal exstrophy, which shows large, skin-covered meningocystocele over back. (Courtesy of Patricia W. Hayden, M.D., University of Washington, Seattle, WA)

hydromyelia of the cervicothoracic spine in 2 (13%) of the 15, and of the lumbar spine in another 2 (13%) children.

Radiographs have identified hemivertebrae in the thoracic and lumbar region, a decreased number of ribs, and often, partial agenesis of the sacrum (102, 114). Defects in cervical vertebrae and spina bifida in the thoracic region were less common than defects in lower vertebrae in four population-based surveys (109).

Anatomic dissections of the pelvis of an affected infant, who had died at 72 days of age, showed abnormalities of the innervation of the bladder (115).

The structural abnormalities in the gastrointestinal tract affect the morbidity and mortality of the affected children. 25 to 50% of affected individuals have had short bowel syndrome, which has highlighted the need, during surgical reconstruction, to preserve as much bowel as possible (106). In a case series of 22 patients (116), two (9%) had duodenal atresia and short bowel syndrome and seven (32%) had had malrotation. Many affected children have either ileostomy or colostomies, as part of the surgical repair. While their birth weights were between 10th and 90th centile of normal, many experienced nutritional losses and showed failure to thrive. Total parenteral nutrition was used on 8 (36%) of the 22 affected children. Defective absorptive function of the bowel, attributed to the associated abnormality of the spine, has contributed to the poor nutritional status (116).

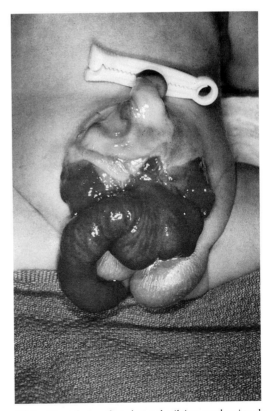

FIGURE 18.8 Frontal view that shows the ileium prolapsing through the open bladder and the omphalocele just above the bladder. (From W. Hardy Hendren, M.D., Massachusetts General Hospital, Boston, MA. Used with permission.)

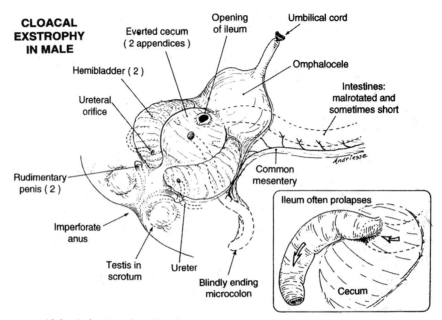

FIGURE 18.9 A drawing that identifies the anatomic structures visible in the frontal view. (From W. Hardy Hendren, M.D., Massachusetts General Hospital, Boston, MA. Used with permission.)

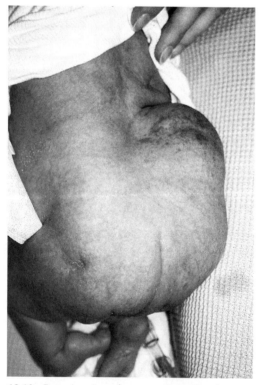

FIGURE 18.10 Posterior view of asymmetric swelling from meningocystocele. (Courtesy of David D. Weaver, M.D., Indiana University School of Medicine, Indianapolis, IN.)

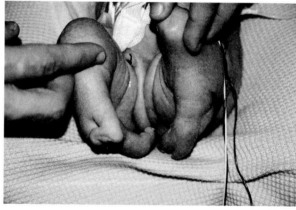

FIGURE 18.11 Terminal transverse and longitudinal deficiencies in the legs of the infant with cloacal exstrophy. Also shown in figure 18-10. (Courtesy of David D. Weaver, M.D., Indiana University School of Medicine, Indianapolis, IN.)

considered initially to be difficult in affected children, have been successful (117).

Limb deficiencies in the legs, but not the arms, have been reported in 17 to 26% of the infants with cloacal exstrophy. Absence of toes and absence of tibia are two of the most common limb deficiencies (118) [Figure 18-11].

Six of 15 affected infants diagnosed prenatally (113) had a club foot deformity.

Developmental Defect

Cloacal exstrophy has been considered the severe end of a spectrum with epispadias and bladder exstrophy

Ureteral reflux is a common finding and a priority in the surgical repair. Absence of one kidney has been observed frequently, specifically, 28% (112) and 21% (129) in two small case series. Kidney transplants,

the mild end of that spectrum. The cellular and molecular basis for the defective development in cloacal exstrophy is not known. It is presumed to involve the narrow band of mesoderm between the genital tubercles and body stalk, cells that are derived from the caudel eminence during the last stages of gastrulation. Between weeks 4 and 8, this mesoderm migrates between the ectoderm and endoderm to form the anterior abdominal muscles and pubic bones. Several theories have been developed for the primary abnormality in this process that causes cloacal exstrophy (119, 120). One theory is that there is a decrease in the development of this mesodermal component, combined with decreased apoptosis at the umbilical ring. Another theory is that cloacal membrane develops more extensively and fails to regress. This thickened membrane serves as a wedge that prevents the invasion of mesoderm.

Serial ultrasound images of two affected fetuses showed that a cloacal abnormality persisted until after 22 (121) and 18 (122) weeks of gestation, respectively, and then "ruptured" to result in the expected "typical" appearance in those affected fetuses at birth.

Another hypothesis is that partial or complete duplication of the organizing center within a single embryonic disc increases the risk of mesodermal deficiency. This leads to a failure of development of the cloacal membrane and, somehow, the occurrence of cloacal exstrophy.

The increased frequency of identical or monozygous twinning, and monozygotic twinning in particular, has been interpreted to mean that the twinning process is a major factor in the occurrence of cloacal exstrophy. This hypothesis was supported by the observation by prenatal ultrasonography that 8 of 11 affected fetuses in one case series (100) had a second fetal heart tone, and a presumed "vanishing twin," in the first trimester of pregnancy. Five of those 8 pregnancies had only a single fetus in the second trimester. Blighted conjoined twinning was postulated to lead to cloacal exstrophy in the surviving twin.

Conjoined twins with cloacal exstrophy have also been described, remarkably with diamniotic placentation in rare instances (123, 124). This observation is consistent with the etiology of conjoining by "primary fusion," as proposed by Spencer (125). By this mechanism, two primitive streaks arise in a single embryonic disc and later ends in incomplete fission of the two embryos.

HLXB9 was considered a candidate gene, as mutations in this gene have been associated with the Currarino Syndrome (MIM #176450) in malformations of the sacrum, rectum, and anterior meningocele occur. However, all exons of the HLXB9 gene from the DNA of five individuals with cloacal exstrophy were analyzed and no obvious mutations or deletions were identified (129). The DNA was obtained from bladder specimens, not peripheral lymphocytes.

Testing for an association with the methylene tetrahydrofolate reductase (MTHFR) polymorphism 677C→T in 91 individuals with either epispadias (n=7) bladder exstrophy (n=72) or cloacal exstrophy (n=12) showed no evidence of significant deviation from random transmission of the 677→T allele from mother to affected child (128).

Experimental exposures or injuries in chick embryos have been shown to cause cloacal exstrophy, but not the associated myelocystocele in the affected fetus (126, 127). Thomalla et al (126) used CO_2 laser to damage the developing tail bud caudal to the omphalon esenetric vessels at 68 to 76 hours of incubation. Five (8%) of the 59 chicks that survived 10 days or longer had cloacal exstrophy, but none had a myelocystocele.

Trypan blue and the anti-trypanosomal drug suramin applied to stage 14 chick embryos produced cloacal exstrophy in 20% and 6.9% of the surviving embryos, respectively. Myelocystocele was present in 31% of the suramin-treated embryos, but not in association with cloacal exstrophy (127).

Prevalence

In Manitoba Province, during the years 1970–1981, the prevalence of cloacal exstrophy was 0.05/1,000 (1:20,000) [105]. In Spain (1976–1999), 11 infants among 1,601,860 consecutive liveborn infants had cloacal exstrophy for a prevalence rate of 0.005/1,000 (1:200,000) [111]. In Iowa between 1972 and 2000, 14 affected infants were identified for a prevalence of 1:82,000 total births (112).

Among 10,017 consecutive stillbirths in Spain (1980–1999), the prevalence rate of cloacal exstrophy was 0.3/1,000 (1:3,333) livebirths and for bladder exstrophy was 0.1/1,000 (1:10,000) [111].

Race/Ethnicity

Data on prevalence rates in different racial and ethnic groups is not available.

Birth Status

In an analysis of the 5,260 malformed infants identified in 5.84 million births, the nonrandom cluster of omphalocele, bladder exstrophy, imperforate anus, and spine malformation was a clearly defined entity. There were 194 probable cases (1:27,134) [109].

An increased frequency among stillbirths was noted in Spain (111). The birth weights and gestational ages of infants with cloacal exstrophy were lower significantly than those of infants with bladder exstrophy (111).

Sex Ratio

The ratio of the number of males to females has been equal in studies of consecutive cases, whereas there was an excess of males with exstrophy of the bladder (111, 129).

Sidedness

This is a midline developmental abnormality.

Parental Age

In a study of 232 families with bladder exstrophy-epispadias, paternal age was increased significantly (129). However, in a population-based series of 11 infants with cloacal exstrophy, paternal age was not increased (112).

Twinning

10% of the infants with cloacal exstrophy are like-sex twins (130). In a series of eight identical twins, 3 (38%) were concordant for cloacal exstrophy. In another review (131) the concordance rates were 45% in monozygous twins and 6% in dizygous twins. The process of monozygous twinning has been postulated to be a risk factor in the occurrence of several malformations (132). Cloacal exstrophy has been attributed to blighted conjoined twinning (100). The high frequency of vanishing twin in the pregnancies of infants with cloacal exstrophy was considered suggestive of transient twinning, followed by an affected singleton (119).

Genetic Factors

In a study of 232 families with bladder exstrophy-epispadias, 15 of the probands had cloacal exstrophy (129). One affected female had a half brother with epispadias. Another affected male had two male second cousins with epispadias. In an analysis of 14 affected individuals identified in a statewide malformations surveillance program (112), one affected female had a maternal grandfather with bladder exstrophy and a bifid penis. In addition, two affected infants had one parent with anal stenosis. In another family (133), unaffected parents had two affected infants.

Several affected individuals have had healthy children.

In general, chromosome analysis has identified no abnormalities. In one case series (129) of 232 infants with the spectrum cloacal exstrophy, epispadias alone and bladder exstrophy-epispadias, two chromosome abnormalities were identified: 47, XYY in one child and a translocation in another: 46, XY (8;9) (p 11.2; q13). One reported infant (134) had a 9q 34.1-qter deletion from a de novo imbalanced translocation between chromosomes 9q and Yq. The steroidogenic factor 1 (SF1) gene is located in the deleted region normally, but no pathogenic mutation was found by direct gene sequencing in this individual.

Another affected infant had an interstitial deletion in chromosome 3, specifically del (3) (q12.2q13.2), but seven other individuals with 3q interstitial deletions (135) did not have cloacal exstrophy.

Environmental Factors

None has been identified. In one epidemiologic study in which the mothers of affected infants were interviewed retrospectively, no associations with teratogenic exposures were identified (129).

Treatment and Prognosis

The condition of cloacal exstrophy appears not to be an intersex condition, but rather a malformation syndrome in which there can be inadequacy of the phallus in the 46,XY male (103). Social and behavioral adaptation, after reconstructive surgeries, is a major challenge, but can go well (136, 137). The risk for neurologic defects and/or developmental delay appears to be low (112, 113), based on the limited information available.

Genetic Counseling

The clinician's diagnostic challenge is to distinguish between cloacal exstrophy, urorectal septum malformation sequence, and the limb-body-wall complex, as there is overlap in their phenotypic features (138).

In discussing the potential cause of cloacal exstrophy, there is a strong association with the twinning process, but the specific developmental abnormality is not known. Fortunately, there is a very low risk (less than 1%) that a subsequent sib will be affected (116). To date, no individual with cloacal exstrophy has had an affected child.

Cloacal exstrophy has been associated with increased nuchal translucency in first trimester screening (113, 139), but the frequency and accuracy of early detection by the prenatal screening has not been determined.

Fetuses with cloacal exstrophy have been identified by ultrasound during pregnancy. However, the extent of the abnormalities of the intestine and genitals has been difficult to establish during pregnancy (113).

ENCEPHALOCELE

Definition

A soft tissue protrusion of cranial contents and meninges through a defect in the cranium.

ICD-9:   742.000   (occipital encephalocele)
             742.085   (frontal encephalocele)
             742.086   (parietal encephalocele)
             742.090   (unspecified encephalocele)

ICD-10:   Q.01   (encephalocele,
                        meningoencephalocele,
                        encephalomyclocele,
                        cerebral meningocele)

Mendelian   None for isolated
Inheritance   encephalocele.
in Man:

Appearance

The protrusion occurs most often in the midline and is skin-covered, except for defects in the skin at the tip of the protrusion. The protrusion or cyst may contain only cerebrospinal fluid, or brain tissue, such as cerebellum, occipital lobe or brain stem, and vascular structures. Protrusions that do not contain brain tissue are sometimes called a "meningocele"; by comparison, the term "encephalocele" (or meningoencephalocele) means that brain tissue is present in the protrusion (140). When the protrusion contains meninges, brain, and ventricles, it is referred to as "meningoencephalocystocele" (Figures 18-13, 18-14 and 18-15).

The relative frequency of each type of encephalocele varies by ethnic group and geographic area (141–152). Among Caucasians, the most common location is the posterior occipital area, typically below the torcula and in the posterior fossa (153). When a hindbrain anomaly is present, the fluid-filled sac is usually midline, caudal to the developing cerebellum, and communicates with the fourth ventricle as a ventriculocele (Figures 18-13, 18-14).

The anterior (frontal) encephalocele (Figure 18-15), the most common location of encephalocele in Asian populations (145, 146, 149), always originates from the midline glabella and protrudes just above the nose. These are called sincipital encephaloceles and are protrusions through the foramen cecum (144) [Figure 18-12].

Nasoethmoid defects originate from the lateral side of the nose (148). The most common sites of protrusion in one series of 25 affected children (142) were nasal orbital and nasoethmoid, and nasoethmoid in another series of 92 infants (147). The skull base defects in frontal, nasal, and ethmoidal encephaloceles can be either a single opening or multiple openings (145).

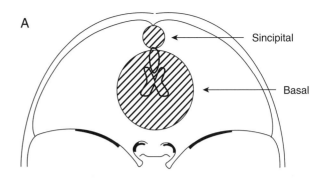

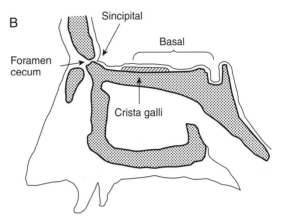

FIGURE 18.12   Shows the location of sincipital and basal encephalocele in a sagittal diagram (5).

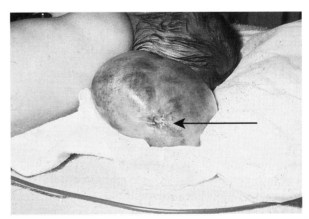

FIGURE 18.13   Posterior view of large occipital encephalocele with skin defect (arrow) at tip of protrusion.

The protrusions in the frontal, nasal, and ethmoid regions vary from mild to huge; from an area of skin thickening to a large disfiguring mass. In a case series of 23 individuals, three-dimensional computed tomography (3D-CT) showed that 61% had more than one external defect (148). The most common type, in Asia, was a combined nasal ethmoid-nasal orbital type. Computed tomography (CT) has identified also "seguestrated cephaloceles," meaning a hernia mass located far from the external bone defect.

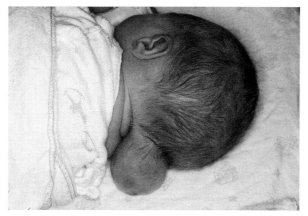

FIGURE 18.14   Posterior view of smaller occipital encephalocele.

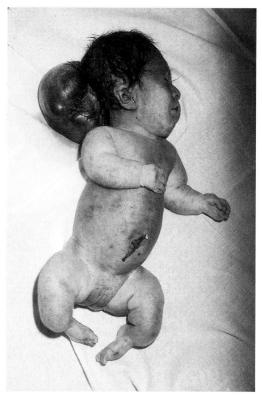

FIGURE 18.16   Shows osteogenesis imperfecta with occipital encephalocele, a rare autosomal recessive phenotype. (173)

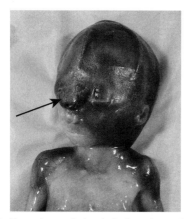

FIGURE 18.15   Frontal encephalocele in fetus (arrow). (Courtesy of Mason Barr, M.D., University of Michigan, Ann Arbor, MI.)

Parietal encephaloceles (Figure 18-16) are not always in the midline. One subgroup is the atretic type in which there is an area of alopecia and, underneath the dura, a dorsal crypt (144, 154, 155). The atretic type often involves the superior sagittal sinus, such as fenestration or splitting it into two venous channels (156). By contrast, the nodular type has an associated dural sinus and no associated cerebral malformation.

Only 74% of 114 encephaloceles in one case series (146) were detected at birth. Occult basal encephaloceles, which protrude either through the crista galli or the sphenoid, are usually not detected at birth, but the symptoms begin in infancy (147, 153). The rare temporal bone encephaloceles herniate into the petrous apex of the temporal bone, the tegmen tympani, or the mastoid cavity (157).

Associated Malformations

Three dimensional (3D) imaging by CT in 23 Asian patients with frontoethmoidal encephaloceles showed that 17% had brain malformations, including arachnoid cysts in two and ventricular dilation in one patient and porencephaly in another (148).

Infants with frontoethmoidal encephaloceles often have hypertelorism (143, 144, 158, 159) and median (154) or lateral cleft lip. Endocrine efficiencies were apparent in many of the 84 individuals with frontoethmoid encephalocele, including short stature, diabetes insipidus, hypothyroidism, and growth hormone deficiency (160).

There is an occasional (about 10%) association of thumb hypoplasia (161) with occipital encephalocele.

Many specific malformation syndromes include encephalocele in the phenotype (162–164) [Table 18-5].

In the United Kingdom, Ireland, and Europe, after excluding infants with chromosome abnormalities, Meckel-Gruber Syndrome, amnion rupture, and cloacal exstrophy, 21 to 24% of the infants with encephalocele had multiple malformations (162). Among 50 liveborn infants with occipital encephalocele in Atlanta, Georgia, excluding infants with chromosome abnormalities and amniotic band syndrome, 22% had multiple malformations; in the same series, only 5% of 20 infants with anterior encephalocele had multiple defects (163).

TABLE 18-5 *Etiologic and Phenotypic Heterogeneity of Encephalocele: Brigham and Women's Hospital: 1972-74, 79-2000.*

	Non-transfer*			Transfer**			
	Isolated	Multiple Anomalies	Phenotype Unknown	Isolated	Multiple Anomalies	Phenotype Unknown	Totals
I. Mendelian Disorders							(3.5%)
a.) Meckel-Gruber (MIM #249000)		1			1		2
b) Osteogenesis imperfecta and occipital encephalocele*** (Figure 18.16)		1					1
II. Specific Syndromes							(10.5%)
a) Amniotic band		1			2	4	7
b) Iniencephaly with encephelocele	1						1
c) Otocephaly					1		1
III. Familial (affected sib)			1				(1.2%) 1
IV. Chromosome Abnormalities							(5.8%)
a) Trisomy 18		2					2
b) 46,XY/47,XY,+8					1		1
c) 47,XXX		1					1
d) 47,XY,+4****		1					1
(unbalanced trans)							
V. Maternal Conditions							(4.7%)
a) Infants of diabetic mothers	2	0	1	0	0	1	4
VI. Twinning					1	3	4 (4.7%)
VII. Unknown etiology	13	3	7	10	6	21	60 (69.8%)
Totals	16	10	9/35	10	12	29/51	86

Legends: The infants with encephalocele were identified in the Active Malformations Surveillance Program of 206,244 liveborn and stillborn infants and elective terminations for fetal anomalies.
 * A non-transfer is an infant born to a woman who had always planned to deliver at Brigham and Women's Hospital (BWH) in Boston;
 ** A transfer is an infant born to a woman who had not planned to deliver at BWH and who transferred her care after the prenatal diagnosis of the fetal abnormality.
 *** An infant with osteogenesis imperfecta and a large occipital encephalocele born to consanguineous parents. A very similarly affected infant has been reported (173) with related parents. This is presumed to be a rare autosomal recessive disorder.
 **** Unbalanced translocation

Developmental Defect

Three different developmental mechanisms have been proposed (153):

1. a mismatch between the growth of the base of the skull (which is reduced) and the structures of the posterior fossa (which are normal) [165];
2. the encephalocele is secondary to the occurrence of hydrocephalus;
3. failure of neural tube closure.

Frontoethmoid encephaloceles have been attributed to a defective separation of neural and surface ectoderm at the site of final closure of the rostral neuropore during the final phase of neurulation in the fourth week of gestation (143).

Prevalence

The overall prevalence rate for all subgroups of encephalocele has been between 0.08 and 1.3/1,000 in different populations (151, 163, 166–169). The lowest frequencies were documented in California (0.08/1,000 [166]), Northern France (0.08/1,000 [167]), and Australia (0.08/1,000 [169]) among predominantly Caucasian populations. The two most common types of encephalocele in Caucasian populations have been occipital encephalocele (70%) [144, 163] and frontal or anterior (15–30%) [144, 163].

Race/Ethnicity

In California, the frequencies among white, black, Hispanic, and Asian were very similar (0.07–0.09/1,000 [166]. In central Nigeria (168) (1987–1990), the prevalence rate of encephalocele was 2.3/1,000 with 57% frontal encephaloceles and 43% occipital.

Anterior encephaloceles are much more common in Southeast Asia, especially in Thailand (146, 170, 171), Pakistan, India (147), Burma, Malaysia, and among aboriginal Australians (142).

Birth Status

The prenatal detection and elective termination of affected fetuses has increased steadily over the past 20 years. In metropolitan Atlanta (1979–1998), 115 index cases included 18 stillbirths and six elective terminations (163). In Europe, 60% of isolated cases were detected prenatally in several medical centers (162). In Australia (169) by 1989, 12.5% of affected infants were diagnosed prenatally and those pregnancies were terminated by choice.

Sex Ratio

The sex ratios differ for each anatomic group.

In an analysis of infants with neural tube defects in the United Kingdom, Ireland, Europe, and Malta (158) in 1980–1987, there were 191 infants with encephalocele. There was an excess of females in the United Kingdom and Ireland and an excess of males in Europe and Malta.

Parental Age

A population-based analysis of the infants born in the years 1961–1999 in the Czech Republic raised the question as to whether encephalocele was significantly more common in the infants of very young (ages 15–16) and older (over 32) mothers (151).

Twinning

An increased frequency of twins has been noted among infants with all types of neural tube defects, including encephalocele (166). In the analysis of 1,041 infants and fetuses with encephalocele in eight malformation registry programs (172), twins concordant for encephalocele usually had a specific syndrome.

In the Boston study (Table 18-5) four (4.7%) of 85 infants with encephalocele were in twin pregnancies. In three, the twins were discordant. In the fourth, the co-twin had anencephaly. Zygosity was not established in any of these four twin pregnancies.

Four sets of monoamniotic (monozygous) twins have been reported (174–177). In one set, one twin had anencephaly and the other, a small occipital encephalocele that was detected only at autopsy (174). In another set, one twin had an occipital encephalocele and the other was found later to have an intracerebellar dermoid tumor with a contiguous occipital dermal sinus (175). In the third set of female twins, both had an occipital encephalocele; one had also hypoplasia of one lung and a single umbilical artery (176). In a discordant set of male MZ twins in Cameroon, one had a frontal encephalocele, but his brother was healthy (177).

Genetic Factors

A rare non-consanguineous family in Vietnam was reported in which individuals with normal development in three generations were born with occipital cephaloceles, presenting primarily as subcutaneous bulges (1.5 × 1.5 cm at birth) in the occipital region (178). The occipital lesions were skin covered, contained meninges or remnants of glial or neural tissues, and were referred to as "atretic cephaloceles." This is a rare, apparently monogenic (autosomal dominant) phenotype.

Many monogenic disorders associated with encephalocele have been identified (140) [Table 18-5], but mutations have been identified in only a few:

1. An ARX (Aristaless-related homeobox genes) poly-alanine expansion has been reported in a mentally retarded boy with transphenoidal encephalocele, agenesis of the corpus callosum, and partial anterior hypopituitarism (179).
2. The autosomal recessive Knobloch Syndrome (MIM #267750), the features of which include occipital encephalocele, high myopia, vitreoretinal degeneration with retinal detachment, has been associated with mutations in COL18A1 gene on 21q22.3 (180). A second unmapped locus for the Knobloch Syndrome has been postulated based on families in which there was no linkage to COL18A1.
3. The autosomal recessive Meckel-Gruber Syndrome (MIM #249000), the features of which include occipital encephalocele, polydactyly (postaxial), polycystic kidneys. This autosomal recessive disorder has been shown to be due to a mutation in a gene encoding a component of the flugellar apparatus basal body proteome TMEM67 (181).

The frequency of associated chromosome abnormalities was 6% (5/86) in the case series in Boston (Table 18-5). No association with a specific chromosome deletion has been identified.

No systematic studies of the empiric recurrence risk for isolated encephalocele have been reported. Careful family studies in Thailand (171) and Australia (142) did not show an increased rate of occurrence of sincipital, i.e., frontal, cephaloceles in the sibs or offspring of affected individuals.

A swine model (182) with a high incidence of meningocele and encephalocele has been reported, but the mutation or other etiologic factors have not been identified.

Environmental Factors

A dramatically higher frequency (ten-fold increase in one series [183] of neural tube defects, primarily spina bifida and anencephaly) has been identified in infants of insulin-dependent diabetic mothers (IDMs).

However, the risk for encephalocele specifically among IDMs has not been established. Some case series (184) [Table 18-5] and case reports (185) have included infants of diabetic mothers with encephalocele.

An association between hyperthermia (defined as prolonged fever of at least 1.5 degrees C above normal early in gestation) and the occurrence of encephalocele has been postulated (186, 187).

Animal models of hyperthermia have been developed. For example, in ICR mice, hyperthermia, such as immersion of pregnant mice in hot water (42°C for 12.5 to 15 minutes), produced a spectrum of anterior neural tube defects, including exencephaly, anencephaly, encephalocele, and neural tube defects with facial cleft (188). In another experimental model (189), triamcinolone acetomide, administered intramuscularly (mg/kg) for five alternate days of pregnancy, beginning on gestational day 23 in nonhuman primates, produced a dorsal protrusion.

Treatment and Prognosis

The prognosis for affected infants has been difficult to predict. Chapman et al. (153) noted that the amount and type of neural tissue present within the encephalocele sac was the best single indicator of prognosis.

Yokota et al. (154) pointed out that a parietal cephalocele associated with an overlying scalp alopecia and porencephalic cysts was usually associated with a poor prognosis.

In a study of 114 children with several types of encephalocele in Toronto (144), 59% had normal psychomotor development, 18% had mild disability, and 23% were impaired to a severe degree.

In a series of infants with meningoencephalocele in Australia (142), the total mortality was 16%; another 18% were totally or severely incapacitated; among the other 56%, some had no disability, others have slight problems or significant complaints.

In metropolitan Atlanta (1979–1998), there were 83 livebirths with encephalocele, 79% of whom had an isolated defect (163). 76% of the deaths occurred during the first day of life; 70.8% survived to one year and 67.3% to age 20 years (163). Factors that increased mortality were low birth weight, the presence of multiple anomalies, and being African American. The overall survival of infants with multiple anomalies was 41.2%, compared to 74.3% for infants with isolated encephalocele.

Genetic Counseling

The empiric recurrence risk for "isolated" encephalocele has not been established.

Several reports have suggested an etiologic relationship between the occurrence of encephalocele, spina bifida, and anencephaly: 1) all are more common among infants of diabetic mothers; 2) rare reports of twins, one with anencephaly and the other with encephalocele (174) [Table 18-5]. However, specific risks of recurrence of either encephalocele or other neural tube defects in subsequent pregnancies after the birth of the index case with encephalocele have not been determined.

Periconceptional supplementation with mulitvitamins, including folic acid, is recommended, although its effect on the occurrence of encephalocele in subsequent pregnancies has not been established.

When encephalocele is part of a genetic syndrome for multiple anomalies, the recurrence risk depends on the specific disorder.

The sensitivity of prenatal screening by ultrasound to detect any type of encephalocele will depend on the size of the protrusion.

INIENCEPHALY

Definition

An extremely retroflexed head with an intact, skin-covered cranium and either an open or closed occipital region (inien = nape of neck; encephaly = brain) [190, 191].

ICD-9	740.2	(iniencephaly
ICD-10:	Q00.2	(iniencephaly)
Mendelian Inheritance in Man:	None	

Appearance

In iniencephaly, there is a confluence of the cavities of the cranium and the spine. The head is retroflexed over the cervico-thoracic spine (190–201) (Figures 18.17, 18.20 and 18.21). The cranial cavity is present and is skin-covered in the retroflexed region (193). There is virtually no neck region. The neck region and back are usually hirsute. The face skin is continuous with the chest skin and the posterior scalp is connected directly with the skin of the back (197). The foramen magnum is enlarged. The cervical region may be covered (clausus type) in which case the occipital bone is not malformed. In the open (apertus) type, the occipital bone is hypoplastic and the cervical area is open, that is not skin-covered (192, 195). The open defect can be an encephalocele or spina bifida (Figures 18.18 and 18.19). There is shortening of the spinal column with marked lordosis and hyperextension of the malformed cervical thoracic spine (198).

Many different malformations of the cerebrum, such as polymicrogyrias, heterotopias, disorganization and agenesis of the vermis of the cerebellum, have been reported, but none is considered distinctive for iniencephaly (194).

Duplication of cervical vertebrae is a distinctive change present in most infants (198). There is incomplete closure of the vertebral arches of many cervical vertebrae (198). Some infants with iniencephaly have an associated spina bifida (201).

Iniencephaly is separate and distinct from anencephaly with craniorachischisis with retroflexion (191, 193). The craniospinal articulation is anterior in iniencephaly and posterior in anencephaly with craniorachischisis (200).

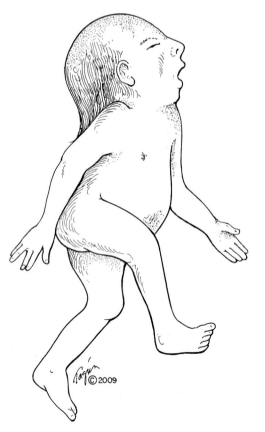

FIGURE 18.17 Diagram of stillborn infant with iniencephaly, which shows retroflexed head and neck, shortened neck, and thorax.

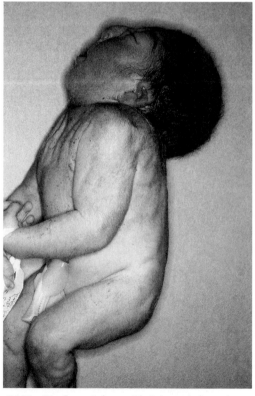

FIGURE 18.18 Newborn infant with iniencephaly and associated thoracolumbar myelomeningocele (see figure 18.19).

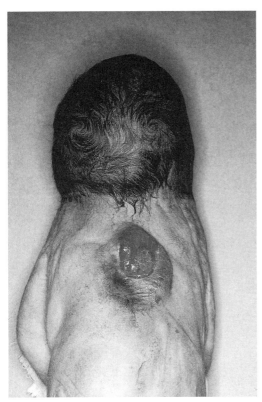

FIGURE 18.19 Newborn infant with iniencephaly and associated thoracolumbar myelomeningocele.

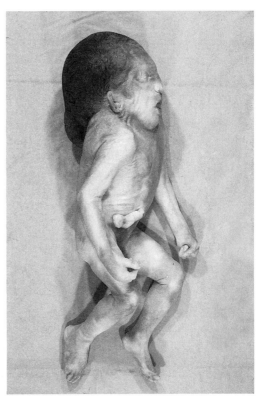

FIGURE 18.21 Side view of stillborn fetus at 26 weeks of gestation with iniencephaly. Phenotype included occipito-cervical encephalocele, polysplenia, malrotation of intestine, atrial septal defect, and infused pancreas. (Courtesy of Mason Barr, M.D., University of Michigan, Ann Arbor, MI)

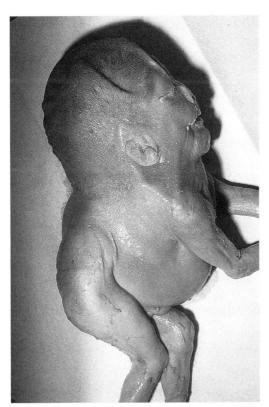

FIGURE 18.20 Side view of stillborn infant with retroflexed head and shortened neck and thorax. (See Figure 18.19)

Associated Malformations

The frequency of associated malformations is higher than in other types of neural tube defects (200–206). In a series of 50 stillborn and liveborn infants with iniencephaly in Bristol, England, 41/50 (82%) had other malformations (202). The most common associated malformations were omphalocele, diaphragmatic hernia, cleft lip and/or palate, and horseshoe kidney. In another series of 39 infants, ascertained in several European countries (203), 69% had associated non-neural malformations: 42% had a diaphragmatic hernia, 21% omphalocele, and 19% cleft palate alone.

Developmental Defect

There is significant reduction of the length of the spine. This shortening has been postulated to alter the development of major organs in the thorax and abdomen and, thereby, to cause associated malformations, such as congenital heart disease, diaphragmatic hernia, and omphalocele (207). By comparison, cleft lip and cleft palate occur in fetuses with neural tube defects that are not associated with shortening of the spine (Figure 18.22).

Prevalence

From 1980 to 1987 among 580,000 births there were 1,830 infants with neural tube defects. Two percent of the infants with a neural tube defect identified in the United Kingdom and Ireland had iniencephaly. In the same study (203), 0.5% of the infants with neural tube defects identified in Continental Europe and Malta had iniencephaly. In East Ireland 1980–1994, the prevalence rate was 0.03 per 1,000 births (208). In Northern China, a region with a total rate of all neural tube defects of 5.7 per 1,000, the rate of iniencephaly was 0.16 per 1,000. By comparison, in Southern China, where the overall rate of neural tube defects was much lower, 0.9 per 1,000, the rate of iniencephaly was 0.02 per 1,000 births (201).

Race/Ethnicity

No racial differences in prevalence rate have been identified, but very little data is available on affected infants from different racial groups.

Birth Status

The majority of the affected infants are stillborn: 87% in a series of 11 (208) and 72% in a series of 50 (201). Most are also born prematurely and weigh less than 2500 grams (206) (Figures 18.20 and 18.21).

Six more mildly affected infants have survived (205, 206, 209, 210). These individuals have a retroflexed head, skin-covered neck, and a posterior spine defect in several cervical vertebrae. One survivor had an associated encephalocele and after several surgeries, had no neurologic abnormalities at age three years (205, 206).

Sex Ratio

Many more affected females than males have been observed in several case series.

Parental Age

There is no information on this aspect of the infants and fetuses with iniencephaly.

Twinning

None of 50 affected fetuses and newborn infants in one series (202) was a twin. One mildly affected male infant had an unaffected twin sister (209).

Genetic Factors

Associated chromosome abnormalities have been identified in about 5 to 10% of the infants with the more common neural tube defects, such as anencephaly, spina bifida, and encephalocele. None of 11 infants with iniencephaly in one series (211) and none of seven fetuses in another series (206) had a visible chromosome abnormality by routine Giemsa banding. A few infants with iniencephaly have had associated chromosome abnormalities: trisomy 2 (212), 46,XY/47,XY+ 13 (214), and 45,X/46,XX (214) and triploidy (214). An infant with 46,XX/ 47,XX+13 had associated holoprosencephaly with cyclopia (214).

In the Boston series (Table 18-6) of 8 infants, chromosome analysis was carried out on only 3 affected fetuses and infants; one abnormality was identified: 46,XY/47,XY, +8.

Multifactorial inheritance is postulated as the basis for the other neural tube defects. However, no published

TABLE 18-6 *Iniencephaly (BWH 1972–1974, 1979–2000*)*

Etiology	Non-transfers**			Transfers***		
	Isolated	MCA	Phenotype Unknown	Isolated	MCA	Phenotype unknown
1. Mendelian						
2. Familial					1****	
3. Chromosome Abnormalities						
a.) 46,XY/47,XY,+8					1	
4. Maternal conditions						
5. Twinning						
6. Unknown etiology	1				3	2

Legends: * Affected infants and fetuses were identified among all livebirths, stillbirths and elective terminations at Brigham and Women's Hospital (BWH). There were 206,244 infants born to non-transferred mothers.
** Non-transfer: correct as written.
*** Transfer: correct as written.
**** Mother's cousin had child with anencephaly.

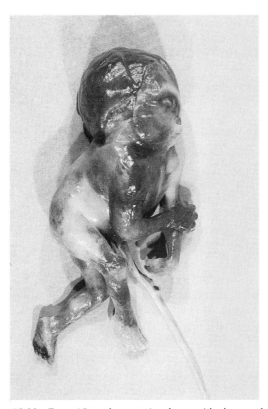

FIGURE 18.22 Fetus 19 weeks gestational age with shortened neck and thorax. Other anomalies included occipital cranium bifidum, diaphragm defect, malrotation of intestine, cleft palate, and lung hypoplasia. (Courtesy of Mason Barr, M.D., University of Michigan, Ann Arbor, MI)

studies have reported the expected characteritics of multifactorial inheritance in the familes of an informative number of infants with iniencephaly.

The basis for the presumed etiologic association and relationship between anencephaly, spina bifida, encephalocele, and iniencephaly are the rare families in which one infant had iniencephaly (Figures 18.18 and 18.19) and a sib had myelomeningocele (215) or one infant had iniencephaly and a cousin had anencephaly (Table 18-6).

Environmental Factors

None has been identified.

Treatment and Prognosis

This is usually a lethal condition.

Genetic Counseling

The phenotype of iniencephaly suggests that it is a rare, usually lethal, type of neural tube defect. There is no data published on the empiric risk that the parents with one affected infant will have another infant with either iniencephaly or another type of neural tube defect.

Likewise, there is no evidence that periconceptional supplementation with multivitamins and folic acid will reduce the risks in subsequent pregnancies.

The affected fetuses are often identified by chance from prenatal screening by ultrasound. Polyhydramnios is a common associated finding (206).

LIPOMYELOMENINGOCELE

Definition

Lipomyelomeningocele is a midline subcutaneous lipoma in the lumbosacral region, which is connected through an underlying defect in the vertebrae by a fibrous stalk to an intradural intramedullary fatty mass.

ICD-9:	741.985	(lipomyelomeningocele)
ICD-10:	Q05.7	(lumbar spina bifida without hydrocephalus)
	Q05.9	(spina bifida, unspecified)
Mendelian Inheritance in Man:	609537	(lipomyelomeningocele)

Appearance

The spinal lipoma is typically a midline soft swelling in the lumbar region, often covered with a hemangioma [217–224] (Figures 18-23, 18-24, 18-25 and 18-26). Skin dimples and tags (Figure 18-25), hair patches, and denuded and hypopigmented skin patches over the lipomas have also been described in many patients (217, 219, 221, 223).

The lipomas can be asymmetric swellings in one buttock (Figures 18-25–18-27).

The lipoma is fat tissue subdivided by fibrous bands. The lipomas are most common in subcutaneous location, but can be intraspinal. Typically, the affected spinal cord is elongated, continuing down into the lumbar and even the sacral canal (224). By comparison, the normal conus ends in the region between T-12 and L-2. At surgery, three types of lipomatous lesions have been described (217): 1) the dorsal lipoma attached by a fatty stalk to the spinal cord; 2) the transitional lipomyelomeningocele that arises from the dorsal and terminal aspects of the spinal cord; 3) the caudal lipomyelomeningocele that is attached to the termination of the spinal cord.

Associated Malformations

In several case series (219–221), very few affected infants had associated major malformations. In one series (219) of 97 children, there were four with genitourinary anomalies, three with dermal sinus, three with epidermoid or dermoid cyst, one with anal stenosis, and one infant with Down Syndrome. There were also anomalies of the spinal cord: split spinal cord (3 infants), diastematomyelia (3), and terminal hyromelia (3). In another series of 80 affected individuals (221), six had amniotic band deformity, four had sacral dysgenesis, two had an anteriorly placed anus with stenosis and two had hydromelia of the spinal cord.

There is usually no associated hydrocephalus. In one series of 73 children (220), one had a Chiari Type I anomaly.

There have been rare reports of infants with either lumbar lipoma or lumbar lipomeningomyelocele (226) having an associated occipital encephalocele.

Resections of the lipomas have identified teratomatous elements, such as bone and cartilage (227), and stomach and testis in a choristoma (224).

Developmental Defect

A lumbosacral spina bifida, in general, is attributed to the failure of closure of that region, which would be visible in the fourth week postfertilization. It has been postulated that lipomeningomyelocele is formed when the neural tube detaches from the cutaneous ectoderm prematurely, which leads to the paraxial mesenchyme invading the neural tube (228).

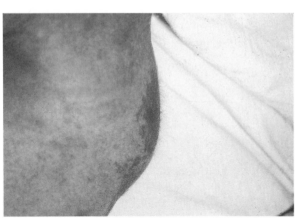

FIGURE 18.23 Lateral view of midline lipoma; tethering of spinal cord present.

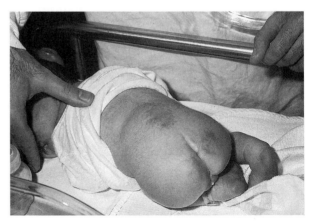

FIGURE 18.24 Posterior view of same infant shown in Figure 18.23, showing overlying hemangioma.

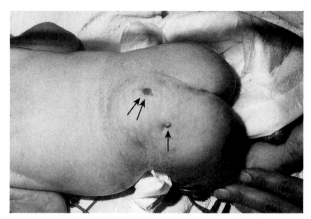

FIGURE 18.25 Lateral view of asymmetrical lipoma, which shows a skin tag (arrow) and a dark red nevus (two arrows) associated with lipomyelomeningocele.

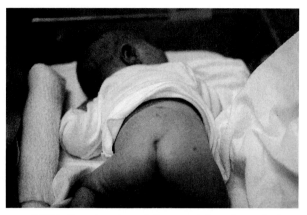

FIGURE 18.27 Posterior view of the same infant shown in figures 18.25 and 18.26.

No similar phenotypes in mouse models of either drug-induced or genetic myelomeningocele have been identified (229).

Prevalence

The frequency of lipomyelomeningocele has been estimated to be 1:4,000. Prevalence rates in specific populations have been 0.5/1,000 (1:2,000) in Hawaii

(1986–2001 [230]) and 0.16/1,000 (1:6,250) in Nova Scotia [1986–2001 (231)].

Racial/Ethnicity

In one statewide analysis of 17 affected infants (230), the prevalence rate was highest in infants with Pacific Islander and Filipino ancestry. More information is needed to establish racial/ethnic differences with certainty.

Birth Status

No increase in the frequency of prematurity, stillbirth, or perinatal mortality has been reported.

Sex Ratio

More affected females than males have been observed in several studies (219, 221, 230).

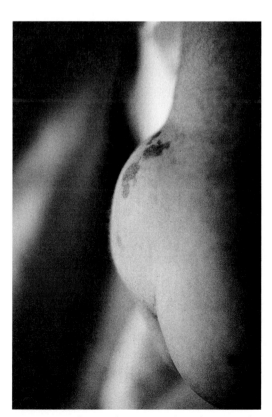

FIGURE 18.26 Lateral view of asymmetric large lipoma with midline hemangioma shown in Figure 18.25.

Parental Age

No abnormal distributions of ages of either the mothers or the fathers have been reported.

Twinning

The rate of twinning in individuals with lipomyelomeningocele and their families has not been reported.

Genetic Factors

The vast majority of the infants with lipomyelomeningocele have no affected siblings or parents. One instance of two siblings with lipomyelomeningocele has been reported (227). Rare families have been reported in which siblings, half-siblings, and cousins have had anencephaly, myelomeningocele, lipoyelomeningocele, and fatty filum, with empiric risks for these other lesions of about 4%

(232, 233) and 3% (234). In a case series of 52 families (233), none of the probands had a sibling with lipomyelomeningocele. In a case series of 20 index cases, one of 32 previous or older siblings had had spina bifida (234).

Environmental Factors

No human teratogen has been shown to cause lipomyelomeningocele. There have been case reports of children with lipomyelomeningocele, who had been exposed during pregnancy to the anticonvulsant drugs phenytoin (Figures 18-23 and 18-24) and valproic acid (235), but these case reports do not establish causality.

Prevention

In a comparison of the prevalence rate in Nova Scotia of lipomyelomeningocele before and after dietary supplementation with folic acid, there was no evidence of effect from that supplementation (231).

Treatment and Prognosis

The infants with transdural adhesion of the lipoma to the spinal cord are at risk of having neurologic complications (217-223). The tethering of the spinal cord produces ischemia and injury to the conus medullaris and lower sacral nerve roots during infancy. Early repair prevents this damage and avoids injury to nerves, which can cause a flaccid bladder and spasticity.

If the lipomyelomeningocele is asymptomatic and is not recognized in infancy, that child, when older, can develop incontinence, urinary tract infections, or leg pain and weakness as the first symptoms.

Genetic Counseling

When an infant is found to have a lipomyelomeningocele, the most urgent need is an evaluation for possible tethering of the spinal cord, as this occurs in many affected infants. Early surgical repair prevents the damage to the spinal cord and nerve roots.

Lipomyelomeningocele is to be distinguished from other closed neural tube defects: myelocystoceles (236), terminal lipomas, fatty filum, and intraspinal lipoma.

The affected infant is not expected to have associated non-neural anomalies, except for a low rate of occurrence of anomalies of the anus and genitourinary tract.

The limited information available suggests an increased risk for having a child with either lipomyelomeningocele or another neural tube defect in subsequent pregnancies. The magnitude of the risk has not been established.

Prenatal screening by ultrasound can identify an affected fetus (226, 237). Usually the lipomyelomeningocele is identified in the scanning of the lumbosacral region. The intracranial contents would be expected to be normal with no sign of an Arnold Chiari malformation (237).

MENINGOCELE

Definition

This is a skin-covered cystic protrusion of the meninges through a posterior defect in the vertebrae, with the spinal cord in its normal location.

ICD-9:   741.080   (other spina bifida, meningocele of a specified site with hydrocephalus)

741.085   (spina bifida, meningocele, cervicothoracic, with hydrocephalus)

741.086   (spina bifida, meningocele thoracolumbar, with hydrocephalus)

741.087   (spina bifida, meningocele lumbosacral with hydrocephalus)

ICD-10:   Q05   (spina bifida, includes meningocele and myelomeningocele)

Mendelian Inheritance in Man: #182940   (neural tube defects, includes spina bifida)

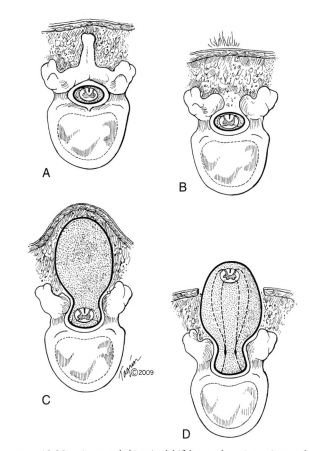

FIGURE 18.28   a) normal; b) spinal bifida occulta; c) meningeocele; d) myelomeningocele.

Appearance

This is a skin-covered protrusion of the meninges, including arachnoid and dura, through a defect in the vertebrae. It contains spinal fluid, but does not contain the spinal cord. Nerve roots may be present (238–242) [Figures 18-29C through 18-31].

Meningoceles have occurred at three levels: cervical, thoracic, and lumbosacral.

Associated Malformations

No case series with descriptions of associated malformations has been published. It would be expected to include an increased additional vertebral anomalies and frequency of kidney malformations, as has been observed in infants with myelomeningocele (243).

Developmental Defect

This is considered a mild defect in the closure of the neural tube, which should be complete in the fourth week post-fertilization. This cystic posterior protrusion would be present at that time.

Theoretically there could be effects on the adjacent spinal cord from the protrusion of a meningocele through the defect in the vertebrae.

Prevalence

Population based surveys of the prevalence of neural tube defects, such as those in Canada (244) and Europe (245), have not tabulated separately the prevalence of meningocele. It is considered a rare type of neural tube defect.

In the Active Malformations Surveillance Program at the Boston Lying-In Hospital, and later, the Brigham and Women's Hospital, ten infants (1:20,624) had meningocele among 206,244 births (including still-births and elective terminations for anomalies) [246]. One of the ten infants with meningocele was an infant with Down Syndrome. Another was an infant of an insulin-dependent diabetic mother. The other 8 were of unknown etiology.

Race/Ethnicity

The prevalence rates in major racial and ethnic groups have not been established.

Birth Status

No information is available on the frequency of prematurity, stillbirth, or neonatal death.

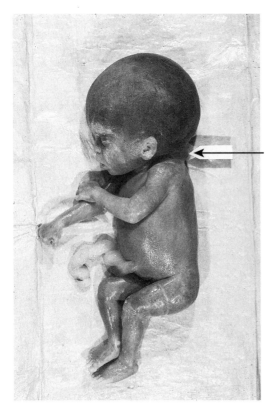

FIGURE 18.29   Fetus with cervical meningocele. (Courtesy of Mason Barr, M.D., University of Michigan, Ann Arbor, MI.)

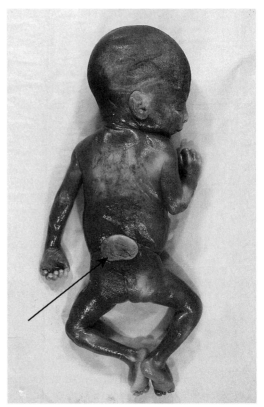

FIGURE 18.31   22-week fetus with meningocele at sacral vertebrae 1-2. (Courtesy of Mason Barr, M.D., University of Michigan, Ann Arbor, MI.)

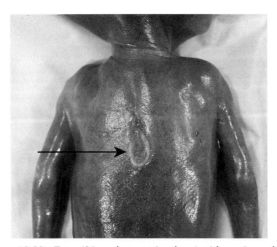

FIGURE 18-30   Fetus (21 weeks gestational age) with meningocele in thoracic region (arrow). (Courtesy of Mason Barr, M.D., University of Michigan, Ann Arbor, MI.)

Sex Ratio

The ratio of affected males to females has not been established.

Parental Age

No changes in the distribution of the ages of the mothers or fathers have been described.

Twinning

There is no information on the frequency of twins among infants with meningocele.

Genetic Factors

One would assume that there is an etiologic relationship between the occurrence of meningocele and the other types of neural tube defects. This relationship is suggested by the reports of adults, who were born with a meningocele, having children with either myelomeningocele or anencephaly (247).

Environmental Factors

The frequency of meningocele could be increased among fetuses exposed to teratogens, such as maternal insulin-dependent diabetes mellitus, the medications valproate and carbamazepine, and maternal obesity, risk factors for the occurrence of myelomeningocele.

Treatment and Prognosis

The examination of the affected infant is not expected to show any neurologic abnormalities or associated hydrocephalus, hip dislocation, or club foot deformity.

Surgery is performed to resect the herniated meninges (238).

Genetic Counseling

The protrusion of a meningocele should contain only arachnoid, dura, and spinal fluid. It will be translucent when transilluminated. Imaging studies will confirm the presence of the defect in the posterior portion of the vertebrae at the level of the protrusion.

The physical examination and imaging will distinguish between the different types of closed (skin-covered) spinal dysraphism:

1. meningocele: no lipoma, no hydrocephalus;
2. lipomyelomeningocele: lipoma is present within the protrusion;
3. meningocystocele: hydromyelia of the spinal cord, with herniations of the meninges through the vertebral defect (248); this condition can occur as an isolated abnormality, separate from cloacal exstrophy;
4. lateral meningoceles: there is no midline protrusion, but laterally and often at several levels;
5. anterior sacral meningocele, a feature of the Currarino Syndrome (MIM 176450); the other features are anorectal malformations and sacral defects.

Meningocele is to be distinguished from spina bifida occulta, which is an abnormality of the posterior arch of one or two vertebrae, most often sacral vertebrae 1 (S1) or S1 and S2 (249). Systematic studies of normal adults have shown the prevalence rate was 23%.

Meningoceles are typically small. Occasional large meningoceles have been reported (250).

In the counseling, the parents of an infant with a meningocele should be told about the presumed relationship between meningocele, myelomeningocele, and anencephaly. In the absence of data from family studies of infants with meningocele, the recurrence risk in a future pregnancy would be similar to the empiric data in that geographic area for infants with anencephaly or myelomeningocele. Supplementation with multivitamins and folic acid would be recommended in the periconceptional period, as well.

MYELOMENINGOCELE

Definition

A localized defect in closure of the neural tube with associated vertebral anomalies, malformed spinal cord, lack of skin covering, and defective function of nerves below level of defect.

ICD-9:	741.010	(spina bifida cystica, any site, with hydrocephalus and Arnold-Chiari malformation)
	741.030	(spina bifida cystica, cervical, with unspecified hydrocephalus)
	741.040	(spina bifida cystica, thoracic, with unspecified hydrocephalus, no mention of Arnold-Chiari)
	741.910	(spina bifida cystica, cervical, without hydrocephalus)
	741.920	(spina bifida cystica, thoracic, without hydrocephalus)
	741.930	(spina bifida cystica, lumbar, without hydrocephalus)
	741.940	(spina bifida, cystica, sacral, without hydrocephalus)
ICD-10:	Q0.5	(includes myelomeningocele, meningocele, and rachischisis)
Mendelian Inheritance in Man:	#182940	(neural tube defects; includes spina bifida)

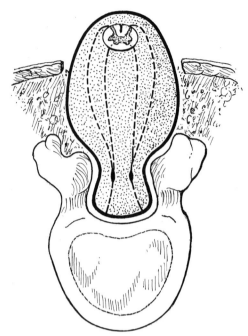

FIGURE 18.32   Diagram of myelomeningocele that shows deficiency of posterior vertebral segment, protrusion of spinal cord and nerves, and lack of skin covering.

Appearance

Myelomeningocele is often in the lumbosacral region, but occurs also at lower and upper thoracic levels. There is a lack of skin covering with the malformed spinal cord protruding through several levels of defective vertebrae (Figures 18-33 and 18-34). The red, serous surface of the spinal cord may be covered by a thin sac.

The most significant associated primary abnormality is another neural tube defect, most often anencephaly (Figure 18-5).

The infant with myelomeningocele often has several different secondary abnormalities, hydrocephalus and Chiari II malformations, and the effects of paralysis, which include hip dislocation, club foot, and ureteral reflux.

Associated Malformations

Among infants with "isolated" myelomeningocele, excluding those with either chromosome abnormalities

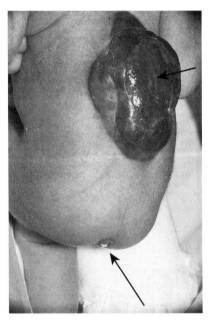

FIGURE 18.33   Large thoracolumbar defect with infant's anus shown at bottom of picture (arrow).

or a specific malformation syndrome, there is an increased frequency of neural and non-neural malformations. The most important neural abnormalities are cerebral heterotopias, partial agenesis of the corpus callosum, and abnormalities of the brain stem (251).

In a series of 312 individuals with myelomeningocele in a provincial registry (1958–1984) in Canada, 10.7% had non-neural anomalies, including cleft-lip and/or palate in 1.3% and heart defects in 2.2% (252).

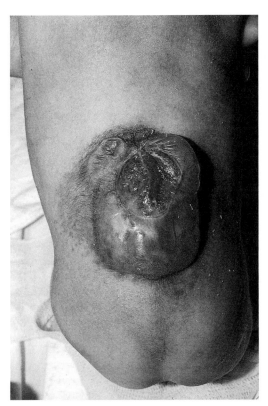

FIGURE 18.34 Thoracolumbar myelomeningocele with associated hemangioma.

The highest association (19.5%) of non-neural anomalies was with the high spina bifida (defined as above thoracic vertebra T10 [252]), in contrast to 6.7% in low spina bifida. An autopsy series (1986–1999) confirmed this pattern (253). The frequency of other malformations may be higher in fetuses with myelomeningocele diagnosed prenatally because of the association of lethal chromosome abnormalities and malformation syndromes that would not be identified in follow-up studies of affected children.

Malformations of the kidneys were identified in 2.1% of a series of 138 children with myelomeningocele and no other vertebral anomalies (254). However, among the 19 children with myelomeningocele and other vertebral anomalies, primarily hemivertebrae, 21% had renal anomalies, such as absence of one kidney and horseshoe kidney (254).

A "schisis-association," meaning a non-random occurrence of neural tube defects with other specific midline malformations, has been postulated (255). In the analysis of all index cases with two or more malformations in a national malformations surveillance program in Hungary (1970–1977), the most common malformations associated with spina bifida were omphalocele, diaphragmatic hernia, and cleft lip/palate.

The association of glandular hypospadias with lumbosacral myelomeningocele (SB) was documented in an analysis of 159 newborn infants with SB and 1,670 with hypospadias in a national malformations registry in Spain (256).

Myelomeningocele, like anencephaly and encephalocele (251), occurs in many phenotypes and has many apparent etiologies (258) [Tables 18-7].

Developmental Defect

The process of neurulation leads to the development of the neural tube and brain. This complex process includes changes in cell differentiation and migration. Primary neurulation occurs in weeks 3–4 postfertilization and includes the formation of the brain and the spinal cord down to the sacral region (259). The process of secondary neurulation leads to the formation of the lowest portion of the spinal cord in the sacral region. The process of forming the neural plate, shaping the neural plate and fusion of the neural plate has been shown in mouse models to involve factors, such as *noggin*, *chordin* and *follistatin*, from the primitive node and several signaling pathways, as well as *wnt* signaling, *insulin-like growth factor* and *fibroblast growth factor*. The formation of the bending points in the neural plate to form the neural tube is controlled by the signal transduction protein *sonic hedgehog*, which originates from the notochord. The cellular and molecular mechanisms that lead to the fusion of the neural folds are not known yet. The closure itself proceeds bidirectionally, like a zipper.

Theoretically a meningomyelocele represents failure of closure of the neural tube that is visible in the fourth week post-fertilization, specifically days 24 to 28. This is the period of stages 11 to 13 (260, 261). Human embryos with open myeloschisis in Carnegie developmental stages 12, 13, and 14 have been identified in a systematic collection of human embryos in Japan (262). The process of normal closure begins in the cervical region. Initially, the sequence of closure events at several sites in the mouse embryo was postulated to occur also in humans, based on correlation of specific types of neural tube defects with closure defects at specific sites (263, 264). However, studies of human embryos with neural tube defects have been interpreted to show a pattern that differs from the pattern in mice, reflecting significant differences between species (259, 265).

Another theory of the development of neural tube defects is that rupture, caused by an air pressure gradient, occurs after the neural tube has closed (266). This could be a mechanism by which a teratogenic exposure after 28 days post-fertilization could cause spina bifida.

The complexity of the molecular basis for myelomeningocele and other neural tube defects in humans has been suggested by the cellular and molecular changes identified in over 190 different mouse models of defects in the closure of the neural tube (267, 268).

TABLE 18-7 *Etiologic and phenotype heterogeneity of infants with myelomeningocele: Brigham and Women's Hospital, Boston, 1972–1974, 1979–2000 (206,244) births, including stillbirths and elective terminations for fetal anomalies).*

Etiology	Non-transfers*			
	Isolated	Multiple Anomalies	Unknown Phenotypes**	
I. Mendelian Inheritance	0	0	0	
II. Syndromes	0	0	0	
III. Chromosome Abnormalities				(9 / 90 : 10%)
a. Trisomy18	0	3	0	
b. Trisomy13	0	1	0	
c. Trisomy9 (see Figure 18-35)	0	1	0	
d. Triploidy	0	2	0	
e. Chromosome deletion (due to) unbalanced translocation***	0	1	0	
	0	<u>1</u>	0	
IV. Exposures toTeratogens				(7 / 90 : 7.8%)
a. valproate	0	1	0	
b. carbamazepine	1		0	
c. Infant of diabetic mother	<u>0</u>	<u>5</u>	0	
	1	6		
V. Twinning (dizygous)	1	0	0	(1 / 90 : 1.1%)
VI. Unknown etiology	<u>35</u>	<u>10</u>	<u>28</u>	(73 / 90 : 81.1%)
	37	25	28	= Total 90 (1:2,291)
	(41.1%)	(27.8%)	(31.1%)	

Legends:

* Non-transfers: mothers who had always planned to deliver at this hospital; the "transfers" were women who transferred their medical care to this hospital after the prenatal diagnosis at another medical facility.

** Pregnancy terminated by destructive procedure, preventing the delineation of phenotypic features.

*** 46,XX,der(18),t(8;18) (q22;q23) mat

Major differences in mechanisms have been determined for the different mutations. While most of the models produce exencephaly in the mouse (analogous to anencephaly in humans), some produce myelomeningocele. Harris and Juriloff (267), in reviewing the mouse mutants, noted that the effects of the mutations often include the pathways of actin function, apoptosis and chromatin methylation and structure. Both genetic and nutritional factors have been identified in several of the mouse mutants. They predicted that the non-syndromic neural tube defects in humans will be attributable primarily to multifactorial inheritance.

Prevalence

Geographic areas of high and low prevalence have been documented all over the world. For example, in the period 1965 to 1968 in London the rate of all types of neural tube defects was 3 per 1,000 births (269). In Newfoundland, the frequency of all neural tube defects over a nine-year period (1976–1984), based on hospital records and death certificates in a provincial registry, showed a high of 4.2/1,000 in Barin peninsula and a low of 1.4/1,000 in Bonavista Bay (270). In Europe, the rate of all neural tube defects was 1.2/1,000 in Belgium

(1980–1987) in comparison to 3./1,000 in Belfast, Ireland, in 1980–1986 (271, 273).

In China in 1986–1987, the prevalence of all types of neural tube defects was 5.2 per 1,000 in rural areas and 1.5 per 1,000 in urban areas; for spina bifida the rates were 1.5/1,000 rural and 0.5/1,000 urban (272).

During the 1980s and 1990s a steady decrease in the occurrence of myelomeningocele was documented in many geographic areas, including Ireland (273) and the United States (274). This occurred before there was an active campaign to encourage women to take a periconceptional supplement of folic acid.

Race/Ethnicity

When population-based statistics have been subdivided by apparent racial/ethnic groups, marked differences were identified. For example, in several states in the United States in the years 1998–2002, the prevalence rate of myelomeningocele was 0.42/1,000 in the infants of Hispanic women, 0.34/1,000 for non-Hispanic whites and 0.29/1,000 of non-Hispanic blacks (274). In California (1983-1987), the highest prevalence rate was among the infants of white Hispanic women and the lowest was among the infants of Asian women (275).

Birth Status

An increased frequency of low birth weight (less than 2,500 grams), prematurity, and stillbirths was documented in the 419 infants with spina bifida in East Ireland (1980–1994) [273].

An increased frequency of premature birth, low birth weight, and breech presentations was also documented in Hungary, 1970–1977 (255).

Sex Ratio

An excess among females has been demonstrated in several population-based studies, such as in Hungary (255) and British Columbia (252).

In an autopsy series, there was an excess of females with cervical lesions and lumbosacral spina bifida, but not in the high thoracic defects (253). But in other countries, there was no excess of females: the sex ratio (F:M) among 419 cases of spina bifida in East Ireland was 1.1:1.0 [273]. There was an excess of males among 184 infants with spina bifida in California (275); this was true for both isolated and multiple anomalies.

In London among 147 affected fetuses (gestational ages 16 to 23 weeks) [1975–1986], the sex ratio varied with the level of the spina bifida: an excess of females among higher defects, but an excess of males with low defects (276). However, among 178 affected liveborn infants and fetal deaths in California (1983–1987), the opposite correlations were made (275).

Parental Age

In East Ireland (1980–1994) [273], younger mothers had a higher rate of births of infants with all types of neural tube defects. However, no pattern of increasing or decreasing risk with younger or older maternal and paternal ages was observed in California, 1983–1987 (275).

In China, in a high prevalence region, the rate of neural tube defects was higher among mothers less than 20 years old and those 30 and older (277).

Twinning

Twinning and neural tube defects occur together more often than would be expected by chance, prompting the suggestion that the two findings are, somehow, causally related (252, 273, 279–282). In a large multinational study (282), the rate of twinning was highest (4.3%) among infants with anencephaly, and at lower rate among infants with encephalocele (3.3%), lumbosacral spina bifida (2.2%), and thoracic spina bifida (1.2%).

An excess of twinning has also been observed among the near relatives of infants with "upper" neural tube defects, defined as at or above the 11th thoracic vertebra (281).

No study of the rate of concordance of myelomeningocele in identical twins has been reported in which molecular methods were used to establish zygosity. Earlier reports of like-sex twins (283) suggested the rate of concordance was low. There have been rare reports of MZ twins with one having anencephaly and the other having myelomeningocele (277).

Genetic Factors

The occurrence of myelomeningocele has been postulated to be the result of both genetic and nongenetic or environmental factors, illustrating the process of multifactorial inheritance (269, 270). In this model, the first degree relatives (sibs and offspring) of the affected individual will have an increased risk of being affected. The risk correlates roughly with the prevalence of the abnormality, i.e., the higher the prevalence rate, the greater the recurrence risk.

Theoretically, in the model of multifactorial inheritance, the parent of an affected infant would have an increased frequency of minor manifestations of the same disorder. Spina bifida occulta (SBO) has been postulated to be an example of this mild expression. If SBO was defined as failure of fusion of one lamina of one vertebra, one study of the parents of 69 children with "open neural tube defects" showed no difference in frequency between those parents and 108 adult controls (284). SBO of one vertebra appears to be a common, normal anatomic variant. However, if the SBO involved several vertebrae, an increased risk of occurrence of myelomeningocele among their siblings has been reported (285, 286).

Individual families with multiple affected individuals have also been identified. In some of those families, X-linked inheritance has been postulated (287) and, in others, autosomal dominant inheritance (288). The phenotype in the latter families ranged from sacral agenesis to spina bifida occulta to myelomeningocele. The presence of the "atypical" phenotypes distinguished these apparent monogenic families from those attributed to multifactorial inheritance.

The new technology of arrayCGH to identify microdeletions and copy number variants has been used to study the rare multigenerational Caucasian family with several individuals with lumbar myelomeningocele (289). Two regions on chromosome 2q and 7p were identified as containing NTD susceptibility genes.

An increased frequency of chromosome abnormalities has also been documented in infants with open neural tube defects. The abnormalities identified by prenatal screening and diagnosed during pregnancy have varied with the specific neural tube defect and whether or not non-neural malformations were also

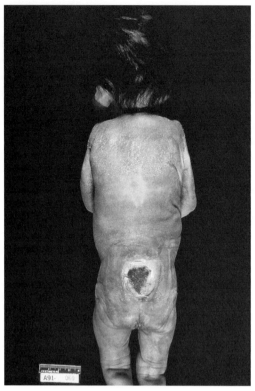

FIGURE 18.35   Infant with lumbosacral myelomeningocele associated with trisomy 9.

present. In one study (290) (1990–1996), 10 (10%) of 98 infants with myelomeningocele had associated chromosome abnormalities; 8 of these 10 infants had additional malformations. The chromosome abnormalities identified were trisomies 18 (4 infants) and 9 (1 infant), triploidy (1), 45, X (1), and chromosome duplications or deletions (3). In another study, 6 (10%) of 66 fetuses with open neural tube defects had chromosome abnormalities: all were trisomies, either 18 (4 infants) and 13 (2 infants) [291].

The demonstration (292, 293) of the decrease in the frequency of the occurrence of myelomeningocele after periconceptional supplementation with folic acid led to many studies of genetic biomarkers of risk in the metabolism of folic acid and related micromutations (294, 295). The studies have included measuring the frequency of associated gene polymorphisms (such as the R653 Q polymorphism of the C1-synthase [296] and the 19-bp deletion polymorphism in intron-1 of dihydrofolate reductase [297]), gene-gene interactions (294), autoantibodies to folate receptors (298), and comparisons of the genotypes of each parent and the affected child in transmission disequilibrium tests (TDT). Studies in several racial/ethnic groups have shown that a mutation at position 677 that changes C to T (designated C677T), in the methylene tetrahydrofolate reductase gene (MTHFR), is relatively common. It is associated with a decrease in the plasma level of

folate and an increase in homocysteine. In some studies (259), the woman homozygous for MTHFR C677T has had an increased risk for having a child with a neural tube defect.

Genetic changes have also been looked for in paired box containing genes, the PAX genes, which encode for DNA-binding transcription factors (299) that are important for specification of neural crest-derived structures during the formation of the neural tube. Candidate genes have been discovered from the studies of animal models. The genes involved in the planar cell polarity pathway, including the *VANGL1* protein and its binding partners disheveled –1, -2 and -3, are promising candidates (259). A small number of silent mutations, some disease-specific, and others not disease-specific, have been identified in *VANGL2* and *VANGL1* in clinical studies (300, 301).

A battery of molecular testing has not developed yet that could be used to explain the occurrence of a neural tube defect in an affected infant.

Two potential etiologies, not yet evaluated systematically (302), are associated mutations in mitochondrial genes and errors in imprinting.

Environmental Factors

One of the first signs of apparent environmental factors as a cause of myelomeningocele and anencephaly was the dramatic epidemic in the 1930s in Providence, Rhode Island, and Boston, Massachusetts (303). The cause of this epidemic was not determined.

The environmental exposure most frequently associated with the occurrence of myelomeningocele is insulin-dependent diabetes mellitus in the pregnant woman (304). The poor control of the mother's diabetes has correlated with an increased risk for a recognizable group of major malformations, including primarily myelomeningocele, anencephaly, renal a/dysgenesis, and vertebral anomalies.

In addition, exposure to two anticonvulsant drugs, including sodium valproate (305) (Figure 18.36) and carbamazepine (306), have been associated with an increased risk for myelomeningocele. The risks for these teratogenic effects of drugs varies by the dose of the drug taken, the mother's blood level and, theoretically, her genetic susceptibility to this teratogenic effect.

Exposure to the antiretroviral drug efavirenz is, also, a potential cause of myelomeningocele (307).

Extreme maternal obesity, especially a BMI (body mass index) above 30, have doubled the rate of spina bifida (308). Obesity together with gestational diabetes have appeared to increase the risk for neural tube defects (309). The gastric bypass procedure is also a risk factor for a woman having a child with myelomeningocele or anencephaly, because it can produce vitamin deficiencies in the mother (310). Maternal hyperthermia has

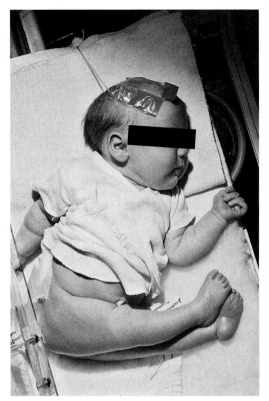

FIGURE 18.36   Infant with stiff legs secondary to myelomeningocele in an infant exposed to valproate as an anticonvulsant during pregnancy.

been shown, also, to correlate with an increased risk in several studies (311).

Many environmental exposures, such as contaminants of drinking water (312) and waste anesthetic genes (313), have been postulated to "cause" neural tube defects, but the findings have not been replicated in subsequent studies. The experience with one of the most widely publicized environmental causes, "blighted potatoes" eaten in early pregnancy (314, 315), showed the importance of careful study design and independent testing of hypothesis in separate populations before a postulated "cause" was publicized. It was shown to be a colorful idea, but not correct.

Prevention

The first dramatic examples of the prevention of major malformations demonstrated was the significant decreases in the recurrence of another infant with a neural tube defect in Great Britain and other countries in 1991(292) and in the first occurrence of an affected infant in Hungary in 1992 (293). Confirmation of these observations was provided in China in 1953–1993 (316). In China, taking a pill containing 400 micrograms of folic acid by 130,142 women in the periconceptional period reduced significantly their chance of

having a child with a neural tube defect in comparison to 117,689 women who did not take the supplement. These observations led to the hypothesis that a relative deficiency of folic acid in the mother and her embryo had "caused" the neural tube defect to occur.

After intense debate in the United States, fortification of enriched grain products with folic acid was authorized by the Food and Drug Administration in March 1996 and required by January 1998. The goal was to reduce the occurrence of all types of neural tube defects. The early studies showed the expected effects: the maternal serum folate concentration increased by 0.94 ng/ml for every 0.1 ng/day increase in intake of folic acid by women between 20 and 35 years old. Each doubling of the level of serum folate decreased by 50% the rate of occurrence of neural tube defects (317). Successes have been reported from the United States (274), Canada (318), Mexico (319), Costa Rica (320), and many other countries. The greater effect would be expected in regions with the highest prevalence rate (274) and among the racial/ethnic groups with the highest prevalence rates (317). Confirming the correlation with race and ethnicity, data from 21 population-based malformations surveillance programs showed in 1995–2002 significant decreases in the prevalence of spina bifida and anencephaly among non-Hispanic white and Hispanic births, but not among non-Hispanic black births (276).

Likewise, with folic acid supplementation, there was a decrease in the severity of the neural tube defects (321). For example, in Ireland, which had been a area with a high prevalence of the occurrence of both anencephaly and spina bifida in the same infant, there was a significant decrease in this more severe phenotype after supplementation (322).

In addition to these decreases in infants with neural tube defects, the folic acid supplementation in the periconceptional period has been shown to be associated with a significant reduction in the occurrence of wide variety of major malformations, including many types of heart defects, cleft lip, cleft palate, limb deficiencies, omphalocele, and imperforate anus (323).

There is a potential for greater prevention if the fortification includes vitamin B12 in addition to folic acid. In a large multicenter case-control study in France, the nutritional and genetic determinants of vitamin B and homocysteine metabolism of 77 pregnant women with an affected fetus (prior to elective termination) were compared to 60 pregnant women with a normal sonogram. There was an association of the risk for having an affected fetus with a decreased erythrocyte level of folate, as well as low blood levels of vitamins B6 and B12 (324).

Unfortunately, mandatory supplementation with folic acid and vitamin B12 has not been implemented in any country in Europe (325). This places a greater burden on education campaigns to convince women in the child-bearing age groups to take these supplements. The voluntary supplementation has not been as successful as having the supplements added to the cereals and grains, as a country-wide mandate (326).

However, myelomeningocele and other types of neural tube defects have occurred in infants born to women who have taken supplements with folic acid and multivitamins before and after conception. Supplements with inositol have been shown to prevent folate resistant neural tube defects in mice (327). Isoforms of protein kinase C have been postulated to be essential for this effect of inositol (328). Inositol supplementation has been used in a few pregnancies at risk for apparent folate-resistant neural tube defects (329).

Other risk factors, such as zinc deficiency, have been identified in developing regions with nutritional deficiencies in Iran (330) and the Amazon region (331).

Treatment and Prognosis

An increasing portion of the infants with myelomeningocele have been identified prenatally by sonography. In systematic evaluations of leg movements, it was noticed that most affected fetuses had normal movement in utero, but very few had normal leg movement postnatally (332). This observation led to the concern that the spinal cord was damaged secondarily throughout pregnancy or during labor and delivery. One proposed solution was to deliver the affected fetuses by cesarean section before the onset of labor. One study of 260 infants with myelomeningocele in Seattle showed that the infants born by cesarean section had better motor function at age two years than those born after vaginal delivery (333).

Observations in an experimental model of myelomeningocele in fetal lambs showed loss of neural tissue, areas of necrosis, and disrupted neural bundles in the exposed spinal cord (334). If the lamb with a spina bifida created at 75 days of gestation (term gestation, 140 days) had a repair with covering of the exposed spinal cord at 100 days of gestation, the spinal cord was better preserved and the repaired lamb, over time, could stand, walk, and climb stairs (335). This apparent benefit of intervention during pregnancy led to trials of fetal surgery for affected human fetuses. The early reports showed a reduction in herniations of the hindbrain and Arnold-Chiari II malformation and an improved neurologic outcome. A randomized trial of fetuses with myelomeningocele, between 19 and 25 weeks six days gestation, was recommended (335).

A multicenter randomized controlled trial is underway at the three medical centers in the United States to evaluate the intrauterine repair of myelomeningocele (336).

For the affected fetus treated at birth with coverage of the open and abnormal spinal cord, the prognosis is guarded. In a follow-up study of 64 affected infants with surgical repair at birth (1981–1990), 98% had a ventriculo peritoneal shunt. 23% developed symptoms of brainstem dysfunction. 14% did not survive to age 5 years, with many of the deaths attributed to brainstem dysfunction (337).

Affected individuals, as adults, continue to require medical and social assistance. In a long-term follow-up study of individuals born between 1963 and 1971, only half were able to live independently (338). In another long-term follow-up study of 904 individuals with myelomeningocele in Seattle (1957–2000), survival was shown to have increased in recent decades (339). However, adults over age 35 with shunts had increased risks and decreased survival. More recent follow-up studies are expected to show continued improvement in survival and the quality of daily activities.

Psychometric testing has shown that the majority of infants with myelomeningocele and hydrocephalus have normal intelligence, although their IQs are lower than those of normal controls (340). Hydrocephalus has been associated with various impairments. Children with spina bifida typically have a lower performance IQ than verbal IQ scores. Non-verbal deficits can be related to lesions in the right hemisphere and white matter, attributed to the hydrocephalus. An MRI morphometric study of 10 adults with myelomeningocele and shunted for hydrocephalus showed the changes associated with the Chiari II malformation and varied changes in the lateral ventricles (341). They did not find a correlation of cognitive function with the dilatation of the ventricles, thickness of the parenchyma or the size of the corpus callosum.

Genetic Counseling

The clinician's first challenge is to determine whether or not the affected infant has an isolated myelomeningocele or a specific multiple malformation syndrome in which myelomeningocele is a component (Table 18-7).

Malformation syndromes to be considered in evaluating the newborn infant with myelomeningocele include:

1. meningocele – distinguished by the fact that the lumbosacral defect is skin-covered;
2. myelocystocele – distinguished by being skin-covered; cystic swelling of the enlarged central canal of the spinal cord (342); also occurs as a component of cloacal exstrophy;
3. anterior spina bifida – distinguished by a presacral mass and imperforate anus; features of the Currarino Syndrome (MIM 176450).

Chromosome analysis is indicated in all phenotypes because of the higher frequency of abnormalities. The medical management and counseling are based on the underlying etiology of the myelomeningomyelocele. For example, when the infant with spina bifida has trisomy 18 or trisomy 9 (Figure 18-35), the prognosis for the infant is determined by the chromosome abnormality. If the infant has meningomyelocele in association with exposure to sodium valproate (Figure 18-36), the clinical evaluation should focus on the potential spectrum of teratogenic effects of that drug which can include multiple anomalies and developmental delay (343).

The prenatal diagnosis, primarily by ultrasound screening, and elective termination of fetuses with meningomyelocele has impacted the portion of affected infants that are born alive since the 1980s (344–349). The frequency of elective termination of the pregnancies with affected (myelomeningocele) fetuses has varied by nationality and religious affiliation: 26.9% in Australia in 1989 (344); 23% in Atlanta in 1980–1991 (346); 30% in 1989–1991 in California (347); 75% in Boston in 1982 to 1992 (349).

If the infant has isolated myelomeningocele with no chromosome abnormality, the child's prognosis will be determined by the associated complications of hydrocephalus, flaccid bladder, hip dislocation, etc. The presence of the non-neural malformations that are more common among affected infants will contribute to that prognosis.

The recurrence risks in subsequent pregnancies have been determined for several high- and low-risk populations and, as expected, show the higher recurrence rate with the higher prevalence rate (Table 18-8). The challenge for the counselor is to identify empiric recurrence risk data appropriate for the geographic area and race of the family.

The relatives of individuals with myelomeningocele have been shown in several studies to have an increased rate of occurrence of both neural tube defects and other non-neural anomalies, such as heart defects and limb defects. This increased risk has been demonstrated in sibs (252, 273), as well as aunts and uncles (355), especially among the relatives of the mother of the affected infant. The basis for this increase in frequency of birth defects has not been determined.

TABLE 18-8 *Empiric data: risks and concordance.*

	Neural Tube Defect	Other Malformations
1. Recurrence/precurrence risk for another affected sib:		
i) East Ireland: Precurrence risk: (1980–1994; Caucasians 821 cases of NID; 419 spina bifida) [25]	2.1%	3.1%
ii) British Columbia: (1958–1984 512 cases of NTD; 307 spina bifida) [4]		
a) if index case had high spina bifida (i.e. above T11 vertebrae):	7.8%	6.1%
b) if index case had low spina bifida:	0.7%	2.2%
c) East Indian Sikhs	4.4%	8.8%
vs. non Sikhs	2.0%	2.4%
iii) Brittany/France (1975–1984; all Caucasians; 449 cases of NTD; 227 spina bifida) [102]	1.8%	0.3%
iv) United States and Michigan (103)		
Sibs	3.2%	
nieces, nephews, aunts, uncles	0.5%	
Cousins	0.17%	
(1983; 204 probands with spina bifida or anencephaly; race not specified.)		
2. Empiric risk for an affected child:		
a) London (104):	2.8%	
(14 affected adults had 35 children, one of whom had myelomeningocele; race/ethnicity not specified.)		

3. Concordance/discordance of NTD:

It is most likely that the second affected sib will have the same level of defect. In a study of 831 pregnancies in which one sibling had either myelomeningocele or anencephaly, there were 41 families in which a second affected infant was born (105). Of the 27 couples whose first child had myelomeningocele, the second affected infant had myelomeningocele in 23 (85%) of those families. In 13 of the 14 families, whose first infant had anencephaly, the second affected infant also had anencephaly.

However, among affected sibs with nonsyndromic myelomeningocele a series of 66 families did not show a consistent pattern of sibs with high lesions (above vertebral level T12) having primarily similarly affected sibs (106).

4. Risk for recurrence of other neural tube defects.

There is insufficient information from family studies to establish the empiric risk, following the birth of a child with myelomeningocele, of having another affected child with less common neural tube defects, such as encephalocele, meningocele, and anencephaly.

Prenatal screening by ultrasound at 15 to 16 weeks of gestation has been shown to be very reliable in detecting the presence of a myelomeningocele (356).

REFERENCES

Reference Books

1. Lemire RJ, Beckwith JB, Warkany J. *Anencephaly*. Raven Press: New York; 1978.
2. Kalousek DK, Fitch N, Paradice BA. *Pathology of the Human Embryo and Previable Fetus: An Atlas*. New York: Springer-Verlag; 1990: 67–73.
3. Elwood JM, Little J, Elwood JH. *Epidemiology and Control of Neural Tube Defects*. New York: Oxford University Press; 1992.
4. Wyszynski DF, ed. *Neural Tube Defects: From Origin to Treatment*. New York: Oxford University Press; 2006.
5. O'Rahilly R, Müller F. Human Embryology & Teratology. 3rd ed. New York: Wiley-Liss; 2001: 442 and 444.
6. Moore KL, Persaud TVN. *The Developing Human: Clinically Oriented Embryology*. 7th ed. Philadelphia: WB Saunder; 2003: 434–442 and 451–453.

Reference Articles

7. Dolk H, DeWals P, Gillerot Y, Lechat MF, Ayme S, Cornel M, Cuschieri A, Garne E, Goujard J, Laurence KM, Lillis D, Lys SF, Nevin N, Owens J, Radic A, Stoll C, Stone D, Ten Kate L. Heterogeneity of neural tube defects in Europe: the significance of site of defect and presence of other major anomalies in relation to geographic differences in prevalence. *Teratology*. 1991;44: 547–559.
8. Seller MJ, Kalousek DK. Neural tube defects: heterogeneity and homogeneity. *Am J Med Genet*. 1986;2:77–87.
9. Sadovnick AD, Baird PA. Congenital malformations associated with anencephaly in liveborn and stillborn infants. *Teratology*. 1985;32:355–361.
10. David TJ, McCrae FC, Bound JP. Congenital malformations associated with anencephaly and iniencephaly. *J Med Genet*. 1983;20:338–341.
11. David TJ, Nixon A. Congenital malformations associated with anencephaly and iniencephaly. *J Med Gen*. 1978;13:263–265.
12. Melnick M, Myrianthopoulos NC. Studies in neural tube defects II. Pathologic findings in a prospectively collected series of anencephalics. *Am J Med Genet*. 1987;26:797–810.
13. David TJ, Parker VM, Illingworth CA. Anencephaly with diaphragmatic hernia in sibs. *J Med Genet*. 1979;16:157–158.
14. Müller F, O'Rahilly R. Cerebral dysraphic (future anencephaly) in a human twin embryo at stage 13. *Teratology*. 1984;30: 167–177.
15. O'Rahilly R, Müller F. The two sites of fusion of the neural folds and the two neuropores in the human embryo. *Teratology*. 2002; 65:162–170.
16. Marin-Padilla M. Study of the skull in human cranioschisis. *Acta Anat (Basel)*. 1965;62:1–20.
17. Lomholt JF, Fischer-Hansen B, Kelling JW, Reintoft I, Kjar I. Subclassification of anencephalic human fetuses according to morphology of the posterior cranial fossa. *Pediatr Develop Path*. 2004;7:601–606.
18. Vukelić Z, Metelmam W, Müthing J, Kos M, Peter-Katalinić J. Anencephaly: structural characterization of gangliosides in defined brain regions. *Bio Chem*. 2001;382:259–274.
19. Harris MJ, Juriloff DM. Mouse models for neural tube closure defects and their role in understanding human neural tube

defects. *Birth Def Res (Part A): Clin Mol Teratol*. 2007;79: 187–210.
20. VanAllen MI, Kalousek DK, Chernoff GF, Juriloff D, Harris M, McGillivray BC, Yong S-L, Langlois S, MacLeod PM, Chitayat D, Friedman JM, Wilson RD, McFadden D, Pantzar J, Ritchie S, Hall JG. Evidence for multi-site closure of the neural tube in humans. *Am J Med Genet*. 1993;47:723–743.
21. Kibor Z, Capra Z, Gros P. Toward understanding the genetic basis of neural tube defects. *Clin Genet*. 2007;71:295–310.
22. Copp AJ, Greene NDE, Murdock JN. The genetic basis of mammalian neurlation. *Nature Reviews*. 2003;4:784–793.
23. Hall JL, Harris MJ, Juriloff DM. Effect of multifactorial genetic liability to exencephaly on the teratogenetic of valproic acid in mice. *Teratology*. 1997;55:306–313.
24. Nishimura H, Takano K, Tanimura T, Yasuda M. Normal and abnormal development of human embryos: first report of the analysis of 1,213 intact embryos. *Teratology*. 1970;1:281–290.
25. Creasy M, Alberman E. Congenital malformations of the central nervous system in spontaneous abortions. *J Med Genet*. 1976; 13:9–16.
26. Byrne J, Warburton D. Neural tube defects in spontaneous abortions. *Am J Med Genet*. 1986;25:327–333.
27. Moore CA, Li S, Liz Z, Hong S-X, Gu H-Q, Berry RJ, Mulinare J, Erickson JD. Elevated rates of severe neural tube defects in a high-prevalence area in Northern China. *Am J Med Genet*. 1997;73:113–118.
28. Cotter AM, Daly SF. Neural tube defects: is a decreasing prevalence associated with a decrease in severity? *Eur J Obst Gynecol Reprod Biol*. 2005;119:161–163.
29. Bower C, Raymond M, Lamley J, Bury G. Trends in neural tube defects 1980–1989. *Med J Australia*. 1993;158:152–154.
30. Shaw GM, Jensvold NG, Wasserman CR, Lammer EJ. Epidemiologic characteristics of phenotypically distinct neural tube defects among 0.7 million California births, 1983–1987. *Teratology*. 1994;49:143–149.
31. Limb CJ, Holmes LB. Anencephaly: changes in prenatal detection and birth status, 1972 through 1990. *Amer J Ob Gyn*. 1994; 170:1333–1338.
32. Stoll C, Alembic Y, Dott B, Roth MP. Impact of prenatal diagnosis on live birth prevalence of children with congenital anomalies. *Ann Genet*. 2002;45:115–121.
33. Coddington DA, Hismanick JJ. Midline congenital anomalies: the estimated occurrence among American Indian and Alaska Native infants. *Clin Genet*. 1996;50:74–77.
34. Cragan JD, Roberts HE, Edmonds LD, Khoury MJ, Kirby RS, Shaw GM et al. Surveillance for an anencephaly and spina bifida and the impact of prenatal diagnosis – United States, 1985–1994. *MMWR CDC Surveill Summ*. 1995;44:1–13.
35. McDonnell RJ, Johnson Z, Delaney V, Dack P. East Ireland 1980–1994: epidemiology of neural tube defects. *J Epidemiol Comm Health*. 1999;53:782–788.
36. Jung SC, Kim SS, Yoon KS, Lee JS. Prevalence of congenital malformations and genetic diseases in Korea. *J Hum Genet*. 1999;44: 30–34.
37. Cherian A, Seena S, Bullock RK, Anthony AC. Incidence of neural tube defects in the least-developed area of India: a population-based study. *Lancet*. 2005;366:930–931.
38. Anyebuno M, Amofa G, Peprah S, Affram A. Neural tube defects at Korle Bu Teaching Hospital, Acra, Ghana. *East Afr Med J*. 1993;70:572–574.
39. Moreno-Fuenmayor H, Valera V, Socorro-Candanoza L, Bracho A, Herrera M, Rodriguez Z, Concho E. Preventive program of birth defects: incidence of anencephaly in Maracaibo, Venezuela, 1993–1996 period. *Invest Clin*. 1996;37:271–278. (In Spanish)
40. Brender JD, Carmichael L, Preece MJ, Larimer GC, Suarez L. Epidemiology of anencephaly in Texas, 1981–1986. *Texas Medicine* 1989; 85: 33–35.

41. Feldman JG, Stein SC, Klein RJ, Kohl S, Casey G. The prevalence of neural tube defects among ethnic groups in Brooklyn, New York. *J Chronic Dis.* 1982;35:53–60.

42. Strassburg MA, Greenland S, Portigal LD, Sever LE. A population-based case-control study of anencephalus and spina bifida in a low-risk area. *Develop Med Child Neurol.* 1983;25:632–641.

43. Knox EG. Twins and neural tube defects. *Br J Prev Soc Med.* 1974;28:73–80.

44. James WH. The sex ratio in anencephaly. *J Med Gen.* 1979;16:129–133.

45. Seller MJ. Neural tube defects and sex ratios. *Am J Med Genet.* 1987;26:699–707.

46. Hall JG, Freidman JM, Kenne BA, Popkin J, Jawanda M, Arnold W. Clinical genetics of epidemiological factors in neural tube defects. *Am J Hum Genet.* 1988;43:827–837.

47. Källén B, Cocchi G, Knudsen LB, Castilla EE, Robert E, Daltvelt AK, Lancaster PL, Mastroiacovo P. International study of sex ratio and twinning of neural tube defects. *Teratology.* 1994;50:322–331.

48. Ben-Ami I, Vaknin Z, Reish O, Sherman D, Herman A, Maymon R. Is there an increased rate of anencephaly in twins? *Prenat Diag.* 2005;25:1007–1010.

49. Lim KI, Dy C, Pergash D, Williams KP. Monoamniotic twins discordant for anencephaly managed conservatively with good outcomes: two case reports and a review of the literature. *Ultrasound Obstet Gynecol.* 2005;26:188–193.

50. Hansen LM, Donnenfeld AE. Concordant anencephaly in monoamniotic twins and analysis of maternal serum markers. *Prenat Diagn.* 1997;17:471–473.

51. Putz B, Rehder H. Anencephaly in one monoamniotic-monochorionic twin and encephalocele in the other. *Am J Med Genet.* 1985;21:631–635.

52. Chan P-C, Hsieh W-S, Peng SSF. Klippel-Feil Syndrome plus atretic meningocele in one identical twin and anencephaly in the other. *J. Formosa Med Assoc.* 2003;102:506–509.

53. Townes PL, Router K, Rosquete EE, Magee BD. XK Aprosencephaly and anencephaly in sibs. *Am J Med Genet.* 1988;29:523–528.

54. Farag TI, Teebi AS, Al-Awadi SA. Nonsyndromal anencephaly: possible autosomal recessive variant. *Am J Med Genet.* 1986;24:461–464.

55. Toriello HV, Warren ST, Lindstrom JA. Possible X-linked anencephaly and spina bifida – report of a kindred. *Am J Med Genet.* 1980;6:119–121.

56. Jensson O, Arnason A, Gunnarsdottir H, Petursdottir I, Fossdal R, Hreidarsson S. A family showing apparent X-linked inheritance of both anencephaly and spina bifida. *J Med Genet.* 1988;25:227–229.

57. Newton R, Stanier P, Loughna S, Henderson DJ, Forbes SA, Farrall M, Jensson O, Moore GE. Linkage analysis of 62 X-chromosomal loci excludes the X chromosome in an Icelandic family showing apparent X-linked recessive inheritance of neural tube defects. *Clin Genet.* 1994;45:241–249.

58. Rogner UC, Danoy P, Matsuda F, Moore GE, Stanier P, Avner P. SNPs in the CpG island of NAP1L2: a possible link between DNA methylation and neural tube defects? *Am J Med Genet.* 2002;110:208–214.

59. Hume RF Jr, Drugan A, Reichler A, Lampinen J, Martin LS, Johnson MP, Evans MI. Aneuploidy among prenatally detected neural tube defects. *Am J Med Genet.* 1996;61:171–173.

60. Kennedy D, Chitayat D, Winsor EJT, Silver M, Toi A. Prenatally diagnosed neural tube defects: ultrasound, chromosome, and autopsy or postnatal findings in 212 cases. *Am J Med Genet.* 1998;77:317–321.

61. Sepulveda W, Corral E, Ayala C, Be C, Gutierrez J, Vasquez P. Chromosomal abnormalities in fetuses with open neural tube defects: prenatal identification with ultrasound. *Ultrasound Obstet Gynecol.* 2004;23:352–356.

62. Hahn GK, Barth RF, Schauer GM, Reiss R, Opitz JM. Trisomy 2p syndrome: a fetus with anencephaly and postaxial polydactyly. *Am J Med Genet.* 1999;87:45–48.

63. Doray B, Favre R, Gasser B, Girard-Lemaire F, Schluth C, Flori E. Recurrent neural tube defects associated with partial Trisomy 2p22-pter: report of two siblings and review of the literature. *Genetic Counseling.* 2003;14:165–172.

64. Botto LD, Olney RS, Erickson JD. Vitamin supplements and the risk for congenital anomalies other than neural tube defects. *Am J Med Genet Part C (Semin Med Genet).* 2004;125C:12–21.

65. Parle-McDermott A, Kirke PN, Mills JL, Molloy AM, Cox C, O'Leary VB et al. Confirmation of the R653Q polymorphism of the trifunctional C1-synthase enzyme as a maternal risk for neural tube defects in the Irish population. *Eur J Hum Genet.* 2006;14:768–772.

66. Parle-McDermott A, Pangilinan F, Mills JL, Kirke PN, Gibney ER, Troendle J et al. The 19-bp deletion polymorphism of intron-1 of dihydrofolate reductase (DHFR) may decrease rather than increase risk for spina bifida in the Irish population. *Am J Med Genet Part A.* 2007;143:1174–1180.

67. Volchik KA, Blanton SH, Kruzel MC, Townsend IT, Tyerman GH, Mier RJ, Northrup H. Testing for genetic associations with the PAX gene family in a spina bifida population. *Am J Med Genet.* 2002;110:195–202.

68. Kibar Z, turban E, McDearmid JR, Reynolds A, Berghout J, Mathieu M et al. Mutations in VANGL1 associated with neural tube defects. *N Engl J Med.* 2007;356:1432–1437.

69. Amorosi S, D'Armiento M, Calcagno G, Russo I, Adriani M, Christiano AM et al. FOXN1 homozygous mutation associated with anencephaly and severe neural tube defect in human athymic Nude/SCID fetus. *Clin Genet.* 2008;73:380–384.

70. McMahon B, Yen S. Unrecognized epidemic of anencephaly and spina bifida. *Lancet.* 1971;i:31–33.

71. Shiota K. Neural tube defects and maternal hyperthermia in early pregnancy: epidemiology in a human embryo population. *Am J Med Genet.* 1982;12:281–288.

72. Renwick JH. Hypothesis: anencephaly and spina bifida are usually preventable by evidence of a specific but unidentified substance present in certain potato tubers. *Brit J Prev Soc Med.* 1972;26:67–88.

73. Greene MF. Spontaneous abortions and major malformations in women with diabetes mellitus. *Sem Reprod Endocrinol.* 1999;17:127–136.

74. Anderson JL, Waller DK, Canfield MA, Shaw GM, Watkins ML, Werler MM. Maternal obesity, gestational diabetes, and central nervous system birth defects. *Epidemiology.* 2005;16:87–92.

75. Rosa FW. Spina Bifida in infants of women treated with carbamazepine during pregnancy. *N Engl J Med.* 1991;324:674–677.

76. Omtzigt JGC, Los FJ, Grobbee DE, Pijpers L, Jahoda MGJ, Brandenburg H, Stewart PA, Gaillard HLJ, Sachs ES, Wladimiroff JW, Lindhout D. The risk of spina bifida aperta after first-trimester exposure to valproate in a prenatal cohort. *Neurology.* 1992;42 (Suppl 5):119–125.

77. Lindhout D, Schmidt D. In-utero exposure to valproate and neural tube defects. *Lancet.* 1986;i:1392–1393.

78. Medical Research Council. Prevention of neural tube defects: results of the Medical Research Council Vitamin Study. MRC Vitamin Study Research Group. *Lancet.* 1991;338:131–137.

79. Czeizel AE, Dudas I. Prevention of the first occurrence of neural-tube defects by periconceptional vitamin supplementation. *N Engl J Med.* 1992;327:1832–1835.

80. Berry RJ, Li Z, Erickson JD. Prevention of neural-tube defects with folic acid in China. China – U.S. Collaborative Project for Neural Tube Defect Prevention. *N Engl J Med.* 1999;341:1485–1490.

81. Williams LJ, Rasmussen SA, Flores A, Kirby RS, Edmonds LD. Decline in the prevalence of spina bifida and anencephaly by race/ethnicity: 1995–2002. *Pediatrics.* 2005;116:580–586.

82. De Wals P, Tairou F, Van Allen MI, Uh SH, Lowry RB, Sibbald B et al. Reduction of neural-tube defects after folic acid fortification in Canada. *N Engl J Med.* 2007;357:135–142.

83. Martínez de Villarreal L, Villarreal Pérez JZ, Vázquez PA, Herrera RH, Velazco Campos M del R, López RA et al. Decline of neural tube defects case after a folic acid campaign in Nuevo León, México. *Teratology.* 2002;66:249–256.

84. Oakley GP Jr. When will we eliminate folic acid-preventable spina bifida? *Epidemiology.* 2007;18:367–368.

85. Ray JG, Wyatt P, Thompson MD, Vermeulen MJ, Meier C, Wong PY, et al. Vitamin B12 and the risk of neural tube defects in a folic-acid-fortified population. *Epidemiology.* 2007;18: 362–366.

86. Cowchock S, Ainbender E, Prescott G, Crandall B, Lau L, Heller R et al. The recurrence risk for neural tube defects in the United States: a collaborative study. *Am J Med Genet.* 1980;5: 309–314.

87. Laurence KM. The recurrence risk in spina bifida cystica and anencephaly. *Devel Med Child Neurol Suppl.* 1969;20:23–30.

88. Byrne J, Cama A, Vigliarolo M, Levato L. Patterns of inheritance in Irish and Italian families with neural tube defects: comparison between high and low rate areas. *Ir Med J.* 1997;90: 32–34.

89. McBride ML. Sib risks of anencephaly and spina bifida in British Columbia. *Am J Med.* 1979;3:377–387.

90. Journel H, Parent P, Roussey M, L Marec B. "Isolated" hydrocephalus in families of spina bifida and anencephaly: a coincidence? *Neuropediatrics.* 1989;20:220–222.

91. Littre A. Diverse observations anatomique. *Mem Acad Roy des Sc.* 1709;4:9.

92. Spencer R. Exstrophia splanchnica (exstrophy of the cloaca). *Surgery.* 1965;57:751–766.

93. Beckwith JB. The congenitally malformed VII. Exstrophy of the bladder and cloacal exstrophy. *Northwest Medicine.* 1966;65: 407–410.

94. Hayden PW, Chapman WH, Stevenson JK. Exstrophy of the cloaca. *Am J Dis Child.* 1973;125:879–883.

95. Carey JC, Greenbaum B, Hall BD. The OEIS Complex (omphalocele, exstrophy, imperforate anus, spinal defects). *Birth Defects.* 1978;14(6B):253–263.

96. Rickham PP. Vesio-intestinal fissure. *Arch Dis Child.* 1960; 35:97–.

97. MacLaughlin KP, Rink RC, Kalsbeck JE, Keating MA, Adams MC, King SJ, Luerssen TG. Cloacal exstrophy: the neurological implications. *J Urol.* 1995;154:782–784.

98. Lattimer JK, Hensel TW, MacFarlane MT, Beck L, Braun E, Esposito Y. The exstrophy support team: a new concept in the care of the exstrophy patient. *J Urol.* 1979;121:472–473.

99. Redman J, Seibert J, Page B. Cloacal exstrophy in identical twins. *Urology.* 17:73–74, 1981.

100. Casale P, Grady RW, Waldhausen JH, Jayna BD, Wright J, Mitchell M. Cloacal exstrophy variants. Can blighted conjoined twinning play a role? *J Urol.* 2004;172:1103–1106.

101. Byrd SE, Harvey C, Daraling CF. MR of terminal myelocystoceles. *Eur J Radiol.* 1995;20:215–220.

102. Dick EA, DeBruyn R, Patel K, Owens CM. Spinal ultrasound in cloacal exstrophy. *Clin Radiol.* 2001;56:289–294.

103. Reiner WG, Gearhart JP. Discordant sexual identity in some genetic males with cloacal exstrophy assigned to female sex at birth. *N Eng J Med.* 2004;350:333–341.

104. McLone DG, Naidich TP. Terminal myelocystocele. *Neurosurgery.* 1985;16:36–43.

105. Evans JA, Darvill KD, Trevenen C, Rockman-Greenberg C. Cloacal exstrophy and related abdominal wall defects in Manitoba: incidence and demographic factors. *Clin Genetics.* 1985;27:241–251.

106. Hurwitz RS, Manzoni GAM, Ransley PG, Stephens FD. Cloacal exstrophy: a report of 34 cases. *J Urol.* 1987;138:1060–1064.

107. Chapman PH. Comment. *Neurosurgery.* 1991;28:843.

108. Cohen AR. The mermaid malformation: cloacal exstrophy and occult spinal dysraphism. *Neurosurgery.* 1991;28:834–843.

109. Källén K, Castilla EE, Robert E, Mastroiacovo P, Källén B. OEIS Complex-a population study. *Am J Med Genet.* 2000;92:62–68.

110. Tubbs RS, Smyth MD, Oakes WJ. Chiari I malformation and cloacal exstrophy: report of a patient with both defects of blastogenesis. *Am J Med Genet.* 2003;119:231–233.

111. Martinez-Frais ML, Bermejo E, Rodriquez-Pinilla E, Frias JL. Exstrophy of the cloaca and exstrophy of the bladder. Two different expressions of a primary development field defect. *Am J Med Genet.* 2001;99:261–269.

112. Keppler-Noreuil KM. OEIS Complex (omphalocele-exstrophy-imperforate anus-spinal defects): A review of 14 cases. *Am J Med Genet.* 2001;99:271–279.

113. Keppler-Noreuil K, Gorton S, Foo F, Yankowitz J, Keegan C. Prenatal ascertainment of OEIS Complex/Cloacal Exstrophy – 15 new cases and literature review. *Am J Med Genet Part A.* 2007;143A:2122–2128.

114. Meglin AJ, Balotin RJ, Jelinek JS, Fishman ER, Jeffs RD, Ghael V. Cloacal exstrophy: radiologic findings in 13 patients. *AJR.* 1990;155:1267–1272.

115. Schlegel PN, Gearhart JP. Neuroanatomy of the pelvis in an infant with cloacal exstrophy: a detailed microdissection with histology. *J Urol.* 1989;141:583–585.

116. McHoney M, Ransley PG, Duffy P, Wilcox DT, Spitz L. Cloacal exstrophy: morbidity associated with abnormalities of the gastrointestinal tract and spine. *J Pediatr Surg.* 2004;39: 1209–1213.

117. Koo HP, Bunchman TE, Flynn JT, Punch JD, Schwartz AC, Bloom DA. Renal transplantation in children with severe lower urinary tract dysfunction. *J Urol.* 1999;161:240–245.

118. Jain M, Weaver DD. Severe lower limb defects in exstrophy of the cloaca. *Am J Med Genet.* 2004;128:320–324.

119. Siebert JR, Rutledge JC, Kapur RP. Association of cloacal anomalies, caudal duplication, and twinning. *Peditric Devel Path.* 2005;8:339–354.

120. Vermeij-Keers C, Hartwig NG, Van der Werff JF. Embryonic development of the ventral body wall and its congenital malformations. *Semin Pediatr Surg.* 1997;6:180–186.

121. Langer JC, Brennan B, Lappalainen RE, Caco CC, Winthrop AL, Hollenberg RD, Paes BA. Cloacal exstrophy: prenatal diagnosis before rupture of the cloacal membrane. *J Pediat Surg.* 1992;27:1352–1356.

122. Bruch SW, Adzick NS, Goldstein RB, Harrison MR. Challenging the embryogenesis of cloacal exstrophy. *J Pediat Surg.* 1996; 31:768–770.

123. Kapur RP, Jack RM, Siebert JR. Diamniotic placentation associated with omphalopagus conjoined twins: implications for a contemporary model of conjoined twinning. *Am J Med Genet.* 1994;52:188–195.

124. Goldfischer ER, Almond PS, Statter MB, Miller G, Arensman RM, Cromie WJ. Omphalopagus twins with covered cloacal exstrophy. *J Urol.* 1997;157:1004–1005.

125. Spencer R. Conjoined twins: theoretical embryologic basis. *Teratology.* 1992;45:591–602.

126. Thomalla JV, Rudolph RA, Rink RC, Mitchell ME. Induction of cloacal exstrophy in the chick embryo using the CO_2 laser. *J Urol.* 1985;134:991–995.

127. Manner J, Kluth D. A chicken model to study the embryology of cloacal exstrophy. *J Pedi Surg.* 2003;38:678–681.

128. Reutter H, Becker T, Ludwig M, Schäfer N, Detlefsen B, Beaudoin S et al. Family-based association study of the MTHFR

Polymorphism C677T in the bladder-exstrophy-epispadias-complex. *Am J Med Genet Part A.* 2006;140A:2506–2509.

129. Boyadjiev SA, Dodson JL, Radford CL, Ashrafi GH, Beaty TH, Mathews RI, Broman KW, Gearhart JP. Clinical and molecular characterization of the bladder exstrophy-epispadias complex: analysis of 232 families. *Brit J Urol Internat.* 2004;94: 1337–1343.

130. Lee DH, Cottrell JR, Sanders RC, Meyers CM, Wolfsberg EA, Sun C-CJ. OEIS complex (omphalocele-exstrophy-imperforate anus-spinal defects) in monozygotic twins. *Am J Med Genet.* 1999;84:29–33.

131. Reutter H, Qi L, Gearhart JP, Boemers T, Ebert A-K, Rösch W, Ludwig M, Boyadjiev SA. Concordance analyses of twins with bladder exstrophy–epispadias complex suggest genetic etiology. *Am J Med Genet Part A.* 2007;143A:2751–2756.

132. Schinzel AAGL, Smith DW, Miller JR. Monozygotic twinning and structural defects. *J Pediatri.* 1979;95:921–930.

133. Smith NM, Chambers HM, Furness ME, Haan EA. The OEIS complex (omphalocele-exsrophy-imperforate anus-spinal defects): recurrence in sibs. *J Med Genet.* 1992;29:730–732.

134. Thauvin-Robinet C, Faivae L, Casin V, Van Kein PK, Callier P, Parker KL, Fellous M, Borgnan J, Gounot E, Huet F, Sapin E, Mugneret F. Cloacal exstrophy in an infant with 9q34.1qter deletion resulting from a *de novo* imbalanced translocation between chromosome 9q and Yqq. *Am J Med Genet.* 2004; 126A:303–307.

135. Kosaki R, Fukuhara Y, Kosuga M, Okuyama T, Kawashima N, Honna T, Ueoka K, Kosaki K. OEIS complex with del(3) (q12.2q13.2). *Am J Med Genet Part A.* 2005;224–226.

136. Mathews RI, Gan M, Gearhart JP. Urogynecological and obstetric issues in women with the exstrophy-epispadias complex. *Brit J Urol Internat.* 2003;91:845–849.

137. Baker Towell DM, Towell AD. A preliminary investigation into quality of life, psychological distress and social competence in children with cloacal exstrophy. *J Urol.* 2003;169: 1850–1853.

138. Heyroth-Griffis CA, Weaver DD, Faught P, Bellus GA, Torres-Martinez W. On the spectrum of limb-body wall complex, exstrophy of the cloaca, and urorectal septum malformation sequence. *Am J Med Genet Part A.* 2007;143A:1025–1031.

139. Schemm S, Grembruch, Germer U, Jänig U, Jonat W, von Kaisenberg CS. Omphalocele-exstrophy-imperforate anus-spinal defects (OEIS) complex associated with increased nuchal translucency. *Ultrasound Obstet Gynecol.* 2003;22:95–97.

140. Norman MG, McGillivray BC, Kalousek DK, Hill A, Poskitt KJ. *Congenital Malformations of the Brain: Pathologic, Embryologic, Clinical and Genetic Aspects.* New York: Oxford University Press; 1995.

141. Flatz G, Sukthomy C. Fronto-ethmoidal encephalomeningoceles in the population of Northern Thailand. *Humangenetik.* 1970; 11:1–8.

142. Simpson DA, David DJ, White J. Cephaloceles: treatment, outcome and antenatal diagnosis. *Neurosurgery.* 1984;15:14–21.

143. Yokota A, Matsukado Y, Fuwa I, Moroki K, Nagahiro S. Anterior basal encephalocele of the neonatal and infantile period. *Neurosurgery.* 1986;19:468–478.

144. Macfarlane R, Rutka JT, Armstrong D, Phillips J, Posnick J, Forte V, Humphreys RP, Drake J, Hoffman HJ. Encephaloceles of the anterior cranial fossa. *Pediatr Neurosurg.* 1995;23:148–158.

145. Boonvisut S, Ladpli S, Sujatanond M, Tandhavadhana C, Tisavipat N, Luxsuwong M et al. Morphologic study of 120 skull base defects in frontoethmoidal encephalomeningoceles. *Plast Reconstr Surg.* 1998;101:1784–1795.

146. Agthong S, Wiwanitkit V. Encephalomeningocele cases over 10 years in Thailand: case series. *BMC Neurology.* 2002;2:3 (http://biomedicalcentral.com/1471-2377/2/3).

147. Mahapatra AK, Suri A. Anterior encephaloceles: a study of 92 cases. *Pediatr Neurosurg.* 2002;36:113–118.

148. Rojvachiranonda N, David DJ, Moore MH, Cole J. Frontoethimoidal encephalomeningocele: new morphological findings and new classification. *J Craniofac Surg.* 2003;14: 847–858.

149. Hunt JA, Hobar PC. Common craniofacial anomalies: facial clefts and encephaloceles. *Plast Reconstr Surg.* 2003;112:606–615.

150. Monteith SJ, Heppner PA, Law AJJ. Encephalocele-epidemiological variance in New Zealand. *J Clin Neuroscience.* 2005;12:557–558.

151. Sípek A, Horácek J, Gregor V, Rychtaríková J, Dzurová D, Masátová D. Neural tube defects in the Czech Republic during 1961–1999: incidences, prenatal diagnosis and prevalences according to maternal age. *J Obstet Gyn.* 2002;22:501–507.

152. Zlotogora J, Amitai Y, Kaluski DN, Leventhal A. Surveillance of neural tube defects in Israel. *Isr Med Assoc.* 2002;J 4: 1111–1114.

153. Chapman PH, Swearingen B, Caviness VS. Subtorcular occipital encephaloceles: anatomical considerations relevant to operative management. *J Neurosurg.* 1989;71:375–381.

154. Yokota A, Kajiwara H, Kohchi M, Fuwa I, Wada H. Parietal cephalocele: clinical importance of its atretic form and associated malformations. *J Neurosurg.* 1988;69:545–551.

155. Patterson RJ, Egelhoff JC, Crone K, Ball WS. Atretic parietal cephaloceles revisited; an enlarging clinical and imaging spectrum. *Am J Neuroradiol.* 1998;19:791–795.

156. Tubbs RS, Doughty K, Smyth MD, Oakes WJ. Parietal cephalocele. *Pediatr Neurosurg.* 2004;40:37–38.

157. Sdano MT, Pensak ML. Temporal bone encephaloceles. *Current Opin Otolaryngol & Head Neck Surg.* 2005;13:287–289.

158. D'Antonio M, Palacios E, Scheuemann C. CSF fistula secondary to sphenoid meningoencephalocele. *ENT-Ear, Nose and Throat Journal.* 2003;82:912–913.

159. Hoving EW, Vermeij-Keers C. Frontoethmoidal encephaloceles, a study of their pathogenesis. *Pediatr Neurosurg.* 1997;27: 246–256.

160. Wacharasindhu S, Asawutmangkul U, Srivuthana S. Endocrine abnormalities in patients with frontoethmoidal encephalomeningocele. *Horm Res.* 2005;64:64–67.

161. Carvalho DR, Rizzo IM, Farage L, Barros ALC, Speck-Martins CE. Occipital encephalocele and hypoplastic thumb: a nonrandom association of malformations. *Clin Dysmorphol.* 2008; 17:273–274.

162. Dolk H, DeWals, P, Gillerot Y, Lechaf MF, Ayme S, Cornel M, Cuschieri Garne E, Goujard J, Laurence KM et al. Heterogeneity of neural tube defects in Europe: the significance of site of defect and presence of other major anomalies in relation to geographic differences in prevalence. *Teratology.* 1991;44:547–559.

163. Siffel S, Wong L-YC, Olney RS, Correa A. Survival of infants diagnosed with encephalocele in Atlanta, 1979–1998. *Paediatr Perinatal Epidemiol.* 2003;17:40–48.

164. Rowland CA, Correa A, Cragan JD. Descriptive epidemiology of encephalocele in Atlanta, Georgia, 1968–2002. *Birth Def Res (Part A): Clin Mol Terat.* 2005;73:304.

165. Marin-Padilla M. Notochordal-basichondrocranium relationships: abnormalities in experimental axial skeletal (dystrophic) disorders. *J Embryol Exp Morphol.* 1979;53:15–38.

166. Feuchtbaum LB, Currier RJ, Riggle S, Roberson M, Lorey FW, Cunningham GC. Neural tube defect prevalence in California (1990–1994): eliciting patterns by type of defect and maternal race/ethnicity. *Genetic Testing.* 1999;3:265–272.

167. Alembik Y, Dott B, Roth MP, Stoll C. Prevalence of neural tube defects in Northeastern France, 1979–1994: Impact of prenatal diagnosis. *Ann Génét.* 1997;40:69–71.

168. Airede KI. Neural tube defects in the middle belt of Nigeria. *J Trop Ped.* 1992;38:27–30.

169. Bower C, Raymond M, Lumley J, Bury G. Trends on neural tube defects 1980–1989. *Med J Aust.* 1993;158:152–154.

170. Suwanwela C, Suwanwela N. A morphological classification of sincipital encephalomeningocele. *J Neursurg.* 1972;36: 201–211.

171. Suwanwela C. Geographical distribution of fronoethmoidal encephalomeningocele. *Br J Prev Soc Med.* 1972;26:193–198.

172. Kallen B, Cocchi G, Knudsen LB, Castilla EE, Robert E, Daltveit AK, Lancaster PL, Mastroiacovo P. International study of sex ratio and twinning of neural tube defects. *Teratology.* 1994; 50:322–331.

173. Ruano R, Picone O, Benachi A, Grebille AG, Martinovic J, Dumez Y, Dommergues M. First trimester diagnosis of osteogenesis imperfecta associated with encephalocele by conventional and three-dimensional ultrasound. *Prenat Diag.* 2003; 23:539–542.

174. Putz B, Rehder H. Anencephaly in one monoamniotic-monochorionic twin and encephalocele in the other. *Am J Med Genet.* 1985;21:631–635.

175. Groen RJM, van Ouwerkerk WJR. Cerebellar dermoid tumor and occipital meningocele in a monozygotic twin: clues to the embryogenesis of craniospinal dysraphism. *Child Nerv Syst.* 1995;11:414–417.

176. Ertunc D, Tok EC, Kaplanoglu M, Polat A, Aras N, Evruke C. Concordant occipital encephalocele in monoamniotic twins. *J Perinat Med.* 2005;33:357–359.

177. Djientcheu V de P, Wonkam A, Njamnshi AK, Ongolo-Zogo P, Rilliet B, Morris MA. Discordant encephalocele in monozygotic twins. *Am J Med Genet.* 2006;140A:525–526.

178. Bassuk AG, McLone D, Bowmen R, Kessler JA. Autosomal dominant occipital cephalocele. *Neurology.* 2004;62:1888–1890.

179. Van Esch H, Poinier K, deZegher F, Holvoet M, Bienvence T, Chelly J, Devriendt K, Fryas J-P. ARX mutations in a boy with transphenoidal encephalocele and hypopituitarism. *Clin Genet.* 2004;65:503–505.

180. Menzel O, Bekkeheien RCJ, Reymond A, Fukai N, Boye E, Kosztolanyi G et al. Knobloch Syndrome: Novel mutations in COL18A1, Evidence for genetic heterogeneity, and a functionally impaired polymorphism in endostatin. *Hum Mutation.* 2004;23:77–84.

181. Consugar MB, Kubly VJ, Lager DJ, Hommerding CJ, Wong WC, Bakker E et al. Molecular diagnostics of Meckel-Gruber syndrome highlights pehenotypic differences between MKS1 and MKS3. *Hum Genet.* 2007;121:591–599.

182. Vogt DW, Ellersieck MR, Deutsch WE, Akremi B, Islam MN. Congenital meningocele-encephalocele in an experimental swine herd. *Am J Vet Res.* 1986;47:188–191.

183. Milunsky A, Albert E, Kitzmiller JL, Younger MD, Neff RK. Prenatal diagnosis of neural tube defects. VII. The importance of serum alpha-fetoprotein screening in diabetic pregnant women. *Am J Obstet Gynecol.* 1982;142(8):103–132.

184. Miller, Hare JW, Cloherty JP, Dunn PJ, Gleason RE, Soedner JS, Kitzmiller JL. Elevated maternal hemoglobin A1C in early pregnancy and major congenital anomalies in infants of diabetic mothers. *N Eng J Med.* 1981;304:1331–1334.

185. Evrard P, Caviness VS Jr. Extensive developmental defect of the cerebellum associated with posterior fossa ventriculocele. *J Neuropath Exper Neurol.* 1974;33:385–399.

186. Fisher NL, Smith DW. Occipital encephalocele and early gestational hyperthermia. *Pediatrics.* 1981;68:480–483.

187. Sandford MK, Kissling GE, Joubert PE. Neural tube defect etiology: new evidence concerning maternal hyperthermia, health and diet. *Devel Med Child Neurol.* 1992;34:661–675.

188. Shiota K. Induction of neural tube defects and skeletal malformations in mice following brief hyperthermia in utero. *Biol Neonate.* 1988;53:86–97.

189. Tarara RP, Wheeldon EB, Hendrickx AG. Central nervous system malformations induced by; triamcinolone acetonide in non-human primates: pathogenesis. *Teratology.* 1988;38:259–270.

190. Coffey VP. Anencephaly or iniencephaly? *J Irish Med Assoc.* 1965;56:96.

191. Blackburn W, Maertens P, Cooley Jr NR, Barr Jr M. Studies of cranioskeletal anomalies associated with iniencephaly. *Proc Greenwood Gen Ctr.* 1995;14:87.

192. Howkins J, Lawrie RS. Iniencephalus. *J Obst Gynaec Brit Empire.* 1939;46:25–31.

193. Lemire RJ, Beckwith JB, Shepard TH. Iniencephaly and anencephaly with spinal retroflexion. A comparative study of eight human specimens. *Teratology.* 1972;6:27–36.

194. Paterson SJ. Iniencephalus. *J Obstet Gynecol Brit Emp.* 1944; 51:330–334.

195. Aleksic S, Budzilovich G, Greco MA, Feigin I, Epstein F, Pearson J. Iniencephaly. A neuropathologic study. *Clin Neuropathol.* 1983;2:55–61.

196. Mórocz I, Szeifert GT, Molńar P, Tóth Z, Csécsei K, Papp Z. Prenatal diagnosis and pathoanatomy of iniencephaly. *Clin Gen.* 1986;30:81–86.

197. Kalousek DK, Fiter N, Paradice BA. *Pathology of the Human Embryo and Previable Fetus: Am Atlas.* New York: Springer Verlag; 1990: 18–20.

198. Scherrer CC, Hammer F, Schinzel A, Briner J. Brain stem and cervical cord dysraphic lesions in iniencephaly. *Pediatr Pathol.* 1992;12:469–476.

199. Norman MG, McGillivray BC, Kalousek DK, Hill A, Poskitt KJ, Becker LE, Cochrane DD, Muenke M. *Congenital Malformations of the Brain. Pathologic, Embryologic, Clinical, Radiologic and Genetic Aspects.* New York: Oxford University Press; 1995: 126–129.

200. Gilbert-Barness E. *Potter's Pathology of the Fetus and Infant.* Vol. 2. St. Louis, MO: Mosby; 1997:1053–1054.

201. Moore CA, Li S, Li Z, Hong S-X, Gu H-Q, Berry RJ, Mulinare J, Erickson JD. Elevated rates of severe neural tube defects in a high-prevalence area in Northern China. *Am J Med Genet.* 1997;73:113–118.

202. David TJ, Nixon A. Congenital malformations associated with anencephaly and iniencephaly. *J Med Genet.* 1976;13:263–265.

203. Dolk H, De Wals P, Gillerot Y, Lechat MF, Ayme S, Cornel M, Cuschieri A, Garne E, Goujard J, Laurence KM, Lillis D, Lys F, Nevin N, Owens J, Radic A, Stoll C, Stone D, Ten Kate L. Heterogeneity of neural tube defects in Europe: the significance of site of defect and presence of other major anomalies in relation to geographic differences in prevalence. *Teratology.* 1991; 44:547–559.

204. Doğan MM, Ekici E, Yapar EG, Soysal ME, Soysal SK, Gökmen O. Iniencephaly: sonographic-pathologic correlation of 19 cases. *J Perinta Med.* 1996;24:501–511.

205. Erdincter P, Kaynar MY, Canbaz B, Kocer N, Kaday C, Ciplak N. Iniencephaly: neuroradiological and surgical features. Case report and review of the literature. *J Neuro Surg.* 1998;89:317–320.

206. Sahid S, Sepulveda W, Dezerega V, Gutierrez J, Rodriguez L, Corral E. Iniencephaly: prenatal diagnosis and management. *Prenat Diag.* 2000;20:202–205.

207. Seller MJ, Kalousek DK. Neural tube defects: heterogeneity and homogeneity. *Amer J Med Genet.* 1986;2:77–87.

208. McDonnell RJ, Johnson Z, Delaney V, Dack P. East Ireland 1980–1994: epidemiology of neural tube defects. *J Epid Comm Health.* 1999;53:782–788.

209. Katz VL, Aylsworth AS, Albright SG. Iniencephaly is not uniformly fatal. *Prenatal Diagnosis.* 1989;9:595–599.

210. Sherk HH, Shut L, Chung S. Iniencephalic deformity of the cervical spine with Klippel-Feil anomalies and congenital elevation of the scapula: report of three cases. *J Bone Jt Surg.* 1974; 56:1254–1259.

211. Sepulveda W, Corrall E, Ayala C, Be C, Gútierrez J, Vasquez P. Chromosomal abnormalities in fetuses with open neural tube

defects: prenatal identification with ultrasound. *Ultrasound Obstet Gynecol.* 2004;23:352–356.

212. Seller MJ, Mazzaschi R, Ogilvie CM, Mohammed S. A Trisomy 2 fetus with severe neural tube defects and other abnormalities. *Clin Dysmorphol.* 2004;13:25–27.

213. Halder A, Agarwal S, Pandey A. Iniencephaly and chromosome mosaicism: a report of two cases. *Cong Anomalies.* 2005;45:102–105.

214. Phadke SR, Thakur S. Prenatal diagnosis of iniencephaly and alobar holoprosencephaly with Trisomy 13 mosaicism: a case report. *Prenat Diag.* 2002;22:1238–1241.

215. Schneider A, Goodwin D, Ug-Putong A. Iniencephaly and thoraco-lumbosacral meningomyelocele in a sibship. *Am J Hum Genet.* 1987;41(Suppl 3): A82.

216. Bryne J, Warburton D. Neural tube defects in spontaneous abortions. *Am J Med Genet.* 1986;25:327–333.

217. Chapman PH. Congenital intraspinal lipomas. Anatomic considerations and surgical treatment. *Child's Brain.* 1982; 9:37–47.

218. Schut L, Bruce DA, Sutton LN. The management of the child with a lipomyelomeningocele. *Clin Neurosurgery.* 1982;30:464–476.

219. Hoffman HJ, Taecholarn C, Hendrick EB, Humphreys RP. Management of lipomyelomeningoceles. Experience at the Hospital for Sick Children, Toronto. *J Neurosurg.* 1985;62:1–8.

220. Pierre-Kahn A, Lacombe J, Pichon J, Givdicelli Y, Renier D, Sainte-Rose C et al. Intraspinal lipomas with spina bifida. Prognosis and treatment in 73 cases. *J Neurosurgery.* 1986;65:756–761.

221. Kanev PM, Lemire RJ, Loeser JD, Berger MS. Management and long-term follow-up review of children with lipomyelomeningocele, 1952–1987. *J Neurosurg.* 1990;73:48–52.

222. Foster LS, Kogan BA, Cogen PH, Edwards MSB. Bladder function in patients with lipomyelomeningocele. *J Urol.* 1990;143:984–986.

223. Kanev PM, Bierbrauer KS. Reflections on the natural history of lipomyelomeningocele. *Pediatr Neurosurg.* 1995;22:137–140.

224. Chapman PH, Davis KR. Surgical treatment of spinal lipomas in childhood. *Pediatric Neurosurg.* 1993;19:267–275.

225. Lorber J. The prognosis of encephalocele. *Dev Med Child Neurol Suppl.* 1967;13:75–86.

226. Tubbs RS, Wellons JC III, Oakes WJ. Occipital encephalocele, lipomeningomyelocele, and Chiari I malformation: case report and review of the literature. *Childs Nerv Syst.* 2003;19:50–53.

227. Seeds JW, Powers SK. Early prenatal diagnosis of familial lipomyelomeningocele. *Obstet Gynecol.* 1988;72:469–471.

228. McLone DG. Congenital malformations of the central nervous system. *Clin Neurosurg.* 2000;47:346–377.

229. Juriloff DM, Harris MJ. Mouse models for neural tube closure defects. *Hum Mol Gen.* 2000;9:993–1000.

230. Forrester MB, Merz RD. Descriptive epidemiology of lipomyelomeningocele, Hawaii, 1986–2001. *Birth Def Res (Part A): Clin Mol Terat.* 2004;70:953–956.

231. McNeely PD, Howes WJ. Ineffectiveness of dietary folic acid supplementation on the incidence of lipomyelomeningocele: pathogenetic implications. *J Neurosurg (Pediatrics 2).* 2004;100:98–100.

232. George TM, Wolpert CM, Worley G, Mackey JF, Fuchs HE, Speer MC. Variable presentation of neural tube defects in three families. *Amer J Hum Genet.* 1996;59:A93.

233. Sebold CD, Melvin EC, Siegel D, Mehltretter L, Enterline DS, Nye JS, et al. Recurrence risks for neural tube defects in siblings in patients with lipomyelomeningocele. *Genet Med.* 2005;7:64–67.

234. Forrester MB, Merz RD. Precurrence risk of neural tube defects in siblings of infants with lipomyelomeningocele. *Genet Med.* 2005;7:457.

235. Carter BS, Steward JM. Valproic acid prenatal exposure: association with lipomyelomeningocele. *Clin Pediatr.* 1989;28:81–85.

236. Gupta DK, Mahapatra AK. Terminal myelocystoceles: a series of 17 cases. *J Neurosurg (Pediatrics 4).* 2005;100:344–352.

237. Kim SY, McGahan JP, Boggan JE, McGrew W. Prenatal diagnosis of lipomyelomeningocele. *J Ultrasound Med.* 2000;19:801–805.

238. McComb JG. Spinal and cranial neural tube defects. *Semin Pediatr Neurol.* 1997;4:156–166.

239. Botto LD, Moore CA, Khoury MJ, Erickson JD. Neural-tube defects. *N Engl J Med.* 1999;341:1509–1519.

240. Tortori-Donati P, Rossi A, Cama A. Spinal dysraphism: a review of neuroradiological features with embryological correlations and proposal for a new classification. *Neuroradiology.* 2000;42:471–491.

241. O'Rahilly R, Müller F. *Human Embryology & Teratology.* New York: Wiley-Liss; 2001: 435–453.

242. Moore CA. Classification of Neural Tube Defects. In: Wyszynski DF, ed. *Neural Tube Defects from Origin to Treatment.* New York: Oxford University Press; 2006: 66–75.

243. Tori JA, Dickson JH. Association of congenital anomalies of the spine and kidneys. *Clin Orthopaed Rel Res.* 1980;148:259–262.

244. Hall JG, Friedman JM, Kenna BA, Popkin J, Jawanda M, Arnold W. Clinical, genetic, and epidemiological factors in neural tube defects. *Am J Hum Genet.* 1988;43:827–837.

245. Dok H, De Wals P, Gillerot Y, Lechat MF, Ayme S, Cornel M et al. Heterogeneity of neural tube defects in Europe: the significance of site of defect and presence of other anomalies in relation to geographic differences in prevalence. *Teratology.* 1991;44:547–559.

246. Nelson K, Holmes LB. Malformations due to presumed spontaneous mutations in newborn infants. *N Engl J Med.* 1989;320:19–23.

247. Carter CO, Evans K. Children of adult survivors with spina bifida cystica. *Lancet.* 1973;ii:924–926.

248. Gupta DK, Mahapatra AK. Terminal myelocystoceles: a series of 17 cases. *J Neurosurg.* 2005;103:344–352.

249. Fidas A, MacDonald HL, Elton RA, Wild SR, Chisholm GD, Scott R. Prevalence and patterns of spina bifida occulta in 2707 normal adults. *Clin Radiol.* 1987;38:537–542.

250. Sanli AM, Kertimen H, Karavelioglu E, Sekerci Z. Giant true dorsal thoracic meningocele in a school-age child. Case report. *J Neurosurg Pediatr.* 2008;1:399–.

251. Dennis M, Landry SH, Barnes M, Fletcher JM. A model of neurocognitive function in spina bifida over the life span. *J Internat Neuropsychol Soc.* 2006;12:285–296.

252. Hall JG, Friedman JM, Kenna BA, Popkin J, Jawanda M, Arnold W. Clinical, genetic, and epidemiological factors in neural tube defects. *Am J Hum Genet.* 1988;43:827–837.

253. Davies BR, Durán M. Malformations of the cranium, vertebral column, and related central nervous system: morphologic heterogeneity may indicate biological diversity. *Birth Def Res (Part A): Clin Mol Terat.* 2003;67:563–571.

254. Tori JA, Dickson JH. Association of congenital anomalies of the spine and kidneys. *Clin Orthopaed Rel Res.* 1980;148:259–262.

255. Czeizel A. Schisis-Association. *Am J. Med Genet.* 1981;10:25–35.

256. Martínez-Frías ML. Spina bifida and hypospadias: a non random association or an X-Linked recessive condition? *Am J Med Genet.* 1994;52:5–8.

257. Holmes LB, Driscoll S, Atkins L. Etiologic heterogeneity of neural tube defects. *N Engl J Med.* 1976;294:365–369.

258. Martin RA, Fineman RM, Jorde LB. Phenotypic heterogeneity in neural tube defects: a clue to causal heterogeneity. *Am J Med Genet.* 1983;16:519–525.

259. Kibar Z, Capra V, Gros P. Toward understanding the genetic basis of neural tube defects. *Clin Genet.* 2007;71:295–310.

260. O'Rahilly R, Müller F. *Developmental Stages in Human Embryos, including a Revision of Streeter's "Horizons" and a Survey of the Carnegie Collection.* Washington, DC: Carnegie Institution of Washington, Publication No. 637, 1987.

261. O'Rahilly R, Müller F. "Neuroschisis" in human embryos. *Teratology.* 1988;38:189.

262. Osaka K, Matsumoto S, Tanimura T. Myeloschisis in early human embryos. *Child's Brain.* 1978;4:374–359.

263. Van Allen MI, Kalousek D, Chernof GF, Juriloff D, Harris M, McGillivray BC, Yong S-L, Langlois S, MacLeod PM, Chitayat D, Friedman JM, Wilson RD, McFadden D, Pandtzan J, Ritchie S, Hall JG. Evidence for multi-site closure of the neural tube in humans. *Am J Med Genet.* 1993;47:723–743.

264. Martínez-Frías M-L, Urioste M, Bermejo E, Sanchis A, Rodriguez-Pinilla E. Epidemiological analysis of multi-site closure failure of neural tubes in humans. *Am J Med Genet.* 1996;66:64–68.

265. Nakatsu T, Uwabe C, Shiota K. Neural tube closure in human initiates at multiple sites: evidence from human embryos and implications for the pathogenesis of neural tube defects. *Anat Embryol.* 2000; 201:455–466.

266. Gardner WJ, Breuer AC. Anomalies of heart, spleen, kidneys, gut, and limbs may result from an over distended neural tube: a hypothesis. *Pediatrics.* 1980; 65:508–514.

267. Harris MJ, Juriloff DM. Mouse mutants with neural tube closure defects and their role in understanding human neural tube defects. *Birth Def Res (Part A): Clin Mol Teratol.* 2007;79:187–210.

268. Copp AJ, Greene NDE, Murdoch JN. The genetic basis of mammalian neurulation. *Nature Reviews Genetics.* 2003;4:784–793.

269. Carter CO, Evans K. Spina bifida and anencephalus in Greater London. *J Med Genet.* 1973; 10:209–234.

270. Frecker M, Fraser FC. Epidemiological studies of neural tube defects in Newfoundland. *Teratology.* 1987; 36:355–361.

271. Dolk H, De Wals P, Gillerot Y, Lechat MF, Ayme S, Cornel M, Cuschieri A, Garne E, Goujard J, et al. Heterogeneity of neural tube defects in Europe: the significance of site of defect and presence of other major anomalies in relation to geographic difference in prevalence. *Teratology.* 1991;44:547–559.

272. Xiao KZ, Zhang ZY, Su YM, Liu FQ, Yan ZZ, Jian AQ et al. Central nervous system congenital malformations, especially neural tube defects in 29 provinces, metropolitan cities, and autonomous regions of China. Chinese Birth Defects Monitoring Program. *Internat J Epid.* 1990;19:978–982.

273. McDonnell RJ, Johnson Z, Delaney V, Dack P. East Ireland 1980–1994: epidemiology of neural tube defects. *J Epidemiol Comm Health.* 1999;53:782–788.

274. Williams LJ, Rasmussen SA, Flores A, Kirby RS, Edmonds LD. Decline in the prevalence of spina bifida and anencephaly by race/ethnicity: 1995–2002. *Pediatrics.* 2005;116:580–586.

275. Shaw GM, Jensvold NG, Wasserman CR, Lammer EJ. Epidemiologic characteristics of phenotypically distinct neural tube defects among 0.7 million California births, 1983–1987. *Teratology.* 1994;49:143–149.

276. Seller MJ. Neural tube defects and sex ratios. *Am J Med Genet.* 1987;26:699–707.

277. Li Z, Ren A, Zhang L, Ye R, Li S, Zheng J et al. Extremely high prevalence of neural tube defects in a 4-county area in Shanxi Province, China. *Birth Def Res (Part A): Clin Mol Teratol.* 2006;76:237–240.

278. Frey L, Hauser WA. Epidemiology of neural tube defects. *Epilepsia.* 2003;44 (Suppl 3): 4–13.

279. Knox EG. Twins and neural tube defects. *Brit J Prev Soc Med.* 1974;28:73–80.

280. Field B, Kerr C. Twinning and neural-tube defects. *Lancet.* 1974;ii:964–965.

281. Garabedian BH, Fraser FC. A familial association between twinning and upper-neural tube defects. *Am J Hum Genet.* 1994;55:1050–1053.

282. Kallen B, Cocchi G, Knudsen LB, Castilla EE, Robert E, Daltveit Ak, Lancaster PL, Mastroiacovo P. International study of sex ratio and twinning of neural tube defects. *Teratology.* 1994;50:322–331.

283. Yens S, MacMahon B. Genetics of anencephaly and spina bifida? *Lancet.* 1968;ii:623–626.

284. Schweitzer ME, Balsam D, Weiss R. Spina bifida occulta. Incidence in parents of offspring with spina bifida cystica. *Spine.* 1993;18:785–786.

285. Carter CD, Evans KA, Till K. Spinal dysraphism: genetic relation to neural tube malformations. *J Med Genet.* 1976;13:343–350.

286. Lendon RG, Wynne-Davies R, Lendon M. Are congenital vertebral anomalies and spina bifida cystica aetiologically related? *J Med Genet.* 1981;18:424–427.

287. Jensson R, Arnason A, Gunnarsdotter H, Petursdottir I, Fossdal R, Hreidarsson S. A family showing apparent X linked inheritance of both anencephaly and spina bifida. *J Med Genet.* 1988;25:227–229.

288. Fellous M, Boué J, Malbrunot C, Wollman E, Saspartes M, Van Cong N, et al. A five-generation family with sacral agenesis and spina bifida: possible similarities with the mouse T-locus. *Am J Med Genet.* 1982;12:465–487.

289. Stamm DS, Siegel DG, Mehltretter L, Connelly JJ, Trott A, Ellis N et al. Refinement of 2q and 7p loci in a large multiple NTD family. *Birth Def Res (Part A): Clin Mol Teratol.* 2008;82:441–452.

290. Kennedy D, Chitayat D, Winsor EJT, Silver M, Toi A. Prenatally diagnosed neural tube defects: ultrasound, chromosome, and autopsy or postnatal findings in 212 cases. *Am J Med Genet.* 1998;77:317–321.

291. Sepulveda W, Corral E, Ayala C, Be C, Gutierrez J, Vasquez P. Chromosomal abnormalities in fetuses with open neural tube defects: prenatal identification with ultrasound. *Ultrasound Obstet Gynecol.* 2004;23:352–356.

292. MRC Vitamin Study Research Group. Prevention of neural tube defects: results of the Medical Research Council Vitamin Study. *Lancet.* 1991;338:131–137.

293. Czeizel AE, Dudas I. Prevention of the first occurrence of neural-tube defects by periconceptional vitamin supplementation. *N Eng J Med.* 1992;327:1832–1835.

294. Relton CL, Wilding CS, Pearce MS, Laffling AJ, Jonas PA, Lynch SA, Tawn EJ, Burn J. Gene-gene interaction in folate-related genes and risk of neural tube defects in a UK population. *J Med Genet.* 2004;41:256–260.

295. Cabrera RM, Hill DS, Etheredge AJ, Finnell RH. Investigations into the etiology of neural tube defects. *Birth Def Res (Part C): Clin Mol Terat.* 2005;72:330–344.

296. Parle-McDermott A, Kirke PN, Mills JL, Molloy AM, Cox C, O'Leary VB et al. Confirmation of the R653Q polymorphism of the trifunctional C1-synthase enzyme as a maternal risk for neural tube defects in the Irish population. *Eur J Hum Genet.* 2006;14:768–772.

297. Parle-McDermott A, Pangilinan F, Mills JL, Kirke PN, Gibney ER, Troendle J et al. The 19-bp deletion polymorphism in intron-1 of dihydrofolate reductase (DHFR) may decrease rather than increase risk for spina bifida in the Irish population. *Am J Med Genet Part A.* 2007;143:1174–1180.

298. Rothenberg SR, daCosta MP, Sequeira JM, Cracco J, Roberts JL, Weedon J. Quadros EV. Autoantibodies against folate receptors in women with a pregnancy complicated by a neural-tube defect. *N Engl J Med.* 2004;350:134–142.

299. Volcik KA, Blanton SH, Kruzel MC, Townsend IT, Tyerman GH, Mier RJ, Northrup H. Testing for genetic associations with the PAX gene family in a spina bifida population. *Am J Med Genet.* 2002;110:195–202.

300. Kibar Z, Turban E, McDearmid JR, Reynolds A, Berghout J, Mathieu M et al. Mutations in VANGL1 associated with neural-tube defects. *N Engl J Med.* 2007;356:1432–1437.

301. Doudney K, Ybot-Gonzalez P, Paternotte C, Stevenson RE, Greene ND, Moore GE et al. Analysis of the planar cell polarity gene Vangl2 and its co-expressed paralogue Vangl1 in neural tube defect patients. *Am J Med Genet A.* 2005;136:90–92.

302. Chatkupt S, Lucek PR, Koenigsberger MR, Johnson WG. Prenatal sex effect in spina bifida: A role of genomic imprinting? *Am J Med Genet.* 1992;44:508–512.

303. MacMahon B, Yen S. Unrecognized epidemic of anencephaly and spina bifida. *Lancet.* 1971;i:31–33.

304. Greene MF. Spontaneous abortions and major malformations in women with diabetes mellitus. *Semin Reprod Endocrinol.* 1999;17:127–136.

305. Omtzigh JGC, Los FG, Grobbee DE, Pijperst, Jahoda MGH, Brandenburg H, Stewart PA, Gaillard HLJ, Sachs ES, Wladimiroff JW, Linddhout D. The risk of spina bifida aperta after first-trimester exposure to valproate in a prenatal cohort. *Neurology.* 1992;42 (Suppl 5): 119–125.

306. Rosa FW. Spina bifida in infants of women treated with carbamazepine during pregnancy. *N Engl J Med.* 1991;324: 674–677.

307. Saitoh A, Hull AD, Franklin P, Spector SA. Myelomeningocele in an infant with intrauterine exposure to Efavirenz. *J Perinatol.* 2005;25:555–556.

308. Waller DK, Mills JL, Simpson JL, Cunningham GC, Conley MR, Lassman MR, Rhoads GC. Are obese woman at higher risk for producing malformed offspring? *Am J Obstet Gynecol.* 1994;170:541–548.

309. Anderson JL, Waller DK, Canfield MA, Shaw GM, Watkins ML, Werler MM. Maternal obesity, gestational diabetes, and central nervous system defects. *Epidemiology.* 2005;16: 87–92.

310. Moliterno JA, DiLuna ML, Sood S, Roberts KE, Duncan CC. Gastric bypass: a risk factor for neural tube defects? Case report. *J Neurosurg Pediatrics.* 2008;1:406–409.

311. Suarez L, Felkner M, Hendricks K. The effect of fever, febrile illnesses, and heat exposures on the risk of neural tube defects in a Texas-Mexico border population. *Birth Def Res (Part A): Clin Mol Terat.* 2004;70:815–819.

312. Croen LA, Todoroff K, Shaw GM. Maternal exposure to nitrate from drinking water and diet and risk for neural tube defects. *Am J Epid.* 2001;153:325–331.

313. Ratzon NZ, Ornoy A, Pardo A, Rachel M, Hatch M. Developmental evaluation of children born to mothers occupationally exposed to waste anesthetic gases. *Birth Def Res (Part A): Clin Mol Terat.* 2004;70:476–482.

314. Renwick JH. Hypothesis: anencephaly and spina bifida are usually preventable by evidence of a specific but unidentified substance present in certain potato tubers. *Brit J Prev Soc Med.* 1972;26:67–88.

315. Clark CA, McKendrick OM, Sheppard PM. Spina bifida and potatoes. *Brit Med J.* 1973;3:251–254.

316. Berry RJ, Li Z, Erickson TD, Li S, Moore CA, Wang H et al. Prevention of neural-tube defects with folic acid in China. *N Engl J Med.* 1999;341:1485–1490.

317. Wald NJ, Law MR, Morris JK, Wald DS. Qualifying the effect of folic acid. *Lancet.* 2001;358:2069–2073.

318. De Wals P, Tairou F, Van Allen MI, Uh S-H, Lowry RB, Sibbald B, Evans JA et al. Reduction in neural-tube defects after folic acid fortification in Canada. *N Engl J Med.* 2007;357: 137–142.

319. Martínez de Villarreal L, Villarreal Pérez JZ, Arrendondo Vázquez P, Hernández Herrera R, Velazco Campos MDR, Ambriz López R et al. Decline in neural tube defects cases after a folic acid campaign in Nuevo León, Mexico. *Teratology.* 2002;66:249–256.

320. Chen LT, Ascencio Rivera M. The Costa Rican experience: reduction of neural tube defects following food fortification programs. *Nutrition Reviews.* 2004;62:S40–S43.

321. Moore CA, Li S, Liz A, Hong S-X, GH-Q, Berry RJ, Mulinare J, Erickson JD. Elevated rates of severe neural tube defects in a high-prevalence area in Northern China. *Am J Med Genet.* 1997; 73:113–118.

322. Cotter AM, Daley SF. Neural tube defects: is a decreasing prevalence associated with a decrease in severity? *Eur J Obst Gynec Reprod Biol.* 2005;119:161–163.

323. Botto LD, Olney RS, Erickson JD. Vitamin supplements and the risk for congenital anomalies other than neural tube defects. *Am J Med Genet Part C (Semin Med Genet).* 2004;125C: 12–21.

324. Candito M, Rivet R, Herbeth B, Boisson C, Rudigov R-C, Luton D et al. Nutritional and genetic determinants of vitamin B and homocysteine metabolism in neural tube defects: a multicenter case-control study. *Am J Med Genet Part A.* 2008; 140A:1128–1133.

325. Busby A, Abramsky L, Dolk H, Armstrong B, Addor MC, Anneren G, et al. Preventing neural tube defects in Europe: a missed opportunity. *Reprod Toxicol.* 2005;20:393–402.

326. Oakley GP Jr. When will we eliminate folic acid-preventable spina bifida? *Epidemiology.* 2007;18:367–368.

327. Greene NDE, Copp AJ. Inositol prevents folate-resistant neural tube defects in the mouse. *Nature Med.* 1997;3:60–66.

328. Cogram P, Hynes A, Dunlevy LPE, Greene NDE, Copp AJ. Specific isoforms of protein kinase C are essential for prevention of folate-resistant neural tube defects by inositol. *Hum Mol Genet.* 2004;13:7–14.

329. Cavelli P, Tedoldi S, Riboli B. Inositol supplementation in pregnancies at risk of apparently folate-resistant NTDs. *Birth Def Res (Part A): Clin Mol Teratol.* 2008;82:540–542.

330. Golalipour MJ, Mansourian AR. Maternal zinc deficiency and neonatal neural tube defects in Gorgan-North of Iran. *Reproduc Toxicol.* 2005;20:453–491.

331. Lehti KK. Stillbirth rates and folic acid and zinc status in low-socioeconomic pregnant women of Brazilian Amazon. *Nutrition.* 1993;9:156–158.

332. Sival DA, Begeer JH, Staal-Schreinemachers AL, Vos-Niël JM, Beekhuis JR, Prechtl HF. Perinatal motor behaviour and neurological outcome in spina bifida aperta. *Early Hum Dev.* 1997; 50:27–37.

333. Luthy DA, Wardinsky T, Sturtleff DB, Hollenbach KA, Hickok DE, Nyberg DA, Benedetti TJ. Cesarean section before the onset of labor and subsequent motor function in infants with meningomyelocele diagnosed antenally. *N Engl J Med.* 1991; 324:662–666.

334. Meuli M, Meuli-Simmen C, Hutchins GM, Yingling CD, Hoffman KM, Harrison MR, Adzick NS. In utero surgery rescues neurological function at birth in sheep with spina bifida. *Nature Medicine.* 1995;1:342–347.

335. Adzick NS, Walsh DS. Myelomeningocele: prenatal diagnosis, pathophysiology and management. *Semin Pediatr Surg.* 2003;12:168–174.

336. Fichter MA, Dornseifer U, Henke J, Schneider KT, Kovacs L, Biemer E et al. Fetal spina bifida repair—current trends and prospects of intrauterine neurosurgery. *Fetal Diagn Ther.* 2008; 23:271–286.

337. Worley G, Schuser JM, Oates WJ. Survival at 5 years of a cohort of newborn infants with myelomeningocele. *Devel Med Child Neurol.* 1996;38:816–822.

338. Hunt GM. Open spina bifida: outcome for a complete cohort treated unselectively and followed into adulthood. *Devel Med Child Neurol.* 1990;32:108–118.

339. Davis BE, Daley CM, Shurtleff DB, Duquay S, Seidel K, Loeser JD et al. Long-term survival of individuals with myelomeningocele. *Pediatr Neurosurg.* 2005;41:186–191.

340. Fletcher JM, Francis DJ, Thompson NM, Thompson NM, Brookshire BL, Bohan TP et al. Verbal and nonverbal discrepancies in hydrocephalic children. *J Clin Exp Neuropsychol.* 1992;14:593–609.

341. Hommet C, Cottier JP, Billard C, Perrier D, Gillet P, DeToffol B et al. MRI morphometric study and correlation of cognitive functions in young adults shunted for congenital hydrocephalus related to spina bifida. *Eur Neurol.* 2002;47:169–174.

342. Gupta DK, Mahapatra AK. Terminal myelocystoceles: a series of 17 cases. *J Neurosurg.* 2005;103:344–352.

343. Ardinger HH, Atkin JF, Blackston RD, Elsas LJ, Clarren SK, Livingstone S, Flannery DB et al. Verification of the fetal valproate syndrome phenotype. *Am J Med Genet.* 1988;29:171–185.

344. Bower C, Raymond M, Lumley J, Bury G. Trends in neural tube defects 1980–1989. *Med J Aust.* 1993;158:152–154.

345. Cragan JD, Roberts HE, Edmonds LD, Khoury MJ, Kirby RS, Shaw GM, Velie EM, Merz RD, Forrester MB, Williamson RA, Krishnamurti DS, Stevenson RE, Dean JH. Surveillance for anencephaly and spina bifida and the impact of prenatal diagnosis. United States, 1985–1994. *MMWR.* 1995;44:1–13.

346. Roberts HE, Moore CA, Cragan JD, Fernhoff PM, Khoury JM. Impact of prenatal diagnosis and the birth prevalence of neural tube defects, Atlanta, 1990–1991. *Pediatrics.* 1995;96:880–883.

347. Velic EM, Shaw GM. Impact of prenatal diagnosis and elective termination in prevalence and risk estimates of neural tube defects in California, 1989–1991. *Am J Epid.* 1996;144:473–479, 1996.

348. Kennedy D, Chitayat D, Winsor EJT, Silver M, Toi A. Prenatally diagnosed neural tube defects: ultrasound, chromosome, and autopsy or postnatal findings in 212 cases. *Am J Med Genet.* 1998;77:317–321.

349. Cromie WJ, Lee K, Houde K, Holmes LB. Implications of antenatal ultrasound screening in the incidence of major genitourinary malformations. *J Urol.* 2001;165:1677–1689.

350. Journel H, Parent P, Roussey M, LeMarec B. "Isolated" hydrocephalus in families and anencephaly: a coincidence? *Neuropediatrics.* 1989;70:220–222.

351. Toriello HV, Higgins JV. Occurrence of neural tube defects among first-, second-, and third-degree relatives of probands: results of a United States Study. *Am J Med Genet.* 1983;15:601–606.

352. Carter Co, Evans K. Children of adult survivors with spina bifida cystica. *Lancet* ii:924–926, 1973.

353. Cowchock S, Ainbender E, Prescott G, Crandall B, Lau L, Heller R et al. The recurrence risk for neural tube defects in the United States: a collaborative study. *Am J Med Genet* 5:309–314, 1980.

354. Drainer E, May HM, Tolmil JL. Do familial neural tube defects breed true? *J Med Genet* 28:605–608, 1991.

355. Byrne J. Birth defects in uncles and aunts from Irish families with neural tube defects. *Birth Def Res (Part A): Clin Mol Teratol* 82:8–15, 2008.

356. Nadel AS, Green JK, Holmes LB, Frigoletto FD Jr, Benacerraf BR. Absence of need for amniocentesis in patients with elevated maternal serum alpha-fetoprotein and normal ultrasonic examination. *N Engl J Med* 323:557–661, 1990.

Chapter 19

Omphalocele

Definition

Herniation of abdominal viscera, especially intestines, through a widened umbilical ring into a translucent sac at the top of which is the umbilical cord (Figure 19–1).

ICD-9:   756.700   (omphalocele)

ICD-10:   Q79.2   (omphalocele)

Mendelian   164750   (omphalocele, isolated)
Inheritance
in Man:

                310980   (omphalocele, X–linked)

Appearance

The abdominal contents have herniated through the umbilical ring and are covered by a translucent membrane that consists of amnion on the outside and Wharton's jelly and peritoneum on the inside (1–3). The umbilical cord is always at the top or vertex of the protrusion.

By comparison, an umbilical hernia is skin-covered and in gastroschisis, the defect is lateral to the umbilical cord, and not covered by a membrane.

There are three locations of omphalocele: a) central (the most common and the focus of this summary); b) epigastric (a high abdominal location that is just below the sternum and a feature of the Pentalogy of Cantrell); c) hypogastric [5, 6]). In a case series of 90 affected fetuses identified by prenatal screening in Norway (1985–1994) [4], there were 58 (64%) central, 32 (36%) epigastric, and none (0%) had a hypogastric omphalocele.

The hypogastric type of omphalocele is located in the lower abdomen just above the exstrophied bladder, as in cloacal exstrophy. Cloacal exstrophy is a rare, multiple anomaly syndrome that may include exstrophy of

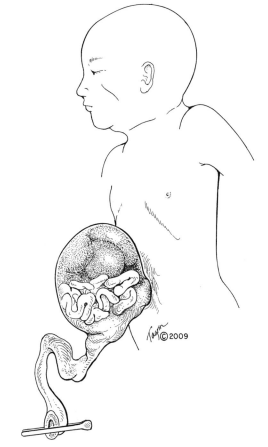

FIGURE 19.1 A diagram of omphalocele that shows intestine and liver in the membrane-covered protrusion. Note the umbilical cord emerges from the top of the omphalocele sack.

the bladder, divided genital structures, imperforate anus, gastrointestinal anomalies, and meningocystocele.

The central omphalocele has been subdivided, by size, into three groups: small, "giant" (over 6 centimeters in diameter), and the common type (Figure 19-1

263

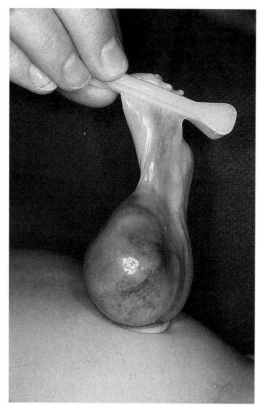

FIGURE 19.2 Shows a newborn infant with an omphalocele just before surgical repair. (Courtesy of W. Hardy Hendren, MD., Massachusetts General Hospital, Boston, MA.)

and 19.2), which is typically at least 4 centimeters in diameter.

The size and contents of the omphalocele are important in establishing prognosis (5–7). The small omphalocele, which contains only intestine, has a good prognosis (7). However, there can be significant complications even in the small omphaloceles. In a series of 45 affected infants (8), there were 8 (18%) with a Meckel diverticulum, 7 (16%) with malrotation, including necrotic bowel in 3 (6%), and ileal atresia in one (2%).

In general, when the omphalocele contains only intestine, there is a higher likelihood of chromosome abnormalities. Combining the findings in four studies, 87% of the fetuses with omphaloceles that contained only bowel had a chromosome abnormality in comparison to 9% when the omphalocele contained liver and intestines (9).

The "giant" omphalocele has the most associated problems, such as respiratory insufficiency requiring ventilation, and is the most difficult type of omphalocele to repair (6).

Associated Malformations

The presence of malrotation of the bowel or bowel atresia, due to vascular occlusion, is related to the occurrence of the omphalocele and is not considered an associated malformation. 30 to 70% of infants with omphalocele have associated major malformations, primarily heart defects, brain anomalies, and neural tube defects (10–22).

In general, the associated anomalies (24) and respiratory insufficiency at birth are the major predictors of the prognosis in the affected infant.

Omphalocele associated with neural tube defects has been reported to be much more common in the British Isles than in European populations. The neural tube defects have included spina bifida, anencephaly, and iniencephaly (14, 15, 25).

Omphalocele occurs in association with several specific phenotypes, including Beckwith-Wiedemann Syndrome (MIM #130650), Cantrell's Pentalogy (ectopia cordis, bifid sternum, anterior diaphragmatic hernia, omphalocele, and heart defects), and cloacal exstrophy (MIM 258040). In a series of 127 affected infants evaluated at a tertiary referral center from 1981 to 1999 in Florida (21), the frequencies were 12% Beckwith-Wiedemann, 9% Pentalogy of Cantrell, and 4% cloacal exstrophy. In Taiwan (1990–2000), among 50 affected infants, 6% had Beckwith-Wiedemann Syndrome and 6% had cloacal exstrophy (26) [Table 19–1].

Omphalocele associated with segmental intestinal dilation appears to be a separate type of omphalocele. In this disorder, the large cystic bowel impedes closure of the normal physiologic umbilical hernia (27). There is a sharp delineation between normal and dilated bowel, as the dilated segments are 3 to 4 times the normal diameter. There is normal intestinal innervation. Resection of the dilated segment is an effective treatment.

Developmental Defect

An omphalocele represents an abnormal persistence of intestine through the umbilical ring (1, 2). Normally, the midgut elongates into the base of the body stalk after six weeks gestation because of the limited amount of intra-abdominal space due to the relatively large liver and kidneys. The herniated intestine returns normally to the abdominal cavity by 12 weeks gestation (1, 2). This ventral wall defect is attributed to failure of migration and fusion of the two lateral embryonic folds of the anterior abdominal wall. The sac covering the herniated intestine is made up of the epithelium of the umbilical cord. The transparent membrane has two layers, peritoneum and amnion.

The experimental knockout of two genes *podocalyxin* and *calreticulin*, in mice (28, 29), has produced phenotypes that include omphalocele. *Podocalyxin* (*podx1*) is a CD34-related sialomucin that is expressed in podocytes, vascular endothelia, and hematopoietic stem cells. *Podx1* (-/-) deficient knockout mice had a high incidence of omphalocele and renal failure (29). Mice deficient in *calreticulin*, a protein implicated in calcium signaling

TABLE 19-1 *Etiologic heterogeneity of omphalocele*

	Eastern France (22) 1979–2003 (334,262 births) n = 86	Taiwan (26) 1990–2000 n = 50	Boston, Brigham and Women's Hospital 1972–1974, 1979–2000 (206,244)* n = 71
I) Mendelian disorders	(4) (4.7%)	0	(4) (5.7%)
1. CHARGE Syndrome	1		
2. Goltz Syndrome	1		
3. Meckel-Gruber Syndrome	1		
4. Oto-palato-digital type II	1		
5. Fanconi Anemia			1
6. Melnick-Needles Syndrome			1 (ref. 23; Figure 19-5)
7. Acrocallosal Syndrome			1
8. Simpson-Golabi-Behuel Syndrome			1
II) Specific Syndromes	(8) (9.3%)	(6) (12%)	(5) (7.1%)
1. Amniotic band syndrome (incl. Limb-Body Wall Syndrome)	1	0	1
2. Beckwith-Wiedemann Syndrome	1	3	1
3. Cloacal exstrophy or bladder exstrophy	3	3	1
4. Pentalogy of Cantrell	2	0	1
5. Marshall-Smith Syndrome	1	0	0
6. Prune-belly Syndrome	0	0	1
III) Chromosome abnormalities	(25) (29%)	(6) (12%)	(14) (20%)
trisomy 18	17	2	6
trisomy 13	5	4	3
45,X	0	0	1
Other	3	0	4
IV) Environmental exposures	(1) (1.2%)	(0)	(4) (5.7%)
valproate	1		
misoprostol			1**
infants of diabetic mothers			3
V) Twinning	0	Not stated	(3) (4.2%) MZ: 1 with acardia (healthy twin with omphalocele); 1 twin with omphalocele and congenital diaphragmatic hernia DZ: 1 discordant
VI) Unknown etiology			
1. isolated	22 (25.6%)	26 (52%)	21 (30%)
2. multiple anomalies	26 (30.2%)	12 (24%)	7 (10%)
3. phenotype unknown			12 (17.1%)
	86 (100%)	50 (100%)	71 (99.8%)

Legends: * The affected infants were identified by the Active Malformations Surveillance Program among 206,244 liveborn and stillborn infants and elective terminations for fetal anomalies at Brigham and Women's Hospital in Boston. Affected infants whose mothers had planned to deliver at another hospital, before the prenatal detection of the anomalies, were excluded.

** Infant reported by Genest DR, Richardson A, Rosenblatt M, Holmes LB. Terminal transverse limb defects with tethering and omphalocele in a 17-week fetus following first trimester misoprostol exposure. *Clinical Dysmorphology.* 1999;8:53–58.

and other cellular functions, develop omphalocele, neural tube defects, and heart defects (29).

Prevalence, Race and Ethnicity

To determine the prevalence of omphalocele, it is essential to identify separately these similar, but different, phenotypes: omphalocele, gastroschisis, and limb-body-wall complex. In addition, pregnancies with affected fetuses that were terminated electively after prenatal diagnosis must be included in the total prevalence rate. Using this approach, the reported prevalence rates have included: 0.29/1,000 in Australia (1980–1990) [13] and 0.25/1,000 in Europe (1980–1990; 2,905,866 births) [15].

There was a somewhat lower prevalence rate of 0.18/1,000 among Pacific Islanders in Hawaii (1986–1997; 61,000 births) [17].

In Japan, the rate was much lower, specifically 0.03/1,000 in the years 1975–1980 and increased to 0.06/1,000 births in 1996–1997 (19).

Birth Status

In a population-based study in France (1979–1998), infants with omphalocele had a decreased head size, length, and weight in comparison to controls (30).

An increased frequency of stillbirths has been observed in infants with all types of omphalocele (18, 22, 31), including the "giant" omphalocele in particular (6).

Sex Ratio

No consistent pattern of the ratio of affected males and females has been observed. In Europe (25) and Taiwan (26), there were more affected males than females (M: F = 1.21 and 2.00 respectively), and in Hawaii (17), more affected females than males (M: F = 0.86).

Parental Age

A U–shaped curve showing a higher rate of occurrence among the infants of both young and older mothers was observed in Finland (11). Omphalocele associated with chromosome abnormalities was highest among mothers over 40. Omphalocele not associated with aneuploidy was most common in the—age group 30–34 years in the North of England (1986–1999) [18]. There was, also, a higher rate of occurrence among young women (<20); this increase was not as dramatic as for gastroschisis.

Twinning

In a case series of 127 affected infants in Florida (1982–1999), 7.1% were twins (8 dizygous [DZ]; 1 monozygous [MZ]). All twin pairs were discordant for omphalocele (21). Both of the MZ twins were malformed: Twin A had omphalocele and twin B had cloacal exstrophy, including bladder exstrophy, imperforate anus, and anomalies of vertebrae.

Genetic Factors

Among the families of 127 affected infants in Florida, two infants (1.6%) had an affected first-degree relative: a mother of one and a sister of the other (21).

A few families have had multiple affected individuals with nonsyndromic omphalocele in successive generations (32). In several other families, there have been affected sibs whose parents were not affected (33). In one

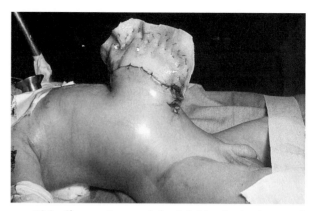

FIGURE 19.3   Shows a giant omphalocele held up by the clamp on the umbilical cord. (Courtesy of W. Hardy Hendren, M.D., Massachusetts General Hospital, Boston, MA.)

family, two affected half-siblings had a healthy father; their mothers were not related (34).

The family studies in two studies (22, 34) showed an increased frequency of major malformations other than omphalocele among the sibs and parents of infants with omphalocele. The basis for this apparent increase has not been established.

Chromosome abnormalities, especially trisomy 18 and trisomy 13, have been present in 10 to 40% of affected infants (Figure 19–4) (5, 9, 22, 36, 37). Infants whose omphalocele does not contain the liver, have been much less likely to have an associated chromosome abnormality. For example, in the series of 58 infants with central omphalocele and 32 with epigastric omphalocele, the frequency of chromosome abnormalities were 69% and 13% respectively (4). In a study of affected fetuses identified prenatally, the frequency of chromosome abnormalities was 39% at 12 weeks gestation, 28% at 20 weeks and 14% in live births (37).

PITX2 is a candidate gene for omphalocele, as mutations in *PITX2* cause the Rieger Syndrome (MIM #180500), one feature of which is abnormalities of the

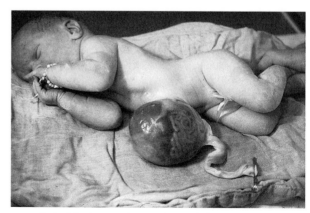

FIGURE 19.4   Newborn infant with omphalocele as a feature of trisomy 13.

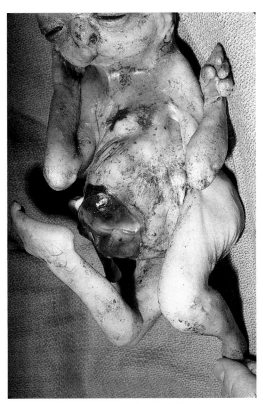

FIGURE 19.5 Stillborn infant with omphalocele as a feature of Melnick-Needles Syndrome (ref 23). Limb contractures due to oligohydramnios.

Prevention

25 children with omphalocele had a higher frequency of polymorphisms of methylene tetrahydrofolate reductase (MTHFR), methylenetetrahydrofolate dehydrogenase (MTHFD1), the reduced folate carrier (SLC19A1) and transcobalamin II (TCN2), than 59 controls, suggesting a mechanism by which periconceptual supplements with multivitamins and folic acid could decrease the occurrence of some cases of omphalocele (42). This hypothesis was tested in a population-based study (43). Periconceptional multivitamin use was associated with a 60% reduction in the risk for nonsyndromic omphalocele.

Treatment and Prognosis

Vaginal delivery has not been shown to affect the outcome of the infant with omphalocele (44, 45).

The repair of "giant" omphalocele remains a challenge. Some surgeons recommend early reconstruction (46), using bipedicled flaps of abdominal skin, and others use the silo technique in delayed closure (47, 48) (Figure 19-3).

The overall survival rate in a population-based survey in eastern France was 24% among 58 affected infants born between 1977 and 1998; 52% of the pregnancies were terminated (30). In a case series of 36 affected infants from North Carolina (1988–2001) and with no chromosome abnormalities (47), the perinatal mortality was 19%. Associated anomalies and chromosome abnormalities were associated with higher morbidity and mortality, as in several previous studies.

The overall prognosis of the affected infant correlates with the presence of respiratory insufficiency at birth in infants with any size omphalocele. Infants who survive long periods of mechanical ventilation after birth have an increased frequency of respiratory problems, including asthma, recurrent infections, and bronchomalacia (6). Feeding problems and gastroesophageal reflux are common in these chronically ill children. There is an increased frequency of developmental delay and learning disabilities, although specific estimates of the frequency have not been established.

abdominal wall (39). In addition, *PITX2* knockout mice have failure of closure of the abdominal wall and evisceration of abdominal contents (39). No mutations that changed amino acid sequence were identified by screening coding and non-coding regions of *PITX2* in 209 patients with omphalocele (40).However, a three nucleotide deletion was found in the *3 UTR* of *PITX2* of a child with omphalocele, esophageal atresia, patent ductus arteriosus, agenesis of the right kidney, and limb deficiencies of the right hand and fingers.

Four individuals with otopalatodigital syndrome (OPD), type 2 (MIM #304120) with an associated omphalocele were found to have a missense mutation in exon 5 of the FLNA gene (40) [Filamin A]. However, no mutations in this exon of FLNA were found in 179 other individuals with omphalocele who did not have OPD, type 2.

Environmental Factors

Maternal insulin-dependent diabetes has been associated with an increased frequency of omphalocele (Table 19–1).

Another risk factor for the occurrence of omphalocele is prepregnancy obesity. In one study (41), women with a body mass index (BMI) over 30 had a two-fold increase risk for having an infant with omphalocele and other anomalies (odds ratio 2.03; 95% CI 1.08–3.81).

Genetic Counseling

Most affected infants are diagnosed during pregnancy, typically by prenatal screening by ultrasound. The counseling during pregnancy should include a discussion of the many potential phenotypes and etiologies (Table 19–1). Chromosome analysis will rule out the important possibility of an associated chromosome abnormality. The high perinatal mortality and complications among survivors makes the prognosis guarded. However, there can be more optimism if the omphalocele is small and there is no associated chromosome abnormality.

The evaluation at birth should include a systematic search for the presence of associated malformations. The features of specific associated syndromes must be looked for and tested for.

The location of the omphalocele predicts the most likely associated syndrome: a central omphalocele with Beckwith-Wiedemann Syndrome, an epigastric omphalocele with the Pentalogy of Cantrell and a low lying omphalocele with cloacal exstrophy.

The empiric recurrence risk after the birth of one affected infant appears to be very low, but no specific rates have been established.

The sensitivity of the prenatal detection of omphalocele by ultrasonography has improved significantly in recent years. In eastern France (22), 52% of the fetuses with omphalocele were identified in prenatal studies in 1982–1989 and 87% between 1990 and 1999.

REFERENCES

1. O'Rahilly R, Muller F. *Human Embryology and Teratology.* New York: Wiley–Liss; 2001: 259.

2. Moore KL, Persaud TVN. *The Developing Human: Clinically Oriented Embryology.* 7th ed. Philadelphia: W.B. Saunders Co.; 2003: 271–275, 282–285.

3. deVries PA. The pathogenesis of gastroschisis and omphalocele. *J Pediat Surg.* 1980;15:245–251.

4. Brantberg A, Blaas H-GK, Haugen SE, Eik-Nes SH. Characteristics and outcome of 90 cases of fetal omphalocele. *Ultrasound Obstet Gynecol.* 2005;26:527–537.

5. Tsakayannis DE, Zurakowski D, Lillehei CW. Respiratory insufficiency at birth: a predictor of mortality for infants with omphalocele. *J Pediatr Surg.* 1996;31:1088–1091.

6. Baird J-M, Wilson RD, Johnson MP, Hedrick HL, Schwarz U, Flake AW et al. Prenatally diagnosed giant omphaloceles: short– and long–term outcomes. *Prenat Diagn.* 2004;24:434–439.

7. Boyd PA, Bhattacharjee A, Gould S, Manning N, Chamberlain P. Outcome of prenatally diagnosed anterior abdominal wall defects. *Arch Dis Child Fetal Neonatal Ed.* 1998;78:F209–F213.

8. Wakhlu A, Wakhlu AK. The management of exomphalos. *J Pediatr Surg.* 2000;35:73–76.

9. Getachew MM, Goldstein RB, Edge VL, Goldberg JD, Filly RA. Correlation between omphalocele contents and karyotypic abnormalities: Sonographic study in 37 cases. *Am J Roentgen.* 1991;158:133–136.

10. Baird P, MacDonald EC. An epidemiologic study of congenital malformations of the anterior abdominal wall in more than half a million consecutive live births. *Am J Hum Genet.* 1981;33:470–478.

11. Hemminki K, Saloniemi I, Kyyrönen P, Kekomäki M. Gastroschisis and omphalocele in Finland in the 1970s: prevalence at birth and its correlates. *J Epid Comm Health.* 1982;36:289–293.

12. Martinez-Frias ML, Salvador J, Prieto L, Zaplana J. Epidemiological study of gastroschisis and omphalocele in Spain. *Teratology.* 1984;29:377–382.

13. Byron–Scott R, Haan E, Chan A, Bower C, Scott H, Clark K. A population-based study of abdominal wall defects in South Australia and Western Australia. *Paediatr Perinat Epidemiol.* 1998;12:136–151.

14. Calzolari E, Bianchi F, Dolk H, Milan M and EUROCAT Working Group. Omphalocele and gastroschisis in Europe: a survey of 3 million births 1980–1990. *Am J Med Gen.* 1995;58:187–194.

15. Calzolari E, Bianchi F, Dolk H, Stone D, Milan M and EUROCAT Working Group. Are omphalocele and neural tube defects related congenital anomalies? Data from 21 registries in Europe (EUROCAT). *Am J Med Genet.* 1997;72:79–84.

16. Morrow RJ, Whittle MJ, McNay MB, Raine PAM, Gibson AAM, Crossley J. Prenatal diagnosis and management of anterior abdominal wall defects in the West of Scotland. Prenat Diag 1 Forrester MB, Merz RD. Epidemiology of abdominal wall defects, Hawaii, 1986–1997. *Teratology.* 1999;60:117–123.

17. Forrester MB, Merz RD. Epidemiology of abdominal wall defects, Hawaii, 1986–1997. *Teratology.* 1999;60:117–123.

18. Rankin J, Dillon E, Wright C. Congenital anterior abdominal wall defects in the North of England, 1986–1996: occurrence and outcome. *Prenat Diag.* 1999;19:662–668.

19. Suita S, Okamatsa T, Yamamoto T, Handa N, Nirasawa Y, Watanbe Y et al. Changing profile of abdominal wall defects in Japan: results of a national survey. *J Pediatr Surg.* 2000;35:66–71.

20. Goldkrand JW, Causey TN, Hull EE. The changing face of gastroschisis and omphalocele in southeast Georgia. *J Mat-Fet Neonat Med.* 2004;15:331–335.

21. Hwang P-J, Kousseff BG. Omphalocele and gastroschisis: an 18 year review study. *Genet Med.* 2004;6:232–236.

22. Stoll C, Almbik Y, Dott B, Roth MP. Omphalocele and gastroschisis and associated malformations. *Am J Med Gen Part A.* 2008;146A:1280–1285.

23. Van Oeyen P, Holmes LB, Trelstad RL, Griscom NT. Omphalocele and multiple severe congenital anomalies associated with osteodysplasty (Melnick–Needles Syndrome). *Am J Med Genet.* 1982; 13:453–463.

24. Tucci M, Bard H. The associated anomalies that determine prognosis in congenital omphaloceles. *Am J Ob Gyn.* 1990;163: 1646–1649.

25. Dolk H, de Wals P, Gillerot Y, Lechat M, Ayme S, Cornel M et al. Heterogeneity of neural tube defects in Europe: the significance of site of defect and presence of other major anomalies in relation to geographic differences in prevalence. *Teratology.* 1991;44: 547–559.

26. Hsu C-C, Lin S–P, Chen C–H, Chi C–S, Lee H–C, Hung H–Y et al. Omphalocele and gastroschisis in Taiwan. *Eur J Pediatr.* 2002;161:552–555.

27. Basaran UN, Sayin C, Oner N, Celtik C. Segmental intestinal dilation associated with omphalocele. *Pediatrics Int.* 2005;47: 227–229.

28. Doyonnas R, Kershaw DB, Duhme C, Merkens H, Chelliah S, Graf T et al. Anuria, omphalocele, and perinatal lethality in mice lacking the cd34-related protein podocalyxin. *J Exp Med.* 2001; 194:13–27.

29. Rauch F, Prud'homme J, Arabian A, Dedhar S, St–Arnaud R. Heart, brain, and body wall defects in mice lacking calreticulin. *Exp Cell Res.* 2000;256:105–111.

30. Stoll C, Alembik Y, Dott B, Roth MP. Risk factors in congenital abdominal wall defects (omphalocele and gastroschisis): a study in a series of 265,858 consecutive births. *Ann de Génét.* 2001; 44:201–208.

31. McKeown T, McMahon BK, Record BG. An investigation of 69 cases of exomphalos. *Am J Hum Genet.* 1953;5:168–175.

32. Kanagawa SL, Begleiter ML, Ostlie DJ, Holcomb G, Drake W, Butler MG. Omphalocele in three generations with autosomal dominant transmission. *J Med Genet.* 2002;39:184–185.

33. DiLiberti JH. Familial omphalocele: analysis of risk factors and case report. *Am J Med Gen.* 1982;13:263–268.

34. Kapur S, Higgins JV, Scott-Emuakpor AB, Dolanski EA. Omphalocele in half-siblings. *Clin Gen.* 1980;18:88–90.

35. Yang P, Beaty TH, Khoury MJ, Chee E, Stewart W, Gordis L. Genetic-epidemiologic study of omphalocele and gastroschisis: evidence for heterogeneity. *Am J Med Gen.* 1992;44:668–675.

36. St-Vil D, Shaw KS, Lallier M, Yazbeck S, Di Lorenzo M, Grignon A, Blanchard H. Chromosomal anomalies in newborns with omphalocele. *J Pediat Surg.* 1996;31:831–834.

37. Snijders RJ, Sebire NJ, Sonka A, Santiago C, Nicolaides KH. Field examphalos and chromosomal defects: relationship to maternal age and gestation. *Ultrasound Obstet Gynecol.* 1995;6: 250–255.

38. Amendt BA, Semina EV, Alward WLM. Rieger syndrome: a clinical, molecular, and biochemical analysis. *CMLS Cell Mol Life Sc.* 2000;57:1652–1666.

39. Kitamura K, Miura H, Miyagawa-Tomita S, Yanasawa M, Katoh–Fukui Y, Suzuki R et al. Mouse PitX2 deficiency leads to anomalies of the ventral body wall, heart, extra and periocular mesoderm and right pulmonary isomerism. *Development.* 1999; 16:5749–5758.

40. Katz LA, Schultz RE, Semina EV, Torfs CP, Kahn KN, Murray JC. Mutations in PITX2 may contribute to cases of omphalocele and VATER-like syndromes. *Am J Med Genet.* 2004;130A: 277–283.

41. Waller DK, Shaw GM, Rasmussen SA, Hobbs CA, Canfield MA, Siego-Riz A–M et al. Prepregnancy obesity as a risk factor for structural birth defects. *Arch Pediatr Adolesc Med.* 2007;161: 745–750.

42. Mills JL, Druschel CM, Pangilinan F, Pass K, Cox C, Seltzer RR et al. Folate-related genes and omphalocele. *Am J Med Genet.* 2005;136A:8–11.

43. Botto LD, Mulinare J, Erickson JD. Occurrence of omphalocele in relation to maternal multivitamin use: a population-based study. *Pediatrics.* 2002;109:904–908.

44. Moretti M, Khoury A, Rodriquez J, Lobe T, Shaver D, Sibai B. The effect of mode of delivery on the perinatal outcome in fetuses with abdominal wall defects. *Am J Ob Gyn.* 1990;163: 833–838.

45. Kitchanan S, Patole SK, Muller R, Whitehall JS. Neonatal outcome of gastroschisis and exomphalos: a 10-year review. *J Paediat Child Health.* 2000;36:428–430.

46. Zama M, Gallo S, Santecchia L, Bertozzi E, Zaccara A, Trucchi A et al. Early reconstruction of the abdominal wall in giant omphalocele. *Brit Assoc Plast Surg.* 2004;57:749–753.

47. Heider AL, Strauss RA, Kuller JA. Omphalocele: clinical outcomes in cases with normal karyotypes. *Am J Obstet Gynecol.* 2004;190:135–141.

48. Pereira RM, Tatsuo ES, Simões e Silva AC, Guimarães JT, Paixão RM, Lanna JCB et al. New method of surgical delayed closure of giant omphaloceles: Lazaro da Silva's technique. *J Pediatr Surg.* 2004;39:1111–1115.

Chapter 20

Renal Agenesis/Dysgenesis

Definition

Absence or severe dysplasia of both kidneys.

ICD-9:   753.000   (bilateral renal agenesis)
            753.003   (bilateral renal agenesis/
                       dysgenesis)
            753.010   (unilateral renal agenesis)
            753.011   (unilateral renal
                       dysgenesis)
ICD-10:   Q60.0   (renal agenesis,
                       unilateral)
            Q60.1   (renal agenesis, bilateral)
            Q60.2   (renal agenesis,
                       unspecified)
            Q60.6   (Potter's Syndrome)
Mendelian   %191830   (heredity urogenital
Inheritance   adysplasia)
in Man:
            %193000   (congenital anomalies of
                       the kidney and urinary
                       tract, including
                       vesicoureteral reflux)

Historical Note

In 1946 Edith Potter (1), a pathologist at the Chicago Lying-In Hospital, published the first of several of her descriptions of the phenotype of infants with bilateral renal agenesis (2, 3). She cited several earlier descriptions of bilateral renal agenesis. She noted that males were affected more frequently, and that the physical features included a "peculiar facies," flattening of the nose, anomalies of derivatives of the Müllerian and Wolffian ducts, absence of the ureters and hypoplasia of the lungs. This was subsequently referred to as "the Potter Syndrome." She commented: "There is no apparent relationship between the embryologic development of the lungs and the ureters and kidneys. The reason for delayed differentiation of pulmonary tissue remains unexplained."

Potter (2–4) contributed further to the classification of kidney malformations by proposing four types:

I) polycystic kidney disease in familiar type, autosomal recessive;
II) multiple dysplastic kidneys;
III) polycystic kidney disease, adult type, autosomal dominant;
IV) urethral obstruction and obstructive renal dysplasia.

Subsequent experience has shown that the external appearance, described by Potter, can be produced by chronic leakage of amniotic fluid and by many conditions that cause decreased renal function, including bilateral renal dysgenesis, hypoplasia, and multicystic dysplastic kidneys.

This summary focuses on two components of this spectrum: absence of both kidneys and severe dysgenesis, referred to as bilateral agenesis/dysgenesis or a/dysgenesis (BRA/D).

Appearance

The absence of the kidney can be associated with absence of the ureter, but presence of the adrenal gland (Figure 20-1). The term severe dysgenesis refers to the presence of only a "remnant" of a kidney with no normal kidney structure on histologic sections (5), the features of the Potter Type II dysplastic kidneys (2). The placenta also has a distinctive appearance in association with the prolonged oligohydramnios (3). Amnion nodosum, the term which refers to nodules of amorphous

270

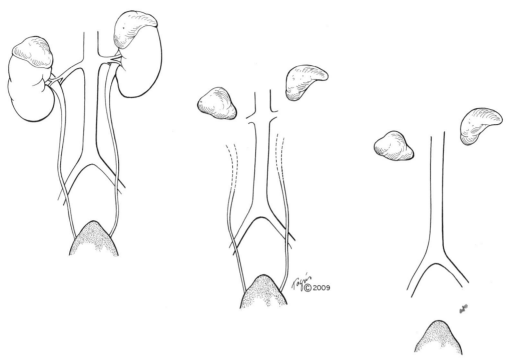

FIGURE 20.1   Diagram showing absence of both kidneys in an affected fetus. Two BRA phenotypes are shown, one with ureters present and the other with no ureters associated with absence of both kidneys.

granular material, is present on the surface of the amnion (Figure 20-2).

Rare features include an apparent phallus in a 46,XX fetus. Another is the presence of a tail (Figure 20-3).

Association Malformations

Most infants with bilateral renal agenesis/dysgenesis (BRA/D) have anomalies only in adjacent anatomic structures, such as the ureters, bladder, and genital structures (1, 5–13). The affected males show absence of the vas deferens and/or seminal vesicles; females

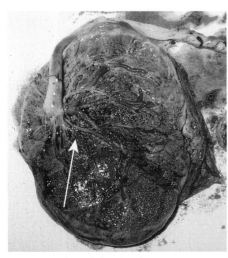

FIGURE 20.2   Fetal surface of placenta showing amnion nodosum.

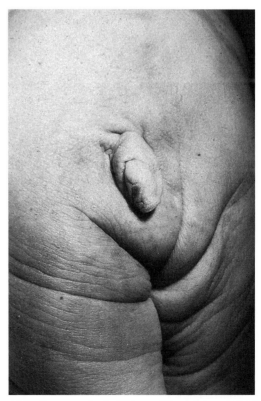

FIGURE 20.3   Presence of a "tail" in a stillborn infant with bilateral renal agenesis and sacral agenesis.

often have absence of a portion of the vagina and anomalies or absence of the uterus.

Among infants with BRA/D, a minority will have anomalies of the sacrum or coccyx, heart defects, imperforate anus, and bowel atresia, primarily esophageal atresia and duodenal atresia. Brain abnormalities, including defects in all migration and formation of gyri, and small size have been reported in most affected infants (14).

Renal anomalies are also associated with myelomeningocele and hemivertbrae (15). Many of these abnormalities are unilateral and include unilateral renal agenesis. Bilateral renal agenesis is associated with two more severe malformations of the sacrum and lumbar vertebrae, including the caudal regression syndrome and sirenomelia. The caudal regression syndrome is a pattern of caudal anomalies with absence of the central portion of the sacrum, hypoplasia of the distal portion of the spinal cord, and associated neurologic deficits and hypoplasia of the buttocks (13, 14, 16).

Sirenomelia is a more severe condition that is almost always lethal and is associated with bilateral renal agenesis (13). There is fusion of the fibular sides of the two legs into a single midline leg, reflecting absence of the midline caudal structures. It has been hypothesized that sirenomelia is due to a "vascular steal" phenomenon, in which nutrients are diverted from the affected regions of the body (17, 18).

A nonrandom association of renal anomalies and limb deficiencies, referred to as the "acro-renal syndrome," has been postulated. However, there is debate (19) as to whether this is a valid pattern. A systematic analysis of 197 infants with limb and renal abnormalities (19), identified in several population-based surveys of over 5 million births, showed that about 50% had a recognized syndrome or chromosome abnormality. Among the infants with no diagnosis, there was no specific pattern of limb deficiency, which argued against the use of the term "acro-renal syndrome."

An association between unilateral renal agenesis and cystic fibrosis gene mutations (cystic fibrosis transmembrane conductance regulator [CFTR]) has been identified in the evaluation of men infertile because of congenital absence of the vas deferens (20, 21). Most of these men have one or two different CFTR mutations. The men with congenital absence of the vas deferens often have unilateral renal agenesis. As a parent, this man, with fertility restored, has an increased risk of having a child with unilateral or bilateral renal agenesis. An increased frequency of unilateral renal agenesis has also been noted in men with a seminal vesicle cyst (22).

Bilateral renal agenesis or renal agenesis/dysgenesis is a feature of many malformation syndromes, as has been illustrated in many case series and surveys (6–8, 10, 11–13) [Table 20-1].

TABLE 20-1 *Etiologic heterogeneity of renal agenesis/dysgenesis**

Apparent etiology	Bilateral renal agenesis	Renal agenesis/dysgenesis
1. Mendelian disorders:		
Cryptophthalmos	1	
Familial autosomal dominant		1
"Private syndrome" (ref. 23)	2**	
2. Chromosome abnormalities:		
Triploidy		1
trisomy 21, mosaic		1
3. Syndromes:	(4)	
sirenomelia	1 (1)**	1
urethral obstruction	1	1
urorectal septum malformation sequence°		1
VACTERL Association	1	1***
4. Environmental		
Infants of diabetic mothers	7	0
5. Twinning	1+	(1)***
6. Unknown etiology	55	21
Total	70 (1:2, 946)	28/(1:7,366/98)

Legends: * Infants identified in survey of 206,244 liveborn and stillborn infants and elective terminations for fetal anomalies in the years 1972–74, 79–2000 at Brigham and Women's Hospital, Boston. These infants were born to women who had planned always to deliver at this hospital. Affected infants have been excluded whose mothers had planned to deliver at another hospital and transferred their care after the prenatal detection of malformations in the fetus.

** "Private syndrome": four affected infants born to parents with normal kidneys by ultrasound: one male infant had bilateral renal agenesis and sirenomelia, another male had bilateral hydronephrosis attributed to posterior urethral valves; a third male had type IV cystic kidney disease; their fourth infant, a female had bilateral renal agenesis.

*** Monoamniotic twins, one with VACTERL Association; co-twin had tetralogy of Fallot.

+ One affected twin in diamniotic, dichorionic twin pair.

°A lethal malformation syndrome of unknown etiology (ref. 24).

( ) = infants listed twice

Developmental Defect

The metanephros in the human embryo appears at five weeks postfertilization and the first layer of glomeruli forms by the ninth week of gestation. The first sign of kidney development is the interaction between the metanephrogenic mesenchyme and the nephric duct, two tissues derived from the intermediate mesoderm (25). Branching and nephrogenesis continue in the nephrogenic cortex until the 34th week of gestation. Two major theories about the failure of the kidney to develop are: 1) a deficiency of induction of the nephron caused by a lack of activity of the ampulla; 2) abnormal budding of the ureteric bud from the mesonephric duct (4). Many genes have been identified as having a crucial role in early kidney development *OddI*, *Wntl*, *PAX 2*,

EYA2, SIX1, SIX2, SALL1, FOXC1, and *HOX11* genes (26–29). These genes are expressed in the mesenchyme and encode transcription factors that are involved in the regulation of the *gdnf* (glial-derived neurotrophic factor).

The findings in experimental studies in mice suggest that mutations in or deletions involving several genes could be causes of renal agenesis. For example, inactivation of both murine *Lim1* (30) and *PAX2* (31) cause bilateral renal agenesis with other related malformations. A homozygous deficiency of *Fras 1* in mice produced cryptophthalmos, renal agenesis, and blebbed phenotype (32), which is a mouse model of the Fraser Syndrome (Mendelian Inheritance in Man #219000) that includes renal agenesis. Targeted mutagenesis of mouse *gdnf* has caused bilateral renal agenesis or severe dysgenesis associated with failure of outgrowth of the ureteric bud (33). A hypomorphic mutation of *Notch 2* caused defects in development of the glomerulus (34).

Theoretically, the lack of (or absence of) kidney tissue could reflect a primary abnormality in the ureteric bud, which should make contact with the metanephric blastema or a lack of responsiveness in the metanephric blastema. Another potential cause could be defective formation of the Wolffian or Müllerian ducts. While there is a wide range of possibilities, no mutation in any gene involved in kidney development has been identified in a significant percentage of infants with BRA/D.

Experimental oligohydramnios, produced by puncturing and draining amniotic fluid in pregnant day16 (but not day 17) Spraque-Dawley rats, produced the non-renal features of bilateral renal agenesis: hypoplastic lungs, cleft palate, and limb deformities (35).

Prevalence

The prevalence rates for bilateral BRA/D in several population-based surveys have been between 1:5,000 to 1:10,000 or 0.2 to 0.1/1,000 (7–12). In British Columbia (10) from 1952 to 1982, there were 92 cases of bilateral renal agenesis among 625,132 births (live and stillbirths) for a prevalence of 0.12/1,000. In Arkansas (12), between 1985 and 1990, the prevalence rate, based on birth and death certificates, was 0.14/1,000. In the Czech Republic (36), from 1961 to 1995, the prevalence rate of renal agenesis was 0.17:1,000, a rate that included affected fetuses diagnosed prenatally and terminated electively. In Boston, in the years 1972–1974 and 1979–2000, the prevalence rate of bilateral renal agenesis was 0.33:1,000 or 1:2,946 (Table 20-1).

Pediatricians performing deep abdominal palpation in the first day of life in routine examinations of 12,160 consecutive newborns showed that several types of renal anomalies could be identified accurately (37). Three of these newborns were confirmed to have unilateral renal agenesis, for a prevalence rate of 1:4, 053 or 0.25/1,000.

Race/Ethnicity

An increased frequency (OR 2.2; 95CI 1.3–4.0) in black infants in comparison to white infants was noted in Colorado (13). However, in California [39] (1989–1998), the frequency of renal agenesis in infants born to African American parents was the same as for white infants. The frequency among U.S.-born Hispanic infants was increased marginally (Adjusted Relative Risk 1.2; 95CI 1.0–1.5).

Birth Status

Infants with BRA/D are often growth-restricted, stillborn, and in a breech presentation with associated oligohydramnios.

Sex Ratio

More affected males than females have been reported in several case series (7, 10, 11, 13) of infants with bilateral renal agenesis or agenesis/dysgenesis.

Sidedness

Absence of the left kidney was present in 56.4% of patients with unilateral renal agenesis and the right kidney in 43.6% in a literature review of 1,498 patients (38).

Parental Age

In a case-control study of infants born with renal agenesis, in Colorado (1989–1998), which did not distinguish between unilateral and bilateral renal agenesis, there were significantly more mothers 18 or younger whose infants had renal agenesis (13).

Twinning

Reported monozygous twins with bilateral renal agenesis have been concordant (40) and, more often, discordant (7, 41, 42) for bilateral renal agenesis. In some monozygous twin pairs, one infant had unilateral renal agenesis and the co-twin had bilateral agenesis/dysgenesis (43, 44). The co-twin with bilateral renal agenesis/dysgenesis did not have any of the secondary signs of the Potter Syndrome, such as lung hypoplasia and deformations of the face and extremities, because the co-twin with unilateral renal agenesis maintained a normal amount of amniotic fluid.

Genetic Factors

BRA/D has many etiologies (Table 20-1). Among the infants with only BRA/D and anatomically adjacent anomalies, an empiric risk of about 4% of having a second affected child was established in family studies (7, 9, 11). In some families in which one parent has unilateral renal agenesis and the affected child has BRA/D (9, 45), autosomal dominant inheritance has been postulated.

Autosomal recessive inheritance has been postulated in rare consanguineous families with two or more affected infants (46).

Multifactorial inheritance also has been postulated (7, 11). The affected close relatives may have BRA/D or unilateral renal agenesis. Consistent with this hypothesis, in one case series (9), the parents with two or more affected infants had a high frequency of associated "silent" renal anomalies, but this was not the case in another publication-based study (11).

Chromosome abnormalities have been identified usually in less than 10% of infants with BRA/D, but no specific abnormalities have been common (6–13; Table 20-1). Bilateral renal dysplasia with no renal structures, but with both ureters present, has been associated with a de novo translocation (1;2) (q32;p25) [47]. Deletions involving 1q31-32 have been reported in association with bilateral (48) and unilateral (49) renal agenesis in addition to other anomalies.

The REN gene maps to 1q32 and encodes renin, a component of the renin-angiotensin system (RAS). Two other more frequent deletions identified have been 5q32-35 and 16q22 (48). Congenital anomalies of the kidney and urinary tract (CAKUT), including vesico-ureteral reflux, have been associated with deletions of chromosome 13q33-34, in children with developmental delay and other anomalies, but not renal agenesis (50).

There are many multiple anomaly syndromes that include renal agenesis, dysplasia, and hypoplasia as part of the Potter's Syndrome phenotype (Table 20-1). Mutations have been identified in a few of these. For example, a mutation in the *PAX2* gene, specifically a deletion of a single nucleotide in exon 5, was identified in one family with an autosomal dominant phenotype that included optic nerve colobomas, renal hypoplasia, proteinuria, and vesicoureteral reflex (51). Another example is the association of EYA1 mutations with the Branchio-Oto-Renal (BOR) Syndrome (MIM #113650), an autosomal dominant disorder that includes renal agenesis and other renal anomalies (52).

Environmental Factors

Among infants of diabetic mothers, renal anomalies, including BRA/D (Table 20-1), are one of the major malformations that are significantly more common than in infants of nondiabetic mothers (36). A 15-fold increase (odds ratio 14.8; 95 CI 3.5–62.1) was identified in one study in Hungary (53).

Renal agenesis was an occasional component of the thalidomide embryopathy (54). Indomethacin has been postulated (55) to be a potential cause of BRA/D, but this has not been confirmed in a large, systematic study.

Treatment and Prognosis

Since BRA/D is associated with a significant degree of oligohydramnios, it is typically fatal in the newborn period. However, theoretically if the affected infant has adequate lung development, it would be possible to use renal dialysis and, later, transplantation of a kidney, to prolong survival.

Genetic Counseling

Because of the significant frequency of associated chromosome abnormalities, the index case should have had these studies. The physical examination will identify significant features of rare phenotypes, such as cryptophthalmos (MIM 21900) or Branchio-Oto-Renal (BOR) Syndrome (MIM #113650).

Case series have shown that some infants with bilateral renal aplasia/dysplasia have absence of the ureters. There can also be other related anomalies of Müllerian duct derivatives, e.g., bicornuate uterus, and Wolffian duct derivatives, e.g., congenital absence of vas deferens. Family studies are needed to determine whether or not the empiric recurrence risk of another affected fetus in the next pregnancy is changed by the presence/absence of associated genitourinary anomalies. Meanwhile, the current empiric risk estimate for bilateral renal agenesis or severe dysgenesis is 4%, based on the risk estimates in three separate family studies in which the rates were 3.5% (9), 3.6% (11), and 4.4% (5), respectively.

Prenatal screening by ultrasound has been successfully to identify the affected fetus by 16 weeks gestation, by which time urine should be present in the bladder (6). The prenatal ultrasound studies are made more difficult by the associated oligohydiamnios; false positive findings have been reported (56). The sonologist can also look for the characteristic "flattened" adrenal gland (57) and, by color flow imaging, absence of the renal arteries (58).

If the diagnosis of "Potter's Syndrome" is based on findings by prenatal ultrasound, it is essential to establish the nature of the presumed kidney abnormalities by autopsy. Experience in a series of 60 fetuses with Potter's Syndrome showed that 50% did not have any renal anomalies (59).

Family studies (9) have also shown that the parents and sibs of an infant with bilateral renal agenesis/dysgenesis have a risk of about 10% of having "silent" renal anomalies or in females, anomalies of the fallopian tube or uterus. The frequency of unilateral absence of the vas deferens in the father and brothers has not been determined.

Because of the relationship between bilateral renal agenesis/dysgenesis and unilateral renal agenesis/dysgenesis, the healthy man or woman with unilateral renal agenesis/dysgenesis should be counseled about a significant risk of either phenotype in her/his offspring. He/she should be evaluated carefully to make certain the single kidney is healthy, as there can be obstructive lesions, like uretero-pelvic junction structure, and associated hypertension (60).

Unilateral multicystic kidney dysplasia can appear to be unilateral renal agenesis by the end of pregnancy. Close relatives of infants with bilateral renal agenesis/dysgenesis have been found to have unilateral multicystic dysplastic kidney (9). More extensive family studies are needed to confirm and establish the genetic relationship between the multicystic dysplastic kidneys and agenesis/severe dysgenesis (61).

REFERENCES

1. Potter EL. Bilateral renal agenesis. *J Pediatri*. 1946;29:68–76.
2. Potter EL. Bilateral absence of ureters and kidneys. A report of 50 cases. *Obstet Gynecol*. 1965;25:3–12.
3. Gilbert-Barness E, ed. *Potter's Pathology of the Fetus and Infant*, Vols. 1 and 2. 4th ed. St. Louis: Mosby; 1997.
4. Shibata S, Nagata M. Pathogenesis of human renal dysplasia: an alternative scenario to the major theories. *Pediatrics International*. 2003;45:605–609.
5. Bernstein J. The morphogenesis of renal parenchymal maldevelopment (renal dysplasia). *Pediatr Clin North Am*. 1971;18:395–407.
6. Buchta RM, Visekul C, Gilbert EF. Familial bilateral renal agenesis and hereditary renal adysplasia. *Z. Kinderheilk*. 1973;115:111–129.
7. Carter CO, Evans K, Pescia G. A family study of renal agenesis. *J Med Genet*. 1979;16:176–188.
8. Curry CJR, Jensen K, Holland J, Miller L, Hall BD. The Potter sequence: a clinical analysis of 80 cases. *Am J Med Genet*. 1984;19:679–702.
9. Roodhooft AM, Birnholz JC, Holmes LB. Familial nature of congenital absence and severe dysgenesis of both kidneys. *N Engl J Med*. 1984;310:1341–1345.
10. Wilson RD, Baird PA. Renal agenesis in British Columbia. *Am J Med Genet*. 1985;21:153–165.
11. Bankier A, de Campo M, Newell R, Rogers JG, Danks DM. A pedigree study of perinatally lethal renal disease. *J Med Genet*. 1985;22:104–111.
12. Cunniff C, Kirby RS, Senner JW. Deaths associated with renal agenesis: a population-based study of birth prevalence, case ascertainment, and etiologic heterogeneity. *Teratology*. 1994;50:200–204.
13. Parikh CR, McCall D, Engelman C, Schrier RW. Congenital renal agenesis: case-control analysis of birth characteristics. *Am J Kid Dis*. 2002;39:689–694.
14. Grunnet ML, Bale JF, Jr. Brain abnormalities in infants with Potter syndrome (oligohydramnios tetrad). *Neurology*. 1981;31:1571–1574.
15. Tori JA, Dickson JH. Association of congenital anomalies of the spine and kidneys. *Clin Orthopaedics Related Res*. 1980;148:259–262.
16. Catala M. Genetic control of caudal development. *Clin Genet*. 2002;61:89–96.
17. Stevenson RE, Jones KL, Phelan MC, Jones MC, Barr M Jr, Clericuzio C et al. Vascular steal: the pathogenetic mechanism producing sirenomelia and associated defects of the viscera and soft tissues. *Pediatrics*. 1986;78:451–457.
18. Drossou-Agakidou V, Xatzisevastou-Loukidou C, Soubasi V, Kostopoulo E, Laporde A, Pantzaki A, et al. Rare manifestations of sireonomelia syndrome: a report of five cases. *Am J Perinat*. 2004;21:395–401.
19. Kroes HY, Olney RS, Rosano A, Liu Y, Castilla EE, Cocchi G, et al. Renal defects and limb deficiencies in 197 infants: is it possible to define the "acrorenal syndrome"? *Am J Med Genet*. 2004;129A:149–155.
20. McCallum TJ, Milunsky JM, Munarriz R, Carson R, Sadeghi-Nejad H, Oates RD. Unilateral renal agenesis associated with congenital bilateral absence of the vas deferens: phenotypic findings and genetic considerations. *Human Reprod*. 2001;16:282–288.
21. Kolettis PN, Sandlow JI. Clinical and genetic features of patients with congenital unilateral absence of the vas deferens. *Urology*. 2002;60:1073–1076.
22. Narlawar RS, Hanchate V, Raut A, Hira P, Nagar A, Chaubal NG. Renal agenesis and seminal vesicle cyst. *J Ultrasound Med*. 2003;22:225–228.
23. Selig AM, Benacerraf B, Greene MF, Garber MF, Genest DR. Renal dysplasia, megalocystis and sirenomelia in four siblings. *Teratology*. 1993;47:65–71.
24. Wheeler PG, Weaver DD, Obeime MD, Vance GH, Bull MJ, Escobar LF. Urorectal septum malformation sequence: report of thirteen additional cases and review of the literature. *Am J Med Genet*. 1997;73:456–462.
25. O'Rahilly R, Müller F. *Human Embryology and Teratology*. New York: Wiley-Liss; 2001:299–308.
26. Stadler HS. Modelling genitourinary defects in mice: an emerging genetic and developmental system. *Nature Reviews/Nature*. 2003;4:1–5.
27. Brodbeck S, Englert C. Genetic determination of nephrogenesis: The Pax/Eya/Six Gene Network. *Pediatr Nephrol*. 2004;19:249–255.
28. Sajithlal G, Zou D, Silvius D, Xu P-X. Eya1 acts as a critical regulator for specifying the metanephric mesenchyme. *Devel Biol*. 2005;284:323–336.
29. James RG, Kamei CN, Wang Q, Jiang R, Schultheiss TM. *Odd-skipped related 1* is required for development of the metanephric kidney and regulates formation and differentiation of kidney precursor cells. *Development*. 2006;133:2995–3004.
30. Shawlot W, Behringer RR. Requirement for *Lim1* in head-organizer function. *Nature*. 1995;374:425–430.
31. Torres M, Gomez-Pardo E, Dressler GR, Gruss P. *Pax-2* controls multiple steps of urogenital development. *Development*. 1995;121:4057–4065.
32. Vrontou S, Petrou P, Meyer BI, Galanopoulos VK, Imai K, Yanagi M, Chowdhury K, Scambler PJ, Chalepakis G. *Fras1* deficiency results in cryptophthalmos, renal agenesis and blebbed phenotype in mice. *Nature Genetics*. 2003;34:209–214.
33. Treanor JJ, Goodman L, de Sauvage F, Stone DM, Poulsen KT, Beck CD et al. Characterization of a multicomponent receptor for GDNF. *Nature*. 1996;382:80–83.
34. McCright B. Notch signaling in kidney development. *Current Opinions in Nephrology and Hypertension*. 2003;12:5–10.
35. Symchych PS, Winchester P. Potters syndrome: Animal model: amniotic fluid deficiency and fetal lung growth in the rat. *Am J Pathol*. 1978;90:779–782.
36. Sipek A, Gregor V, Horacek J, Chudobova M, Korandova V, Skibova J. Incidence of renal agenesis in the Czech Republic from 1961 to 1995. *Ceska Gynekol*. 1997;62:340–343.

37. Sherwood DW, Smith RC, Lemmon RH, Vrabel I. Abnormalities of the genitourinary tract discovered by palpation of the abdomen of the newborn. *Pediatrics*. 1956;18:782–789.

38. Doroshow LW, Abeshouse BS. Congenital unilateral solitary kidney: report of 37 cases and a review of the literature. *Urol Surv*. 1961;11:219–229.

39. Carmichael SL, Shaw GM, Kaidarova Z. Congenital malformations in offspring of Hispanic and African-American women in California, 1989–1997. *Birth Def Res (Part A): Clin Mol Teratology*. 2004;70:382–388.

40. Yates JR, Mortimer G, Connor JM, Duke JE. Concordant monozygotic twins with bilateral renal agenesis. *J Med Genet*. 1984;21:66–67.

41. Cilento BG, Jr., Benacerraf BR, Mandell J. Prenatal and postnatal findings in monochorionic, monoamniotic twins discordant for bilateral renal agenesis-dysgenesis (perinatal lethal renal disease). *J Urol*. 1994;151:1034–1035.

42. Perez-Brayfield MR, Kirsch AJ, Smith EA. Monoamniotic twin discordant for bilateral renal agenesis with normal pulmonary function. *Urology*. 2004;64:589.e1–589.e2.

43. Mauer SM, Dobrin RS, Vernier RL. Unilateral and bilateral renal agenesis in monoamniotic twins. *J Pediatr*. 1974;84:236–238.

44. Kohler HG. An unusual case of sirenomelia. *Teratology*. 1972;6:295–301.

45. Kohn G, Borns PF. The association of bilateral and unilateral renal aplasia in the same family. *J Pediatr*. 1973;83:95–97.

46. Bromiker R, Glam-Baruch M, Gofin R, Hammerman C, Amitai Y. Association of parental consanguinity with congenital malformations among Arab newborns in Jerusalem. *Clin Genet*. 2004;66:65–66.

47. Joss S, Howatson A, Trainer A, Whiteford M, FitzPatrick DR. De novo translocation (1; 2)(q32; p25) associated with bilateral renal dysplasia. *Clin Genet*. 2003;63:239–240.

48. Brewer C, Holloway S, Zawalnyski P, Schinzel A, FitzPatrick D. A chromosomal deletion map of human malformations. *Am J Hum Genet*. 1998;63:1153–1159.

49. Steinbach P, Wolf M, Schmidt H. Multiple congenital anomalies/mental retardation (MCA/MR) syndrome due to interstitial deletion 1q. *Am J Med Genet*. 1984;19:131–136.

50. Guron G, Friberg P. An intact renin-angiotensin system is a prerequisite for normal renal development. *J Hypertens*. 2000;18:123–137.

51. Sanyanusin P, Schimmenti LA, McNoe LA, Ward TA, Pierpont ME, Sullivan MJ, Dobyns WB, Eccles MR. Mutation of the PAX2 gene in a family with optic nerve colobomas, renal anomalies and vesicoureteral reflux. *Nat Genet*. 1995;9(4):358–364.

52. Ruf RG, Xu PX, Silvius D, Otto EA, Beekmann F, Muerb UT, et al. SIX1 mutations cause branchio-oto-renal syndrome by disruption of EYA1-SIX1-DNA complexes. *Proc Natl Acad Sci USA*. 2004;101:8090–8095.

53. Nielsen GL, Norgard B, Puho E, Rothman KJ, Sorenson HT, Czeizel AE. Risk of specific congenital abnormalities in offspring of women with diabetes. *Diabetic Medicine*. 2005;22:693–696.

54. Smithells RW. Defects and disabilities of thalidomide children. *Brit Med J*. 1973;1:269–272.

55. Restaino I, Kaplan BS, Kaplan P, Rosenberg HK, Witzleben C, Roberts N. Renal dysgenesis in a monozygotic twin: association with in utero exposure to indomethacin. *Am J Med Genet*. 1991;39:252–257.

56. Sgro M, Shah V, Barozzino T, Ibach K, Allen L, Chitayat D. False diagnosis of renal agenesis on fetal MRI. *Ultrasound Obstet Gynecol*. 2005;25:197–200.

57. Hoffman CK, Filly RA, Callen PW. The "lying down" adrenal sign: a sonographic indicator of renal agenesis or ectopia in fetuses and neonates. *J Ultrasound Med*. 1992; 11:533–536.

58. Sepulveda W, Stagiannis KD, Flack NJ, Fisk NM. Accuracy of prenatal diagnosis of renal agenesis with color flow imaging in severe second-trimester oligohydramnios. *Am J Obstet Gynecol*. 1995;173:1788–1792.

59. Scott RJ, Goodburn SF. Potter's syndrome in the second trimester-prenatal screening and pathological findings in 60 cases of oligohydramnios sequence. *Prenat Diagn*. 1995;15:519–525.

60. Argueso LR, Ritchey ML, Boyle ET Jr, Milliner DS, Bergstralh EJ, Kramer SA. Prognosis of patients with unilateral renal agenesis. *Pediatr Nephrol*. 1992;6:412–416.

61. Mesrobian HJ, Rushton HJ, Bulas D. Unilateral renal agenesis may result from in utero regression of multicystic renal dysplasia. *J Urol*. 1993;150:793–794.

Chapter 21

Skeletal Dysplasias

Definition

A group of genetic disorders characterized by abnormal growth and development of bone and cartilage.

ICD-9:	756.1 to 756.591	(spondylocostal dyostosis) (other osteo dystrophies)
ICD-10:	M80-M94	(osteopathies and chondropathies)
Mendelian Inheritance in Man:		See Table 21-1

Appearance

The skeletal dysplasias identified at birth are a very heterogenous group of genetic disorders (Tables 21-1 and 21-2; 1–6). They have a spectrum of physical abnormalities (7, 8):

- disproportionate short stature (Figure 21-1);
- altered upper (U)-to-lower (L) segment ratio (U/L):

  ex. with a short trunk, the U/L ratio is lower than expected;

  ex. with short limbs, the U/L ratio is higher than expected;

- the shortening can affect primarily the proximal (humerus/femur) segments, called rhizomelic shortening, as in achondroplasia (MIM #100800);
- shortening of the middle portion of arms or legs, called mesomelic shortening, as in Leri-Weill Syndrome (MIM #127300); in this disorder there

can also be a dorsal sub-luxation of the distal ulna, the Madelung deformity;

- shortening of the distal (hands/feet) segments, called acromelic shortening, as in the hereditary brachydactylies;
- an enlarged head with a depressed nasal bridge, as in achondroplasia and hypochondroplasia (MIM #146000);
- a large fontanel, which reflects defective ossification in several disorders;
- the cloverleaf skull deformity (or Kleeblattschädel) [Figure 21-2] with craniosynostosis, a feature of thanatophoric dysplasia, type II;
- the flattening of the midface with a short nasal columella is a feature of the many types of chondrodysplasia punctata and the Stickler Syndrome (MIM #108300 [type II], #604841 [type I] and #184840 [type III]);
- a small chin, cleft palate and retinal detachment are features of Stickler syndrome;
- polydactyly is a feature of several skeletal dysplasias, such as the short rib-polydactyly group [Figure 21-3];
- the "hitch-hiker" thumb is a distinctive feature of diastrophic dysplasia;
- the dimple over the mid-portion of the tibia is a feature of campomelic dysplasia (MIM #114290) [Figure 21-4];
- cystic swelling of the ears, which is not tender, a distinctive features of diastrophic dysplasia;
- sparse hair is a feature of cartilage–hair hypoplasia (MIM #250250) and the trichorhinophalangeal dysplasia syndromes (MIM #190350 and 190351 [types I/III] and MIM #150230 [type II]);
- hypoplastic nails are features of the Ellis-Van Creveld Syndrome (MIM #225500) and the chondrodysplasia punctatas.

TABLE 21-1 *Common skeletal dysplasias detected in newborn infants*

Mendalian Inheritance in Man number	Condition	Gene affected	Gene Product Function	Inheritance Pattern
#187600 (type I) #187601 (type II)	Thanatophoric dysplasia, types I & II	FGFR3	Tyrosine kinase transmembrane receptor for FGFs	AD
#100800	Achondroplasia	FGFR3	Tyrosine kinase transmembrane receptor for FGFs	AD
#166210	Osteogenesis imperfecta, type II	Type I collagen	Genes encoding type I collagen (COL1A1, COL1A2)	AD
%200600 (type IA) #600972 (type IB) #200610 (type II)	Achondrogenesis, type I, A, B type II	DTDST COL1A1	Extracellular protein	AR AD
#114290	Campomelic dysplasia	SOX9	Transcription factor	AD
#183900	Spondyloepiphyseal dysplasia congenital	COL2A1	Extracellular matrix protein	AD

Legend: FGFR3: Fibroblast growth factor
DTDST: Diastrophic dysplasia sulfate transporter
SOX9: SRY-related box genes, a trans-acting regulatory factor
COL1A1: Collagen, type I
AD: Autosomal dominant; AR: Autosomal recessive

TABLE 21-2 *Birth prevalence rates for skeletal dysplasias*

	South America (20) 1978–1983 3349, 470 LB, SB		France (21) 1979–1986 105, 374 LB, SB and Elect Ab		Brigham & Women's Hospital, Boston (22) 1972–74,79–2000 206,244, LB, SB, Elect Ab***	
	# Rate/1,000		# Rate/1,000		# Rate/1,000	
Achondroplasia*	33*		7		7	
Thanatophoric dysplasia	3		3		6	
Osteogenesis all types imperfecta, type II imperfecta, type III imperfecta, type I	15		7		7	
Spondyloepiphyseal dysplasia congenita	0		1		3	
Achondrogenesis	1 + 4**		3		3	
Campomelic dysplasia	3		1		2	
Chondroectodermal dysplasia	2		1		0	
Chondrodysplasia punctata Conrad-Hünerman Rhizomelic type	1 1		2 1		0 0	
Desbuquois syndrome	0		0		1	
Diastrophic dysplasia	1		1		0	
Engelman disease	0		1		0	
Fibrous dysplasia	1		1		0	
Jeune thoracic dystrophy	0		1		0	
Larsen Syndrome	0		0		1	
Melnick-Needles	0		0		1	
Multiple exostoses	0		2		0	
Osteopetrosis	0		2		0	
Pfeiffer Syndrome	0		0		1	
Short rib polydactyly, type I type II	0 0		0 0		1 1	
Stickler syndrome	0		0		1	
Unknown	0		0		3	
Total	65	0.23/1,000	34	0.32/1,000	38	0.18/1,000

Legends: LB = liveborn; SB = stillborn
Elect Ab: elective termination
* = includes 16 infants with achondroplasia and 17 "questionable" achondroplasia
** = includes one infant with achondrogenesis and four with either achondrogenesis or thanatophoric dysplasia.
*** = includes the findings described by Rasmussen et al. (22) which have been extended through 2000, an additional 10 years.

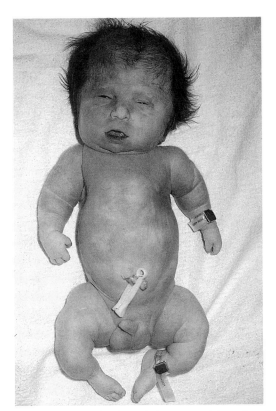

FIGURE 21.1   Shows the bending of the arms and legs of an infant with osteogenesis imperfecta, type II. (Courtesy of Frederick R. Bieber, Ph.D., Brigham and Women's Hospital, Boston.)

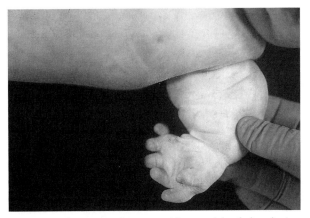

FIGURE 21.3   Shows very short arm with postaxial polydactyly, in an infant with short-rib polydactyly, type II.

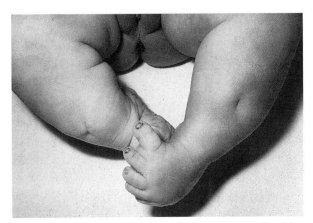

FIGURE 21.4   Shows the dimpling in the midportion of the tibia, a feature of campomelic dysplasia.

Associated Malformations

Some of the skeletal dysplasias identified in newborn infants have common and significant associated malformations. For example, infants with the Jeune asphyxiating thoracic dystrophy (MIM %208500) have cystic changes in the kidney and fibrosis of the liver and pancreas. Infants with Jarcho-Levin spondylocostal dyostosis (MIM #277300) may have imperforate anus and anomalies of the uterus (9). Severe heart defects are a feature of the Ellis-Van Creveld Syndrome. Males with campomelic dysplasia (MIM #114290) may have sex reversal, caused by mutations in the SRY-related gene SOX9. In general, only specific disorders have patterns of associated malformations, rather than there being a nonspecific increase in the occurrence of nonskeletal malformations.

Developmental Defects

In the developing fetus the vertebrate skeleton is formed by two processes: a) bone formation by endochondral ossification, which leads to the development of long

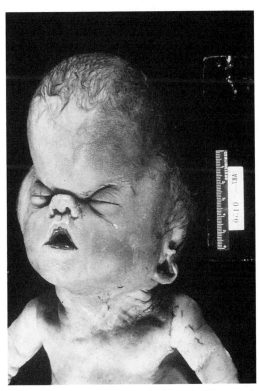

FIGURE 21.2   Shows the skull shape Kleeblattschädel anomaly in an infant with thanatophoric dysplasia. (Courtesy of Frederick R. Bieber, Ph.D., Brigham and Women's Hospital, Boston.)

bones in the skeleton; b) intramembranous ossification, whereby the flat bones of the cranial vault, mandible, and parts of the clavicle are formed (11–19).

During the fifth week of development postfertilization, mesenchymal cells condense in the limbs to form unmineralized and vascular models of developing bones. The mesenchymal cells produce types I and III collagen and differentiate into chondrocytes, which produce type II collagen, the major collagen of cartilage. The chondrocytes in the developing growth plate from the epiphysis to the diaphysis form discrete regions of the growth plate: resting zone, proliferative zone, maturation zone, metaphysis, and hypertrophic zone (Figure 21-5).

The reserve zone contains spherical cells and exhibits cell divisions only occasionally. By contrast, the cells in the proliferative zone are dividing rapidly and make extracellular matrix.

The maturing cells differentiate into hypertrophic cells, which show an increase in cell volume. These cells are a major factor in longitudinal bone growth until puberty.

Abnormalities in mesenchymal cell differentiation and condensation lead to the structural changes recognized as skeletal dysplasias. The cellular and molecular basis for these changes (Figures 21-6, 21-5) have included:

- transcription factors:

    ex. Mutations in the SHOX (short stature homeobox) are associated with the Leri-Weill dyschondrosteosis;

    ex. Mutations in the cartilage-derived morphogenetic protein-1 (CDMP-1) have been identified in several skeletal dysplasias, including chondrodysplasia, Grebe type [formerly achondrogenesis, type II] (MIM #200700).

- matrix in the growth plate:

    ex. Mutations in COL2A1 cause several different disorders, including lethal achondrogenesis, type II, SED congenita and Stickler Syndrome (MIM +120140);

- disruption of the fibroblast growth factor receptors (FGFRs):

    ex: mutations in the transmembrane domain of FGFR3 cause achondroplasia.

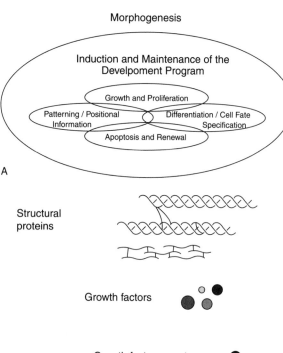

A

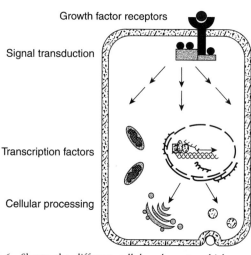

B

FIGURE 21.6 Shows the different cellular elements which can be affected by mutations that cause a specific skeletal dysplasia. (From Dreyer SD et al.: *Clin Genet.* 1998;54:465. Figure 1b. Used with permission).

Zone	Gene	Dysplasia
Resting	SOX9	Campomelic dyslasia
Proliferation	FGFR3	Achondroplasia
Hypertrophy	PTHR1	Metaphyseal dysplasia
Terminal differentiation	RUNX2	Cleidocranial dysplasia

FIGURE 21.5 A diagram of the growth plate which shows the genes that affect specific cell types and the skeletal dysplasias caused by mutations in those genes. (From Alman BA: *Clin Genet.* 2008;73:25. Figure 1. Used with permission).

- disruption of chondrocyte maturation:
  ex: mutations in the human parathyroid hormone related peptide (PTHrP) and its receptor cause the Blomstarnd lethal skeletal dysplasia (MIM #215045).
- generalized undermineralization is a feature of osteogenesis imperfecta (MIM #166221), hypophosphatasia (MIM #241500), and achondrogenesis, types I and II.

Prevalence

In the 1980s fetuses with severe skeletal dysplasias began to be identified prenatally by ultrasound. Those pregnancies were often terminated by choice. After this became possible, the most accurate estimates of prevalence rates of specific disorders were those that identified the fetuses with lethal skeletal dysplasias in elective terminations (20–23).

The prevalence rates of skeletal dysplasias identified at birth, in different studies, have been between 0.2 and 0.3/1,000 infants (including liveborn, stillborn, and elective terminations of affected fetuses) [20–22].

Prevalence rates are available for some of the most common skeletal dysplasias (Table 21-2). For example, population-based surveillance of 10,876,099 births showed that the prevalence rate of achondroplasia ranged between 0.04 and 0.06/1,000 livebirths (1:27,780 to 1:16,670). The prevalence of thanatophoric dysplasia was from 0.02 to 0.03/1,000 livebirths (1:33,330 to 1:47,620) [24]. Among the 79 infants with achondroplasia identified in Texas, one was an elective termination. 9 (20.9%) of the 29 cases of thanatophoric dysplasia were elective terminations.

Race/Ethnicity

There have not been enough diagnostic evaluations in diverse populations to determine whether or not there are distinctive ethnic differences in prevalence rates for specific skeletal dysplasias.

Birth Status

The fetuses with lethal skeletal dysplasias may be stillborn or die soon after birth.

Sex Ratio

The disorders attributed to either autosomal dominant or autosomal recessive inheritance exhibit the expected equal sex ratios. The only exceptions are: a) the rare X-linked disorders, such as chondrodysplasia punctata, X-linked recessive type (MIM #302940), which have only affected males, and b) 46,XY infants with campomelic dysplasia, who may have sex reversal, i.e., female or ambiguous external genitals.

Parental Age

One contributing factor for a spontaneous mutation is paternal age. A higher paternal age, and presumably a paternal age effect, has been documented for infants with thanatophoric dysplasia. For example, in a series of 34 infants in South America (1967–1992), the average paternal age was 36.4 ± 9.4 years and maternal age was 28.7 ± 5.6 years in comparison to the average paternal and maternal ages of 28.8 ± 6.2 and 25.2 ± 5.2 years respectively in 66 controls (p-value = < 0.01)) [25].

In Texas, where 79 infants with achondroplasia and 43 with thanatophoric dysplasia were identified among 2,042,554 births (1996–2002), a significant paternal age effect was apparent (24). For fathers of infants with achondroplasia, the odds ratio for men 40 and older was 5.0 (95 CI 1.5-16.1) and progressively less at younger ages, with OR 2.8 (95 CI 1.2-6.7) for men 25–29. For fathers of the infants with thanatophoric dysplasia, the odds ratios were higher: 10.2 (95 CI 2.6–17.8) for men 40 and older, decreasing to 5.8 (95 CI 1.7–9.8) for men 25–29 years old.

Twinning

The monozygous twins with genetic disorders attributed to autosomal recessive or dominant inheritance will both be affected, i.e., concordant. However, identical twins may not be concordant for associated features. For example, in one set of identical twins with thanatophoric dysplasia, only one infant had the cloverleaf skull deformity (26) [Figure 21-3].

Genetic Factors

Many of the skeletal dysplasias identifiable either prenatally or at birth are attributed to autosomal dominant inheritance.

Since some of these autosomal dominant disorders are lethal, like thanatophoric dysplasia, the affected child is the result of a new or spontaneous mutation. The causes of these spontaneous mutations have not been determined.

Another potential characteristic of conditions attributed to autosomal dominant inheritance is gonadal mosaicism in one of the parents, who is unaffected. This has caused the recurrence risk in subsequent pregnancies to be about 6% after the birth of a newborn infant with osteogenesis imperfects (OI), type II (27). Evidence of mosaicism was provided by mutation analysis of sperm from the father of a child with OI, type II which identified two populations of sperm, one group containing the OI, type II mutation and the other group of sperm containing no OI, type II mutations (27).

With the identification of the underlying mutations for many skeletal dysplasias, some surprising observations have been made (8). First, mutations in the same gene can cause very different and distinctive skeletal dysplasias. For example, separate mutations in the FGFR3 gene cause achondroplasia, hypochondroplasia, and thanatophoric dysplasia. A second striking finding is the fact that mutations in three different genes cause the same phenotype. For example, mutations in the genes COMP, COL9A2 and COL9A3 all produce multiple epiphyseal dysplasia.

As more associated mutations have been identified, the classification of the skeletal dysplasias has been a combination of molecular analysis, the pattern of radiographic changes, and the clinical phenotype (16).

Environmental Factors

A few teratogens produce a distinctive skeletal dysplasia. For example, exposure to the anticoagulant warfarin, an inhibitor of vitamin K reductase (28), produces marked hypoplasia of the nose cartilage, stippled epiphyses, and shortening of the distal phalanges of the fingers. Exposure to the anticonvulsant drug phenytoin can produce a phenotype referred to as chondrodysplasia punctata, characterized by a depressed bridge of the nose, short nose, shortened distal phalanges of the fingers, and punctata calcifications (29).

Treatment and Prognosis

For infants with skeletal dysplasias diagnosed at birth, the treatment focuses on the features of each condition. For example, the management of the newborn with achondroplasia has included surgery to relieve cervicomedullary compression of the brainstem and spinal stenosis, treatment for recurrent otitis media, osteotomy to treat bowing of the tibia, and treatment for restrictive lung disease (30–32).

Genetic Counseling

A significant portion of the fetuses with skeletal dysplasias are identified during pregnancy in screening by ultrasound. Experience has shown that the detection of the general features of skeletal dysplasia is accurate, but it has been very difficult to establish the specific disorder accurately (15, 17, 18). Hopefully the new techniques, such as three-dimensional imaging, will improve the accuracy of diagnoses suggested during pregnancy (33–35).

The evaluation of the affected infant at birth begins with the physical examination and radiographic images to establish the phenotype. Then, the clinician and family often have the option of molecular testing at a laboratory to identify the associated mutation.

www.genetests.org is a resource for identifying laboratories inside and outside of the United States where either extracted DNA, white blood cells, or skin fibroblasts can be sent for testing.

Another option is to obtain a diagnostic evaluation at the International Skeletal Dysplasia Center (www.csmc.edu/3805.html) at Cedars-Sinai Hospital in Los Angeles. A clinical summary, clinical photographs, images (prenatal and postnatal), and tissues for histology and molecular testing are submitted for a thorough evaluation.

The counseling of the parents follows the diagnostic evaluation. An empiric recurrence risk has been established for many disorders. Prenatal by ultrasound has been used to determine whether or not the subsequent fetus is affected. For some conditions, DNA obtained by chorionic villus sampling at 10 or 12 weeks of gestation can be used to determine whether or not the fetus has the same mutation as was found in the first affected infant or fetus.

For couples who choose to continue the pregnancy with an affected fetus, it is very helpful to outline the expected natural history of the disorder. The psychosocial aspects of nonlethal skeletal dysplasias vary for the affected individual, and their unaffected parents (36). Guidelines for clinical management are available for some disorders, such as achondroplasia (30–32).

Little People of America (www.lpaonline.org) is a nonprofit organization that provides support and information to the families of infants with all types of dwarfism.

REFERENCES

I. General Reference

1. Taybi H, Lachman RS, eds. *Radiology of Syndromes, Metabolic Disorders, and Skeletal Dysplasias.* 4th ed. St. Louis, MO: Mosby; 1996.
2. McKusick VA, Amberger JS, Francomano CA. Progress in Medical Genetics: Map-based gene discovery and the molecular pathology of skeletal dysplasias. *Am J Med Genet.* 1996;63: 98–105.
3. Dugoff L, Thieme G, Hobbins JC. Skeletal anomalies. *Clinics in Perinatology.* 2000;27:979–1005.
4. Wynne-Davies R, Hall C, Hurst J. An approach to the radiological diagnosis of the lethal and other skeletal dysplasias presenting at birth. Skeletal Dysplasia Group. Occasional Publications No. 8d. Available from: Churchill Hospital, Oxford, OX37LJ: Skeletal Dysplasia Group, Membership Secretary, Department of Clinical Genetics; 2004.
5. Adelson BM. *Dwarfism: Medical and Psychosocial Aspects of Profound Short Stature.* Baltimore, MD: Johns Hopkins University Press; 2005.

II. Articles

6. Superti-Furga A, Unger S. Nosology and classification of genetic skeletal disorders: 2006 revision. *Am J Med Genet A.* 2007;143: 1–18.
7. Macpherson RI, Pai GS. Evaluation of newborns with skeletal dysplasias. *Ind J Ped.* 2000;67:907–913.

8. Mortier GR. The diagnosis of skeletal dysplasias: a multidisciplinary approach. *Eur J Radiol.* 2001;40:161–167.

9. Poor MA, Alberti O Jr, Griscom NT, Driscoll SG, Holmes LB. Non-skeletal malformations in one of three siblings with Jarcho-Levin syndrome of vertebral anomalies. *J Pediatr.* 1983;103:270–272.

10. Kwok C, Weller PA, Guioli S, Foster JW, Mansour S, Zuffardi O, et al. Mutations in SOX9, the gene responsible for Campomelic Dysplasia and Autosomal Sex Reversal. *Am J Hum Genet.* 1995;57:1028–1036.

11. Horton WA. Molecular Genetics of Human Chondrodysplasias. *Growth Genetics and Hormones.* 1997;13:49–55.

12. Dreyer SD, Zhou G, Lee B. The long and the short of it: developmental genetics of the skeletal dysplasias. *Clin Genet.* 1998;54:464–473.

13. Unger S. A genetic approach to the diagnosis of skeletal dysplasia. *Clin Orthopaedics Rel Res.* 2002;Number 401: 32–38.

14. Cole WG. Skeletal dysplasias reveal genes of importance in skeletal development and structure. *Conn Tissue Res.* 2003;44 (Suppl):246–249.

15. Newman B, Wallis GA. Skeletal dysplasias caused by a disruption of skeletal patterning and endochondral ossification. *Clin Genet.* 2003;63:241–251.

16. Savarirayan R, Rimoin DL. The skeletal dysplasias. *Adv Pediat.* 2004;51:209–229.

17. Hurst JA, Firth HV, Smithson S. Skeletal dysplasias. *Semin Fetal Neonatal Med.* 2005;10:233–241.

18. Cohen MM Jr. The new bone biology: pathologic, molecular, and clinical correlates. *Am J Med Genet.* 2006;A 140:2546–2706.

19. Alman BA. Skeletal dysplasias and the growth plate. *Clin Genet.* 2008;73:24–30.

20. Orioli IM, Castilla EE, Barbosa-Neto JG. The birth prevalence rates for the skeletal dysplasias. *J Med Gen.* 1986;23:328–332.

21. Stoll C, Dott B, Roth M-P, Alembik Y. Birth prevalence rates of skeletal dysplasias. *Clin Genet.* 1989;35:88–92.

22. Rasmussen SA, Bieber FR, Benacerraf BR, Lachman RS, Rimoin DL, Holmes LB. Epidemiology of osteochondrodysplasias: Changing trends due to advances in prenatal diagnosis. *Am J Med Genet.* 1996;61:49–58.

23. Tretter AE, Saunders RC, Meyers CM, Dungan JS, Gumbach K, Sun C-CJ et al. Antenatal diagnosis of lethal skeletal dysplasias. *Am J Med Genet.* 1998;75:518–522.

24. Waller DK, Correa A, Vo TM, Wang Y, Hobbs C, Langlois PH et al. The population-based prevalence of achondroplasia and thanatophoric dysplasia in selected regions of the US. *Am J Med Genet Part A.* 2008;146A:2385–2389.

25. Orioli IM, Castilla EE, Scarano G, Mastroiacovo P. Effect of paternal age in achondroplasia, thanatophoric dysplasia, and osteogenesis imperfecta. *Am J Med Genet.* 1995;59:209–217.

26. Horton WA, Harris DJ, Collins DL. Discordance for the Kleeblattschädel anomaly in monozygotic twins with thanatophoric dysplasia. *Am J Med Genet.* 1983;15:97–101.

27. Cohen DH, Starman BJ, Blumberg B, Byers PH. Recurrence of lethal osteogenesis imperfecta due to parental mosaicism for a dominant mutation on a human type I collagen gene (COL1A1). *Am J Hum Genet.* 1990;46:591–601.

28. Shaul WL, Hall JG. Multiple congenital anomalies associated with oral anticoagulants. *Am J Ob Gyn.* 1977;127:191–198.

29. Howe AM, Lipson AH, Sheffield LJ, Haan EA, Halliday JL, Jenson F et al. Prenatal exposure to phenytoin, facial development, and a possible role for vitamin K. *Am J Med Gen.* 1995;58:238–244.

30. Seashore MR, Cho S, Desposito F, Sherman J, Wappner RS, Wilson MG. Committee on Genetics. Health Supervision for Children with Achondroplasia. *Pediatrics.* 1995;95:443–451.

31. Ho NC, Guarnieri M, Brant LJ, Park SS, Sun B, North M, Francomano CA, Carson BS. Living with achondroplasia: quality of life following cervico-medullary decompression. *Am J Med Genet.* 2004;131A:163–167.

32. Carter EM, Davis JG, Raggio CL. Advances in understanding etiology of achondroplasia and review of management. *Curr Opin Pediatr.* 2007;19:32–37.

33. Krakow D, Williams J, Poehl M, Rimoin DL, Platt LD. Use of three-dimensional ultrasound imaging in the diagnosis of prenatal-onset skeletal dysplasias. *Ultrasound Obstet Gynecol.* 2003;21:467–472.

34. Gonçalves LF, Espinoza J, Mazor M, Romero R. Newer imaging modalities in the prenatal diagnosis of skeletal dysplasias. *Ultrasound Obstet Gynecol.* 2004;24:115–120.

35. Ruano R, Molho M, Roume J, Ville Y. Prenatal diagnosis of skeletal dysplasias by combining two-dimensional and three-dimensional ultrasound and intrauterine three-dimensional helical computer tomography. *Ultrasound Obstet Gynecol.* 2004;24:115–120.

36. Hunter AGW. Some psychosocial aspects of non lethal chondrodysplasias: I. Assessment using a life-styles questionnaire. *Am J Med Genet.* 1998;78:1–8.

Chapter 22

Vertebral Anomalies: Hemivertebra

HEMIVERTEBRAE

Definition

A deformity of one or more vertebrae in which only half of a single vertebra has been formed.

ICD-9:   756.145   (hemivertebrae, cervical)
              756.150   (hemivertebrae, thoracic)
              756.165   (hemivertebrae, lumbar)
              756.185   (hemivertebrae, not
                         otherwise specified)
ICD-10:   Q76.4   (other congenital
                         malformations of spine:
                         hemivertebra)

Mendelian   None
Inheritance
in Man:

Appearance

A hemivertebra can be at any level of the spine: cervical, thoracic or lumbar. The hemivertebra may have an associated rib.

Hemivertebrae have been subdivided into three types (1–3) [Figure 22-1]:

1. fully segmented (non-incarcerated hemivertebrae), which have disc spaces above and below (Figure 22-1); this type of hemivertebrae is usually equal or nearly equal in height to the adjacent vertebrae; some extend across the midline; those in the thoracic spine have a single pedicle and an associated rib; fully segmented hemivertebrae occur throughout the thoracic and lumbar regions.
2. semi-segmented (non-incarcerated hemivertebrae), which are similar in shape to the fully segmented type, but have no intervening disc space and are synostosed to one of the adjacent vertebrae; this type cannot be distinguished until the spine has ossified.

3. incarcerated hemivertebrae are usually ovoid in shape, smaller than a fully segmented hemivertebrae and most common in the thoracic region; they are located in a niche in the adjacent vertebrae, which compensate for the hemivertebra; therefore, there is more normal alignment of the spine; these are the least common type of hemivertebra; typically one is present.

The hemivertebra is to be distinguished from the butterfly vertebra (Figure 22-2), the vertebra with a coronal cleft (Figure 22-3), and a hypoplastic vertebra. Each of these other malformations affects the entire vertebra and, unlike the hemivertebrae, is not caused by the formation of only half of a vertebra.

Hemivertebrae can be an isolated, single deformity or part of a series of adjacent hemivertebrae with other anomalies of the spine and ribs. The most common site of vertebral anomalies is either the mid-thoracic or lower lumbar area (1).

A hemivertebra can act as an enlarging wedge and force the spine into a curve.

Associated Malformations

Several case series (1, 2, 4) and one population-based study (5) have shown that vertebral anomalies, in general, and hemivertebrae in particular, can be either isolated defects or, more often, associated with other vertebral anomalies or nonskeletal malformations.

Some of associated abnormalities are in adjacent structures and include: fused posterior processes, and malformed or fused adjacent ribs. These abnormalities are attributed to the same developmental error that produced the hemivertebra.

There are also several well-established associations with visceral anomalies, including urinary tract anomalies (6), anorectal anomalies (7), esophageal atresia (8),

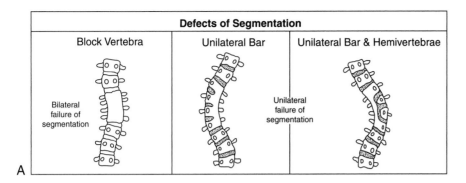

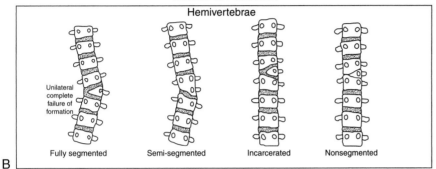

FIGURE 22.1A & 22.1B   The different types of hemivertebrae. (Reproduced with permission from Green DW: Current Opinion, 2000)

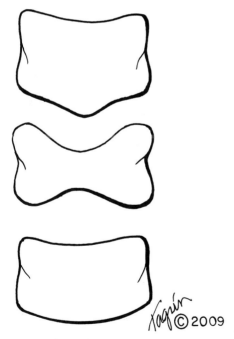

FIGURE 22.2   Butterfly vertebra

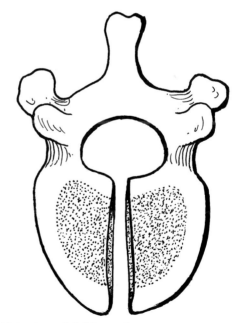

FIGURE 22.3   Coronal cleft in vertebra

heart defects (9), duodenal atresia (10), and the VACTERL Association (11).

The association of vertebral anomalies with renal anomalies is one of the most frequent associations. In a survey of 202 individuals with vertebral abnormalities, 26.7% had at least one genitourinary abnormality, often unilateral renal agenesis (2). Fetuses with hemivertebrae

identified by prenatal screening with ultrasound have been found to have a high frequency of nonskeletal anomalies (12). In a series of 27 fetuses, 11 (40%) were considered isolated. Seven of the 16 with multiple anomalies had Potter's Syndrome of renal a/dysgenesis.

The vertebral anomalies identified in association with esophageal atresia and anorectal malformations have included defects in the formation of vertebrae, including hemivertebrae and segmentation defects, such as fusion of vertebrae (6).

Congenital unilateral absence of the first cervical vertebra, called a hemi-atlas, has been associated with torticollis and, occasionally, esophageal atresia (13).

In a case series of 218 individuals with vertebral anomalies evaluated at an orthopedic center (excluding those with spina bifida cystica) (2), 61% had an associated nonskeletal abnormality. The most common finding was cranial nerve palsy. In this case series, the most common vertebral anomaly was hemivertebrae, either single or multiple. The frequency of associated malformations was similar for individuals with a single affected vertebra in comparison to those with multiple spine abnormalities.

In the only population-based analysis of all infants with hemivertebrae among 316,508 liveborn and stillborn infants and elective terminations in Hawaii (1986–2002) [5], 41 affected infants were identified. 8 (20%) of the 41 had a specific malformation syndrome, with the VACTERL Association the most common (4/8; 50%).

Developmental Defect (14–17)

The axial skeleton, all skeletal muscles and tendons, and the dorsal dermis are all derived from the presomitic mesoderm. During the weeks after gastrulation, the mesenchymal cells from the presomitic mesoderm form the paired blocks of mesoderm, which become the somites. During this process of somitogenesis, the presomitic mesoderm is constantly renewed at its caudal end by cell proliferation in the tail bud.

The "clock and wavefront" model, first proposed over 30 years ago (18), is the current model of how the development of somites occurs. All cells in the presomitic mesoderm oscillate between two internal states, prior to being incorporated into a somite. The number of genes exhibiting oscillatory expression has been estimated to be 50 to 100. One group is involved in the Notch and fibroblast growth factor (FGF)-mitogen-activated protein kinase (MAPK) signaling pathways. The other group of genes is expressed in WNT signaling pathways.

The "wave front" is generated by two opposing gradients of signaling activity in the presomitic mesodermal. One gradient is with retinoic acid in the nostral region and the other is FGF and WNT signaling from the caudal PSM. The wave front proceeds slowly. A single wave front moves through the entire region of somites in the time it takes to form all somites.

In humans the first somite begins to be formed at 20 days post-fertilization. 38 pairs of somites form during the next 10 days, with a total of 42–44 forming (4 occipital, 8 cervical, 12 thoracic, 5 lumbar, 5 sacral and 10 coccygeal) [15]. The number of vertebrae is fixed in the species. In humans, variation in the number of vertebrae is uncommon and is often associated with nonskeletal malformations (19).

The cause of one or more isolated hemivertebrae has not been determined. It has been noted that the vertebral body forms as a cartilaginous anlage and that defective development would be present at that time, not occurring later (20). A hemivertebra has been identified in an 11.5 week human fetus (20).

Hemivertebrae are also part of several phenotypes of multiple vertebral anomalies that include also several fused vertebrae and ribs. The preferred terminology is in flux. One system is to subdivide into subdivisions of spondylocostal dysplasias (SCD), types I-III (21). Another classification system focuses on the major gene mutations, such as DLL3 mutations in SCD1 and MESP2 for SCD2 (16, 21). The expectation is that many more mutations will be identified in individuals with hemivertebrae and other vertebral anomalies. These could be genes active in each step in the formation of somites and, subsequently, the axial skeleton.

Experimental models of exposure-induced vertebral anomalies in mice and rats have been developed using maternal carbon monoxide exposure (22) and 1% ethylenethiourea (ETU [23]. The acute exposures for seven hours to moderate and high doses of carbon monoxide showed that day 9.5 of gestation was a more sensitive time than either day 8.5 or 10.5. The higher the dose, the greater the frequency of anomalies. There was no correlation between the gestational day of exposure and the level of vertebral abnormality. The high dose (125 mg/kg) exposure to 1% ETU was administered by gavage on day 10 in Sprague-Dawley rates (23). 98.5% of the exposed pups had anorectal malformations. The vertebral anomalies were more severe in pups with an unfused neural tube, that is, rachischisis.

Prevalence

Screening in pregnancy by ultrasound increases the number of affected infants with hemivertebrae identified in comparison to clinical examinations at birth, as the milder phenotypes would be identified. In prenatal screening in Israel of 78,500 liveborn infants between 15 and 22 weeks of gestation, the prevalence rate was 0.33/1,000 (24). In a population-based birth defects registry in Hawaii (1986–2002) [5], the prevalence of hemivertebra was 0.13/1,000 among 316,508 liveborn and stillborn infants and elective terminations. The identification of newborn infants with hemivertebrae in Hawaii included a review of medical records that included the findings in prenatal screening.

Race/Ethnicity

The prevalence rates were similar among infants with Caucasian, Far East Asian, Pacific Islander, and Filipino ancestry in Hawaii (5).

Birth Status

The prevalence rate of hemivertebrae was higher in the lower birth weight (less than 2,500 grams) and premature infants (less than 38 weeks of gestation) in Hawaii (5).

Sex Ratio

More affected males than females have been observed in case series (1, 2) and in one population-based study (5).

Parental Age

In the population-based survey in Hawaii (5), the prevalence rate of hemivertebrae was lower with increasing maternal age (35 or older).

Twinning

No increased frequency of twins has been reported in individuals with hemivertebrae in comparison to unaffected individuals.

In one case series of infants with congenital scoliosis, all five sets of identical twins had only one affected twin, i.e., were discordant (25).

In one set of concordant female identical twins (26), one had hemivertebra from T7 to T9 and the co-twin had a left hemivertebra at T5-T6. Both twins had also paired butterfly vertebra in the lower cervical spine.

Concordance has been reported in one pair of identical twins for other changes in vertebrae: one twin had a butterfly vertebra of the eighth thoracic vertebra (T8) and the other had a coronal cleft of one vertebra, also T8 (27).

Genetic Factors

While significant progress has been made in identifying gene mutations in individuals with multiple hemivertebrae and anomalies of segmentation of the axial spine (16, 21), the cause of a single hemivertebra has not been determined.

The family studies by Ruth Wynne-Davies (28) showed that there was no risk of occurrence among siblings of individuals with a solitary hemivertebrae. She evaluated 337 individuals with scoliosis with several types of skeletal abnormalities in Edinburgh and London and their families. None of the 45 children with isolated hemivertebrae had a sibling with either a vertebral anomaly or a neural tube defect.

Environmental Factors

The most common environmental factor associated with the occurrence of any type of vertebral anomaly is insulin-dependent diabetes in the mother (11, 29, 30). In the analysis of the 26 malformed infants of diabetic mothers (IDM) among 4,929 infants with major malformations identified in the Metropolitan Atlanta Congenital Defects Program (1968–1980), the combination of vertebral and cardiovascular anomalies had the highest predictive value (6.5%) [29]. 8 (31%) of the 26 malformed infants had multiple anomalies. In an analysis of the malformed IDM among 19,039 pregnancies surveyed in Spain (1976–1992), 36% had malformations of the vertebrae, primarily infants with multiple anomalies. The most distinctive pattern of vertebral anomalies described was caudal dysgenesis, a severe abnormality of the sacral vertebrae.

Isolated hemivertebra also occur in IDM. 4 (25%) of 16 infants with one or two hemivertebra identified in the surveillance of 206,244 infants in Boston were infants of a diabetic mother (Table 22-1).

Treatment and Prognosis (31–35)

The treatment of hemivertebrae can be fusion of the vertebral deformity or excision of the hemivertebrae.

The hemivertebra can act as an enlarging wedge, forcing the spine into a curve. Multiple hemivertebrae produce faster progression (35). The treatment of multiple hemivertebrae may be required before age five years. However, treatment of a single hemivertebra may be delayed until the preadolescent growth spurt.

The prognosis for the complications from hemivertebrae are determined by the site of the affected vertebra, the number of affected vertebrae, and the presence of associated nonskeletal anomalies. Whether or not the congenital scoliosis associated with a single hemivertebrae will progress has been extremely difficult to predict. Some progress severely, others slowly and some not at all (25).

Genetic Counseling

Vertebral anomalies are heterogenous in phenotype and in apparent etiology, as are all common malformations. The group of phenotypes includes variation in the number of vertebrae (19), transformation in the morphology of vertebrae, changes over time (such as in the flattening or platyspondyly that develops in individuals with skeletal dysplasias [35, 36]) and congenital developmental abnormalities, such as the hemivertebrae.

A hemivertebra is to be distinguished from other structural abnormalities of vertebrae, such as the butterfly vertebra (Figure 22-2), the vertebra with a coronal

TABLE 22-1 *Hemivertebrae identified in the surveillance for congenital malformations at Brigham and Women's Hospital in Boston*.

Apparent Etiology	Isolated	Multiple anomalies
1. Mendelian disorders		
a) spondyloepiphyseal dysplasia	-0-	1 (T7)
2. Chromosome abnormalities	-0-	0
3. Specific syndromes		
a) diaphragmatic hernia with limb defect		1 (T3; plus T3 & T4 coronal cleft)
b) renal agenesis, bilateral		1 (T11-12)
c) anencephaly		1 (T2 and L3)
d) anotia		1 (multiple hemivertebrae)
e) VACTERL Association		3 (multiple hemivertebrae)
4. Exposures		
a) dilation and curettage (ref; patient #2)		1 (T2 and T9; plus L3-4 block vertebra)
b) insulin-dependent diabetes mellitus in mother	1 (L5)	4 (1:T10) (1:T11) (1:L4) (1:multiple)
5. Twinning:		1 (T6)** 1 (infant with VACTERL Association**)
6. Unknown etiology	4 (1:T4) (1:T4-T8) (1:T5, T11) (bifid T1, T2)	7 (1:T11-L2) (1:T11-12) (1:T multiple) (1:T8-9) (1:L2-3) (1:T7-9) (1:T5)
TOTAL	5	22

Legends: * The affected infants were identified in the survey at birth of 206,244 live births, stillbirths and elective terminations for fetal anomalies in the years 1972–1974, 1979–2000.

The detection of hemivertebrae was impacted by routine prenatal screening in the third trimester of pregnant women with diabetes mellitus.

** = twin pairs, only one twin affected.
T = thoracic vertebra
L = lumbar vertebra

cleft (Figure 22-3), and a hypoplastic vertebra. A hemivertebra is often associated with abnormalities of adjacent structures, such as ribs. These rib anomalies are attributed to the same developmental process that led to the occurrence of the hemivertebra.

An isolated single hemivertebrae appears to be a nonfamilial abnormality, based on the limited information available.

Hemivertebra associated with either an omovertebra or with a unilateral bar are considered separate and distinct from isolated hemivertebra. An omovertebra is an ectopic, extra band of bone between a cervical vertebra and the scapula (37). Multiple hemivertebrae with a unilateral bar is associated with intraspinal anomalies,

such as diastematomyelia and changes in the overlying skin (e.g. having patch or red nevus) and neurologic abnormalities. Treatments include excision of the diastematomyelia and fusion of the vertebrae before age five. The prognosis for correction with a short, relatively straight spine is limited (38).

Several phenotypes, referred to as spondylocostal dysplasias (SCD) and which include multiple hemivertebrae, segmentation defects, and fused ribs, have been described. Many of these are attributed to autosomal dominant or recessive mutations. If the infant with hemivertebrae has these additional spine anomalies, the diagnostic evaluation must focus on the clinical diagnosis, and, if possible, the mutation analyses. The genetic counseling will be based on the specific diagnosis established.

1. SCD, type 1: Mendelian Inheritance in Man: #277300; due to mutation in delta-like 3 gene (DLL3); autosomal recessive.

2. SCD, type 2: Mendelian Inheritance in Man: #608681; due to mutation in mesoderm posterior 2 homolog gene (MESP2); autosomal recessive.

3. SCD, type 3: Mendelian Inheritance in Man: #609813; due to mutation in LFNG0-fucosylpeptide 3-beta-N-acetylglucosaminyl-transferase gene (LFNG); autosomal recessive.

4. Spondylospinal thoracic dysostosis: Mendelian Inheritance in Man 601809; short curved spine, fused spinous processes and "crab-like" configuration of ribs, arthrogryposis and hypoplastic mandible and maxilla; autosomal recessive.

5. Spondylocostal dysostosis with anal atresia and urogenital anomalies: Mendelian Inheritance in Man: 271520; severe vertebral and rib dysplasia with associated malformations; autosomal recessive.

6. Spondylocostal dysplasia, autosomal dominant form: Mendelian Inheritance in Man: %122600; shortening in thorax; 11 pairs of ribs; hemivertebrae and vertebral fusion.

7. Spinal dysplasia in father and son (39); severe kyphoscoliosis; multiple segmentation anomalies; decreased anterior-posterior diameter of affected vertebrae. Autosomal dominant.

REFERENCES

1. McMaster MJ, David CV. Hemivertebrae as a cause of scoliosis. *J Bone Jt Surg.* 1986;68B:588–595.

2. Beals RK, Robbins JR, Rolfe B. Anomalies with vertebral malformations. *Spine.* 1993;18:1329–1332.

3. Tortori-Donati P, Fondelli MP, Rossi A, Rayband CA, Cama A, Capra V. Segmental spinal dysgenesis: neuroradiologic findings with clinical and embryologic correlation. *Am J Neuroradiol.* 1999;20:445–456.

4. Erol B, Tracy MR, Dormans JP, Zackai EH, Maisenbacher MK, O'Brien ML, Turnpenny PD, Kusumi K. Congenital scoliosis and vertebral malformations. Characterization of segmental defects for genetic analysis. *J Pediatr Orthop.* 2004;24:674–682.

5. Forrester MB, Merz RD. Descriptive epidemiology of hemivertebrae, Hawaii, 1986–2002. *Congenital Anomalies.* 2006;46: 172–176.

6. Rai AS, Taylor TKF, Smith GHH, Cumming RG, Plunkett-Cole M. Congenital abnormalities of the urogenital tract in association with congenital vertebral malformations. *J Bone Jt Surg.* 2002;[B] 84-B:891–895.

7. Heij HA, Nievelstein RAJ, de Zwart I, Verbeeten BW, Volk J, Vos A. Abnormal anatomy of the lumbosacral region imaged by magnetic resonance in children with anorectal malformations. *Arch Dis Childh.* 1996;74:441–444.

8. Chetcuti P, Dickens DRV, Phelan PD. Spinal deformity in patients born with oesophageal atresia and tracheo-esophageal fistula. *Arch Dis Childh.* 1989;64:1427–1430.

9. Weston AD, Ozolins TR, Brown NA. Thoracic skeletal defects and cardiac malformations: a common epigenetic link? *Birth Def Res (Part C).* 2006;78:354–370.

10. Atwell JD, Klidjian AM. Vertebral anomalies and duodenal atresia. *J Pediatr Surg.* 1982;17:237–240.

11. Martinez-Frias ML, Bermejo E, Rodriguez-Pinilla E. Anal atresia, vertebral, genital, and urinary tract anomalies: a primary polytopic developmental field defect identified through and epidemiological analysis of associations. *Am J Med Genet.* 2000; 95:169–173.

12. Zelop CM, Pretorius DH, Benacerraf BR. Fetal hemivertebrae: associated anomalies, significance, and outcome. *Obstet Gynecol.* 1993;81:412–416.

13. Dubousset J. Torticollis in children caused by congenital anomalies of the atlas. *J Bone Jt Surg Am.* 1986;68:178–188.

14. Theiler K. Vertebral malformations. *Adv Anat Embryol Cell Biol.* 1988;112:1–99.

15. Sparrow DB, Chapman G, Turnpenny PD, Dunwoodie SL. Disruption of the somatic molecular clock causes abnormal vertebral segmentation. *Birth Def Res (Part C): Clin Mol Terat.* 2007;81:93–110.

16. Martinez-Frias ML. Segmentation anomalies of the vertebras and ribs: one expression of the primary developmental field. *Am J Med Genet.* 2004;128A:127–131.

17. O'Rahilly R, Müller F. *Human Embryology and Teratology.* 3rd ed. New York: Wiley-Liss; 2001: 362–374.

18. Cooke J, Zeeman EC. A clock and wavefront model for control of the number of repeated structures during animal morphogenesis. *J Theoret Biol.* 1976;58:455–476.

19. Bates AW, Nale K. Segmentation defects of the human axial skeleton without dysostoses or skeletal dysplasias. *Fetal and Pediatric Pathology.* 2005;21:121–127.

20. Tanaka T, Uhthoff HK. The pathogenesis of congenital vertebral malformations. A study based on observations made in 11 human embryos and fetuses. *Acta Orthop Scand.* 1981;52: 413–425.

21. Sewell W, Kusumi K. Genetic analysis of molecular oscillators in mammalian somitogenesis: clues for studies of human vertebral disorders. *Birth Defects Res (Part C): Clin Mol Terat.* 2007;81: 111–120.

22. Loder RT, Hernandez MJ, Lerner AL, Winebrener DJ, Goldstein SA, Hensinger RN et al. The induction of congenital spinal deformities in mice by maternal carbon monoxide exposure. *J Pediatr Arthop.* 2000;20:662–666.

23. Qi BQ, Beasley SW, Arsic D. Abnormalities of the vertebral column and ribs associated with anorectal malformations. *Pediatr Surg Int.* 2004;20:529–533.

24. Goldstein I, Makhoul IR, Weissman A, Drugan A. Hemivertebra: prenatal diagnosis, incidence and characteristics. *Fetal Diagn Ther.* 2005;20:121–126.

25. Winter RB, Lonstein JE, Boachie-Adjei O. Instructional Course Lectures, The American Academy of Orthopaedic Surgeons. *J Bone Jt Surg [Am].* 1996;78-A:300–311.

26. Sturm PF, Chung R, Bomze SR. Hemivertebra in monozygotic twins. *Spine.* 2001;26:1389–1391.

27. van den Bos RW, Vielvoye GJ, Blickman JG. Vertebral anomalies in monozygotic twins. *Diagn Imag Clin Med.* 1984;53:259–261.

28. Wynne-Davies R. Congenital vertebral anomalies: aetiology and relationship to spina bifida cystica. *J Med Genet.* 1975;12: 280–288.

29. Khoury MJ, Vecerra JE, Cordero JF, Erickson JD. Clinical-epidemiologic assessment of patterns of birth defects associated with human teratogens: application to diabetic embryopathy. *Pediatrics.* 1989;84:658–665.

30. Martínez-Frias ML. Epidemiological analysis of outcomes of pregnancy in diabetic mothers: identification of the most characteristic and most frequent congenital anomalies. *Am J Med Genet.* 1994;51:108–113.

31. Winter RB, Moe JH. The results of arthrodesis for congenital spinal deformity in patients younger than five years old. *J Bone Jt Surg (Am).* 1982;64:419–432.

32. Thompson AG, Marks DS, Sayampanathan SRE, Piggott H. Long-term results of combined anterior and posterior convex epiphysiodesis for congenital scoliosis due to hemivertebrae. *Spine.* 1995;20:1380–1385.

33. Goldberg CJ, Moore DP, Fogarty EE, Dowling FE. Long-term results from In Situ fusion for congenital vertebral deformity. *Spine.* 2002;27:619–628.

34. Weisz B, Achiron R, Schindler A, Eisenberg VH, Lipitz S, Zalel Y. Prenatal sonographic diagnosis of hemivertebra. *J Ultrasound Med.* 2004;23:853–857.

35. Jaskwhich D, Ali RM, Patel TC. Congenital scoliosis. *Curr Opin. Pediatr.* 2000;12:61–66.

36. Vanhoenacker FM, De Schepper AM, Parizel PM. Congenital abnormalities of the osseous spine: a radiological approach. *JBR-BTR.* 2005;88:37–41.

37. Azouz EM. CT demonstration of omovertebral bone. *Pediatr Radiol.* 2007;37:404.

38. McMaster MJ. Congenital scoliosis caused by a unilateral failure to vertebral segmentation with contra lateral hemivertebra. *Spine.* 1998;23:998–1005.

39. Auhalt H, Parker B, Paranjpc DV, Neely EK, Silverman FN, Rosenfeld RG. Novel spinal dysplasia in two generations. *Am J Med Genet.* 1995;56:90–93.

Chapter 23

Patterns of Malformations: Non-Random Clusters

CANTRELL PENTALOGY

Definition

The association of a bifid lower end of the sternum, deficiency of the anterior and pericardial portion of the diaphragm, a midline abdominal wall defect above the umbilicus, and an ectopic beating heart.

ICD-9:	756.680	(other specified anomalies of diaphragm)
	756.700	(omphalocele)
	756.790	(other and unspecified anomalies of abdominal wall)
ICD-10:	Q79.1	(other congenital malformations of diaphragm)
	Q79.2	(omphalocele)
	Q79.5	(other congenital malformations of abdominal wall)
Mendelian Inheritance in Man:	None	

Historical Note

In 1958 three surgeons at the Johns Hopkins Hospital in Baltimore, Drs. James R Cantrell, J. Alex Haller, and Mark M. Ravitch, reported having treated several patients with "an unusual combination of congenital defects," which they considered a clinical syndrome. Each patient had "1) a midline, supraumbilical abdominal wall defect; 2) a defect in the lower sternum; 3) a deficiency of the anterior diaphragm; 4) a defect in the

disphragmatic pericardium; 5) congenital intracardiac defects" (1) [Figure 23-1].

They noted that this phenotype was different from ectopia cordis, because of the associated anomalies. They credited Byron (2) as having first reported in 1948 the association of ectopia cordis and other anomalies.

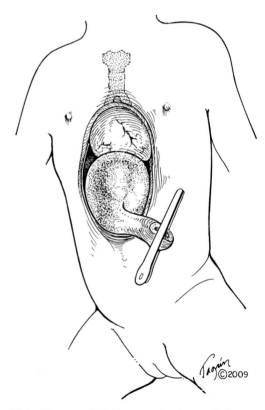

FIGURE 23.1 Diagram which illustrates the phenotypic features of the Pentalogy of Cantrell: bifid sternum, ectopic heart, deficiency of pericardium, and high abdominal omphalocele.

They listed the patients with this phenotype that had been reported between 1734 and 1948 and added five of their own affected patients. They described the diaphragm defect as a partial or total failure of the transverse septum to develop. The portion of the pericardium affected was the section adjacent to the transverse septum of the diaphragm. They noted that, while the associated heart defects varied, all infants had defects in the cardiac septa. The defects of the sternum (bifid) and abdominal wall were attributed to a developmental defect. Unrelated anomalies outside of the anatomic area of the defects were uncommon. Among the 21 affected infants they reviewed from previous publications, two had malrotation of the intestines, one had absence of the left lung, and one had anencephaly.

Appearance

The affected infant has a normal appearance, except for closure defects in the lower sternum and upper abdomen. There may be a membrane-covered omphalocele (Figures 23-1 and 23-3) and a beating ectopic heart in the upper abdomen, just below the edge of the ribs and sternum (3–12).

There can be herniations into the pericardial sac of an omental tab (5), the small and large intestine (4), and the appendix of the large intestine (1).

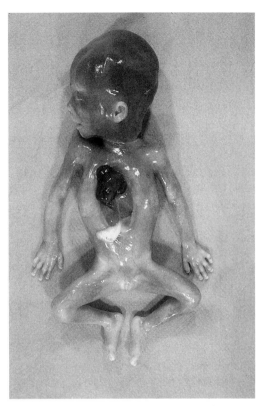

FIGURE 23.3 20-week gestational age fetus with cleft sternum, ectopia cordis, double outlet right ventricle, transposition of great arteries, pulmonary atresia, pulmonary situs inversus, anorectal atresia, and renal duplication. (From Mason Barr, M.D., University of Michigan, Ann Arbor, MI. Used with permission.)

In the original description (1), "intracardiac defects" were one of the five cardinal factors of the Cantrell Pentalogy. In a review of 50 affected individuals (11), after excluding those with chromosome abnormalities and amniotic band syndrome, 42% had conotruncal heart defects. Other associated heart defects included atrial and ventricular septal defects and single ventricle with double outlet and pulmonary and tricuspid atresia (12).

Associated Malformations

The reviews (5, 8, 9) of the many reports of infants with this pattern of malformations have shown that only some have the five cardinal features. Some do not have a heart defect. Some do not have a diaphragm defect (12). Some have diastasis recti instead of omphalocele or complete absence of the pericardium rather than a defect in the pericardium (5).

In addition to variations in the core phenotype, several affected infants have had additional malformations, such as cleft lip, myelomeningocele, encephalocele, and malrotation of the colon (5). Three of the five infants with the Pentalogy of Cantrell identified in the Baltimore-Washington Infant Cardiovascular Malformation Study (1981–1989) had cleft lip deformity with or without cleft palate (8).

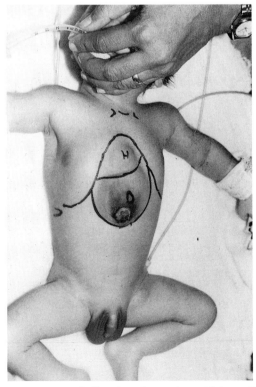

FIGURE 23.2 Picture of affected newborn infant with heart (H) and abdominal defect (O) covered by skin. (From Agrawal N et al: *Anaesth Intensive Care.* 200331:120.)

Developmental Defect

This group of non-randomly associated malformations is localized primarily to structures in the lower sternum, upper abdomen, diaphragm, and heart. It has been called a ventral midline developmental field (8), but the underlying cellular or molecular abnormality has not been determined.

A sequence of abnormal development between days 14 and 18 after fertilization has been postulated (13). There is failure of the lateral fusion of the ectomesodermal folds, causing thereby the omphalocele. A deficient fusion of the cephalic ectomesodermal fold causes the ectopic heart and the defects in the sternum and anterior portion of the diaphragm.

Another hypothesis suggested (14) has been that the ectopic heart, seen in a 28 day human embryo, reflected "an arrest of cardiac descent at 3 weeks of development. . . ." The authors postulated that early rupture of the chorion and/or yolk sac could have produced mechanical distortion of the abnormalities of the heart and sternum.

Animal models of defective abdominal closure have been described in mouse knockouts for the genes Tcfap2a (15) and Pitx2 (16). The genes A-P2 and bicoid type homeobox gene Pitx2 affect closure of the ventral body wall. However, the phenotypes produced, specifically a completely open thorax and abdomen, are much more severe than that of the Pentalogy of Cantrell.

Prevalence

In Atlanta, two affected infants (1:250,000) were identified in the metropolitan Atlanta Congenital Defects Program (MACDP) among 508,949 births (1968–1986) [7]. In the Baltimore-Washington series (8), the prevalence rate was 1:181,810 live births over a ten-year period.

Race/Ethnicity

There is insufficient information on the occurrence in different racial, ethnic groups.

Birth Status

Death soon after birth was common before the advent of modern surgical and anesthesia care (5). Two of the five infants identified in the Baltimore-Washington area in the 1980s died in the first day of life (8).

Sex Ratio

No large case series established the sex ratio.

Sidedness

This is a midline defect.

Twinning

One of the five cases in the Baltimore-Washington series (8) was a male twin, with an unaffected co-twin (zygosity not provided). One set of monozygous twins concordant for Cantrell Pentalogy has been reported (17).

Genetic Factors

One instance of affected brothers has been reported (18). The empiric recurrence risk has not been established.

No associated chromosome abnormalities have been reported.

Environmental Factors

No exposures in pregnancy have been shown to cause the Cantrell Pentalogy. No systematic studies evaluating the exposures in a significant number of affected infants have been published.

Treatment and Prognosis

Usually, these interrelated and associated malformations are repaired in the newborn period or in early infancy. Sometimes a staged repair of the chest, abdominal, and heart defects is necessary (10, 19).

Only 5 of 59 affected infants, as of 1996, had survived (10). A major complication during the surgical repair is compression of the heart and kidney of major vessels after intra-thoracic relocation of the heart (20).

Experience with surgical repair has shown the importance of performing echocardiography to confirm the findings suggested in prenatal studies, as the distortions of the anatomy can obscure significant abnormalities (21). The presence of an intracardiac anomaly is the best predictor of neonatal mortality (22).

Genetic Counseling

There have been rare instances of individual families with two brothers with Pentalogy of Cantrell and a third brother with a diaphragmatic hernia (18). However, there has been no evidence of mendelian inheritance pattern for this syndrome, except for these rare families.

Two rare and separate disorders to be considered in establishing the clinical diagnosis of Pentalogy of Cantrell are:

a) MIM %313850 Thoracoabdominal Syndrome. This is an X-linked dominant disorder, linked to Xq25-q26 (23). The features include ventral hernias, heart defects, diaphragmatic hernias and hypoplastic lungs.

b) MIM 606519 PHACES Association. This syndrome includes clefting of the sternum (sometimes only the upper sternum), large and complex hemangiomas of the face, heart defects, eye abnormalities and sometimes a supraumbilical septa (24).

Since the Pentalogy of Cantrell has occurred as a sporadic condition, the empiric recurrence risk is very low.

It will be particularly important to establish that an affected male infant does not have the features of the X-linked thoracoabdominal syndrome.

The occurrence of Pentalogy of Cantrell may be identified during pregnancy by ultrasonography (25). The variability of the phenotype observed postnatally will make it more difficult to be certain of the diagnosis and the differentiation from rare, but similar, disorders.

C.H.A.R.G.E. ASSOCIATION

Definition

The occurrence of this non-random cluster of malformations: ocular coloboma (C), heart defects (H), choanal atresia (A), retarded growth (R), genital anomalies (G), and ear anomalies (E). Most affected infants do not have each of these abnormalities.

ICD-9:	759.800	(congenital malformation syndrome affecting facial appearance)
ICD-10:	Q87.0	(congenital malformation syndromes prdominantly affecting facial appearance)
Mendelian Inheritance in Man:	#214800	(Choanal atresia; CHARGE Association)

Historical Note

The term "Association" was suggested from nonrandom clusters of malformations that appeared to have a common etiology. The first reports of infants with CHARGE Association were in 1979 by Bryan Hall (26), a clinical geneticist, and HM Hintner, an ophthalmologist and his associates (27). Hall's 17 patients all had choanal atresia and were identified in a retrospective review of patients whom he had evaluated. Hintner et al. (27), writing for an ophthalmology journal, described 10 patients with microphthalmia and a pattern of anomalies similar to those noted by Hall. In 1981 (28), Pagon, Graham, Zonana, and Young, clinical geneticists, described 21 children from three medical centers with either a coloboma of the eye or choanal atresia and other anomalies. They suggested the acronym CHARGE for this nonrandom cluster for anomalies. Clinical experience has shown subsequently that most affected infants had no affected sibs or parents and no visible chromosome abnormalities with the techniques of analysis that had been used.

Several etiologies were postulated, including a "teratogenic insult" in 1988 (29) and a microdeletion in 1994 (30). Several patients with different unbalanced chromosome translocations have been reported (31). A genome wide screen with 811 microsatellite markers for loss of expected heterozygosity failed to identify a deletion (32).

The first success in identifying related mutations was from using the new technique of comparative genomic ˙dization (CGH). Abnormalities were identified in the gene known as CDH7 (33, 34, 36), which is one of the chromodomain helicase DNA-binding genes. Molecular studies of regions affected by chromosome translocations led to the identity of other candidate genes, such as SEMA3E (Semaphorin 3E) and associated mutations (35). Semaphorin proteins are involved in a variety of cellular processes, including exon guidance and cell migration. On-going research is expected to identify causative mutations in additional genes.

Appearance

Many of the affected children have dysmorphic facial features, are growth restricted, have multiple anomalies and functional deficits, such as cranial nerve deficiencies and hearing loss (37).

Major and minor criteria for diagnosis have been suggested (37–39). The major criteria that occur commonly in children with CHARGE Association are coloboma of iris, retina, choroids and/or optic disc, choanal atresia (unilateral or bilateral), cranial nerve deficiencies, and lop or cup-shaped external ears.

The obstruction of the upper airway can be life-threatening in the affected newborn. The abnormalities identified by fiber optic laryngoscopy include anterior posterior flattening of the larynx and short vocal cords; tall and hypertrophic arytenoids that are positioned anteriorly and obscure the glottis; a coordinated movement of the vocal cords, epiglottis and arytenoids and pooling of saliva (40).

The affected children may have abnormal postural behavior, which could reflect their vestibular anomalies. In a series of 17 affected children with the CHARGE Association (41), a CT scan of the inner ear showed anomalies of the semicircular canals in 94%. These children showed no response in testing of the function of the vestibular canal. In postmortem studies of the temporal bones, absence or hypoplasia of the semicircular canal has been a distinctive finding that is associated with hearing loss (39, 41).

Cranial nerve (CN) dysfunction, especially involving CN V (weak chewing or sucking), CN VII (facial palsy), (hearing loss and balance vestibular problems), have been identified in most patients. In a survey of 99 affected individuals in Canada (42), 92% had at least one CN dysfunction and 72% had one or more.

Among older children with CHARGE Association, signs of hypogonadotropic hypogonadism and a defective sense of smell are common. The signs in boys are micropenis and undescended testes. Girls show a lack of spontaneous puberty over age 12. The children with a defective sense of smell in one case series (43) showed abnormal olfactory bulbs in all cases by magnetic resonance imaging.

Associated Malformations

Cleft lip or cleft palate, esophageal atresia with a tracheoesophageal fistula, and renal abnormalities are additional malformations that have been present in 15 to 25% of affected children (37, 38).

Limb malformations were not considered part of this phenotype initially. However, three children with the CHARGE phenotype also had a wide variety of abnormalities, specifically monodactyly, absent tibia, and bifid femurs, were shown to have truncating mutations in CHD7 and gene (44, 45). Further analyses have shown that 30% of the infants with the CHARGE Association have limb anomalies.

Developmental Defect

The underlying abnormality (ties) that cause all of the associated malformations has not been determined. The genes in which associated and presumably causative mutations and deletions have been identified, specifically CDH7 (33, 34, 36, 46) and SEMA3E (35), a semaphoring protein, are involved in basic embryologic processes. The malformations produced arise during a limited time period early in pregnancy (47).

Prevalence

The prevalence of the CHARGE Association has been estimated to be 1:10,000 to 1:15,000 live births (37). In a three-year national survey among pediatricians in Canada, the highest prevalence rate was 1:8,500 live births in the Atlantic Province and no (0%) cases were identified in Alberta (47). Among four large European malformations registries, there were 106 infants (1:55,904) with two or three of the features of CHARGE Association among 5,260 infants with multiple malformations out of 5.84 million births (48).

Sex Ratio

More affected males than females have been identified in several case series (31, 37).

Parental Age

Advanced paternal age has been observed among children with CHARGE Association who have no affected relatives (31, 37).

Twinning

Several sets of concordant identical twins have been reported (29, 49, 36). The pattern of anomalies in the co-twins has been similar, but not identical.

Birth Status

The more severely affected infants are more often born prematurely and have a low birth weight for gestational age (37, 38).

Genetic Factors

The process of identifying mutations in candidate genes in affected children has just begun, with the findings in CDH7 gene (33, 34, 36, 46, 49) and SEMA3E (35). The frequency of associated heterozygous mutations in CDH7 has been over 60% (36). In affected infants with no mutation in the CDH7 gene, MLPA (multiplex ligation-dependent probe amplification) has identified additional intragenic deletions. The mutations identified have been scattered throughout the gene and have included nonsense, frameshift, missense, and truncating mutations.

The technique of comparative genomic hybridization led to the identity of mutations in CDH7 in chromosome 8. An interstitial deletion that included the same region (8q11.2-q13) had been reported in another affected infant (50).

Most affected children have no affected sibling or parent. However, there have been a few reports of affected siblings (36, 51->53), affected half-siblings (28, 54) and affected parent and child (27).

Environmental Factors

No teratogenic exposure has been identified as a cause of the CHARGE Association.

Treatment and Prognosis

The infant with CHARGE Association may require intensive care at birth, if he/she has bilateral choanal atresia. The associated anomalies, such as that of the eyes, heart, genitals, or kidneys, necessitate separate evaluations. The high frequency of CNS malformations (55) and hearing loss (37) make the search for these associated problems essential to optimal care and for estimating the prognosis of the infant. Development is often delayed. Evaluation is difficult in the child who is deaf and blind. An increased frequency of autism has also been observed (47).

Genetic Counseling

A clinical guidance review, developed by experienced clinicians (37, 38), has provided a comprehensive evaluation format to use in establishing the diagnosis of CHARGE Association. The diagnostic evaluation should include chromosome analysis and array CGH with close attention to regions in which causative deletions have been observed, such as 8q11.2-q13 (50). The most informative testing is for mutations in CDH7 (33, 34, 36) and SEMA3E (35). Presumably additional associated mutations will be identified in on-going research.

Because of the overlap in phenotypes, it would be helpful to rule out the 22q11.2 deletions of the velocardiofacial syndrome.

Based on the findings in the affected child, the parents should be screened for chromosome translocations or to confirm that neither has a specific deletion or mutation.

If the abnormality identified in the affected infant appears to be a new event, and is a de novo change not seen in either parent, the risk for a second affected infant appears to be very low.

The affected child with an identified mutation, when a parent, theoretically, has a 50% risk that each child will inherit the causative molecular abnormality. More empiric recurrence risk data is needed to confirm these estimates.

HEMIFACIAL MICROSOMIA

Definition

This multiple anomaly syndrome affects usually one side of the face. The most common features on that side are: hypoplasia of the mandible and a wide mouth (macrostomia), which extends laterally, a malformed ear, an epibulbar dermoid on the lateral edge of the cornea of the eye, soft tissue deficiency, and a facial nerve palsy.

ICD-9:	744.910	(Congenital anomaly of face, not otherwise specified)
ICD-10:	Q18.9	(Congenital malformation of face and neck, unspecified)
	Q87.0	(Malformation syndromes affecting facial appearance)
Mendelian Inheritance in Man:	%164210	(hemifacial microsomia; HFM)
	141400	(hemifacial microsomia with radial defects)

Historical Note

Several different terms and eponyms have been proposed for this phenotype: a) Goldenhar Syndrome, reflecting the original report by Maurice Goldenhar in 1952 (56); b) oculo-auriculo-vertebral dysplasia (OAVS) in 1963, suggested by Robert Gorlin (57); c) facial-auriculo-vertebral spectrum in 1982, suggested by David Smith (58); and d) hemifacial microsomia with the O.M.E.N.S. Classification (O=orbital distortion; M=mandibular hypoplasia; E=ear anomaly; N=nerve involvement, and S=soft tissue deficiency) in 1991, suggested by Mulliken and his collaborators (59). Each clinician emphasized different features, such as the presence of epibulbar dermoid by Goldenhar and the unilateral hypoplasia of the mandible by Mulliken et al. Characteristics of the abnormality of the mandible in radiographs have added to the specificity of the findings (60), but have not identified any "pathognomonic" features.

A consensus has developed that there are many causes of this phenotype. The recognized etiologies have been genetic factors (61, 62), subtle chromosome duplications (63) and deletions (64, 65), mutations in transcription factors (66, 67), the process of vascular disruption (68, 69), insulin dependent diabetes in the mother (70), and exposure to vasoactive medications (71). Overripeness of the eggs fertilized has been a postulated cause that is related to the excess of twins and the association with assisted reproductive techniques, like IVF and ICSI (intracytoplasmic sperm injection) [72].

Initially, the repair of the craniofacial abnormalities was postponed until the affected individual was older and the deformity had reached the "end stage." More recently surgical treatments have begun early with correction of the deformity of the mandible improving the growth of the maxilla, orbits, and nose (73).

Appearance

Most affected infants have a unilateral deformity of the face with obvious asymmetry in the size of the mandible (59, 61, 74–76) [Figures 23-4 to 23-9].

The corner of the mouth extends further laterally on the smaller size of the face and produces the appearance of an asymmetric and widened mouth (macrostomia) [Figures 23-4, 23-6 and 23-8]. There is a range of severity of all features of hemifacial microsomia, including severe hypoplasia of the mandible with absence of the

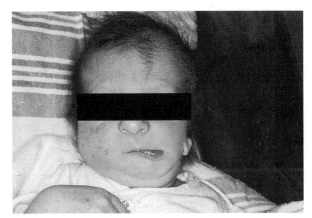

FIGURE 23.4 Shows macrostomia, with the opening of the mouth extending further to the left.

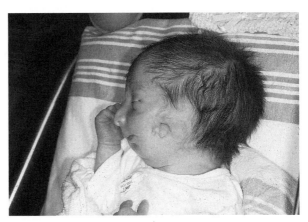

FIGURE 23.5 The lateral view of the infant in Figure 23-4, showing severe microtia.

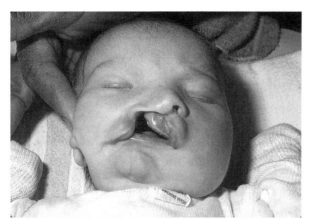

FIGURE 23.6   Shows macrostomia, extending to right, with unilateral cleft lip deformity.

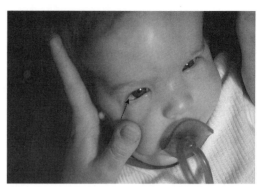

FIGURE 23.8   Close-up view of eyes of an infant with hemifacial microsomia, showing epibulbar dermoid on cornea of right eye.

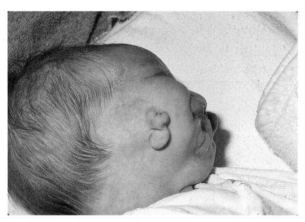

FIGURE 23.7   The lateral view of the infant in Figure 23-6, showing severe microtia.

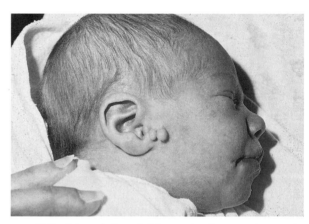

FIGURE 23.9   A lateral view of right ear showing posterior rotation, normal external ear shape and preauricular tag.

ramus, condyle, and temperomandibular joint which makes intubation very difficult (77).

The ear deformities vary from a mild deformity of the pinna with preauricular tags, to a low-set poorly developed ear or microtia (Figures 23-5, 23-7, 23-9).

The epibulbar dermoid is visible on the lateral aspect of the cornea (Figure 23-8).

The facial palsy is typically unilateral, ipsilateral, and associated with the more severe ear deformity and hypoplasia of the mandible.

The presence of multiple accessory tragi of the ear has been noted to be a distinctive feature of this phenotype (74).

Vertebral anomalies are considered part of this disorder. They are more common in the children with the more severe craniofacial abnormalities (72). A wide variety of vertebral anomalies, such as hemivertebrae and fused vertebrae, have been observed with no distinctive anomaly considered characteristic of hemifacial microsomia.

Associated Malformations

Since the diagnosis of this condition is a clinical judgment and since most affected individuals have no other affected relatives, the inclusion under the same diagnosis of infants with associated malformations is arbitrary.

Several individuals with hemifacial microsomia have had heart defects (78, 79), especially conotruncal defects, esophageal atresia (75, 80), and anomalies of the genitourinary system. In the review of 60 children with hemifacial microsomia evaluated at a referral center in Tampa (1985–1993), 3 had esophageal atresia (75). In a review of published reports of 247 infants with hemifacial microsomia (80), 13% had esophageal atresia with or without a tracheoesophageal fistula.

Developmental Factors

Hemifacial microsomia has been attributed to errors in the development of structures formed by the first and second branchial arches (81).

Naora et al. (82) created a transgenic mouse model hemifacial microsomia (hfm), producing a phenotype that included microtia and jaw asymmetry and hypoplasia of the second branchial arch. In addition, there were anomalies of the middle ear, cranial base, maxilla, and pharyngeal structures (83). In the more recent model (83) only hfm heterozygotes were viable. The trait in the hemizygote was transmitted as an autosomal dominant mutation with 25% penetrance.

Experimental induction of hemorrhage by administering triazine to fetal CSI mice produced hemorrhage in the area of the first and second branchial arches. Poswillo (84) noted that the hemorrhage produced was asymmetric and varied in severity, similar to the variability of these craniofacial anomalies in humans.

Prevalence

In the National Collaborative Perinatal Project (85), in which 53,394 singleton infants were examined at birth and followed for seven years, two infants with hemifacial microsomia were identified for a prevalence rate of 1:27,500.

In the years 1972–1974 and 1979–2000 at the Brigham and Women's Hospital in Boston, 8 affected infants were identified in the first five days of life by the Active Malformations Surveillance Program among 206,244 livebirths, stillbirths, and elective terminations for fetal anomalies (86). The prevalence was 1:25,781 or 0.04/1,000 (Table 23-1).

Race/Ethnicity

Information on the rate of occurrence of hemifacial microsomia has not been reported for different racial and ethnic groups.

Birth Status

Hemifacial microsomia has many causes. Among affected twins, prematurity and low birth weight are common, as expected. Some more severely affected twins show signs of growth restriction at birth.

Sex Ratio

A greater number of affected males than females has been shown in several studies (74).

Sidedness

A predominance of right sidedness was observed in one large study (61), but not in another (59).

Parental Age

In one analysis of 101 affected children there was no difference between the ages of the mothers and fathers in comparison to the general population (72).

Twinning

An increased frequency of twins has been noted in case series: 10% of 87 infants in Italy (78) and 7.5% of 67 infants in Germany (72).

The possibility that the twinning process can cause hemifacial microsomia has also been postulated (87, 88). The hemifacial microsomia in the surviving twin could have been caused by embolization of necrotic tissue from a deceased twin (68) or from a placental hematoma (69). An association of the oculo-auriculo-vertebral spectrum with assisted reproductive technology has also been postulated (72).

24 monozygous twins have been reported in which one had hemifacial microsomia. In 20 of the 24 MZ twin pairs, only one was affected (72). In four MZ twin pairs, both were affected.

Genetic Factors

Most affected infants have no affected relatives.

Family studies have suggested that hemifacial microsomia is hereditary (61). Rollnick, Kaye, and their associates evaluated 433 first-degree relatives of 97 probands. 8% had a similar anomaly. 6% of 176 siblings were considered "affected." The findings were interpreted as consistent with multifactorial inheritance. However, it should be noted that some probands had only unilateral microtia and some individuals considered "affected" had only a preauricular tag.

Single families with an affected parent and child in one (62, 90) and two affected sisters with healthy unrelated parents (91) in another.

Individuals with hemifacial microsomia have been included in family studies for specific mutations. SALL1 mutations were identified in one family (67) and SALL4 mutations in another (66). A missense mutation in exon 9 of the TCOF1, the mutation in Treacher Collins Syndrome, and two silent mutations in exons 10 and 23

TABLE 23-1 *Pattern of anomalies of newborn infants with hemifacial microsomia identified at Brigham and Women's Hospital (1972–1974, 1979–2000) among 206,244 livebirths, stillbirths, and elective terminations for fetal anomalies.*

	Year	Twin	Non-transfer	Maternal transfer	Sex	Race	Microtia	Small mandible	Macro-stomia	Preaur. tags	Vertebral Anomaly	Heart Defect	Other anomalies	Karyotype
1.	1979	S		MT	M	W	Rt	Rt	Rt	–	?		Cleft lip, Rt	46,XY
2.	1979	S	NT		M	W	Lt	Lt	Lt	+	?		Sinus in cheek (Rt)	
3.	1980	S		MT	M	W	Rt (severe)	Rt (severe)	Rt	–	+		IUFD clavicle absent, cleft palate	
4.	1982	S	NT		M	W	–	Rt (mild)	Rt	–	–			
5.	1985	S		MT	M	W	Lt (severe)	Lt	Lt	+	+		Epibulbar dermoid (rt) aqueductal stenosis	46,XY
6.	1986	S		MT	F	W	–	Rt	Rt	+ (bilat)	?	VSD	Imperforate anus	46,XX
7.	1987	S		MT	F	W	Rt	Rt	Bilat	+	?		Cleft lip bilateral, facial nerve palsy, left	46,XX
8.	1992	S	NT		F	Mixed	–	Lt	Lt	–	?		Cleft lip, left	46,XX
9.	1993	T	NT		F	W	Lt	Lt	Lt	+	?		Coloboma upper eyelid (lt)	46,XX
10.	1993	T	NT		M	W	–	Lt	Lt	+	?		Cleft lip, left; club foot, left; narrow palpebral fissures, left	46,XY
11.	1995	S		MT	F	W	–	–	Bilat	+	+	ASD	Omphalocele, cleft lip, bilat; infant of diabetic mother	46,XX
12.	1997	S	NT		F	W	Rt	?	Bilat	–	+		Dandy-Walker Syndrome; unilobular lung, Rt	
13.	1998	S	NT		M	W	Lt	Lt	Lt	–	+	VSD; membranous atrial septal defect, bicuspid aortic valve		46,XY
14.	1998	S	NT		M	H	Lt	Lt	Lt	–	?	–		
15.	1999	S	T		M	W	Rt	Rt	Rt	–	?	Tricuspid stenosis		46,XY

NT = Non-transfer (Mother had planned all along to deliver at BWH.)
MT = Maternal transfer (mother had planned to deliver at another hospital, but transferred to BWH after the prenatal detection of fetal anomalies.)
Sex: M = male; F = female
Race: W = Caucasian; B = Black; H = Hispanic
Lt = left; Rt = right
Heart defects: VSD = ventricular septal defect; ASD = atrial septal defect
T = twin; #9 dizygous; #10 diamniotic monochorionic; both sets of twins discordant for hemifacial microsmia.
S = singleton.

in another individual were identified in an individual with "typical" hemifacial microsomia (92).

Several different associated chromosome abnormalities have been reported (63–65). A deletion of the terminal 5p has been identified in several children with hemifacial microsomia (93). An interstitial 1p22.2-p31.1 deletion was identified recently by microarray analysis in a mentally retarded individual with craniofacial features of hemifacial microsomia (65).

Kelberman and associates (94) postulated that the goosecoid gene was an excellent candidate gene for hemifacial microsomia. They searched for mutations in the goosecoid gene coding regions in two families with multiple affected individuals and in 120 sporadic cases. No abnormalities were identified. A related member of the NK2 class of homeobox gene _BAPX1_ has also been identified as a candidate gene (95). No mutations were identified in 105 patients, but epigenetic dysregulation of _BAPX1_ was postulated as the underlying developmental abnormality.

An epidemiologic analysis of 5,260 infants with multiple malformations in large population-based registries showed a relationship between the features of the oculo-auriculo-vertebral syndrome (or hemifacial microsomia) and the CHARGE Association (96). This association suggested that these disorders could have a common pathogenetic mechanism.

Environmental Factors

Hemifacial microsomia has been attributed to maternal insulin-dependent diabetes mellitus (70), chorionic villus sampling (69) and vasoactive agents taken during the first trimester of pregnancy (74).

Hemifacial microsomia has been observed among infants exposed to the prenatal diagnosis procedure chorionic villus sampling, which has been postulated to be caused by a secondary vascular event, such as embolization (74).

An increased rate of exposure to vasoactive compounds, such as pseudoephedrine, ibuprofen, and cocaine, was revealed in interviews of the 230 mothers of children with hemifacial microsomia in comparison to 678 controls (97). There was a higher association when these exposures occurred in mothers who smoked cigarettes or took vasoactive medications. This analysis also showed a significant association of infants with hemifacial microsomia and twinning, as well as maternal diabetes mellitus.

An increased frequency of hemifacial microsomia has been alleged to be more common among infants born to men and women who had served in the Persian Gulf combat operations between 1990 and 1993. However, a systematic review of 75,414 infants conceived after this conflict and born in medical treatment facilities of the U.S. Department of Defense did not support this

theory (98). The biologic plausibility of this postulated male-mediated effect has not been established.

Treatment and Prognosis

Initially, philosophy of surgical repair was to wait for the deformity to reach the "end stage" when the affected child was older (73). However, longitudinal studies showed that the deformities were progressive and were more difficult to repair if not corrected in childhood. In addition, the child benefited significantly in social interactions from having less visible abnormalities. Mulliken and Kaban (73) recommended a systematic approach to the early correction of the hypoplastic mandible. They noted that, if unrepaired, this deformity restricts the vertical growth of the midface.

In a multidisciplinary evaluation of 18 affected individuals, Stromland and her associates (99) documented a high frequency of functional deficits, including hearing loss, impaired vision, difficulties in eating, speech impediments, mental retardation and significant risk of autism. Similar studies are needed on a larger, unselected sample of affected children to establish the natural history of hemifacial microsomia and to establish correlations, if any, of the presence of specific craniofacial abnormalities with each potential deficit.

Genetic Counseling

Since the diagnosis of hemifacial microsomia is based on clinical findings, rather than mutation analysis, the clinician must have her or his own minimal criteria for using this diagnosis.

While examples of affected sibs and parents have been reported, many of these descriptions include "atypical" features. How relevant are these observations to the healthy parents with one affected child?

More experience is needed with arrayCGH to determine how often duplications or deletions are present. Likewise, more experience is needed to determine the findings in mutation analysis of SALL1, SALL4 and TCOF1 genes.

An empiric recurrence risk of 2 to 3% for the sib of an affected child was suggested by the findings of Rollnick and Kaye (100). More family studies are needed of infants with craniofacial abnormalities of varied severity who have no abnormalities identified by both mutation analysis and arrayCGH testing.

The clinician must also consider similar phenotypes, which have been considered separate from hemifacial microsomia: Three examples are:

1. Axial mesodermal dysplasia, first described in 1981 by Russell, Weaver, and Bull (101), is a more severe phenotype that includes the features of hemifacial microsomia. It has also been associated with maternal diabetes mellitus (102).

2. Hemifacial microsomia with radial defects (MIM 141400). Is this a separate disorder that shares some of the features of hemifacial microsomia, or is it part of the same clinical spectrum? The associated features, such as hearing loss and inner ear abnormalities, are more severe than in individuals with hemifacial microsomia (103).

3. Oculo-auriculo-vertebral syndrome with ocular coloboma, ptosis, and microphthalmia (104). Is this part of the spectrum of hemifacial microsomia or a separate autosomal dominant disorder?

While the risk of recurrence is very low, parents may rely on prenatal screening by ultrasound for reassurance. A few more severely affected fetuses have been identified prenatally (105). However, the accuracy of this prenatal screening has not been determined.

OTOCEPHALY

Definition

Otocephaly is a rare, lethal craniofacial malformation with dramatic facial features, including a midline malposition (melotia) or fusion (synotia) of the ears, a very small mouth with hypoplasia or absence of the tongue, and a hypoplastic or absent mandible.

ICD-9:   756.046   (other craniofacial syndromes)

ICD-10:   Q75.9   (congenital malformation of the skull and face bones, unspecified)

Mendelian Inheritance in Man: %202650   (dysgnathia complex; agnathia holoprosencephaly; holoprosencephaly-agnathia-otocephaly)

Appearance

The abnormal appearance and location of the ears is the most striking abnormality (106–111). In some affected infants, the ears are oriented horizontally and are adjacent to the very small mouth. In others, the horizontal ears are fused inferiorly (Figures 23-10 and 23-11).

On the less severe end of the spectrum, the ears are low-set and malformed.

The oral cavity is usually very small (microstomia). There is choanal atresia and hypoplasia of the larynx and trachea, which makes intubation at birth very difficult, if not impossible.

The mandible is either very small or absent. With the very small chin, the face has a triangular shape. The nasal bridge may be broad and the palpebral fissures slope downward, sometimes dramatically (107).

There can also be dramatic facial features, such as fusion of the nose and mouth, a proboscis, or a proboscis-like mass in the midline.

Associated Malformations

The severe forebrain malformation holoprosencephaly is the most common associated malformation. Sometimes there is an associated cyclopia.

The other common associated malformations are situs inversus totalis, and anomalies of the kidneys, müllerian duct derivatives, vertebrae, lungs, and brain. Essentially, otocephaly can be multiple malformation syndrome or confined to the craniofacial features and brain, such as an uncovered brain mass (Figures 23-10 and 23-12) and encephalocele (Figures 23-11 and 23-13) [112].

The relationship with regard to etiology has not been determined for the different phenotypes, such as otocephaly, otocephaly with holoprosencephaly, and agnathia-holoprosencephaly-situs inversus (113).

Developmental Defect

The primary developmental defect is not known. This deficiency is due to deficient migration or proliferation of neural crest cells, arising from the dorsal region of the neural epithelium. In a mouse mutant with autosomal recessive otocephaly (oto), the primary abnormality was postulated to be mesodermal deficiencies, which were present as early as the time of the induction of the anterior neural plate, and were expressed in the anterior midline (114).

In 1934, Wright (115) had studied the occurrence of otocephaly in the guinea pig. His findings suggested that otocephaly was a threshold trait with an associated major recessive factor and a secondary dominant factor. Wright and Wagner had postulated (116) that otocephaly occurs because of defective development from the neural portion of the first brandial arch.

Most knock-out mice deficient in PGAP1 (post-glycosylphosphatidyfinosilol attachment to proteins 1) show otocephaly and die soon after birth. Those which survive show growth retardation and severely reduced fertility (117).

Otx2 is a bicoid-class homeobox gene, which is expressed in the cephalic mesenchyme of the mouse before gastrulation. Mice with haplo-insufficiency for Otx2 (Otx2+/–) have otocephaly (118, 119). The expression varies with the genetic background. No studies of the Otx2 gene in humans with otocephaly have been reported.

Prevalence

Limited information is available. A prevalence rate of less than 1:70,000 newborn infants has been estimated (108, 110).

In the Active Malformations Surveillance Program at Brigham and Women's Hospital in Boston, no affected infants were identified among 206,224 livebirths, stillbirths, and elective terminations among women who had always planned to deliver at that hospital. However, two affected infants (Figures 23-10 to 23-13) were born to women who had transferred for care after the prenatal detection of the fetal anomalies.

Race/Ethnicity

No data is available on prevalence rates among different racial/ethnic groups.

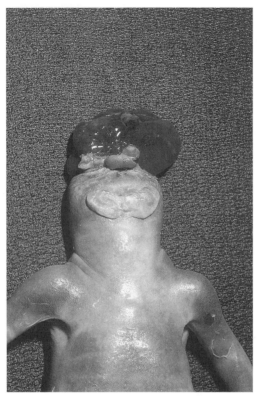

FIGURE 23.10 Shows facial features of otocephaly with ears formed poorly, no mouth, and protruding uncovered brain structures in a stillborn female at 23 weeks gestational age. (Courtesy of Frederick R. Bieber, PhD, Brigham and Women's Hospital, Boston, MA).

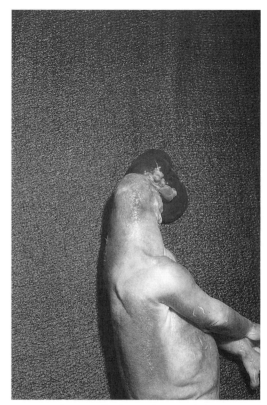

FIGURE 23.12 Side view of infant with otocephaly in Figure 23-10. (Courtesy of Frederick R. Bieber, PhD, Brigham and Women's Hospital, Boston, MA.)

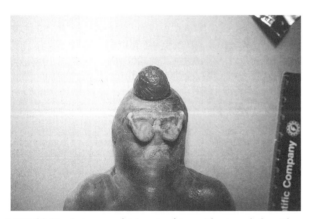

FIGURE 23.11 Late second trimester fetus with otocephaly with no mouth and skin covered brain protrusion (encephalocele) [Ref. 112]. (Courtesy of Frederick R. Bieber, PhD, Brigham and Women's Hospital, Boston, MA.)

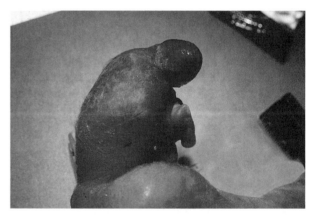

FIGURE 23.13 Posterior view of infant in Figure 23-12. (Courtesy of Frederick R. Bieber, PhD, Brigham and Women's Hospital, Boston, MA.)

Birth Status

An increased frequency of prematurity and intrauterine growth restriction have been noted (111).

Sex Ratio

An equal number of males and females were identified in one review (111).

Parental Age

Information on the ages of a significant number of mothers and fathers and an appropriate comparison group are not available.

Twinning

In two sets of identical twins only one had otocephaly and holoprosencephaly (120, 121). The affected twin had no chromosome abnormality (46,XY) in one of these sets of twins (121).

Genetic Factors

Two affected stillborn sisters were reported initially as a familial occurrence, possibly reflecting autosomal recessive inheritance (122). However, these sisters were shown subsequently to be affected by an unbalanced chromosome translocation:t (6;18) [123].

Environmental Factors

No environmental exposure in human pregnancies has been shown to cause otocephaly. Case reports (108, 124) have suggested environmental causes, but case reports cannot establish causality.

Treatment and Prognosis

Otocephaly has been considered a lethal condition, because the associated otolaryngeal anomalies usually prevent effective intubation and resuscitation. A few affected infants have been treated successfully at birth and have survived (125). These survivors have been infants who could be intubated and who did not have holoprosencephaly.

Genetic Counseling

Otocephaly occurs as a malformation of craniofacial structures or as part of multiple anomalies.

Chromosome analysis is an essential part of the evaluation. Studies with microarrays have not been reported, to date.

No increased risk of recurrence has been established in the sibs of infants with otocephaly.

A potential exception to the apparent lethality of otocephaly was reported by Ehrlich (126), who reported an affected mother with severe micrognathia and microglossia who had an affected daughter. However, she appears to have another non-lethal disorder, the auriculocondylar syndrome (MIM 602483) [127].

Otocephaly has been identified by prenatal screening by ultrasound (128, 129). However, the specific diagnosis has been made using 3-D imaging (128), in prenatal studies only a few times.

POLAND ANOMALY

Definition

Absence of sternal head of pectoralis major chest muscle and hypoplasia of the hand on the same side of the body, usually with shortening of the fingers with syndactyly (symbrachydactyly).

ICD-9:	756.800	(Poland syndrome or anomaly)
ICD-10:	Q79.8	(congenital malformations of musculoskeletal system, including Poland anomaly)
Mendelian Inheritance in Man:	%173800	Poland Syndrome
	^173750	Poland-Möebius Syndrome

Historical Note

Alfred Poland was a student demonstrator of anatomy in 1841, when he described in a cadaver: partial deficiency of the external oblique muscle, absence of the sternal and costal portions of the pectoralis major, absence of the pectoralis minor, and absence of substantial portions of the serratus magnus muscle (130). He described the thoracic vessels supplying the intercostal spaces as hypoplastic. The hand on the same side as the pectoral abnormality showed syndactyly between the proximal phalanges and absence or shortening of the middle phalanges.

Ravitch (131) asked whether Patrick Clarkson (132), in suggesting this eponym in 1962, may have given credit to Alfred Poland for his original description, in deference to him as an older alumnus of the same institution (Guy's Hospital, London).

He identified, also, earlier descriptions of the same abnormalities in 1826 and 1839 (131). Poland (130), and the earlier authors, had noted that the affected individual also had a deficiency of: i) hair in the mammary and axillary regions; ii) subcutaneous fat over the pectoralis muscle; iii) the nipple(s); iv) the muscles adjacent to the pectoralis major and v) costal cartilages and the anterior ends of ribs.

Ravitch, commenting on the inaccuracies of eponyms in general, noted that the individual memorialized was often not the first person to describe the condition, often did not understand fully what he/she had described, and often was either misrepresented or misquoted. Nevertheless, it is now customary to refer to the pattern of abnormalities described by Poland, Clarkson, and many others as the Poland Anomaly. Absence of the pectoral muscle alone occurs also, and is presumed to reflect the same, but less severe, developmental abnormality, but is usually not referred to as the Poland Anomaly.

Appearance

There is depression of the soft tissues in the area where the sternal head of the pectoral muscle is missing (Figures 23-14 to 23-16).

The adjacent areolae and breast may be absent, small, or displaced. The clavicle may be shortened. Sometimes there are gaps in the ribs in the same area (Figures 23-14 and 23-15), with the overlying skin moving in and out with breathing (133–141).

In a series of surgical repairs on 75 individuals (142) each had absence of the pectoralis minor and the costal portion of the pectoralis major.

More extensive absence of adjacent muscles, such as the trapezius (143) and latissimus dorsi (144) and the posterior shoulder girdle (137), has been reported. The association of cranial nerve deficiencies, such as the Möebius Syndrome (145) and constriction rings on shortened fingers (146), has been attributed to the same underlying process of vascular disruption that caused the Poland Anomaly (147, 148).

The hand and forearm on the same side of the body, i.e., ipsilateral, are smaller and shorter by several centimeters than those portions of the other, unaffected arm. There is shortening of the fingers in varying combinations with syndactyly between the shortened fingers (Figure 23-14). Typically, the middle phalanges are abnormal, varying from mild to complete absence (141). The syndactyly varies from proximal (Figure 23-17) to complete. The changes in the dermal ridge patterns on the small, shortened fingers are nonspecific, and include reduced pattern intensity. There is also an abnormal

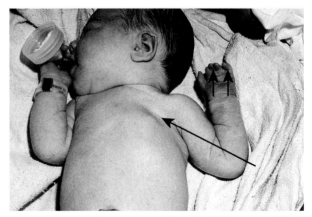

FIGURE 23.14 A newborn infant with marked deformity of left side of chest with absence of nipple and pectoral muscle with depressed appearance (arrow) due to deficiency of ribs. The left hand shows short fingers and syndactyly (two arrows).

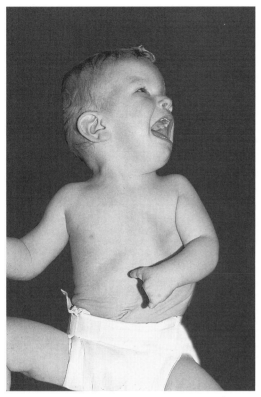

FIGURE 23.15 Another infant with depression of left side of chest, absence of nipple and pectoral muscle. The left hand shows absence of fingers 2, 3 and 4 and hypoplastic fifth finger. This infant also had facial diplegia due to cranial nerve deficiencies (Möebius Syndrome).

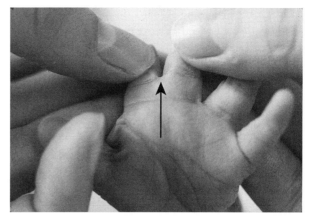

FIGURE 23.17 Mild syndactyly (arrow) in the left hand of the infant in Figure 23-16.

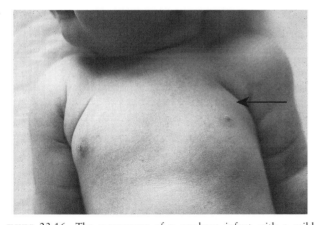

FIGURE 23.16 The appearance of a newborn infant with a mild deformity on left side of chest with deficiency of pectoral muscle (arrow).

palm print pattern with a distally placed triradius (149).

Associated Malformations

Dextrocardia [150, 151] (or more specifically dextroposition [152]), has been observed in many individuals with the Poland Anomaly, primarily involving the left side of the thorax.

A variety of other associated limb, body wall, and kidney malformations have been reported (153–157). Associated ocular anomalies, including coloboma of the optic disk (158), juxtafoveal telangiectasia (159) and hamartoma of the retina (160), have been reported in individuals with the Poland Anomaly. Whether or not these are different phenotypes cannot be determined until a biomarker specific to the Poland Anomaly has been identified.

There have been reports of several children with the Poland Anomaly who developed acute leukemia in childhood (154). It has not been determined whether these are chance associations or not.

Developmental Defect

Disruption of the internal mammary artery at 6 to 8 weeks gestation has been postulated to be the primary event that causes absence of the sternal head of the pectoralis major muscle (148). Hypoplasia of the ipsilateral subclavian artery has also been postulated to be the primary abnormality (147). It has been noted (138) that at days 44 to 48 postfertilization there is close proximity of structures destined to form the hand and the pectoral muscles, suggesting that a localized abnormality or insult could affect both structures at that time.

While vascular disruption and decreased blood flow are the most frequently postulated mechanisms for the occurrence of the Poland anomaly, there is limited proof of these events. One relevant observation was stenosis of the left subclavian artery identified in one child with a left Poland Anomaly (147). Hypoplasia of the internal thoracic artery was described in another affected individual (148). However, other reports have shown that hypoplasia of the internal thoracic artery is not a consistent finding on the affected side. For example, during surgery on an affected 70-year-old man, it was noted that his left subclavian artery and left internal thoracic arteries were wide and normal in association with affected left pectoral muscle (161). A second contrary observation was in using contrast-enhanced MR-angiography, which showed no difference in the diameter of the left and right subclavian arteries (162). The failure to find abnormalities of the subclavian artery could mean that the postulated decrease in blood flow was a temporary transient phenomenon or that there was another etiology. Another postulated

explanation was a disruption of the lateral plate mesoderm between 16 and 28 days postfertilization (163).

Prevalence

1 in 32,000 in liveborn infants in British Columbia (1952–1975) [137];
1 in 22,189 among 599,109 livebirths in South America (1967–1977) [139];
1 in 87,550 births in Hungary (1975–1984) [164];
1 in 34,394 at Brigham and Women's Hospital in Boston (Table 23-2).

TABLE 23-2 *Infants with Poland Anomaly or only absence of pectoralis major identified at Brigham and Women's Hospital (1972–1974, 1979–2000)*

	Year	Sex/Race	N/T	Affected Side of Chest	Ribs	Hand Malformation	Möebius	Other Malformations
I) Poland Anomaly								
1.	1972	M, W	N	Lt.		Lt: shortened 2-5; syndactyly 2-3		
2.	1973	M, W	N	Lt.		Lt: absence of fingers 2-4 hypoplasia 1, 5 hypoplasia metacarpals 1-5		Absent left nipple Multicystic dysplasia right kidney
3.	1984	M, W	N	Rt.		Rt. syndactyly 1-2, 3-4, complete Rt. stiff thumb	Affected	
4.	1992	M, W	N	Lt.	Hypoplastic Lt. 4th rib	Lt: Hypoplasia of digits		Heart dextroposition Torticollis, right
5.	1993	F, W	N	Rt.		Rt. syndactyly and shortened fingers 2-5		
6.	1993	F, B	T	Rt.		Rt. shortened fingers 2-5; absent right thumb		Hypoplastic right nipple
7.	1994	M, H	N	Rt.		Rt. hypoplasia of forearm, hand and thumb; flexicon contracture fingers		Synostosis of radius and ulna; Undescended testicle, left
8.	1998	M, B	T	Rt. & Lt.		None		Trisomy 13
9.	1999	M, O	T	Rt.	Hypoplasia Rt. 3rd rib	Rt. hypoplasia of arm and hand		
II) Absence of pectoralis major only (normal hand)								
10.	1972	M, W	N	Rt.	Fusion 6-7, Rt.	None		Nipple absent; hip dysplasia
11.	1973	F, W	N	Rt.		None		
12.	1974	M, W	N	Rt.		None		
13.	1983	M, W	N	Lt.		None		Absent left nipple
14.	1984	M, W	N	Lt.		None		Asymmetrical nipples
15.	1985	F, A	N	Rt.		None		
16.	1995	M, W	N	Rt.	Hypoplastic Rt. 3rd, 4th, & 5th ribs	None		
17.	1996	F, B	N	Rt.		None		

Totals: 12 males, 5 females; 11 right side, 5 left side, 1 bilateral

Legends: °Infants identified in surveillance of 206,244 liveborn and stillborn infants and elective terminations for fetal anomalies.
Prevalence rate among infants of non-transferred mothers = 6/206,244 or 1:34,374.
Sex: M = male, F = female
Race: W = white, A = Asian, B = Black, H = Spanish-speaking; Hispanic; O = Other (mixed ancestry)
Transfer Status: N = nontransfer; T = mother transferred for care after prenatal detection of anomalies in fetuses.

Race/Ethnicity

The data on the frequency of the Poland Anomaly in different racial/ethnic groups has not been established yet.

Birth Status

There has been no evidence of an increased frequency of miscarriages, stillbirth, or premature birth.

Sex Ratio

Several case series have shown that most (over 70%) affected infants are males (134, 135, 138).

Sidedness

The right pectoralis muscle and right arm and hand have been reported affected much more often than the left (134–136, 138).

Parental Age

Whether or not the average ages of the mothers and fathers of affected individuals differ from a comparison group has not been determined.

Twinning

Discordance has been reported in one monozygous twin pair (165).

Genetic Factors

Affected siblings (166, 167) with unaffected parents, affected second cousins (168, 169), and an affected parent and child (170, 171) have all been reported. However, these are rare occurrences. The empiric recurrence has not been established in a large sample. In Hungary (1975–1984), one of 18 affected infants had an affected parent (164).

The occurrence among relatives of the Poland Anomaly in one and, among other relatives, other similar "vascular defects" (172–174), such as Poland-Möebius (145) and Adams-Oliver Syndrome (173), suggests an underlying predisposition to the process of vascular disruption in all of these phenotypes, but the molecular basis has not been established. The postulated molecular markers have not been identified.

To explain these familial clusters, Happle (175) proposed that the Poland Anomaly could be a paradominant trait, hypothesizing that the heterozygote is phenotypically normal and that a postzygotic mutation causes allele loss and expression of the phenotype in a clone of cells. This would mean the Poland Anomaly is a mosaic phenotype, which makes unilaterality less relevant and variability of associated features to be expected (176).

The occurrence of absence of the pectoral muscles, without an associated ipsilateral hand malformation, has been reported in sibs (177) and in parent and child (178), and in several members of one family (179).

Environmental Factors

David (133) observed an association of the occurrence of the Poland Anomaly with exposures, such as vasoconstrictive agents, taken to terminate a pregnancy.

Poland Anomaly has also been observed in children born after exposure to chorionic villus sampling (180) the prostaglandin E_1 misoprostol (181), cocaine abuse (182), and cigarette smoking (183), each association presumably affecting blood flow and the development of the pectoral muscle and the ipsilateral limb.

Treatment and Prognosis

Imaging by computerized tomography (CT) or magnetic resonance imaging (MRI) can be used to determine the extent of the muscle abnormalities prior to reconstructive surgery (184). One critical finding is whether the latissimus dorsi muscle is missing, as this muscle can be used to reconstruct the missing pectoral muscle (185).

Techniques for the reconstruction of the chest wall deformity, and breast reconstruction in females, have been developed (142, 186). Critical to a good result is correction of the rotation of the sternum toward the involved side and the contralateral carinate deformity (142).

Genetic Counseling

This localized abnormality occurs almost always as a surprise. Relatives with the same or related abnormalities are rare. The risk of recurrence in siblings of the first affected member of the family is very low, but not 0%. Whether or not it is a "genetic" abnormality has not been determined.

Similar, and potentially related, phenotypes, in individuals with absence of the sternal portion of the pectoralis major have included: unilateral gluteal hypoplasia with brachysyndactyly (187), symbrachydactyly involving both the hand and foot (188), below-the-knee leg hypoplasia and ipsilateral toe brachysyndactyly (189), and symbrachydactyly of one foot (190) have been reported. Their relevance to the Poland Anomaly has not been determined.

The occurrence of bilateral absence of the pectoral muscles and brachydactyly in both hands has been reported (191), but it is debatable whether this is an instance of bilateral Poland Anomaly (192).

The examining clinician should also consider the possibility of similar, but different phenotypes, such as thoracic hypoplasia. This phenotype includes depression of the anterior portion of the thorax, hypoplasia of the breast, a superiorly placed nipple-areola complex, and normal pectoralis muscle (193, 194).

URETHRAL OBSTRUCTION: PRUNE BELLY SYNDROME

Definition

Obstruction of the urethra by any of several mechanisms early in pregnancy which is associated with absence / hypoplasia of abdominal muscle and dysplasia of kidneys, primarily in males.

ICD-9:	753.600	(congenital posterior urethral valves or posterior urethral obstruction)
	753.610	(other atresia, or stenosis of bladder neck)
	753.620	(obstruction, atresia, or stenosis of anterior urethra)
	753.690	(other and unspecified atresia and stenosis of urethra and bladder neck)
ICD-10:	Q64.2	(congenital posterior urethral valves)
	Q64.3	(other atresia and stenosis of urethra and bladder neck)
Mendelian Inheritance in Man:	100100	(abdominal muscles, absence of, with urinary tract abnormality and cryptorchidism)

Historical Note

Frederick Eagle and George Barrett, two urologists, drew attention in 1950 (195) in a case series of 9 malformed infants to the association of the absence of abdominal musculature, genitourinary anomalies, and undescended testicles. Subsequently, this triad was referred to as the Eagle-Barrett Syndrome. The unusual appearance of the abdomen with the wrinkled skin and a lack of muscles prompted the designation as "the prune belly syndrome" (196). Initially, it was postulated that the deficiency of the abdominal muscles reflected a primary defect in muscle development (197). Later, several clinicians showed the association with developmental abnormalities of the prostatic urethra, including posterior urethral valves, anterior obstruction of the urethra, and compression of the urethra as a secondary effect of the dilated distal urethra (198–204). This sex-specific basis for the abnormality explained the predominance of affected males.

When affected females were identified (205, 206), other mechanisms, such as ascites in the fetus, were suggested for the deficiency of the muscles of the abdomen (205).

With the advent of prenatal detection by ultrasound, apparent urethral obstruction was identified that could be transient (207). Instances of apparent urethral obstruction were documented, but no abnormality of the urethra was identified and there was no abnormality of the abdominal muscles (200).

Over time, it had become apparent that there are many causes of the "prune belly" or "Eagle-Barrett" syndrome. And the review of early publications (208) identified a much earlier report of this phenotype by Froehlich in 1839 (209). Pagon et al, (199) had noted that Stumme in 1903 and Housden in 1934 had postulated the primary mechanism of urethral obstruction. Nevertheless, Eagle and Barrett (19) deserve credit for having brought this pattern of abnormalities to much wider attention.

Appearance

The lower abdomen may be protuberant because of the distended bladder (Figure 23-18 to 23-21). If the abdominal muscles are deficient, the skin of the abdomen is wrinkled or prune-like (Figures 23-18 and 23-20). The abdomen is lax and viscera are palpated easily.

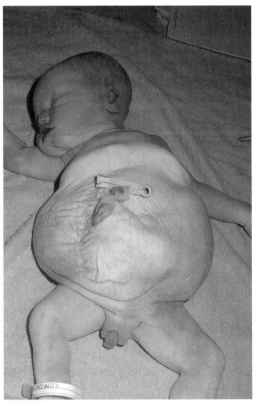

FIGURE 23.18 Shows distended abdomen with wrinkled skin and poor muscle tone in a male new born due to a deficiency of abdominal muscles caused *in utero* by distension of the bladder by urethral obstruction (Prune belly syndrome).

The testes are not palpable. The penis maybe normal in appearance or enlarged due to distension of the distal portion of the urethra.

Associated Malformations

The associated malformations reflect the primary abnormality. Infants with "prune belly syndrome" associated with persistence of the cloaca often have imperforate anus.

In a case series of 3 male and 3 female infants with urethral atresia and "the prune belly syndrome," the females had complex genital anomalies, such as bicornuate uterus, atresia of the vagina, and imperforate anus in females and the males had renal dysplasia and cryptorchidism (208).

A wide variety of associated anomalies and deficiencies of the legs have been reported (210–214), including atrophy and gangrene of one leg (210), terminal transverse limb defects with necrotic tissue at the end of the malformed limb (212), severe hypoplasia of the right leg (Figures 23-19 and 23-21), and club foot deformity of the left leg (213). In a review of 28 associated limb deficiencies, it was noted (214) that all affected the lower limbs and that there were no associated amniotic bands or constriction rings and no prenatal exposures to recognized teratogens. The most common abnormalities were terminal transverse limb defects and hypoplasia of the leg. More were unilateral than bilateral. The overall frequency of deficiency of the lower limb in

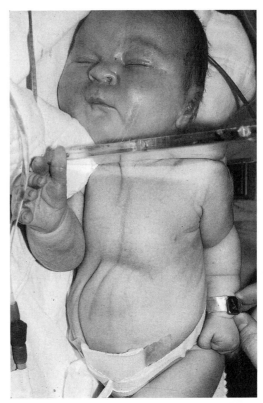

FIGURE 23.20   Distended abdomen and excessive wrinkling of skin over abdomen in affected newborn infant.

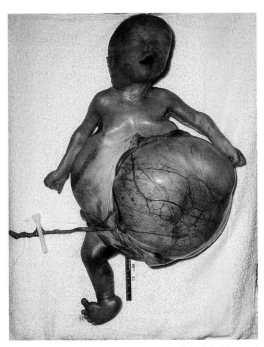

FIGURE 23.19   Shows massive enlargement of the bladder and abdomen in association with marked underdevelopment of the right leg. (Courtesy of Frederick R. Bieber, Ph.D., Brigham and Women's Hospital, Boston, MA.)

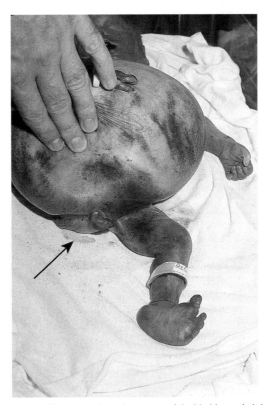

FIGURE 23.21   Shows massive enlargement of the bladder and abdomen in association with marked underdevelopment of the right leg (arrow). (Courtesy of Frederick R. Bieber, Ph.D., Brigham and Women's Hospital, Boston.)

infants with urethral obstruction, of any cause, was estimated to be 5.5%.

Developmental Defects

The primary underlying cellular and molecular events that cause urethra obstruction or maldevelopment of the prostatic portion of the urethra have not been determined (Figure 23-22).

Two major theories have been proposed. 1) the mesendymal defect theory (197); 2) the degeneration of the prostatic portion of the urethra by the obstruction, particularly if early and persistent.

The mesenchymal injury was postulated to have occurred between the 6th and 10th weeks of gestation. This is consistent with the deficiency of the outer peripheral zone of the prostate (204). The bladders of affected fetuses have had thinned muscle layers and increased connective tissue, suggestive of a primary mesenchymal effect (Figure 23-22).

The clinical findings have been considered (203) most consistent with obstruction distal to the bladder. The effects of this distal obstruction are: dilation and dysplasia of the upper renal tract; the deficiency of the muscles of the abdominal wall secondary to the dramatic distention of the bladder early in development; the testes are prevented by the dilated bladder from entering the inguinal gland. The junction of the glandular and penile urethra has been considered the most likely site of the obstruction.

A model of posterior urethral valves has been developed in fetal lambs, by producing complete urethral obstruction at 43 to 45 days of gestation (full term is 140 days) [215]. The phenotypic features produced included a wrinkled and distended abdomen, deficient muscles in the abdomen, limb deformities, and undescended testes.

Prevalence

In a population-based study in British Columbia (1904–1978) of 526,166 live births, the prevalence rate of "prune belly syndrome" was 1:29,231 (216).

A survey of malformations in Saskatchewan Province in the 1960s showed a prevalence rate of 1:35,000 (217).

In an analysis of 1,168 stillborn infants in Utah (1999–2003), 158 had major anomalies, one of which had urethral obstruction (218).

Race/Ethnicity

No data on the prevalence rates among different racial or ethnic groups has been published.

Birth Status

Some of the conditions associated with urethral obstruction are associated with an increased frequency of premature birth and stillbirth.

Sex Ratio

There are many more affected males, than females, because an abnormality of the male-specific anatomy, that is, the prostatic urethra, is the most very common abnormality that leads to obstruction of the urethra.

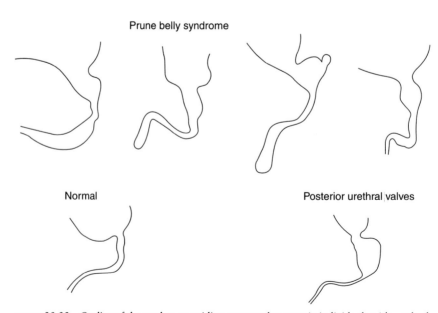

FIGURE 23.22   Outline of the urethra on voiding cystourethrogram in individuals with urethral obstruction (and prune belly syndrome) in comparison to normal and posterior urethral valves. (From Beasley SW et al.: *Pediatr Surg Int.* 1988;3:169–172. Used with permission.)

Sidedness

The abnormality of the urethra is a midline defect. However, the associated defects in the legs are more often unilateral than bilateral (214). In the 20 infants with unilateral limb defects in one review (214), 17 involved the right leg and only 3, the left leg.

Parental Age

No differences in the ages of the mothers or fathers in comparison to the general population have been reported.

Twinning

An increased frequency of twinning has been suggested, but not established.

In the surveillance of the population of Saskatchewan Province over ten years in the 1960s, 10 affected infants were identified (217). Three of the 10 affected infants were like-sex male twins. In each of these sets of twins, only one had the syndrome of urethral obstruction.

Identical twins have been reported in which only one had urethral and anal atresia (219).

Genetic Factors

The findings in family studies have not shown evidence of mendelian inheritance (204, 217). There have been rare reports of families in which two or more individuals were affected (220–222). No distinctive phenotypic features were described in these individuals with affected relatives.

In a series of 22 affected infants with megacystis, diagnosed during pregnancy, three (18.8%) of the 16 who had chromosome analysis had abnormalities: trisomy 18 (1), trisomy 21 (1), and 47, XXY (1)[207].

Environmental Factors

No teratogens have been identified that have caused urethral obstruction. In a population-based case-control study of infants with renal anomalies in 1968–1980, there were 134 with obstruction defects. There was no increase in the frequency of a flu-like illness. However, there was a significant increase in the use of antibiotics and aspirin-containing medication (223).

Treatment and Prognosis

The treatment of the affected infant with multiple anomalies requires systematic approaches, involving several disciplines. Renal insufficiency, which may necessitate kidney transplant, is a common complication in childhood.

Affected men, as adults, have been considered infertile (224).

There have been rare, successful reports of prenatal intervention in the second trimester, but this treatment during pregnancy has been discouraged because of the poor prognosis (225).

Genetic Counseling

The first step for the clinician is to establish the primary cause of the urethral obstruction. Is it an isolated abnormality or one of multiple anomalies? Chromosome analysis is indicated if there are multiple abnormalities.

There have not been careful family studies that have established the empiric recurrence risk in subsequent pregnancies. While there have been rare reports of affected siblings (220–222), the risk of recurrence in subsequent sibs is considered to be very low.

With the widespread use of prenatal screening with ultrasound, detection during pregnancy will be common. However, establishing the specific phenotype will only be possible through a physical examination at birth and postnatal imaging.

Detection by ultrasound has been reported at 12 weeks of gestation in a fetus with massive enlargement of the bladder and distension of the abdomen (226).

VACTERL (VATER) ASSOCIATION

Definition

The association in an infant of malformations of vertebrae, anus, cardiac structures, tracheoesophageal fistula with esophageal atresia, renal and limb anomalies. While it is a non-random association, the number of structural abnormalities varies among affected individuals. Since the underlying developmental defect has not been determined, the minimum number of phenotypic features needed to establish this diagnosis has not been determined.

ICD-9:	759.840	(congenital malformation syndromes involving limbs)
ICD-10:	Q87.2	(congenital malformation syndromes predominantly involving limbs, including VATER syndrome)
Mendelian Inheritance in Man:	174100	(polydactyly, imperforate anus, vertebral anomalies syndrome)
	192350	(VACTERL Association)

Historical Note

The recognition of the VACTERL or VATER Association began with the descriptions of Burnham Say and Park Gerald in 1968 (227) and Linda Quan and David Smith (228) in 1973. In a case series of 186 infants with polydactyly (1946 to 1967), Say and Gerald (227) noted that 10 infants had polydactyly and imperforate anus, with 8 of those 10 infants having rib and vertebral (lumbar and thoracic) anomalies, as well. In their case series, Quan and Smith (228) identified seven infants with vertebral, anus, tracheoesophageal fistula, radius and renal defects and suggested the designation of VATER Association. They noted that the pattern of associated anomalies was broader than had been suggested initially by Say and Gerald (227). They also pointed out that additional anomalies, such as heart defects and ear deformities, were often present, as well. Later, Temtamy and Miller (229) in 1974, Khoury et al. in 1983 (230), and others expanded the acronym to VACTERL to include heart (cardiac) and limb defects.

In 1996, a similar, but separate, phenotype was delineated and referred to as VACTERL Association with hydrocephalus or VACTERL-H (MIM #314390 and MIM #276950).

Appearance

Since the associated anomalies are internal, the affected infant can appear, in the initial examination, to have only anomalies of the thumb or radius.

Several observations have been made about the expected anomalies:

- hemivertebrae are a frequent vertebral anomaly;
- the thumb deformity is often unilateral and on the same side of the body as the associated kidney malformations (232);
- the thumb anomaly can be either hypoplasia or preaxial polydactyly. (Figures 23-23 and 23-24);
- the spectrum of kidney malformations is wide and includes agenesis, multicystic dysplasia, and hydronephrosis (Table 23-3).

Associated Malformations

Several population-based studies (230–237) have confirmed that these interrelated malformations occur in

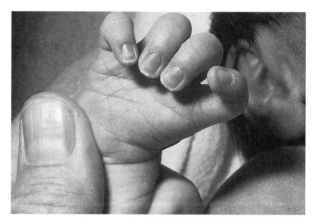

FIGURE 23.23 Absence of thumb in infant with choanal atresia and imperforate anus.

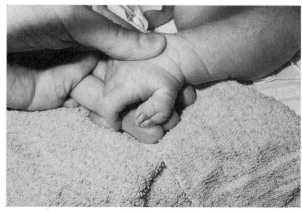

FIGURE 23.24 Preaxial polydactyly of right thumb of infant with imperforate anus.

TABLE 23-3 *Pattern of anomalies in a consecutive population of newborn infants**

Number of infants with	Vertebral		Anus	Cardiac	Tracheo-esophageal TE	Renal		
	hemi-vertebrae	other rib or sacral anomalies	imperforate anus; anal stenosis	heart defects	Tracheo-esophageal anomalies	absence of kidney	horse-shoe kidney	cystic dysplastic kidney
6 of these anomalies (1)	1	1	1	1	1	1		
5 of these anomalies (1)			1	1		1		
4 of these anomalies (6)	2	4	4	5	5	2		2
3 of these anomalies (9)	5	0	6	5	3	3	3	1
2 of these anomalies (17)	<u>10</u>	<u>3</u>	<u>7</u>	<u>1</u>	<u>8</u>	<u>3</u>		<u>2</u>
Totals	18	8	19	13	17	10	3	5

	Limb Malformations			Other anomalies		
	absent/hypoplastic radius	absent fingers or toes	polydactyly, preaxial	single umbilical artery	Genito-urinary anomalies	multiple anomalies
6 or more					1	1
5 or more	1	1				
4 or more					2	2
3 or more	2		1	2	1	3
2 or more	<u>2</u>	<u>3</u>	<u>1</u>	<u>0</u>	<u>3</u>	<u>3</u>
Totals	5	4	2	2	7	9

Legend: *The infants with the features of VACTERL Association identified among 206,224 liveborn and stillborn infants and elective terminations for fetal anomalies at Brigham and Women's Hospital (1972–1974, 1979–2000). Excludes infants with trisomy 18 and those with cloacal exstrophy. Only infants born to woman who had always planned to deliver at this hospital. Excludes infants born to mothers who transferred to BWH for care after the prenatal detection of fetal anomalies at another hospital.

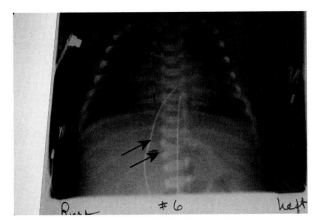

FIGURE 23.25 Hemivertebrae at T11 and T12 in infant with imperforate anus (arrows).

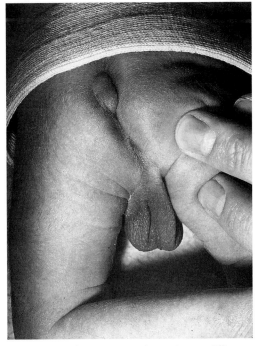

FIGURE 23.26 Imperforate anus and prominent midline raphe in male infant with VACTERL Association.

the same infant much more often than would be predicted by chance. Each study has identified several other disorders with the same malformations:

1. chromosome abnormalities, such as trisomy 18 and 13q-deletion syndrome;
2. Mendelian disorders, like the autosomal dominant Holt-Oram Syndrome (MIM #142950) with heart defects and preaxial forearm anomalies, and the autosomal recessive Fanconi Anemia (MIM #227650) with microcephaly, café au lait spots and kidney and preaxial forearm defects and the Okihiro Syndrome (MIM 607323) with hearing loss, ear deformities, and anomalies of thumbs and kidneys;
3. other syndromes, such as cloacal extrophy, the MURCS (Müllerian duct aplasia, renal aplasia, and cervicothoracic somite dysplasia) [MIM 601076], hemifacial microsomia (MIM %164210) [238], axial mesodermal dysplasia, sirenomelia (MIM %19183) and Pallister-Hall Syndrome (MIM 146510).

The clinician is challenged to recognize and separate out these phenotypes with some of the same abnormalities, which makes the VACTERL Association a diagnosis by exclusion. Further complicating the establishing of this diagnosis is the fact that many individuals with the anomalies of the VACTERL Association have additional anomalies, such as cleft lip and/or palate, genito-urinary anomalies, single umbilical artery, and laryngeal anomalies (230, 234, 239).

Developmental Defects

General underlying abnormalities, such as "defective mesodermal development" (228) and "a primary polytopic developmental field defect" (236), have been suggested.

Several different associated molecular changes have been reported. Studies of a larger number of affected individuals with VACTERL Association are needed to determine whether these findings are co-incidental or an occasional finding. A novel missense mutation in one allele of the PTEN gene was reported in an infant with the VATER Association, macrocephaly, and ventriculomegaly (240). The mitochondrial NP3243 point mutation was identified in the malformed kidney of an infant who also had vertebral anomalies, bilateral absence of radius, and radial digits (241). This infant's mother and sister had the classical mitochondrial cytopathy with the same mitochondrial mutation, but no structural anomalies. An infant of a diabetic mother with anal atresia, vertebral anomalies, and multicystic dysplastic kidneys has also been reported to have this NP 3243 point mutation (242). Several other close relatives had other symptoms of mitochondrial disease. However, subsequent studies of 62 children with the

VACTERL Association showed that NP3243 mutation is "not a common cause of the malformations seen in the VACTERL Association (243). Decreased expression of PAX1, determined by immunochemical analysis, was demonstrated in cultured fibroblasts from two infants with the VATER Association (244).

Knockout mice, deficient in GLI2 and GLI3 genes, have had several of the phenotypic features of the VACTERL Association [245]. Complex genetic interactions involving the GLI signaling pathway are one potential site of the primary molecular defect.

Adriamycin administered on gestational days 6–9 in rat pups produced many of the VACTERL anomalies [246]. It has been postulated that mutations induced by adriamycin could result from the breakdown of the shh (sonic hedgehog) signaling pathway (247).

Prevalence

The estimates of prevalence rates have varied from 0.163 per 1,000 in Atlanta (1968 to 1979) [230] to 0.048 per 1,000 in Hungary (1970–1980) [231]. The rates depend on the definition of the disorder. In the analysis of the 2,295 infants with three or more of 25 selected malformations among 9,995,151 births in 17 birth defect registries, 1 in 34,948 had 3 of the 5 components of the VACTERL Association [234]. Three combinations—VAR, ATER and VATER—accounted for 52.8% of these affected individuals.

The most distinctive components of this association, in an analysis of 5,260 infants with multiple anomalies, are esophageal and anal atresia, preaxial forearm defects, and costovertebral anomalies [239].

Race/Ethnicity

A higher frequency in white infants in comparison to black infants was observed in a population-based study in Atlanta (230).

Sex Ratio

There were more affected males than females in several studies (230, 231). In a population-based study in Hungary (231), there were 30 affected males and 13 affected females.

Sidedness

The sidedness of the common unilateral thumb and kidney malformations has not been established.

Birth Status

An increased frequency of breech presentation, low birth weight (less than 2,500 grams at birth), stillbirth, and neonatal death have been reported in population-based studies (230, 231, 233).

Parental Age

No definite correlations with maternal or paternal age have been reported (230, 235).

Twins

An increased frequency of twinning has been reported: 4.7% of 43 patients in Hungary (231) and 6.1% in a review of 180 affected infants (238) compared to a rate of 1% in the general population.

In one monozygous female twin pair, both twins had esophageal atresia, but only one had vertebral anomalies, absence of vagina, uterus, and fallopian tubes and a pelvic kidney (248). In another set of identical twins, both had lung sequestration and esophageal atresia, but only one had rib and vertebral anomalies and dextrocardia (249).

Genetic Factors

A "genetic" basis for the occurrence of the VACTERL Association has not been determined. There are several published reports from family studies (231, 250) and distinctive families with affected close relatives (247–250) to consider. In a study in Hungary (1973–1982), none of 143 first-degree relatives (parents and siblings) of 43 affected children had any of the features of the VACTERL Association. In a family study of 140 individuals with esophageal atresia, a component of the VACTERL Association, only 0.3% of sibs had esophageal atresia (250). However, 4 (1.2%) of 347 siblings of the affected index cases had at least one of the VACTERL Association anomalies other than esophageal atresia.

The affected close relatives, include brothers (251, 252) and parent-child (253, 254). For example, in one family (254) the mother had an H-type tracheoesophageal fistula, imperforate anus, triphalangeal thumb, hypoplastic kidney (left), and vertebral anomalies. Her son had preaxial polydactyly (right hand), cleft T3 vertebra, incomplete development of the sacrum, and a small ventricular septal defect.

In a genome-wide microsatellite screen in six affected individuals to identify subtle chromosome abnormalities, none were found (255).

To date, no associated subtle chromosome deletions or instances of uniparental disomy have been reported in individuals with the VACTERL Association.

After the VACTERL Association had been established as a recognizable non-random association, several clinicians reported children with VACTERL plus hydrocephalus (256–260). The patterns of recurrence

suggested X-linked inheritance in some (256), autosomal recessive inheritance in others (257), and in others no conclusions could be made (258).

Environmental Factors

Early studies (259) raised the question as to whether exposure to exogenous sex hormones caused the VACTERL pattern of anomalies. However, more extensive and better designed studies (231, 260) did not confirm this association. Laboratory studies showed that the fetal tissues (heart, limbs, vertebrae) allegedly affected by the exogenous sex hormones did not have the cellular receptors that would be essential for the exposure to affect these structures.

The most common association with environmental factors has been insulin-dependent diabetes mellitus in the mother (261).

Treatment and Prognosis

The associated malformations of the heart are a major reason for the increased perinatal mortality rate. Surgical repair of the associated malformations is the primary treatment.

Genetic Counseling

The first question for the clinician is whether the affected infant has several of the core components of the VACTERL Association (Table 23-3) or has those features plus other non-VACTERL major malformations. The number of components that must be present to establish the diagnosis of VACTERL Association has not been established. However, the greater the number and the absence of other major malformations makes this designation more reasonable.

The presence of hydrocephalus should shift the focus to whether the infant has the VACTERL-H Syndrome, which appears to be a separate disorder that shares many phenotypic features with the VACTERL Association.

Since the diagnosis of VACTERL Association is a diagnosis after the exclusion of several other disorders with similar features, both laboratory studies and clinical evaluations are essential in this process. Chromosome analysis helps to rule out conditions, such as the 13q deletion syndrome. When the infant has preaxial limb anomalies, including either hypoplasia or polydactyly, these disorders are to be considered:

1. Holt-Oram Syndrome (MIM #142900): when the infant is old enough to have ossified carpal bones,

the presence of the extra os centrale and abnormal scaphoid bone and shallow glenoid fossa are very distinctive findings (262); the current molecular testing for mutations in TBX5 gene does not identify a mutation in each child with the Holt-Oram phenotype;

2. Fanconi Anemia (MIM #227650): the chromosome breakage studies, using diepoxybutane (DEB)are indicated, as about 5% of individuals with Fanconi Anemia in case series have had the VACTERL phenotype (263). Mutation analysis for the Fanconi Anemia complex can be used to confirm this diagnosis (264).

3. Okihiro Syndrome (MIM: 607343): Theoretically the identification of the associated Duane anomaly could suggest this diagnosis clinically. Mutation analysis for SALL4 mutations will confirm this clinical diagnosis (265).

4. Thrombocytopenia-radial aplasia (TAR) [MIM 274000] will be distinctive in the preaxial anomaly. Unlike the other disorders listed here, the hypoplasia of the radius occurs with the thumbs still present. The associated thrombocytopenia is also a distinguishing feature. Molecular confirmation is possible through the identification of the associated microdeletion 1q21.1 (266).

Having established the clinical diagnosis of VACTERL Association, the empiric recurrence risk in the subsequent pregnancy of the healthy parents of an affected child appears to be very low, but not 0%. At this time, this condition should be considered a "genetic" abnormality, but the specific genetic abnormality has not, yet, been identified.

Affected fetuses have been diagnosed in prenatal ultrasonography (267), based on the presence of hemivertebrae, preaxial anomalies, and kidney malformations. However, the accuracy of prenatal diagnosis has not been determined.

REFERENCES

1. Cantrell JR, Haller JA, Ravitch MM. A syndrome of congenital heart defects involving the abdominal wall, sternum, diaphragm, pericardium, and heart. *Surg Gyn Obstet.* 1958;107:602–614.
2. Byron F. Ectopia cordis. *J Thorac Surg.* 1948;17:717–722.
3. Blatt ML, Zeldes M. Ectopia cordis: Report of a case and review of the literature. *Am J Dis Child.* 1942;63L:515–529.
4. Scott GW. Ectopia cordis: Report of a case successfully treated by operation. *Guys Hospital Report.* 1955;104:55–?.
5. Toyama WM. Combined congenital defects of the anterior abdominal wall, sternum, diaphragm, pericardium and heart: a case report and review of the syndrome. *Pediatrics.* 1972;50:778–792.
6. Leca F, Thibert M, Khoury W. Extrathoracic heart (ectopia cordis). Report of two cases and review of the literature. *In J Cardiol.* 1989;22:221–228.
7. Khoury MJ, Cordero JF, Mulinare J, Opitz JM. Association of selected midline defects: a population study. *Pediatrics.* 1989;84: 266–272.
8. Carmi R, Boughman JA. Pentalogy of Cantrell and associated midline anomalies: a possible ventral midline developmental field. *Am J Med Genet.* 1992;42:90–95.
9. Hornberger LK, Colan SD, Lock JE, Wessel DL, Mayer JE Jr. Outcome of patients with ectopia cordis and significant intracardiac defects. *Circulation.* 1996;94 (Suppl II): II-32–II-37.
10. Fernandez MS, Lopez A, Villa JJ. Cantrell's Pentalogy, Report of four cases and their management. *Pediatr Surg Int.* 1997;12: 428–431.
11. Thakuria JV, Jennings R, Geva T, Tworetsky W, Levine J, Barnewolt CE et al. Phenotypic analysis of ectopia cordis: emphasis on etiology, prenatal diagnosis and cardiovascular malformations. *Proc Greenwood Genetics Center.* 2007;26: 161–162.
12. Song A, McLeary MS. MR imaging of pentalogy of Cantrell variant with an intact diaphragm and pericardium. *Pediatr Radiol.* 2000;30: 638–639.
13. Egan JFX, Petrikovsky BM, Vintzileos AM, Rodis JF, Campbell WM. Combined Pentalogy of Cantrell and sirenomelia: a case report with speculation about a common etiology. *Am J Perinatology.* 1993;10: 327–329.
14. Kaplan LC, Matsuoka R, Gilbert EF, Opitz JM, Kurnit DM. Ectopia cordis and cleft sternum: evidence for mechanical teratogens following rupture of the chorion or yolk sac. *Am J Med Genei.* 1985;21: 187–199.
15. Zhang J, Hagopian-Donaldson S, Serbedzija G, Elsemore J, Plehn-Dujowich D, McMahon AP et al. Neural tube, skeletal and body wall defects in mice lacking transcription factor AP-2. *Nature.* 1996;381:238–241.
16. Kitamura K, Miura H, Miyagawa-Tomita S, Yanazawa M, Katoh-Fukui Y et al. Mouse Pitx2 deficiency leads to anomalies of the ventral body wall, heart, extra- and periocular mesoderm and right pulmonary isomerism. *Development.* 1999;126: 5749–5758.
17. Baker ME, Rosenberg ER, Troffater KF, Inber MJ, Bowie JD. The *in utero* findings in twin Pentalogy of Cantrell. *J Ultrasound Me.* 1984;3:525–527.
18. Martin RA, Cunniff C, Erickson L, Jones KL. Pentalogy of Cantrell and ectopia cordis, a familial developmental field complex. *Am J Med Genet.* 1992;839–841.
19. Mulder DG, Crittenden IH, Adams FH. Complete repair of a syndrome of congenital defects involving the abdominal wall, sternum, diaphragm, pericardium, and heart; excision of left ventricular diverticulum. *Ann Surg.* 1960;151: 113–122.
20. Agrawal N, Sehgal R, Kumar R, Bhadoria P. Cantrell's Pentalogy. *Anaesth Intensive Care.* 2003;31:120–123.
21. Saito T, Suzuki A, Takahata O, Iwasaki H. Anesthetic management of a patient with Cantrell's pentalogy diagnosed prenatally. *Canadian J Anesthesia.* 2004;51: 946–947.
22. Leon G, Chedraui P, San Miguel G. Prenatal diagnosis of Cantrell's Pentalogy with conventional and three-dimensional sonography. *J Maternal-Fetal and Neonatal Medicine.* 2002;12: 209–211.
23. Parvari R, Weinstein Y, Ehrlich S, Steinitz M, Carmi R. Linkage localization of the thoraco-abdominal syndrome (TAS) gene to Xq25-26. *Am J Med Genet.* 1994;49:431–434.
24. Poetke M, Frommeld T, Berlien HP. PHACE Syndrome: new views on diagnostic criteria. *Eur J Pediatr Surg.* 2002;12: 366–374.

25. Onderoglu L, Baykal G, Tulunary G, Talim B, Kale G. Prenatal diagnosis of Cantrell's pentalogy: a case report. *Turk J Pediatr.* 2003;45: 357–358.

26. Hall BD. Choanal atresia and associated multiple anomalies. *J Pediatr.* 1979;95:395–398.

27. Hintner HM, Hirsch NJ, Kreh GM, Rudolph AJ. Colobomatous microphthalmia, heart disease, hearing loss and mental retardation: a syndrome. *J Pediatr Ophthalmol Strabismus.* 1979;16: 122–128.

28. Pagon RA, Graham JM, Zonana J, Yong S-L. Coloboma, congenital heart disease and choanal atresia with multiple anomalies: CHARGE Association. *J Pediatr.* 1981;99: 223–227.

29. Oley CA Baraitser M, Grant DB. A reappraisal of CHARGE Association. *J Med Genet.* 1988;25:147–156.

30. Lubinsky MS. Properties of associations: Identify, nature, and clinical criteria, with a commentary on why CHARGE and Goldenhar are not associations. *Am J Med Genet.* 1994;49: 21–25.

31. Tellier AL, Cormier-Daire V, Abadie V, Amiel J, Sigaudy S, Bonnet D, et al. CHARGE Syndrome: report of 47 cases and review. *Am J Med Genet.* 1998;76:402–409.

32. Lalani SR, Stockton DW, Bacino C, Molinari LM, Glass NL, Fernbach SD, et al. Toward a genetic etiology of CHARGE Syndrome: I. A systematic scan for submicroscopic deletions. *Am J Med Genet.* 2003;118A:260–266.

33. Sanlaville D, Romana SP, Lapierre JM, Amiel J, Genevieve D, Ozilou C, et al. A CGH study of 27 patients with CHARGE Association. *Clin Genet.* 2002;61:131–138.

34. Vissers LELM, Conny MA von Ravenswaaij, Admiraal R, Hurst JA, deVries BBA, Janssen IM et al. Mutations in a new member of the chromodomain gene family cause CHARGE syndrome. *Nature Genetics.* 2004;36:955–957.

35. Lalani SR, Safiullah AM, Molinari LM, Fernbach SD, Martin DM, Belmont JW. SEMA3E mutation in a patient with CHARGE syndrome. *J Med Genet.* 2004;41:e94 (http://www.jmedgenet.com/cgi/content/full/41/7/e94).

36. Wincent J, Holmberg E, Strömland K, Soller M, Mirzaei L, Djureinovic T et al. CHD7 mutation spectrum in 28 Swedish patients diagnosed with CHARGE syndrome. *Clin Genet.* 2008; 74:31–38.

37. Blake KM, Davenport SLH, Hall BD, Hefner MA, Pagon RA, Williams MS, Lin AE, Graham JM Jr. CHARGE Association: an update and review for the primary pediatrician. *Clin Pediatr.* 1998;37:159–174.

38. Graham JM Jr. A recognizable syndrome within CHARGE Association: Hall-Hittner Syndrome. *Am J Med Genet.* 2001;99:120–123.

39. Amiel J, Attié-Bitach T, Marianowski R, Cormier-Daire V, Abadie V, Bonnet D, et al. Temporal bone anomaly proposed as a major criteria for diagnosis of CHARGE Syndrome. *Am J Med Genet.* 2001;99:124–127.

40. Naito Y, Higuchi M, Koinuma G, Aramaki M, Takahashi T, Kosaki K. Upper airway obstruction in neonates and infants with CHARGE Syndrome. *Am J Med Genet.* 2007;Part A 143A: 1815–1820.

41. Abadie V, Wiener-Vacher S, Morisseau-Durand M-P, Porée C, Amiel J, Amanou L et al. Vestibular anomalies in CHARGE syndrome: investigations on and consequences for postural development. *Eur J Pediatr.* 2000;159:569–574.

42. Blake KD, Hartshorne TS, Lawand C, Dailor AN, Thelin JW. Cranial nerve manifestations in CHARGE Syndrome. *Am J Med Genet.* 2008;Part A 146A:585–592.

43. Pinto G, Abadie V, Mesnage R, Blustajn J, Cabrol S, Amiel J et al. CHARGE Syndrome includes hypogonadotropic hypogonadism and abnormal olfactory bulb development. *J Clin Endocr Metab.* 2005;90:5621–5626.

44. Brock KE, Mathiason MA, Rooney BL, Williams MS. Quantitative analysis of limb anomalies in CHARGE syndrome: correlation with diagnosis and characteristic CHARGE anomalies. *Am J Med Genet Part A.* 2003;123A:111–121.

45. Alazami AM, Alzahrani F, Alkuraya FS. Expanding the "E" in CHARGE. *Am J Med Genet.* 2008;Part A 146A:1890–1892.

46. Sanlaville D, Etchevers HC, Gonzale M, Martinovic J, Clément-Ziza M, Delezoide A-H et al. Phenotypic spectrum of CHARGE syndrome in fetuses with CHD7 truncating mutations correlates with expression during human development. *J Med Genet.* 2006; 43:211–217.

47. Issekutz KA, Graham JM Jr, Prasad C, Smith IM, Blake KD. An epidemiological analysis of CHARGE Syndrome: preliminary results from a Canadian Study. *Am J Med Genet.* 2005;133A: 309–317.

48. Källén K, Robert E, Mastroiacovo P, Castilla EE, Källén B. CHARGE Association in newborns: a registry-based study. *Teratology.* 1999;60:334–343.

49. Johnson D, Morrison N, Grant L, Turner T, Fantes J, Connor JM et al. Confirmation of CHD7 as a cause of CHARGE association identified by mapping a balanced chromosome translocation in affected monozygotic twins. *J Med Genet.* 2006;43:280–284.

50. Arrington CB, Cowley BC, Nightingale DR, Zhou H, Brothman AR, Viskochil DH. Interstitial deletions 8q11.2-q13 with congenital abnormalities of CHARGE Association. *Am J Med Genet.* 2005;133A:326–330.

51. Ho CK, Kaufman RL, Podos SM. Ocular colobomata cardiac defects and other anomalies: a study of seven cases including two sibs. *J Med Genet.* 1975;12:289–293.

52. Meinecke P, Blunck W. Unknown syndrome: congenital heart disease, choanal stenosis, short stature, developmental delay and dysmorphic facial features in a brother and a sister. *J Med Genet.* 1989;26:407–409.

53. Awrich PD, Flannery DB, Robertson L, Mamunes P. CHARGE Association anomalies in siblings. *Am J Hum Genet.* 1982;34: 80A.

54. Hall BD, Blunberg BD. Familial CHARGE Association: affected half-siblings through a normal mother. *Am J Hum Genet.* 1988;43:54A.

55. Lin AE, Siebert JR, Graham JM Jr. Central nervous system malformations in the CHARGE Association. *Am J Med Genet.* 1990;37:304–310.

56. Goldenhar M. Associations malformatives de l'oeil et de l'oreille: en particulier, le syndrome: dermoide epibulbaire-appendices auriculaires-fisulta auris congenita et ses relations avec la dysostoses mandibulo-faciale. *J Genet Hum.* 1952;1:243–282.

57. Gorlin RJ, Jue KL, Jacobsen U, Goldschmidt E. Oculoauriculovertebral dysplasia. *J Pediatr.* 1963;63:991–999.

58. Smith DW. *Recognizable Patterns of Human Malformation,* 3rd ed. Philadelphia: WB Saunders; 1982: 497–500.

59. Vento AR, LaBrie RA, Mulliken JB. The O.M.E.N.S. classification of hemifacial microsomia. *Cleft palate-Craniofacial J.* 1991; 28:68–77.

60. Pruzansky S. Not all dwarfed mandibles are alike. *Birth Defects: Original Article Series.* 1969;1(2):120–129.

61. Rollnick BR, Kaya CI, Nagatoshi K, Hauck W, Martin AD. Oculoauriculovertebral dysplasia and variants. Phenotypic characteristics of 294 patients. *Am J Med Genet.* 1987;26: 361–375.

62. Stoll C, Viville B, Treisser A, Gasser B. A family with dominant oculoauriculovertebral spectrum. *Am J Med Genet.* 1998;78: 345–349.

63. Dabir TA, Morrison PJ. Trisomy 10p with clinical features of facio-auriculo-vertebral spectrum: a case report. *Clin Dysmorph.* 2006;15:25–27.

64. Derbent M, Yilmaz Z, Baltaci V, Saygili A, Varan B, Tokel K. Chromosome 22q11.2 deletion and phenotypic features in 30 patients with conotruncal heart defects. *Am J Med Genet.* 2003;116A:129–135.

65. Callier P, Faivre L, Thauvin-Robinet C, Marle N, Mosca AL, D'Athis P et al. Array-CGH in a series of 30 patients with mental retardation, dysmorphic features, and congenital malformations detected an interstitial 1p22.2-p31.1 deletion in a patient with features overlapping the Goldenhar syndrome. *Am J Med Genet.* 2008;Part A 146A:2109–2115.

66. Terhal P, Rösler B, Kohlhase J. A family with features overlapping Okihiro Syndrome, hemifacial microsomia and isolated Duane anomaly caused by a novel SALL4 mutation. *Am J Med Genet.* 2006;140A:222–226.

67. Kosaki R, Fujimaru R, Samejima H, Yamada H, Izumi K, Iijima K, Kosaki K. Wide phenotypic variations within a family with SALL1 mutations: isolated external ear abnormalities to Goldenhar syndrome. *Am J Med Genet.* 2007; Part A 143A: 1087–1090.

68. Schinzel AAGL, Smith DW, Miller JR. Monozygotic twinning and structural defects. *J Pediatr.* 1979;95:921–930.

69. Schinzel A. Possible vascular disruptive origin of hemifacial microsomia? *Am J Ob Gyn.* 1987;157:1319.

70. Ewart-Toland A, Yankowitz J, Winder A. Oculoauriculovertebral abnormalities in children of diabetic mothers. *Am J Med Genet.* 2000;14:303–309.

71. Werler MM, Sheehan JE, Hayes C, Mitchell AA, Mulliken JB. Vasoactive exposures, vascular events, and hemifacial microsomia. *Birth Defects Research (Part A): Clin Mol Teratology.* 2004;70:389–395.

72. Wieczorek D, Ludwig M, Boehringer S, Jongbloet PH, Gillessen-Kaesbach G, Horsthemke B. Reproduction abnormalities and twin pregnancies in parents of sporadic patients with oculo-auriculo-vertebral spectrum/Goldenhar syndrome. *Hum Genet.* 2007;121:369–376.

73. Mulliken JB, Kaban LB. Analysis and treatment of hemifacial microsomia in childhood. *Clinics Plast Surg.* 1987;14: 91–100.

74. Miller TD, Metry D. Multiple accessory tragi as a clue to the diagnosis of the oculo-auriculo-vertebral (Goldenhar) syndrome. *J Am Acad Dermatol.* 2004;50:511–513.

75. Sutphen R, Galan-Gomez E, Cortada X, Newkirk PN, Koussef BG. Tracheoesophageal anomalies in oculoauriculovertebral (Goldenhar) spectrum. *Clin Genet.* 1995;48:66–71.

76. Tasse C, Bohringer S, Fischer S, Ludecke HJ, Albrecht B, Horn D et al. Oculo-auriculo-vertebral spectrum (OAVS): clinical evaluation and severity scoring of 53 patients and proposal for a new classification. *Eur J Med Genet.* 2005;48:397–411.

77. Nargozian C, Ririe DG, Bennun RD, Mulliken JB. Hemifacial microsomia: anatomical prediction of difficult intubation. *Paediatric Anaesthesia.* 1999;9:393–398.

78. Kumar A, Friedman JM, Taylor GP, Patterson MWH. Pattern of cardiac malformation in oculoauriculovertebral spectrum. *Am J Med Gen.* 1993;46:423–426.

79. Digilio MC, Calzolari F, Capolino R, Toscano A, Sarkozy A, de Zorzi A et al. Congenital heart defects in patients with oculo-auriculo-vertebral spectrum (Goldenhar Syndrome). *Am J Med Genet.* 2008;Part A 146A:1815–1819.

80. Duncan PA, Shapiro LR. Interrelationship of the hemifacial microsomia-VATER, VATER, and Sirenomelia phenotypes. *Am J Med Genet.* 1993;47:75–84.

81. Johnston MC, Bronsky PT. Animal models for human craniofacial malformations. *J Craniofac Genet Devel Biol.* 1991;11: 227–291.

82. Naora H, Kimura M, Otani H, Yokoyama M, Koizumi T, Katsuki M, Tanaka O. Transgenic mouse model of hemifacial microsomia: cloning and characterization of insertional mutation region on chromosome 10. *Genomics.* 1994;23: 515–519.

83. Cousley R, Naora H, Yokoyama M, Kimura M, Otani H. Validity of the Hfm transgenic mouse as a model for Hemifacial Microsomia. *Cleft Palate Craniofac J.* 2002;39:81–92.

84. Poswillo D. The pathogenesis of the first and second branchial arch syndrome. *Oral Surg Orgal Med Oral Pathol.* 1973;35: 302–308.

85. Melnick M. The etiology of external ear malformations and its relation to abnormalities of the middle ear, inner ear and other organ systems. *Birth Defects.* 1980;16(4):303–331.

86. Nelson K, Holmes LB. Malformations due to presumed spontaneous mutations in newborn infants. *N Engl J Med.* 1989;320: 19–23.

87. Keusch CF, Mulliken JB, Kaplan LC. Craniofacial anomalies in twins. *Plast Reconstr Surg.* 1991;87:16–23.

88. Lawson K, Waterhouse N, Gault DT. Is hemifacial microsomia linked to multiple maternities? *Br J Plast Surg.* 2002;55: 474–478.

89. Ryan CA, Finer NN, Ives E. Discordance of signs in monozygotic twins concordant for the Goldenhar anomaly. *Am J Med Genet.* 1988;29:755–761.

90. Hermann J, Opitz JM. A dominantly inherited first arch syndrome. *Birth Defects: Orig Art Series.* 1969;5(2):110–112.

91. Saraux H, Grignon JL, Dhermy P. A propos d'une observation. Familiale de syndrome de Franceschetti-Goldenhar. *Bull Soc Ophthalmol Fr.* 1963;63:705–707.

92. Su P-H, Yu J-S, Chen J-Y, Chen S-J, Li S-Y, Chen H-N. Mutations and new polymorphic changes in the TCOF1 gene of patients with oculo-auriculo-vertebral spectrum and Treacher-Collins syndrome. *Clin Dysmorphol.* 2007;16:261–267.

93. Ala–Mello S, Siggberg L, Knuutila S, von Koshull H, Taskinen M, Peippo M. Further evidence for a relationship between the 5p15 chromosome region and the oculoauriculovertebral anomaly. *Am J Med Genet Part A.* 2008;146A:2490–2494.

94. Kelberman D, Tyson J, Chandler DC, McInerney AM, Slee J, Albert D. Hemifacial microsomia: progress in understanding the genetic basis of a complex malformation syndrome. *Hum Genet.* 2001;109:638–645.

95. Fischer S, Lüdecke HJ, Wieczorek D, Böhringer S, Gillessen-Kaesbach G, Horsthemke B. Histone acetylation dependent allelic expression imbalance of BAPX1 in patients with the oculo-auriculo-vertebral spectrum. *Hum Mol Genet.* 2006;15: 581–587.

96. Källén K, Robert E, Castilla EE, Mastroiacovo P, Källén B. Relation between oculo-auriculo-vertebral (OAV) dysplasia and three other non-random associations of malformations (VATER, CHARGE, and OEIS). *Am J Med Genet.* 2004;127A: 26–34.

97. Werler MM, Sheehan JE, Hayes C, Mitchell AA, Mulliken JB. Vasoactive exposures, vascular events, and hemifacial microsomia. *Birth Def Res (Part A): Clin Mol Teratol.* 2004;70: 389–395.

98. Araneta MR, Moore CA, Olney RS, Edmonds LD, Karcher JA, McDonough C et al. Goldenhar Syndrome among infants

born in military hospitals to Gulf War Veterans. *Teratology.* 1997;56:244–251.

99. Strömland K, Miller M, Sjögreen L, Johannsson M, Joelsson BM, Billstedt E et al. Oculo-auriculo-vertebral spectrum: associated anomalies, functional deficits and possible developmental risk factors. *Am J Med Genet.* 2007;143A:1317–1325.

100. Kaye CI, Rollnick BR, Hauck WW, Martin AO, Richtsmeier JT, Nagatoshi K. Hemifacial microsomia: statistical analysis. *Am J Med Genet.* 1989;34:574–578.

101. Russell LJ, Weaver DD, Bull MJ. The axial mesodermal dysplasia spectrum. *Pediatrics.* 1981;67:176–182.

102. Dinleyici EC, Tekin N, Dinleyici M, Kilic Z, Adapinar B, Aksit MA. Severe fatal course of axial mesodermal dysplasia spectrum associated with complex cardiac defect in an infant of a mother with insulin dependent diabetes. *Am J Med Genet Part A.* 2007;143A:2156–2159.

103. Vendramini S, Richieri-Costa A, Guion-Almeida ML. Oculoauriculovertebral spectrum with radial defects: a new syndrome or an extension of the oculoauriculovertebral spectrum? Report of fourteen Brazilian cases and review of the literature. *Eur J Hum Genet.* 2007;15:411–421.

104. Beck AE, Hudgins L, Hoyme HE. Autosomal dominant microtia and ocular coloboma: new syndrome or an extension of the oculo-auriculo-vertebral spectrum? *Am J Med Genet.* 2005; Part A 134A:359–362.

105. Hattori Y, Tanaka M, Matsumoto T, Uehara K, Ueno K, Miwegishi K et al. Prenatal diagnosis of hemifacial microsomia by magnetic resonance imaging. *J Perinat Med.* 2005;33:69–71.

106. Carles D, Serville F, Mainguené M, Dubecq JP. Cyclopia-otocephaly association: a new case of the most severe variant of agnathia-holoprosencephaly complex. *J Craniofac Gen Develop Biol.* 1987;7:107–113.

107. Hersh JH, McChane RH, Rosenberg EM, Powers WH Jr, Corrigan C, Pancratz L. Otocephaly-midline malformation association. *Am J Med Gent.* 1989;34:246–249.

108. Ibba RM, Zoppi MA, Floris M, Putzolu M, Monni G, Todde PF, Sardu G. Otocephaly: prenatal diagnosis of a new case and etiopathogenic considerations. *Am J Med Genet.* 2000;90:427–429.

109. Utkus A, Kazakevičius R, Ptašekas R, Kučinskas V, Beckwith JB, Opitz JM. Human anotocephaly (aprosopus, acrania-synotia) in a Vilnius anatomical collection. *Am J Med Genet.* 2001;101:163–171.

110. Schiffer C, Tariverdian G, Schiesser M, Thomas MC, Sergi C. Agnathia-otocephaly complex: report of three cases with involvement of two different carnegie stages. *Am J Med Genet.* 2002;112:203–208.

111. Faye-Petersen O, David E, Rangwala N, Seaman JP, Hua Z, Heller DS. Otocephaly: report of five new cases and a literature review. *Fetal and Ped Pathol.* 2006;25:277–298.

112. Cayea PD, Bieber FR, Ross MJ, Davidoff A, Osathanondh R, Jones TB. Sonographic findings in otocephaly (synotia). *J Ultrasound Med.* 1985;4:377–379.

113. Özden S, Fiçicioğlu C, Mustafa K, Özay O, Remziye B. Agnathia-holoprosencephaly-situs inversus. *Am J Med Gen.* 2000;91:235–236.

114. Juriloff DM, Sulik KK, Roderick TH, Hogan BK. Genetic and developmental studies of a new mouse mutation that produces otocephaly. *J Craniofac Gen Develop Biol.* 1985;5:121–145.

115. Wright S. On the genetics of subnormal development of the head (otocephaly) in the guinea pig. *Genetics.* 1934;19:471–505.

116. Wright S, Wagner K. Types of subnormal development of the head from inbred strains of guinea pigs and their bearing on the classification and interpretation of vertebrate monstrosities. *Am J Anat.* 1934;54:383–448.

117. Ueda Y, Yamaguchi R, Ikawa M, Okabe M, Morii E, Maeda Y, Kinoshita T. PGAP1 knock-out mice show otocephaly and male infertility. *J Biol Chem.* 2007;282:30373–30380.

118. Suda Y, Nakabayashi J, Matsuo I, Aizawa S. Functional equivalency between Otx2 and Otx1 in development of the rostral head. *Development.* 1999;126:743–757.

119. Hide T, Hatakeyama J, Kimura-Yoshida C, Tian E, Takeda N, Ushio Y et al. Gene modifiers of otocephalic phenotypes in Otx2 heterozygous mutant mice. *Development.* 2002;129:4347–4357.

120. Machin GA, Sperber GH, Wootliffe J. Monozygotic twin aborted fetuses discordant for holoprosencephaly/synotia. *Teratology.* 1985;31:203–215.

121. Reinecke P, Figge C, Majewski F, Borchard F. Otocephaly and holoprosencephaly in only one monozygotic twin. *Am J Med Genet.* 2003;119A:395–396.

122. Pauli RM, Pettersen JC, Arya S, Gilbert E. Familial agnathia-holoprosencephaly. *Am J Med Genet.* 1983;14:677–698.

123. Krassikoff N, Sekhon GS. Familial agnathia-holoprosencephaly caused by an inherited unbalanced translocation and not autosomal recessive inheritance. *Clin Genet.* 1989;34:255–257.

124. Khan A, Bourgeois J, Mohide P. Agnathia-otocephaly complex in a fetus with maternal use of topical 1% salicylate. *Clin Dysmorph.* 2008;17:75–76.

125. Shermak MA, Dufresne CR. Nonlethal case of otocephaly and its implications for treatment. *J Craniofacial Surg.* 1996;7:372–375.

126. Erlich MS, Cunningham ML, Hudgins L. Transmission of the dysgnathia complex from mother to daughter. *Am J Med Genet.* 2000;95:269–274.

127. Guion-Almeida ML, Zechi-Ceide RM, Vendramini S, Kokitsu-Nakata NM. Auriculo-condylar syndrome: additional patients. *Am J Med Genet.* 2002;112:209–214.

128. Ducarme G, Largilliere C, Amarenco B, Davitian C, Bucourt M, Vazquez M-P et al. Three-dimensional ultrasound in prenatal diagnosis of isolated otocephaly. *Prenatal Diagn.* 2007;27:479–487.

129. Umekawa T, Sugiyama T, Yokochi A, Suga S, Uchida K, Sagawa N. A case of agnathia-otocephaly complex assessed prenatally for ex utero intrapartum treatment (EXIT) by three-dimensional ultrasonography. *Prenat Diagn.* 2007;27:679–681.

130. Poland A. Deficiency of the pectoralis muscles. *Guy Hosp Rep.* 1841;6:191–193.

131. Ravitch MM. Poland's Syndrome - a study of an eponym. *Plastic Reconstr Surg.* 1977;59:508–512.

132. Clarkson P. Poland's syndactyly. *Guy's Hosp Rep.* 1962;111:335–346.

133. David TJ. Nature and etiology of the Poland Anomaly. *N Engl J Med.* 1972;287:487–489.

134. Mace JW, Kaplan JM, Schanberger JE, Gotlin RW. Poland's Syndrome: Report of seven cases and review of the literature. *Clin Pediatr.* 1972;11:98–102.

135. Beals RK, Crawford S. Congenital absence of the pectoral muscles. A review of twenty-five patients. *Clin Orthop Relat Res.* 1976;119:166–171.

136. Ireland DC, Takayama N, Flatt AE. Poland's syndrome. *J Bone Jt Surg.* 1976;58–A:52–58.

137. McGillivray BC, Lowry RB. Poland syndrome in British Columbia: incidence and reproductive experience of affected persons. *Am J Med Genet.* 1977;1:65–74.

138. Goldberg MJ, Mazzei RJ. Poland Syndrome: A concept of pathogenesis based on limb bud embryology. *Birth Defects: Orig Art Series XIII*. 1977;(3D):103–115.

139. Castilla EE, Paz JP, Orioli IM. Pectoralis major muscle defect and Poland complex. *Am J Med Genet*. 1979;4:263–269.

140. Wilson MR, Louis DS, Stevenson TR et al. Poland's Syndrome: variable expression and associated anomalies. *J Hand Surg Am*. 1988;13:880–882.

141. Al-Qattan MM, Thunayan AA. The middle phalanx in Poland Syndrome. *Ann Plast Surg*. 2005;54:160–164.

142. Shamberger RC, Welch KJ, Upton J III. Surgical treatment of thoracic deformity in Poland's syndrome. *J Pediatr Surg*. 1989; 24:760–766.

143. Debeer P, Brys P, De Smet L, Fryns JP. Unilateral absence of the trapezius and pectoralis major muscle: a variant of Poland Syndrome. *Genetic Counseling*. 2002;13:449–453.

144. Hegde HR, Shokeir MHK. Posterior shoulder girdle abnormalities with absence of pectoralis major muscle. *Am J Med Genet*. 1982;13:285–293.

145. Larrandaburu M, Schüler L, Ehlers JA, Reis AM, Lemos Silveira E. The occurrence of Poland and Poland-Möebius syndromes in the same family: further evidence of their genetic component. *Clin Dysmorphol*. 1999;8:93–99.

146. Nachnani JS, Supe AN. A variant of Poland Syndrome. *J Postgrad Med*. 2001;47:131–132.

147. Bouvet JP, Leveque D, Bemetieres F, Gros J-J. Vascular origin of Poland syndrome? A comparative rheographic study of the vascularization of the arms in eight patients. *Eur J Pediatr*. 1978;128:17–26.

148. Bouwes Bavinck JN, Weaver D. Subclavian artery supply disruption sequence: hypothesis of a vascular etiology for Poland, Klippel-Feil and Möbius anomalies. *Am J Med Genet*. 1986;23:903–918.

149. David TJ, Saad MN. Dermatologlyphic diagnosis of the Poland Anomaly in the absence of syndactyly. *Human Heredity*. 1974;24:373–378.

150. Bosch-Banyeras JM, Zuasnabar A, Puig A, Catala M, Cuatrecasas JM. Poland-Möbius syndrome associated with dextrocardia. *J Med Genet*. 1984;21:70–71.

151. Hazir T, Malik MS. Poland anomaly with dextrocardia: a case report. *J Pak Med Assoc*. 1996;46:181–182.

152. Fraser FC, Teebi AS, Walsh S, Pinsky L. Poland sequence with dextrocardia: which comes first? *Am J Med Genet*. 1997;73:194–196.

153. Hegde HR, Leung AKC. Aplasia of pectoralis major muscle and renal anomalies. *Am J Med Genet*. 1989;32:109–111.

154. Miller RA, Miller DR. Congenital absence of the pectoralis major muscle with acute lymphoblastic leukemia and genitourinary anomalies. *J Pediatr*. 1975;87:146–147.

155. Bamforth JS, Fabian C, Machin G, Honore L. Poland anomaly with limb body wall disruption defect: case report and review. *Am J Med Genet*. 1992;43:780–784.

156. Frias JL, Felman AH. Absence of the pectoralis major, with ipsilateral aplasia of the radius, thumb, hemidiaphragm and lung: an extreme expression of Poland anomaly? *Birth Defects: Original Article Series*. 1974;X(5):55–59.

157. Kabra M, Suri M, Jain A, Verma IC. Poland Anomaly with unusual associated anomalies: case report of an apparent disorganization defect. *Am J Med Genet*. 1994;52:402–405.

158. Pišteljíc DT, Vranješvíc D, Apostolski D, Pišteljíc DD. Poland syndrome associated with 'morning glory' syndrome (coloboma of the optic disc). *J Med Genet*. 1986;23:364–366.

159. Gomez-Ulla F, Gonzalez F. Retinal vascular abnormality in Poland's syndrome. *Brit J Ophthal*. 1999;83:1092.

160. Stupp T, Pavlidis M, Buchner T, Thanos S. Poland anomaly associated with ipsilateral combined hamartoma of retina and retinal pigment epithelium. *Eye*. 2004;18:550–552.

161. Ailiwadi M, Arildsen RC, Greelish JP. Poland Syndrome: a contraindication to the use of the internal thoracic artery in coronary artery bypass grafting? *J Thor Cardiovas Surg*. 2005;130:578–579.

162. Mentzel H-J, Seidel J, Sauner D, Vogt S, Fitzek C, Zintl F, Kaiser WA. Radiological aspects of the Poland Syndrome and implications for treatment: a case study and review. *Eur J Pediatr*. 2002;161:455–459.

163. Bamforth JS, Fabian C, Machin G, Honore L. Poland Anomaly with a limb body wall disruption defect: a case report and review. *Am J Med Genet*. 1992;43:780–784.

164. Czeizel A, Vitéz M, Lenz W. Birth prevalence of Poland sequence and proportion of its familial cases. *Am J Med Genet*. 1990;36:524.

165. Stevens DB, Fink BA, Prevel C. Poland's Syndrome in one identical twin. *J Pediatric Orthopaedics*. 2000;20:392–395.

166. Cohen A, Zecca S, Dassori A, Pelegrini M, Parodi L, Romano C. Poland sequence in two siblings suggesting an autosomal inheritance transmission. *Clin Genet*. 1996;50:93–95.

167. Sujansky E, Riccardi VM, Matthew AL. The familial occurrence of Poland Syndrome. *Birth Defects: Original Article Series XIII*. 1977;(3A):117–121.

168. David TJ. Familial Poland anomaly. *J Med Gen*. 1982;19:293–296.

169. Fraser FC, Ronen GM, O'Leary E. Pectoralis major defect and Poland sequence in second cousins: extension of the Poland sequence spectrum. *Am J Med Genet*. 1989;33:468–470.

170. Cobben JM, Robinson PH, van Essen AJ, van der Wiel HL, ten Kate LP. Poland anomaly in mother and daughter. *Am J Med Genet*. 1989;33:519–521.

171. Shalev SA, Hall JG. Poland Anomaly – report of an unusual family. *Am J Med Genet*. 2003;118A:180–183.

172. Soltan HD, Holmes LB. Familial occurrence of malformations possibly attributable to vascular abnormalities. *J Pediatr*. 1986;108:112–114.

173. Der Kaloustian VM, Hoyme HE, Hogg H, Entin MA, Guttmacher AE. Possible common pathogenetic mechanisms for Poland sequence and Adams-Oliver Syndrome. *Am J Med Genet*. 1991;38:69–73.

174. Parano E, Falsaperla R, Pavone V, Toscano A, Bolan EA, Trifiletti RR. Intrafamilial phenotypic heterogeneity of the Poland complex: a case report. *Neuro Pediatrics*. 1995;26:217–219.

175. Happle R. Poland anomaly may be explained as a paradominant trait. *Am J Med Genet*. 1999;87:364–365.

176. Van Steensel MAM. Poland Anomaly: not unilateral or bilateral but mosaic. *Am J Med Genet*. 2004;125A:211–212.

177. Lowry RB, Bouvet JP. Familial Poland anomaly. *J Med Genet*. 1983;20:152–154.

178. David TJ, Winter RM. Familial absence of the pectoralis major, serratus anterior, and latissimus dorsi muscles. *J Med Genet*. 1985;22:390–392.

179. Darian VB, Argenta LC, Pasyk RA. Familial Poland's Syndrome. *Ann Plast Surg*. 1989;23:531–537.

180. Firth HV, Boyd PA, Chamberlain P, MacKenzie IZ, Lindenbaum RH, Huson SM. Severe limb abnormalities after chorion villus sampling at 56–66 days' gestation. *Lancet*. 1991;337:762–763.

181. Gonzalez CH, Marques-Dias M-J, Kim CA, Sugayama SMM, DaPaz JA, Huson SM, Holmes LB. Congenital abnormalities in Brazilian children associated with misoprostol

misuse in first trimester of pregnancy. *Lancet.* 1998;351: 1624–1627.

182. Puvabanditsin S, Garrow E, Augustin G, Titapiwatanakul R, Kuniyoshi KM. Poland-Möbius syndrome and cocaine abuse: a relook at vascular etiology. *Pediatr Neurol.* 2005;32: 285–287.

183. Martínez-Frías ML, Czeizel AE, Rodríguez-Pinilla E, Bermejo E. Smoking during pregnancy and Poland sequence: results of a population-based registry and a case-control registry. *Teratology.* 1999;59:35–38.

184. Wright AR, Milner RH, Bainbridge C, Wilsdon JB. MR and CT in the assessment of Poland Syndrome. *J Computerized Assisted Tomography.* 1992;16:442–447.

185. Beer G. The clinical findings of a missing latissimus dorsi muscle in Poland's syndrome. *Plast Reconst Surg.* 1997;99: 926–927.

186. Liao H-T, Cheng M-H, Ulusal BG, Wei F-C. Deep inferior epigastric perforator flap for successful simultaneous breast and chest wall reconstruction in a Poland anomaly patient. *Ann Plast Surg.* 2005;55:422–426.

187. Riccardi VM. Unilateral gluteal hypoplasia and brachysyndactyly: lower extremity counterpart of the Poland Anomaly. *Pediatrics.* 1978;61:653–654.

188. De Smet L, Fryns JP. Synbrachydactyly involving both the hand and foot. *Clin Genet.* 1999;56:176–177.

189. Silengo M, Lerone M, Seri M, Boffi P. Lower extremity counterpart of the Poland syndrome. *Clin Genet.* 1999;55:41–43.

190. Silva EO, Leal GF, Carvalho VN. Poland Anomaly with foot symbrachydactyly. *Am J Med Genet.* 2002;109:333–334.

191. Karnak I, Tanyel FC, Tunçilek E, Ünsal M, Büyükpamukçu N. Bilateral Poland Anomaly. *Am J Med Genet.* 1998;75: 505–507.

192. Shipkov CD, Anastassov YK. Bilateral Poland anomaly: does it exist? *Am J Med Genet.* 2003;118A:101.

193. Spear SL, Pelletiere CV, Lee ES, Grotting JC. Anterior thoracic hypoplasia: a separate entity from Poland Syndrome. *Plast Reconstr Surg.* 2004;113L:69–77.

194. Hodgkinson DJ. Anterior thoracic hypoplasia: a separate entity from Poland Syndrome. *Plast Reconstr Surg.* 2005;115: 960–962.

195. Eagle JF, Barrett HGS. Congenital deficiency of abdominal musculature with associated genito-urinary abnormalities: a syndrome, Report of nine cases. *Pediatrics.* 1950;6: 721–736.

196. Williams DI, Burkholder GV. The prune belly syndrome. *J Urol.* 1967;98: 244–251.

197. Nunn In, Stephens FD. The triad syndrome: a composite anomaly of the abdominal wall, urinary system and testes. *J Urol.* 1961;86: 782–794.

198. Dekletk DP, Scott WW. Prostatic maldevelopment in the prune belly syndrome: a defect in prostatic stromal-epithelial interaction. *J Urol.* 1978;120: 341–344.

199. Pagon R, Smith DW, Shepard TH. Urethral obstruction malformation complex: a cause of abdominal muscle deficiency and the "prune belly." *J Pediatr.* 1979;94:900–906.

200. Monie IW, Monie BJ. Determinants of the prune belly syndrome. *J Pediatr.* 1979;94:1084.

201. Nakayama DK, Harrison MR, Chinn DH, Lorimer AA. The pathogenesis of prune belly. *An J Dis Child.* 1984;138: 834–836.

202. Moerman P, Fryns J, Godderis P, Lauweryns JM. Pathogenesis of the prune belly syndrome: a functional urethral obstruction caused by prostatic hypoplasia. *Pediatrics.* 1984;73: 470–475.

203. Beasley SW, Bettenay F, Huston JM. The anterior urethra provides clues to aetiology of prune belly syndrome. *Pediatric Surg Internat.* 1988;3: 169–172.

204. Sutherland RS, Mevorach RA, Kogan BA. The prune-belly syndrome: current insights. *Pediatr Nephrol.* 1995;9: 770–778.

205. Lubinsky M, Rapoport D. Transient fetal hydrops and "prune belly" in one identical female twin. *N Engl J Med.* 1983;308: 256–257.

206. Reinberg Y, Shapira E, Manivel JC, Manley CB, Pettinato G, Gonzalez R. Prune belly syndrome in females: a triad of abdominal musculature deficiency and anomalies of the urinary and genital systems. *J Pediatr.* 1991;118:395–398.

207. Abbott JF, Levine D, Wapner R. Posterior urethral valves: inaccuracy of prenatal diagnosis. *Fetal Diagn Ther.* 1998;13: 179–183.

208. Reinberg Y, Chelimsky G, Gonzalez R. Urethral atresia and the prune belly syndrome. Report of 6 cases. *Brit J Urology.* 1993;72:112–114.

209. Platt WB. Rare case of deficiency of the abdominal muscles. *Philadelphia Med J.* 1898;1:738–739.

210. Radis Z, Forbes M. Intrauterine atrophy and gangrene of the lower extremity of a fetus caused by megacystis due to urethral atresia. *J Pathol.* 1971;104:31–35.

211. Graham JM, Miller ME, Stephan MJ, Smith DW. Limb reduction anomalies and early in utero limb compression. *J Pediatr.* 1980;96:1052–1056.

212. Carey JC, Eggert L, Curry CJR. Lower limb deficiency and the urethral obstruction sequence. *Birth Defects: Original Article Series.* 1982; 18(3B):19–28.

213. Genest DR, Driscoll SG, Bieber FR. Complexities of limb anomalies: the lower extremity in the "prune belly" phenotype. *Teratology.* 1991;44:365–371.

214. Perez-Ayks A, Graham JM, Hersh JH, Hoyme HE, Aleck K, Carey JC. Urethral obstruction sequence and lower limb deficiency: evidence for the vascular disruption hypothesis. *J Pediatr.* 1993;123:398–405.

215. Gonzalez R, Reinberg Y, Burke B, Wells T, Vernier RL. Early bladder outlet obstruction in fetal lambs induces renal dysplasia and the prune-belly syndrome. *J Pediatr Surg.* 1990;25: 342–345.

216. Baird PA, MacDonald EC. An epidemiologic study of congenital malformations of the anterior abdominal wall in more than half a million consecutive live births. *Am J Hum Genet.* 1981; 33:470–478.

217. Ives EJ. The abdominal muscle deficiency triad syndrome: experience with 10 cases. *Birth Defects: Original Article Series.* 1974;10(4):127–131.

218. Botto LD, Feldman M, Opitz JM, Krikov S, Johnson J, Byrne JLB, Carey JC. Congenital anomalies and stillbirths: a population-based study, Utah 1999–2003. *Proc Greenwood Center.* 2007;26:60.

219. Livoti G, Vitalis SM, Corsello G. Monozygotic monoamniotic twins discordant for urethral and anal atresia with vesicorectal fistula: a favourable combination of defects. *Clin Genet.* 1998;54:164–165.

220. Ricardi VM, Gunn CM. The prune belly anomaly: heterogeneity and superficial X-linkage mimicry. *J Med Genet.* 1977;14: 266–270.

221. Adeyokunner AA, Familus JB. Prune belly syndrome in two siblings and a first cousin. Possible genetic implications. *Am J Dis Child.* 1982;136:23–25.

222. Gaboardi F, Sterpa A, Thiebat E, Cornal R, Manfredi M, Brandi C et al. Prune belly syndrome: report of three siblings. *Helv Paediat Acta.* 1982;37:283–288.

223. Abe K, Honein MA, Moore CA. Maternal febrile illnesses, medication use, and the risk of congenital renal anomalies. *Birth Defects Res (Part A): Clin Mol Teratol.* 2003;67: 911–918.

224. Greskovich FJ, Nyberg LM Jr. The prune belly syndrome: review of its etiology, defects, treatment and prognosis. *J Urol.* 1988;140:707–712.

225. Herndon CDA, Casale AJ. Early second trimester intervention in a surviving infant with postnatally diagnosed urethral atresia. *J Urol.* 2002;168:1532–1533.

226. Shigeta M, Nagata M, Shimoyamada H, Shibata S, Okuno S, Hamada H, Watanabe T. Prune-belly syndrome diagnosed at 14 weeks' gestation with severe urethral obstruction but normal kidneys. *Pediatr Nephrol.* 1999;13:135–137.

227. Say B, Gerald PS. A new polydactyly/imperforate-anus/vertebral-anomalies syndrome? *Lancet.* 1968;ii:688.

228. Quan L, Smith DW. The VATER Association. Vertebral defects, anal atresia, T-E fistula with esophageal atresia, radial and renal dysplasia: a spectrum of associated defects. *J Pediatrics.* 1973; 82:14–107.

229. Temtamy SA, Miller JD. Extending the scope of the VATER Association: definition of the VATER Syndrome. *J Pediatrics.* 1974;85:245–349.

230. Khoury MJ, Corero JF, Greenberg F, James LM, Erickson JD. A Population study of the VACTERL association: evidence for its etiologic heterogeneity. *Pediatrics.* 1983;71:815–820.

231. Czeizel A, Ludányi I. An aetiological study of the VACTERL-association. *Eur J Pediatr.* 1985;144:331–337.

232. Evans JA, Vitez M, Czeizel A. Patterns of acrorenal malformation associations. *Am J Med Gen.* 1992;44:413–419.

233. Schüler L, Salzano FM. Patterns in multimalformed babies and the question of the relationship between sirenomelia and VACTERL. *Am J Med Genet.* 1994;49:29–35.

234. Botto LD, Khoury MJ, Mastoiacovo P, Castilla EE, Moore CA, Skjaerven R et al. The spectrum of congenital anomalies of the VATER Association: an international study. *Am J Med Genet.* 1997;71:8–15.

235. Rittler M, Paz JE, Castilla EE. VACTERL: An epidemiologic analysis of risk factors. *Am J Med Genet.* 1997;73:162–169.

236. Martínez-Frías ML, Frías JL. VACTERL as primary, polytopic developmental field defects. *Am J Med Genet.* 1999;83:13–16.

237. Martínez-Frías ML, Bermejo E, Rodriguez-Pinilla E. Anal atresia, vertebral, genital, and urinary tract anomalies: a primary polytopic developmental field defect identified through an epidemiological analysis of associations. *Am J Med Gen.* 2000; 95:169–173.

238. de Jong EM, Felix JF, Deurloo JA, van Dooren MF, Aronson DC, Torfs CP, Heij HA, Tibboel D. Non-VACTERL-type anomalies are frequent in patients with esophageal atresia/tracheoesophageal fistula and full or partial VACTERL association. *Birth Def Res (Part A): Clin Mol Teratol.* 2008;82:92–97.

239. Källén K, Mastroiacovo P, Castilla EE, Robert E, Källén B. VATER non-random association of congenital malformations: study based on data from four malformation registers. *Am J Med Gen.* 2001;101:26–32.

240. Reardon W, Zhou XP, Eng C. A novel germline mutation of the PTEN gene in a patient with microcephaly, ventricular dilatation and features of VATER association. *J Med Genet.* 2001; 28:820–823.

241. Damian MS, Seibel P, Schachennayr W, Reichmann H, Dorndorf W. VACTERL with the mitochondrial NP 3243 point mutation. *Am J Med Genet.* 1996;62:398–403.

242. Feigenbaum A, Chitayat D, Robinson B, MacGregor D, Myint T, Arbus G, Nowaczyk MJ. The expanding clinical phenotype of the tRNA(Leu(UUR)) A– >G mutation at np 3243 of mitochondrial DNA: diabetic embryopathy associated with mitochondrial cytopathy. *Am J Med Gent.* 1996;62:404–409.

243. Stone DL, Biesecker LG. Mitochondrial NP 3243 point mutation is not a common cause of VACTERL Association. *Am J Med Genet.* 1997;72:237–238.

244. Vaux KK, Masliah E, Crews L, Jones KJ. Abnormal PAX1 expression is a factor in vertebral and rib anomalies seen in VATER association. *Proc Greenwood Ctr.* 2004;8–67.

245. Kim JH, Kim PCW, Hui C-C. The VACTERL association: Lessons from the Sonic Hedgehog pathway. *Clin Genetics.* 2001;59:306–315.

246. Orford JE, Cass DT. Dose response relationship between adriamycin and birth defects in a rat model of VATER association. *J Pediatr Surg.* 1999;34:392–398.

247. Arsic D, Qi BQ, Beasley SW. Hedgehog in the human: a possible explanation for the VATER association. *J Paediatr Child Health.* 2002;38:117–121.

248. King SL, Ladda RL, Schochat SJ. Monozygotic twins concordant for tracheo-oesophageal fistula and discordant for the VATER association. *Acta Paediatr Scand.* 1977;66: 783–785.

249. Becker J, Hernandez A, Dipietro M, Coran AG. Identical twins concordant for pulmonary sequestration communicating with the esophagus and discordant for the VACTERL association. *Pediatr Surg Int.* 2005;21:541–546.

250. McMullen KP, Karnes PS, Moir CR, Michels VV. Familial recurrence of tracheoesophageal fistula and associated malformations. *Am J Med Genet.* 1996;63:525–528.

251. Fuhrman W, Riger A, Vogel F. Beobachtungen zum genetic. Genetik der atresia ani. *Arch Kinderheilk.* 1958;158: 264–270.

252. Auchterlonie LA, White MP. Recurrence of the VATER association within a sibship. *Clin Genet.* 1982;21:122–124.

253. Say B, Balci S, Pirnar T, Hi Csönmez A. Imperforate anus (polydactyly) vertebral anomalies syndrome: a hereditary trait? *J Pediatr.* 1971;79:1033–1034.

254. Nezarati MM, McLeod DR. VACTERL manifestations in two generations of a family. *Am J Med Genet.* 1999;82:40–42.

255. Rosenberg MJ, Vaske D, Killoran CE, Ning Y, Wargowski D, Hudgins L et al. Detection of chromosomal aberrations by a whole-gamma microsatellite screen. *Am J Hum Genet.* 2000; 66:419–427.

256. Hunger AGW, MacMurray B. Malformations of the VATER-association plus hydrocephalus in male infant and his maternal uncle. *Proc Greenwood Genet Ctr.* 1987;6:146–174.

257. Sujansky E, Leonard C. VACTERL association with hydrocephalus – a new recessive syndrome? *Am J Hum Genet.* 1983;35:119A.

258. Evans JA, Stranc LC, Kaplan P, Hunter AG. VACTERL with hydrocephalus: further delineation of the syndrome(s). *Am J Med Genet.* 1981;34:177–182.

259. Nora AH, Nora JJ. A syndrome of multiple congenital anomalies associated with teratogenic exposure. *Arch Environ Health.* 1975;30:17–21.

260. Lammer EJ, Cordero JF, Koury MJ. Exogenous sex hormone exposure and the risk for VACTERL Association. *Teratology.* 1986;34:165–169.

261. Castori M, Rinaldi R, Capocaccia P, Roggini M, Grammatico P. VACTERL association and maternal diabetes: a possible causal relationship? *Birth Def Res (Part A): Clin Mol Teratol.* 2008;82:169–172.

262. Pozmanski AK, Gall JC Jr, Stern AM. Skeletal manifestations of the Holt-Oram syndrome. *Radiology.* 1970;94:45–53.

263. Esmer C, Sánchez S, Ramos S, Molina B, Frias S, Carnevale A. DEB test for Fanconi Anemia detection in patients with atypical phenotype. *Am J Med Genet.* 2004;124A:35–39.

264. Alter BP, Rosenberg PS, Brody LC. Clinical and molecular features associated with biallelic mutations in FANCD1/BRCA2. *J Med Genet.* 2007;44:1–9.

265. Kohlhase J, Schubert L, Liebers M, Rauch A, Becker K, Mohammed SN et al. Mutations at the SALL4 locus on

chromosome 20 result in a range of clinically overlapping phenotypes, including Okihiro syndrome, Holt-Oram syndrome, acro-renal-ocular syndrome, and patients previously reported to represent thalidomide embryopathy. *J Med Genet.* 2003; 40:473–478.

266. Klopocki E, Schulze H, Straus G, Oh C-E, Hall J, Trotier F et al. Complex inheritance pattern resembling autosomal recessive inheritance involving a microdeletion in thrombocytopenia – absent radius syndrome. *Am J Hum Gen.* 2007;80: 232–240.

267. Miller OF, Kolon TF. Prenatal diagnosis of VACTERL Association. *J Urology.* 2001;166:2389–2391.

Chapter 24

Twinning

INTRODUCTION

Mendelian   276410   (monozygotic twinning)
Inheritance
in Man:

%276400   (dizygotic twinning)

Twinning in pregnancy occurs in about 1 in 80 live-births (1). The prevalence rates vary significantly among racial and ethnic groups, from a high of 45-50/1,000 in Nigeria to 10–20/1,000 in the United States and Europe to 6/1,000 in Asia.

Monozygotic twins are, by definition, two individuals who were derived from one sperm and one egg. The separation of the monozygotic twins occurs early. Separation in the first three days after fertilization leads to separate amnion and chorion for each twin, the diamniotic dichorionic placenta. If separation occurs in the period of blastocyst formation, days 4 to 6 after fertilization, there is a monochorionic diamniotic placenta. The placenta with a single set of membranes, that is, monoamniotic monochorionic, occurs at 7 to 9 days after fertilization [1] (Figure 24-1).

The advent of prenatal screening by vaginal sonography early in pregnancy has introduced the term "the vanishing twin" and has raised the question as to whether many twin pregnancies do not survive (2).

Clinicians were taught, in the past, that identical twins share all of the same genes and genetic differences and would be expected to be genetically "identical." However, experience has shown otherwise. Geoffrey Machin (3) has noted that "most monozygotic twin pairs are not identical." He described several post-zygotic genetic events that can lead to striking within pair dissimilarity. Studies of epigenetic differences in adult monozygotic twins (4) and DNA copy-number-variation in phenotypically concordant and discordant monozygotic twins (5) have provided more detailed documentation of the potential bases for phenotypic differences between identical twins.

The increased frequency of congenital malformations was highlighted in 1979 by Drs. Albert Schinzel, David Smith, and James Miller (6) for three types of structural defects: 1) early malformation complexes, such as cloacal exstrophy and sirenomelia; 2) vascular disruptions,

TABLE 24-1 *Increased frequency of major malformations in twins in comparison to singletons.*

	Relative Risk
Central nervous system:	
encephalocele	2.21 (1.66–2.96)
Eye:	
anomalies of posterior segment	3.05 (1.49–6.23)
Heart:	
single ventricle	3.41 (1.84–6.33)
single anomalies of pulmonary artery	2.24 (1.67–3.00)
Respiratory system:	
agenesis/hypoplasia and dysplasia of lung	2.21 (1.52–3.21)
Digestive system:	
esophageal atresia, tracheo-esophageal fistula	2.56 (2.01–3.25)
atresia and stenosis of large intestine, rectum and anus	2.05 (1.71–2.45)
anomalies of intestine	2.36 (1.32–4.21)
Genital system:	
indeterminate sex	2.13 (1.54–2.93)
Urinary system:	
renal agenesis and dysgenesis	2.17 (1.66–2.85)
other, specified of ureter	2.06 (1.05–4.01)
atresia and stenosis of urethra and bladder neck	3.20 (1.82–5.63)
Musculo skeletal deformities:	
other and unspecified anomalies of limb	2.26 (1.56–3.26)
anomalies of spine	2.78 (2.06–3.75)
anomalies of abdominal wall	2.03 (1.69–2.43)

Legend: Shows from Table III (pages 120–121 in ref. 7) those malformations in excels in twins, with an adjusted relative risk greater than 2 (with 95 confidence interval) in comparison to singletons, using the Mantel Haenszel method.

caused by vascular interconnections within the shared placenta, such as aplasia cutis and hydranencephaly; 3) constraint deformations, due to crowding in utero, such as club foot deformity and dislocation of the hip. These observations have been extended to an analysis of 5,572 malformations among 260,865 twins identified in nine population-based malformations registries in Europe and Latin America (7). Several types of malformations were shown to be over twice as common among twins than among singletons (Table 24-1).

We present here these four examples of twin-associated major malformations:

acardia
conjoined twins
sirenomelia
twin-twin transfusion

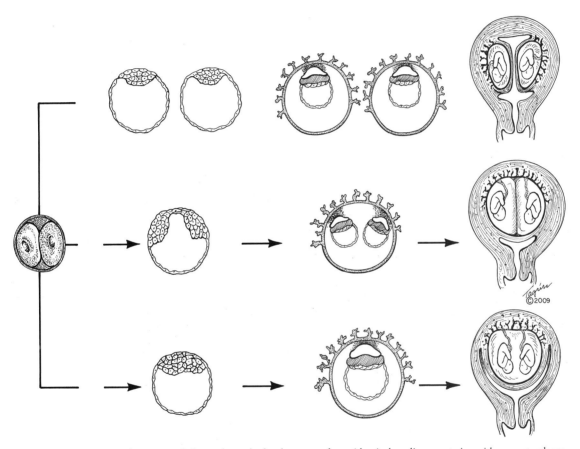

FIGURE 24.1 Twinning. The top panel shows the early development of non-identical or dizygous twins with separate placentas, chorion and amnion. The middle panel shows the development of diamniotic, but monochorionic, identical twins. The bottom panel shows the development of the rare monoamniotic, monochorionic type of identical twins.

ACARDIA

Definition

A severe developmental abnormality in one of a monozygous twin pair, who survives without essential heart function because of blood flow through artery-to-artery and vein-to-vein anastomoses in the monochorionic placenta. This abnormality occurs only in identical twins.

ICD-9:	759.700	(multiple congenital anomalies, not otherwise specified) (twinning, identical)
ICD-10:	Q89.7	(multiple congenital malformations, not elsewhere classified)
Mendelian Inheritance in Man:	276410	(twinning, monozygotic)

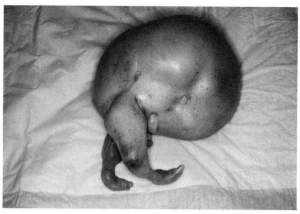

FIGURE 24.2   Shows an amorphous acardiac twin with partial development of two legs. (Courtesy of Frederick R. Bieber, Ph.D., Brigham and Women's Hospital, Boston, MA)

Appearance

There is a dramatic and varied extent of development of the acardiac twin. The potential anatomic findings have been subdivided into four groups:

1. acardius anceps: a partially developed head and brain tissue;
2. acardius acephalus: a trunk with recognizable lower limbs, a defective thorax, and arms and no head; this is the most common type (Figure 24-2);
3. acardius acormus: a head without a body
4. acardius amorphus: the most severe type in which the fetus is a ball of skin without head or limbs.

The findings in several case series (8–17) have shown that there is a varied disorganization of development. Essentially no two acardiac twins are alike.

The placentation is almost exclusively monochorionic: 24% monochorionic, monoamniotic; 74% monochorionic, diamniotic; 2% dichorionic, diamniotic (13). In a review of the blood vessels in the umbilical cord of 90 acardiac twins, 66% had one artery and one vein, 2% had 2 arteries and one vein and 8% had other variations (15).

Associated Malformations

Acardia is a malformed twin fetus. There are many and varied structural abnormalities, all of which are attributed to the primary abnormality. None would be considered an associated malformation.

For example, in a series of 26 acardiac fetuses (17), 6 (50%) of the 12 with facial structures had a cleft lip or cleft palate deformity. The oral cleft deformities were attributed to decreased blood flow and hypoxia.

Developmental Defect

Monozygous twins are derived from one oocyte and develop from one zygote. The twinning process begins usually at the end of the first week postfertilization. The embryoblast is divided into two embryonic primordia. Subsequently each of the two embryos has its own amniotic sac, develop within the same chorionic sac, and share a common placenta.

The acardiac twin does not have a functioning heart. Its survival during pregnancy depends on blood flow through vascular anastomoses (artery-to-artery; vein-to-vein) through the common placenta with the normal "pump" twin. The circulation in the acardiac twin is the reverse of normal, which is the basis for the descriptive term "twin reversed arterial perfusion" or TRAP Sequence (11, 14). The preferential blood flow is through the umbilical arteries to the iliac arteries of the acardiac fetus, perfusing the lower part of the body more than the upper part.

The primary developmental abnormality that leads to the TRAP Sequence has not been established. Several hypotheses have been developed:

1. the heart either fails to develop or its development stops ("arrests") during development (8);
2. degeneration of tissues after their initial formation (9, 18);

3. one tissue type is lost in preference to others (18);
4. an amniotic band compressing the heart (19);
5. the disrupted vascular supply leads to disruption of early events in development (14);
6. the single umbilical artery is common in monochorionic twinning; acardia is a random, coincidental event of the single umbilical artery and monochorionic parabiosis (20).

While the primary abnormality is not known, several observations have been made on the anatomic findings. The structural abnormalities in the acardiac fetus have been attributed primarily to its altered circulation. For example, the extent of heart development has been correlated with the fetal age when the reverse perfusion begins to occur. In one theoretical model (21) (Figure 24.3), it was noted that both the acardiac twin and the pump twin have reduced oxygen saturation. They postulated that the hypoxia leads to neovascularization that increases the capillary density in the acardiac twin and increases the demands on the heart of the pump twin. In an analysis of the central nervous system of the acardiac twin, it was noted that the encephaloclastic changes were caused by the hypoxia (22). In an analysis (16) of the pattern of development in 18 affected fetuses, it was noted that: 1) the number of altered organs decreased in a cranio-caudal direction; the development and weight of the head and thoracic organs are diminished in comparison to the abdominal organs; 2) the symmetry of the abnormalities in bilateral organs and long bones is consistent with a major alteration of the flow in the aorta; 3) the distal long bones are absent more often than the proximal bones, consistent with decreased perfusion in each limb.

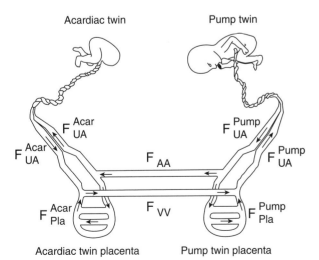

Acardiac twin   Pump twin

F_{UA}^{Acar} F_{UA}^{Pump}
F_{UA}^{Acar} F_{AA} F_{UA}^{Pump}
F_{Pla}^{Acar} F_{VV} F_{Pla}^{Pump}

Acardiac twin placenta   Pump twin placenta

FIGURE 24.3 Schematic flow of the circulation between the pump twin and the acardiac twin. (From De Groot R, Van Den Wijngaard JP, Umur A, Beek JF, Nikkels PG, Van Gemert MJ. Modeling acardiac twin pregnancies. Ann NY Acad Sci 2007; 1101;235–249. Redrawn with permission.).

About 10% of the normal pump twins have associated major abnormalities (11, 12), including anencephaly (23), gastroschisis (24), and amniotic band syndrome (19). These structural abnormalities have been attributed to vascular disruption in the structures that had formed normally (25).

Prevalence

Acardia occurs in about 1% of identical or monozygous twins (11). It is more common in triplets: 1 in 30 (3.3%) [26].

In 109,000 consecutive births in Tunis (1993–2001), the prevalence rate of acardia was 1:18,000 (17). From an early literature review (8), the prevalence rate was estimated to be 1:35,000. In Melbourne (1960–1991) the frequency was 1:39,000 ± 9,000 (15).

Ethnicity/Race

Differences in the prevalence rate of acardia among ethnic/racial groups have not been established.

Birth Status

The perinatal mortality for the acardiac twin is 100%, while the mortality rate for the pump twin has been 30 to 35% (15). Common complications of pregnancy in case series were preterm labor in 79%, polyhydramnios in 51%, congestive heart failure in 28% of the pump twins, and intrauterine fetal demise in 25% of the pump twins.

The weight of the acardiac twin varies significantly, reflecting in part the gestational age at delivery. The occurrence of adverse outcomes, such as premature delivery, polyhydramnios, and congestive heart failure in the pump twin, correlate with the larger (>50%) weight ratio between the acardiac twin and the pump twin (21). In a review of 49 acardiac twin pregnancies (12), the mean gestational age was 29 ± 7.3 weeks; the birth weight of the acardiac twin was 651 ± 571 grams, and the normal twin was 1378 ± 1047 grams. Among those heavier acardiac twins, the sensitivity for detecting hydramnios and preterm delivery was over 80%.

Sex Ratio

Among 184 documented cases of acardia in one series in Australia (1960 to 1991), there were more males than females: 54:46 (15), a difference that was not significant in comparison to the general population in that area.

Paterental Age

No studies of maternal or paternal age have been reported.

Twinning

Acardia is a phenomenon that occurs almost always in monochorionic twin or triplet pregnancies. A few instances of conjoined twins, one with acardia, have been described. There have been rare reports of diamniotic, dichorionic placentas (25, 27).

Genetic Factors

There have been no reports of acardia occurring in the pregnancies of close relatives.

Several types of chromosome abnormalities have been identified in the acardiac fetuses including trisomies, deletions, and mosaicism (28). The overall frequency was 9% in one series (15). No specific chromosome abnormality has been more common. Subtle abnormalities have been reported, such as a skewed pattern of X-inactivation (29) and fertilization of a polar body (30). There have been rare reports (31) of aneuploidy in both the acardiac twin and the normal twin, such as 47,XXY in the pump twin and 94,XXXXYY in the acardic fetus.

Environmental Factors

No exposures in pregnancy have been shown to cause acardia.

Treatment of Prognosis

Experience has shown that the fetus with acardia can be identified by prenatal ultrasound at 10 to 12 weeks of gestation (32). Because of the high risk of death by the normal or "pump" twin, there is urgency in treating the affected co-twin (33–36). The treatments that have been used include:

1. ligation of the umbilical cord of the acardiac twin (37);
2. hysterotomy to remove the acardiac twin (38);
3. removal of amniotic fluid to reduce temporarily the amount of amniotic fluid;
4. laser treatment.

The "pump" twin may develop high-output congestive heart failure, which can be treated with digoxin via his mother (35, 36).

Genetic Counseling

The counseling focuses on the prognosis for the pump twin and options in treatment. There are some families with a high frequency of monozygous twins. Theoretically such a family could have a second affected pregnancy, although that has not been reported.

CONJOINED TWINS

Definition

Two separate fetuses with separate heads and vertebral columns that are joined together at one anatomic site.

ICD-9:	759.4	(conjoined twins)
	759.410	(craniopagus twins; joined at head)
	759.420	(thoracopagus; twins joined at thorax)
	759.430	(xiphopagus; twins joined at xiphoid and ischiopagus; twins joined at pelvis)
	759.440	(pygopagus; twins joined at buttocks)
	759.480	(other specified conjoined twins)
	759.490	(unspecified conjoined twins)
ICD-10:	Q89.4	(conjoined twins; includes craniophagus, dicephaly, pygopagus, thoracopagus, and "double monster")
Mendelian Inheritance in Man:	None	

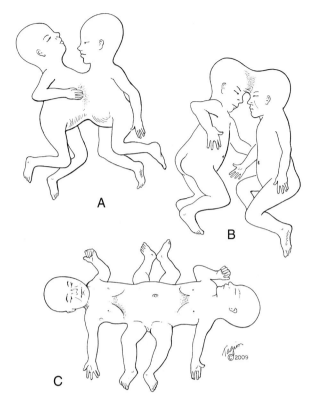

FIGURE 24.4 Drawings of three types of conjoining: (A) thoracoomphalopagus; (B) craniopagus; (C) ischiopagus

Historical Note

Conjoined twins have been described over many centuries and have been the subject of much speculation (39–46). For example, statues of parapagus twins and thorapagus twins, dating from the years before Christ, are housed in museums in Turkey (46, 47). The first successful separation of conjoined twins was in 1689, when the isthmus between a pair of omphalogus twins was ligated in Basel, Switzerland.

Two conflicting theories of the cause of conjoining have been proposed: 1) they represent abnormal early fusion of two separate monovular embryonic discs, or 2) conjoining reflects a failure of the complete separation of two embryonic discs at about days 15–17 postfertilization.

Appearance

The classification of the conjoining is based on the most prominent site of fusion. The term "pagus" is the Greek work for "fixed." Thus, thoracopagus, omphalopagus, prypagus, ischiopagus, and craniopagus are the terms for fusion at, respectively, the thorax, umbilicus, perineum, pelvis, and head (39–41) [Figures 24-4 and 24-5, 24-6].

The most prominent sites of the union, according to Spencer (42), are:

Ventral union (87%)
    Rostral: thoracopagus (19%) [joined heart]
              omphalopagus (18%)
              cephalopagus (11%) [top of head]
    Caudal: ischiopagus (11%) [lower abdominal genito-urinary system]
    Lateral: parapagus (28%) [pelvis and variable trunk]
Dorsal union (13%)
    craniopagus (5%) [cranial vault]
    rachipagus (2%) [vertebral column]
    pygopagus (6%) [sacrum]
    total: 100%

Associated Malformations

Conjoined twins can be discordant for the presence of abnormalities in organs that are not shared (48). For example, in the series of 24 sets of conjoined twins treated at the Great Ormond Street Hospital, 1985–2004, 11 (45.8%) had additional anomalies, excluding heart defects. The anomalies include imperforate anus, omphalocele, bowel atresia, bladder extrophy, cloacal anomaly and renal agenesis, (42) and cleft lip (Figure 24-6).

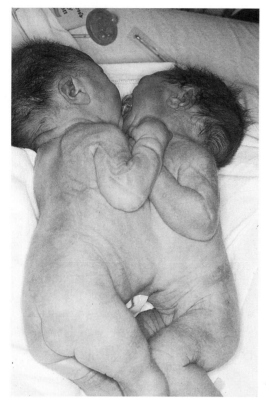

FIGURE 24.5   Twins joined in the thorax and abdomen: thoracopagus twins.

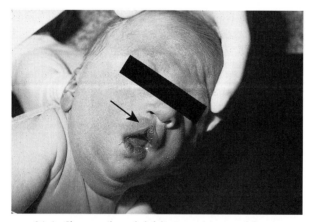

FIGURE 24.6   Shows unilateral cleft lip (arrow) in one of thoracopagus conjoined twins.

The infant with minimally conjoined omphalopgus type of attachment may have a distinctive pattern of associated anomalies (49). Typically, there is an omphalocele (Figure 24-7), imperforate anus with cloacal anomalies, urachal anomalies, and intestinal connection between the co-twins. The vascular supply of the intestinal bridge may include the persistence of a vitelline artery.

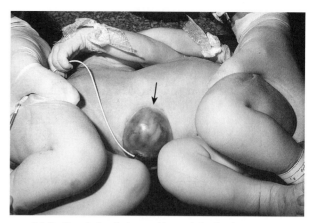

FIGURE 24.7   Omphalocele (arrow) in conjoined twins.

Developmental Defect

Conjoined twins develop from a single fertilized ovum.

Two theories, "fission" and "fusion," have been developed to explain the occurrence of conjoining. In the "fission theory," there is a failure of complete separation of the embryonic disc at about the 15th to the 17th day of gestation. Spencer (39, 47, 48) and others (50, 51) have postulated the "fusion theory" in which fusion occurs between two originally separate monovular embryonic discs.

According to Spencer's model (39, 42, 43), conjoined twins arise when more than one primitive streak (organizing center) is formed in a single embryonic disc during gestation. The orientation and the proximity of the streaks to one another determine the type of conjoining that occurs. For example, head-to-head arrangements of the two primitive streaks produce cephalopagus twins. When the two primitive streaks are parallel and have similar polarity, omphalopagus twins are produced.

The omphalopagus type of conjoined twins has been associated occasionally with diamniotic placentation (52). It has been postulated that the two parallel streaks are produced in the process of folding two amniotic cavities. It seems very unlikely that this could occur in any other type of conjoining.

In the conjoining process, the organs that are normally asymmetrical, such as heart, great vessels, lungs, liver, spleen, and gastrointestinal tract, are usually made more symmetrical. The symmetrical structures, such as the brain, urinary tract, and skeleton are less severely affected (53).

Using twin chick embryos as an experimental model, Levin and his associates (54) suggested that the interrelationship of the genes activin, Sonic hedgehog (Shh), and nodal (f) in determining the orientation of the heart was interrupted by the presence of two parallel primitive streaks. As a result, the lack of expression of nodal leads to randomness of the situs of the heart in the embryo on the left. To test their hypothesis they analyzed the patterns in 69 sets of thoracopagus twins, and found that almost half (33 of 69) had a reversal of heart situs, i.e., situs inversus. However, this reversal was not observed in any of the 98 sets of conjoined twins that had been joined at the head (craniopagus) or pelvis (ischiopagus).

Prevalence

Estimates of the prevalence rate in population-based surveillance programs have shown that conjoined twins are rare. For example, in a survey of 5 counties in greater Atlanta in the years 1965 to 1972, before the use of ART (assisted reproductive technology), there were 7 conjoined twins for a prevalence rate of 1:70,084 total births (55). Similarly, the survey of 7,903,000 births in the period 1970–1977 in the United States showed that the prevalence rate of conjoined twins was between 1 in 30,000 and 1 in 100,000 (56). Thoracopagus and omphalopagus conjoined twins accounted for 56% of all conjoined twins.

In Boston, the Active Malformations Surveillance Program at the Boston Lying-In Hospital (and later, Brigham and Women's Hospital) among 206,244 live births, still births, and elective terminations for fetal anomalies (1972–1974, 1979–2000), identified 29 conjoined twins. However, only two sets were born to women who had always planned to deliver at that hospital for a prevalence rate of 1:103,122. The mothers of the other 27 sets of conjoined twins were transferred for care after the prenatal diagnosis at another facility.

The widespread use of assisted reproductive technologies worldwide has produced an increasing number of multiple gestation pregnancies. It has not been determined whether or not this increase will be associated with an increased rate of occurrence of conjoined twins.

Birth Status

In the survey of 7,903,000 births (1970–1977) (56), there were 81 sets of conjoined twins: 39.5% were stillborn and another 38.3% died between birth and 30 days of life, most on the first day of life.

Sex Ratio

Most surveys have shown an excess of affected females, such as M:F 1:3 (44).

Race/Ethnicity

There is limited information on the occurrence of conjoined twinning in different racial and ethnic groups. No significant differences have been identified consistently (56).

Parental Age

No significant differences in the maternal or paternal ages have been identified. Among the 81 sets of conjoined twins identified among 7,903,000 births in the United States (1970–1977), the age distributions of the mothers were similar to those in the general population (56).

Genetics

While the twinning process can be familial, a genetic basis for the conjoining process has not been established.

Environmental Factors

No environmental factors have been identified that cause twinning, in general, or conjoined twins, in particular, in humans. The role of assisted reproductive technologies remains to be established.

Treatment and Prognosis

The first phase of management is the evaluation after detection in utero. Increasingly, the diagnosis is being made earlier in pregnancy as more imaging is carried out in routine screening.

Before 10 weeks of gestations false positive diagnoses are a concern (57). Once the diagnosis has been established, imaging studies are essential to characterize the site of fusion and the extent of associated anomalies. The parents are to be counseled about options in treatment.

Termination has been a common choice, if the conjoined twins were diagnosed before 24 weeks gestation in the United States.

If the decision is made to continue the pregnancy, the delivery is by caesarean section at 36 to 38 weeks gestation (44, 59, 60).

If there is complex heart fusion or another severe deformity, surgery is not recommended (53).

If one twin is dead or dying and is threatening the survival of the co-twin, emergency separation has been attempted to treat correctable anomalies, such as omphalocele, bowel atresia, or imperforate anus.

If the conjoined twins can be stabilized and the fusion can be corrected, an elective separation has been carried out typically at two to four months of age. Very careful planning is essential to the success of the surgery and the postoperative care.

Genetic Counseling

The first sign of conjoined twins may be increased nuchal translucency at 11 to 13 weeks of gestation in a conjoined twin pregnancy (57). The presence of conjoining has been recognized at 12 weeks gestation and even earlier.

With imaging early in pregnancy a common practice in routine prenatal care, this is the typical setting for counseling about the process of conjoining. Sonologists have established the distinctive features seen by ultrasound: two inseparable bodies; both fetal heads are consistently at the same level; the position of the fetuses does not change over time (61).

The focus in the second trimester of pregnancy will be on the type of conjoining, the possibility of surgical repair and the prospects for survival (59, 60).

After the pregnancy, there may be discussion of the risk of recurrence. No increased risk for a second effected pregnancy has been established.

SIRENOMELIA

Definition

Sirenomelia is a lethal malformation syndrome in which the lower legs are fused and rotated with the fibula on the medial side; there is absence of the anus, genital structures, and sacrum, no true pelvic cavity, and renal agenesis. It has been referred to as the "mermaid syndrome."

ICD-9:   759.840   (congenital malformation syndromes involving limbs; includes sirenomelia)

ICD-10:   Q87.2   (congenital malformations syndromes predominantly involving limbs; includes sirenomelia)

Mendelian   %191830   (urogenital adysplasia, hereditary)
Inheritance
in Man:

Historical Note

Sirenomelia was first characterized in Homer's *Odyssey* with the depictions of Mermaids (62). In Greek mythology, a siren had the upper torso of a woman and the lower legs of a fish. She lured mariners to their destruction by singing seductive melodies (63). St. Hilaire's report was in 1836 (64).

Otto Kampmeier in 1927 (65) noted the historic early descriptions of sirenomelia beginning in 1542. He described the occurrence of one "umbilical" artery as having "outstanding significance." He noted the lack of the normal umbilical arteries and the thin aorta below the point of origin of the single large umbilical artery (Figure 24-9).

He suggested that "the faulty development of the caudal half of the body might be the effect of nutritional want." This hypothesis was pursued subsequently by Stevenson and his colleagues (66) in their presentation of the concept of "vascular steal," as the primary mechanism of the poor development of the caudal structures in fetuses with sirenomelia.

Some affected infants, at the milder end of the spectrum of the phenotype, have separate legs with terminal transverse deficiencies (67) [Figure 24-10].

The term sirenomelia has been considered the more severe form of caudal regression syndrome, a malformation first described by Duhamel in 1961 (68). Recent studies (69) of five infants with caudal regression showed that they also had an aberrant abdominal umbilical artery, similar to that seen in sirenomelia. The authors suggested that sirenomelia and caudal regression have a common pathogenetic basis.

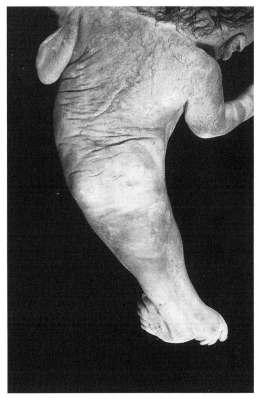

FIGURE 24.8   Posterior view of fused legs with separate toes on each foot in an infant with sirenomelia.

Another major development in the understanding of the occurrence of sirenomelia was the observation of an increased frequency of monozygous twinning among the affected infants (70). The mechanism by which the process of twinning can "cause" sirenomelia remains an intriguing mystery.

Appearance

The fused legs are the predominant feature of sirenomelia (Figures 24-8 and 24-11).

The spectrum of these features has been extended from the earlier classification of three types (64, 65) to seven (71) (Table 24-2):

TABLE 24-2 *Types of leg fusion in infants with sirenomelia*

Type	Characteristics
I	All bones in the upper and lower leg are present.
II	Single fibula
III	Absent fibula
IV	Femurs fused partially; fibulas are fused
V	Femurs fused partially
VI	Single femur and single tibia
VII	Single femur, absent tibia

From Stocker JT et al; ref. 71.

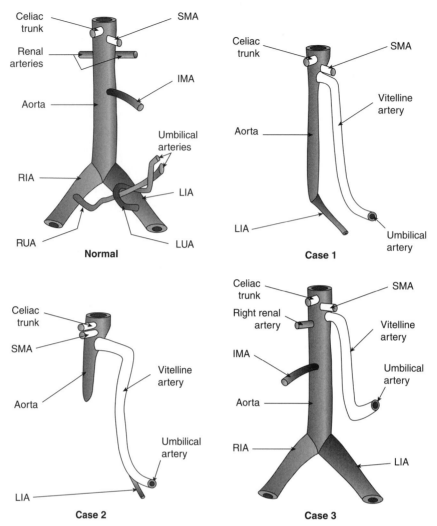

FIGURE 24.9 Vascular patterns in three fetuses with sirenomelia in comparison to normal. (IMA, inferior mesenteric artery; LIA, left iliac artery; LUA, left umbilical artery; RIA, right iliac artery; RUA, right umbilical artery; SMA, superior mesenteric artery). (From Patel S, Suchet I: *Ultrasound Obstet Gynecology.* 2004;24:690; Figure 4. Used with permission.)

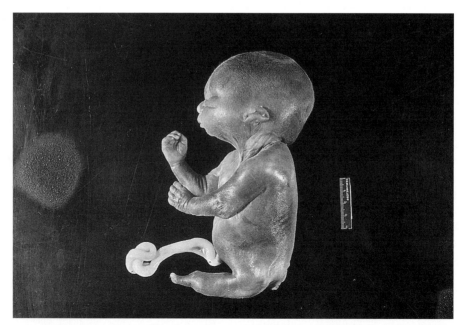

FIGURE 24.10 Fetus with fused legs that end in terminal deficiency. (Courtesy of Fedrick R. Bieber, PhD, Brigham and Women's Hospital, Boston, MA.)

The external appearance of the soft tissues, such as the Potter facies, lung hypoplasia, and amnion nodosum, reflect the effects of oligohydramnios, caused by the absence of both kidneys. In identical twin pregnancies, the healthy co-twin maintains a normal amount of amniotic fluid and, thereby, prevents the fetus with sirenomelia from having these signs of oligohydramnios (72).

The most common anatomic findings are: a large, single umbilical artery that originates from an aberrant major abdominal artery (Figure 24-10), absence of both kidneys, a blind-ending colon with atresia of the rectum, absence of external genital structures, uterus, vagina, prostate and anus, and agenesis or dysplasia of the sacrum (63, 71, 73–75). There is variation in the extent of these anatomic findings, such as the presence of a small poorly functioning kidney instead of renal agenesis.

It has been proposed that the severity of the malformations of the pelvis correlates with the severity of the defects in the legs. Measurements in affected fetuses have shown that the longer the distance between the ilia and the cranial edge of the first sacral vertebral body, the more severe the abnormalities of the legs (76).

Arteriography of the abdominal vasculature of 11 fetuses with sirenomelia showed the presence of a single large artery that arose from high in the abdominal cavity and assumed the function of the umbilical arteries (66) [Figure 24-9]. It was postulated that this artery was derived from the vitelline artery complex, an early embryonic vascular network that supplies the yolk sac.

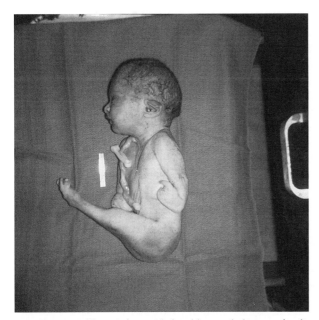

FIGURE 24.11   Stillborn infant with fused legs and absence of radius in each arm.

Associated Malformations

Many additional malformations have occurred in fetuses with sirenomelia (71), including anencephaly (71, 77), anencephaly with rachischisis (78), spina bifida, esophageal atresia, holoprosencephaly (79), omphalocele (80), and absence of the radius (Figure 24-10) and thumb (71, 78, 81).

In a series of 11 fetuses with sirenomelia, one had spina bifida, three had anomalies of the radius or thumb, and one had persistence of the cloaca and hypoplastic left heart deformity (66).

In a series of 80 affected infants, 25% had heart defects (71).

Among the 97 infants with sirenomelia identified in malformation monitoring systems (78), the most common associated malformations were neural tube defects (7.2%), esophageal atresia (8.2%), malrotation of intestine (4.1%), and deficiency of radius (6.2%).

Developmental Defect

The primary defect is not known. Several theories have been suggested:

1. a defect in or injury to the caudal mesoderm between 28 and 32 days of fetal development produces defective midline structures and destruction of cloacal and urogenital derivatives (70);
2. a teratogenic event in the third gestational week interferes with the formation of the notochord, which results in abnormal development of caudal structures (82);
3. the presence of the large intra-abdominal artery and the atretic or absent distal aorta leads to a diversion of blood flow ("vascular steal") from caudal structures of the embryo to the placenta and produces poor perfusion to the lower structures; this loss of blood flow leads to severe maldevelopment of the caudal portion of the embryo (66) (Figure 24-9);
4. the process of monozygotic twinning can cause sirenomelia by interfering with the determination or differentiation of caudal embryonic structures (70, 83).
5. the developmental arrest of the primitive streak initiates formation of a second primitive streak, giving rise to a second normal embryo; this would account for the high frequency of twinning with sirenomelia.

There are animal models of sirenomelia. The srn mutation in the mouse produces sireniform abnormalities in the srn/srn homozygotes (84). The single large umbilical artery appears to have been formed from fusion of the paired primitive umbilical arteries.

Mouse knockouts that are Tsg/Bmp7 compound mutants have sirenomelia (85). (Tsg is twisted gastrulation and bmp7 is bone morphogenetic protein 7.)

Prevalence

Fetuses with sirenomelia have appeared to be more common among spontaneous abortions than in full-term infants (86, 87).

There were 5 infants (1:84,356) with sirenomelia among the 421,781 consecutive births (1:84,356) in the World Health Organization (WHO) survey in 1966 (88).

In eight malformation monitoring systems, primarily in the 1970s and 1980s and including 10,097,383 births, the prevalence of sirenomelia was 1.03/100,000 births or 1:97,087 (78).

Three infants (1:68,741) with sirenomelia have been identified at Brigham and Women's Hospital in Boston among 206,244 livebirths, stillbirths, and elective terminations for fetal anomalies.

Race/Ethnicity

No significant differences among racial/ethnic groups have been identified.

Birth Status

Sirenomelia has been considered a lethal malformation, although occasional survivors have been reported (89–91). More than half of the 80 cases in one review (71) were stillborn, and the remainder died soon after birth. Among 97 infants with sirenomelia identified in eight different malformation monitoring systems, 35 (36%) were stillborn and the 62 liveborn infants died soon after birth. Among 25 infants born at term in one center (71), only 2 (87%) had a birth weight of 2,500 grams or more.

Sex Ratio

Several case series have shown many more affected males than females.

In a review of 80 cases (71), sex could be determined in 62: 37 (60%) had testes and 25 (40%) had ovaries; the sex ratio was: M:F = 1.48. Among the 97 infants in malformation surveillance programs, 17 females and 15 males were identified, but for most of the infants the sex was not determined (78).

Parental Age

In the eight malformation surveys in the 1970s and 1980s, there were small deviations from the expected maternal age distribution with an increased rate among young women (<23) and older women (>40).

Twinning

A significant increase in the frequency of twinning has been observed in all reports. The overall frequency of twinning in several case series were: 7% (70), 16% (71), and 3% (78) in comparison to the expected rate of about 1%.

The twins were usually monozygous and only one twin had sirenomelia. There have been rare reports of malformations in the co-twin without sirenomelia, such as imperforate anus (92). In the case series of 80 infants with sirenomelia, one set of female twins was concordant for sirenomelia (71). In three of the 13 twin pregnancies, one twin had sirenomelia and the co-twin was an acardiac twin.

Two (40%) of the 5 infants with sirenomelia identified among 421,781 pregnancies at 24 centers were twins, both presumed to be monozygotic (88). In that analysis sirenomelia was 150 times more frequent in one of identical twins than in singletons.

Genetic Factors

Associated chromosome abnormalities have not been reported. No molecular basis for this severe malformation syndrome has been established. The findings from new diagnostic techniques, such as aCGH, have not been reported.

In general, the parents with one infant with sirenomelia have not had a second affected infant. However, families have been reported (93, 94) in which siblings had either sirenomelia or severe renal anomalies. No molecular diagnostic studies were carried out. However, these reports suggest that the recurrence risk, while low, is not 0%.

Environmental Factors

Infants of diabetic mothers have a significant risk of having a fetus with sirenomelia (95–99). Passarge and Lenz (97) estimated that the syndrome of caudal regression, including sirenomelia, occurred in about 1% of infants of insulin-dependent diabetic mothers.

Kucera (98) reviewed the specific malformations in 340 affected fetuses among 7,101 fetuses born to women with diabetes mellitus. He estimated that the caudal regression syndrome occurred 211.7 times more frequently among the offspring of diabetics than in the infants of non-diabetic mothers. Mills and his associates (99) reviewed the findings of Kucera and estimated the risk ratio to be 252 for caudal regression among infants of diabetic mothers.

Case reports (100) have suggested that exposure to cocaine might have produced vascular disruption, which led to the occurrence of sirenomelia. However intriguing, no causal relationship to exposure to vasoactive substances, like cocaine, has been established in systematic studies.

A cluster of four infants with sirenomelia and another four with cyclopia was identified over a 165 day period in Cali, Colombia, in 2004–2005 (101). No potentially causative exposure was identified.

Treatment and Prognosis

Variation in the phenotype is expected for each malformation syndrome. As a result, a few infants with sirenomelia have not had bilateral renal agenesis and have survived (89–91). Their cognitive development has not been established.

Genetic Counseling

In general, sirenomelia has not been considered an hereditary disorder. Associated chromosome abnormalities have not been identified. However, two exceptional families have been reported (93, 94). Rudd and Klimer (93) described a family in which two female sibs had sirenomelia. A third healthy sister had a single umbilical artery with an eccentric placental insertion. A brother and the father's half sister had an imperforate anus. These findings were attributed to an autosomal dominant gene with reduced penetrance.

In the family reported by Selig et al. (94), healthy parents with normal kidneys by ultrasound screening had four children with renal anomalies: bilateral renal agenesis (1 female infant), bilateral hydronephrosis attributed to posterior urethral valves (1 male infant), type IV cystic kidney disease (1 male infant), and sirenomelia (1 male infant). Unfortunately neither of these families with multiple affected children had diagnostic molecular studies, such as chromosome microarrays.

If caudal regression is considered part of the spectrum, this abnormality has occurred in siblings born to healthy parents.

Källén et al (79) reported empiric risk data from the findings in the families of 98 infants with sirenomelia identified in the 1970s and 1980s in eight malformation surveys. Among 41 sibs born before the index case with sirenomelia, none had sirenomelia, but one sib had a persistent cloaca. None of the 10 sibs born after the proband with sirenomelia had a major malformation.

Another relevant observation was the fact that the parents of an infant with bilateral renal agenesis or renal dysgenesis did not have an increased risk for having a subsequent infant with sirenomelia (102).

The prenatal detection of sirenomelia has been described in several reports (75, 103–105), some as early as 14 and 16 weeks of gestation (104). The accuracy of this diagnosis by ultrasound is made difficult by the associated oligohydramnios. The major distinction is between bilateral renal agenesis (BRA) and BRA as part of the sirenomelia phenotype. Two common iliac arteries are always present in fetuses with renal agenesis; absence of the distal branching of the main abdominal vessel is characteristic of sirenomelia (105). Color contrast has been very helpful in identifying the distinctive single abnormal umbilical artery, which occurs in most fetuses with sirenomelia (75, 103) [Figure 24-9].

TWIN-TWIN TRANSFUSION

Definition

An excessive amount of blood flow through the vascular anastomoses of the shared placenta. This produces anemia in one twin (donor) and polycythemia in the co-twin (recipient).

ICD-9:	762.3	(placental transfusion syndromes)
ICD-10:	Q43.0	(placental transfusion syndromes, includes twin-to-twin transfusion)
Mendelian Inheritance in Man:	276410	(twinning, monozygotic)

Historical Note

It has long been recognized that there are more congenital malformations in monozygous twins than in either dizygous twins or singletons (106, 107). One reason is that monochorionic, monoamniotic twins almost always share a placenta and are at risk for the problems produced by the vascular interconnections of the shared placenta. About 20% of twin pregnancies are monochorionic and 10% of all monozygous twins with monochorionic placentas have twin-twin transfusion syndrome [TTTS] (107).

Clinical follow-up showed that TTTS was associated with significant perinatal mortality. The death in utero of one twin was shown by the mechanisms of embolization and ischemia to produce a distinctive group of defects, such as bowel atresia, brain damage, and aplasia cutis (108, 109). Among the survivors, many significant medical problems, such as cardiomyopathy and renal failure, occurred (110).

The advent of prenatal screening by ultrasound in the second trimester of pregnancy led to a dramatic increase in the identification of affected pregnancies. Criteria for diagnosis were developed (111, 112). Innovative therapies, such as endoscopic laser treatment to occlude some of the vascular anastomoses, began to be tried (113).

We present here complications of the twin-twin transfusion syndrome that can produce structural abnormalities in a fetus.

Appearance

Based on many case series (114, 115) and case reports (116–126), criteria have been developed for making the

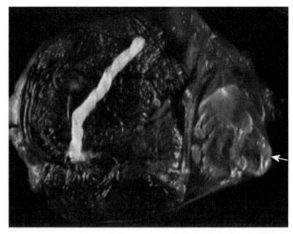

FIGURE 24.12   Placenta of identical twins that shows the normal size left half with white umbilical cord and smaller right half with smaller, darker umbilical cord (arrow) . (Courtesy of John M. Graham Jr., M.D., Sc.D., Cedars-Sinai Medical Center, Los Angeles, CA.).

diagnosis of twin-twin transfusion syndrome (TTTS) [111, 112]:

1. significant disparity in size of fetuses of the same sex;
2. disparity of size between the two amniotic sacs;
3. two separate umbilical cords with disparity in size or in the number of vessels; (Figure 24-12).
4. a single placenta with areas of disparity in echogenicity of the cotyledons supplying the two umbilical cords;
5. hydrops in either fetus or congestive heart failure in the recipient twin.

If a co-twin dies in the second trimester in a monochorionic monoamniotic pregnancy, there can be serious consequences in the surviving twin from the fetal demise. The potential effects include:

1. brain cyst and hydranencephaly (116);
2. multicystic encephalomalacia (117, 118);
3. microcephaly (119);
4. bowel atresia, including multiple atresias (120, 121);
5. gangrenous limb, hand or foot (122–125) [Figures 24-13 and 24-14];
6. terminal transverse limb defect (126);
7. constriction rings in digits and limbs and reduced digits, consistent with the features of the amniotic band syndrome (127, 128); (Figure 24-15)
8. skin defects (Figure 24-16).

There is limited information on the frequency of these fetal effects. For example, in a series of 112 instances of twin-twin transfusion, 3 (2.6%) of the infants had severe ischemia of the lower limbs (114).

In a series of 346 twins, 78% (182 recipients and 164 donors) were born alive (115). Two infants (one recipient and one donor) had amputation of one foot. Two males (both donors) had hypospadias.

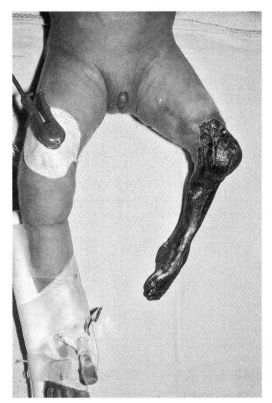

FIGURE 24.13 Embolization: shows gangrene of left leg of newborn whose identical twin had died at 26 weeks of gestation. (Courtesy of W. Hardy Hendren, MD, Childrens Hospital, Boston, MA.)

The associated limb defects have occurred primarily in the legs. They include necrosis in the recipient twin with a surviving donor, as well as an apparent embolization after fetal demise (Figures 24-12, 24-13). Some fetuses with limb defects have been exposed to treatments with amnio drainage (129), others to laser treatment of placental anastomoses and a third group, to no treatment during pregnancy (129).

Developmental Defects

The primary problem is the excessive blood flow through unidirectional AV connections for which the recipient twin cannot compensate. As a result, there is a decompensation of heart function, hydrops, and poly-hydramnios in the recipient twin and oligohydramnios in the donor twin. These physiologic changes have been shown to be associated with an increased level of vaso-active mediators in both the donor and the recipient twins (131). Studies have shown that the renin-angiotensin system (RAS) was unregulated in the kidneys of the recipient. Plasma levels of renin and angiotensin II were elevated in both twins. The source of the RAS components was postulated to be the kidney of the donor and the placenta of the recipient.

Several hypotheses have been developed to explain the fetal effects of the twin-twin transfusion syndrome (TTTS) [132–134].

1. Embolism theory: After the death in utero of the co-twin in the second trimester of pregnancy, necrotic tissue from the dead twin, presumably a thrombo-plastin-like material, passes through the vascular

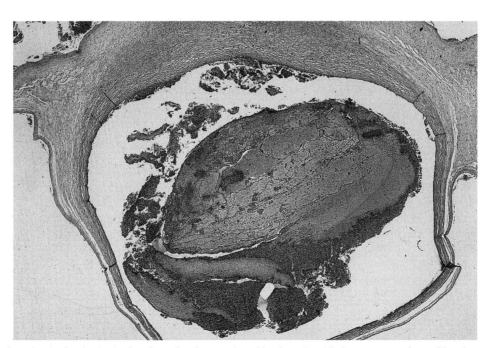

FIGURE 24.14 A thrombus in the chorionic plate from the placenta shared by the twin with the gangrenous leg and her deceased twin.

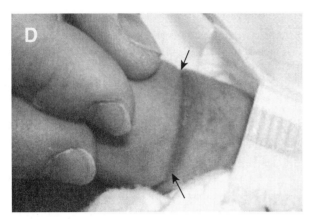

FIGURE 24.15   Amniotic band limb deformity with constriction rings (Reproduced with permission from Winer N et al *Am J Obstet Gynecol.* 2008;198:393e1-e5.)

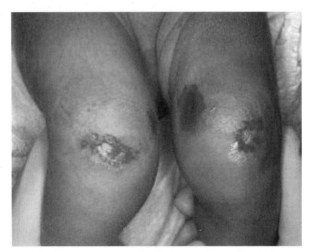

FIGURE 24.16   Shows skin defects over the knees of a liveborn infant whose identical twin died in utero. (Courtesy of John M. Graham Jr., M.D., Sc.D., Cedars-Sinai Medical Center, Los Angeles, CA)

connection in the placenta into the survivor's circulation. The emboli into the mesenteric artery cause bowel atresia. The emboli into the renal arteries causes renal agenesis. The emboli into the peripheral vessels in the skin produce skin defects (Figure 24-16).

2. Ischemia theory: The blood is shunted through the anastomoses in the placenta into the low resistance vascular system of the dead fetus. This shunting produces acute hypovolemia, ischemia, and injury to the end organs.

3. Placentation theory: There is a much higher frequency of velamentous insertion of the umbilical cord in the placenta of the pregnancies with TTTS. The mechanism by which this leads to fetal damage for TTTS has not been determined.

Prevalence

In general, it has been estimated that TTTS occurs in 10 to 15% of all monozygotic twin pregnancies (107).

Specific prevalence data was established in a population-based survey of perinatal centers in Western Australia and in New Zealand (1995–1998). Among 175,152 pregnancies (1992–1999) with deliveries after 20 weeks of gestation, 2,433 twin pairs were born in Western Australia among which 1 in 58 of the twin pairs had twin-twin transfusion syndrome (114).

Birth Status

Over 90% of the sets of twins with twin-twin transfusion syndrome are born prematurely. These twins have many of the complications of prematurity. In a case series (114) of 112 sets of twins with TTTS, those frequencies were: 10.8% had periventricular leukomalacia, 33% had necrotizing enterocolits, and 7.8% had patent ductus arteriosus.

Parental Age

No correlations of the occurrence of TTTS with the age of the mother or father have been established.

Sex Ratio

In the case series of 112 twin pairs with TTTS, there were 64 male (57.1%) and 48 female (42.9%) fetuses (114).

Treatment and Prognosis

Without treatment, only 21% of TTTS pregnancies diagnosed before 28 weeks gestational age survived, in a survey of 27 pregnancies in Houston (1985–1989) [135]. Among the survivors of TTTS serious medical complications are common: neonatal renal failure in 7%, necrotizing enterocolitis in 3.3%, patent ductus arteriosus in 7.8%, and hypertrophic cardiomyopathy in 3.3% in one follow-up study (114).

Several factors correlate with the abnormal outcomes of pregnancy with TTTS:

• Gestational age at delivery;
• Absence of end-diastolic forward flow in the umbilical artery;
• The presence of hydrops in the fetus.

Cerebral palsy and IQ deficits are a serious complication of TTTS (108, 132–134, 136). Immediate effects from the death of the co-twin is one potential cause. This mechanism was suggested in one dramatic case report (117), which described a surviving co-twin who was delivered by cesarean section 30 minutes after the death of the co-twin at the 30th week of gestation. The surviving twin developed disseminated intravascular coagulation and multicystic encephalomalacia. Another postulated cause is the "vanishing twin," whereby the apparent singleton infant has been affected by early demise of a co-twin (136).

One of the first treatments was the removal of amniotic fluid several times during pregnancy. A more recent treatment has been to use endoscopic laser treatment to obliterate the anastomoses between the twins (133, 131). The goal is to create from a monochorionic placenta a dichorionic placenta. The effectiveness of amnio reduction in comparison to laser treatment were compared in the Eurofetus trial (137). While there was initial support for the benefits of laser therapy, experienced maternal-fetal medicine specialists have urged continued, careful analysis before considering the issue settled (133). To guide treatment programs a staging system was developed by Quintero et al. (138). A separate cardiovascular score with different criteria for the severity of the complications of twin-twin transfusion was developed by the staff at the Children's Hospital of Philadelphia (139).

Genetic Counseling

Twinning is a familial condition. Many families with several sets of monozygous twins have been observed. Theoretically families with one set of MZ twins with TTTS have an increased risk for having another set of MZ twins and with TTTS. However, the empiric risk of this occurrence has not been established.

REFERENCES

1. Hall JG. Twinning. *Lancet.* 2003;362:735–743.
2. Landy HJ, Keith LG. The vanishing twin: a review. *Hum Reprod Update.* 1998;4:177–183.
3. Machin GA. Some causes of genotypic and phenotypic discordance in monozygotic twin pairs. *Am J Med Genet.* 1996;61: 216–228.
4. Fraga MF, Ballestar E, Paz MF, Ropero S, Setien F, Ballestar ML et al. Epigenetic differences arises during the lifetime of monozygotic twins. *PNAS.* 2005;102:10604–10609.
5. Bruder CEG, Piotrowski A, Gijsbers AACJ, Andersson R, Erickson S, Diaz de Stohl T et al. Phenotypically concordant and discordant monozygotic twins display different DNA copy-number-variation profiles. *Am J Hum Gen.* 2008;82: 763–771.
6. Schinzel AAGL, Smith DW, Miller JR. Monozygotic twinning and structural defects. *J Pediatr.* 1979;95:921–930.
7. Mastroiacovo P, Castilla EE, Arpino C, Botting B, Cocchi G, Goujard J et al. Congenital malformations in twins: an international study. *Am J Med Genet.* 1999;83:117–124.
8. Napolitani FD, Schreiber I. The acardiac monster. A review of the world literature and presentation of 2 cases. *Am J Obstet Gynecol.* 1960;80:582–589.
9. Benirschke K, Des Roches Harper V. The acardiac anomaly. *Teratology.* 1977;5:311–316.
10. Lachman R, McNabb M, Furmanski M, Karp L. The acardiac monster. *Eur J Pediatr.* 1980;134:195–200.
11. Van Allen MI, Smith DW, Shepard TH. Twin reversed arterial perfusion (TRAP) sequence: a study of 14 twin pregnancies with acardius. *Semin Perinatal.* 1983;7:285–293.
12. Moore TR, Gale S, Benirschke K. Perinatal outcome of forty-nine pregnancies complicated by acardiac twinning. *Am J Obstet Gynecol.* 1990;163:907–912.
13. Nerlich A, Wisser J, Draeger A, Nathrath W, Remberger K. Human acardiac anomaly: a report of three cases. *Eur J Obstet Gynecol Reprod Biol.* 1990;38:79–85.
14. Stephens TD. Muscle abnormalities associated with the twin reversed-arterial-perfusion (TRAP) sequence (Acardia). *Teratology.* 1984;30:311–318.
15. Healey MG. Acardia: predictive risk factors for the Co-twin's survival. *Teratology.* 1994;50:205–213.
16. Jimenez-Scherer JA, Davies BR. Malformations in acardiac twins are consistent with reversed blood flow: liver as a clue to their pathogenesis. *Pediatr Develop Pathol.* 2003;6:520–530.
17. Jones KL, Webster WS, Vaux KK, Beninschke K. Acardiac fetus: evidence in support of a vascular/hypoxia pathogenesis for isolated oral clefting. *Birth Def Res (Part A): Clin Mol Teratol.* 2008;82:597–600.
18. Fujikura T, Wellings SR. A teratoma-like mass on the placenta of a malformed infant. *Am J Obstet Gynecol.* 1964;89:824–825.
19. Draeger A, Nerlich A. Syndrome des bandes amniotiques associé à une malformation acardiaque observé dans une grossesse gémellaire. A propos d'un cas. (Amniotic band syndrome associated with an acardiac malformation in a twin pregnancy. Apropos of a case). *Ann Pathol.* 1988;8:317–320.
20. Kyriazis A, Areán V, Shanklin D. Placental-radiographic analysis of parasitic acardiac fetus: partially common umbilical circulation. *J Reprod Med.* 1974;12:74–81.
21. de Groot R, van den Wijngaard J PHM, Umur A, Beek JF, Nikkels PGJ, van Gemert MJC. Modeling acardiac twin pregnancies. *Ann NY Acad Sci.* 2007;1101:235–249.
22. Sergi C, Schmitt HP. Central nervous system in twin reversed arterial perfusion sequence with special reference to examination of the brain in Acardius Anceps. *Teratology.* 2000;61:284–290.
23. Pavone L, Laurence KM, Mattina T, Nuciforo G, Mollica F. Twins with acardia and anencephaly. *Acta Genet Med Gemellol.* 1985;34:89–93.
24. Habbal OA, Kenue RK, Venugopalan P. Acardia syndrome coexisting with gastroschisis in the co-twin. *Clin Dysmorphol.* 2005;14:45–47.
25. Schinzel AA, Smith DW, Miller JR. Monozygotic twinning and structural defects. *J Pediatr.* 1979;95:921–930.
26. Hanafy A, Peterson CM. Twin-reversed arterial perfusion (TRAP) sequence: case reports and review of literature. *Aust NZJ Obstet Gynaecol.* 1997;37:187–191.
27. Gewolb IH, Freedman RM, Kleinman CS, Hobbins JC. Prenatal diagnosis of a human pseudocardiac anomaly. *Obstet Gynecol.* 1983;61:657–662.
28. Blaicher W, Repa C, Schaller A. Acardiac twin pregnancy: associated with trisomy 2: case report. *Hum Reprod.* 2000;15:474–475.
29. Masuzaki H, Miura K, Yoshimura S, Yoshiura K, Ishimaru T. A monozygotic twin pregnancy discordant for acardia and X-inactivation pattern. *Eur J Obstet Gynecol Reprod Biol.* 2004; 117:102–104.
30. Bieber FR, Nance WE, Morton CC, Brown JA, Redwine FO. Genetic studies of an acardia monster: evidence of polar body twinning in man. *Science.* 1981;213:775–777.
31. Moore CA, Buehler BA, McManus BM, Harmon JP, Mirkin LD, Goldstein DJ. Acephalus-acardia in twins with aneuploidy. *Am J Med Genet Suppl.* 1987;3:139–143.
32. Stiller RJ, Romero R, Pace S, Hobbins J. Prenatal identification of twin reversed arterial perfusion syndrome in the first trimester. *Am J Obstet Gyncol.* 1989;160:1194–1196.
33. Simpson PC, Trudinger BJ, Walker A, Baird PJ. The intrauterine treatment of fetal cardiac failure in a twin pregnancy with an acardiac, acephalic monster. *Am J Obstet Gynecol.* 1983;147: 842–844.

34. Donnenfeld AE, Van de Woestijne J, Craparo F. The normal fetus of an acardiac twin pregnancies: Prenatal management based on echocardiographic and sonographic evaluation. *Prenat Diagn.* 1991;11:235–244.

35. Arias F, Sunderji S, Gimpelson R, Colton E. Treatment of acardiac twinning. *Obst Gynecol.* 1998;91:818–821.

36. Wong AE, Sepulveda W. Acardiac anomaly: current issues in prenatal assessment and treatment. *Pren Diagn.* 2005;25:796–806.

37. McCurdy CM Jr, Childers JM, Seeds JW. Ligation of the umbilical cord of an acardiac-acephalus twin with an endoscopic intrauterine technique. *Obstet Gynecol.* 1993;82:708–711.

38. Fries MH, Goldberg JD, Golbus MS. Treatment of acardiac-acephalus twin gestations by hysterotomy and selective delivery. *Obstet Gynecol.* 1992;79:601–604.

39. Spencer R. *Conjoined Twins: Developmental Malformations and Clinical Implications.* Baltimore, MD: Johns Hopkins Press; 2003.

40. Machin GA, Keith LG, Bamforth F. *An Atlas of Multiple Pregnancy: Biology and Pathology.* New York: CRC Press, Pantheon Publishers; 1999.

41. Machin GA. *Birth Defects: Original Article Series.* 1993;29: 141–179.

42. Spencer R. Anatomic description of conjoined twins: a plea for standardized terms. *J Pediatr Surg.* 1996;31: 941–944.

43. Spencer R. Theoretical and analytical embryology of conjoined twins. *Clin Anat.* 2000;13: 36–53; 97–120.

44. Spitz L, Kiely EM. Conjoined twins. *JAMA.* 2003;289: 1307–1310.

45. Kaufman MH. The embryology of conjoined twins. *Childs Nerv Syst.* 2004;20: 508–525.

46. Spitz L. Conjoined twins. *Prenat Diagn.* 2005;25: 814–819.

47. Geroulanos S, Jaggi F, Wydler J. Thoracopagus symmetries. *Gesnerus.* 1993;50: 179–200.

48. Ornoy A, Navot D, Menashi M, Laufer N, Chemke J. Asymmetry and discordance for congenital anomalies in conjoined twins: a report of six cases. *Teratology.* 1980;22: 145–154.

49. Poenaru D, Uros-Tristan J, Leclerc S, Murphy S, Dickens S-V, Youssef S, Blanchard H. Minimally conjoined omphalopagi: a consistent spectrum of anomalies. *J Pediatr Surg.* 1994;29: 1236–1238.

50. Lograno R, Garcia- Lithgow C, Harris S, Kent M, Meisner L. Heteropagus conjoined twins due to fusion of two embryos: Report and review. *Am J Med Genet.* 1997;73: 239–143.

51. Machin GA. Herteropagus conjoined twins due to fusion of two embryos. *Am J Med Genet.* 1998;78: 388–389.

52. Kapur RP, Jack RM, Siebert JR. Diamniotic placentation associated with omphalopagus conjoined twins: Implications for a contemporary model of conjoined twinning. *Am J Med Genet.* 1994;52: 188–198.

53. Gilbert-Barness E, Debich-Spicer D, Opitz JM. Conjoined twins: morphogenesis of the heart and a review. *Am J Med Genet Part A.* 2003;120 A: 568–582.

54. Levin M, Roberts DJ, Holmes LB, Tabin C. Laterality defects in conjoined twins. *Nature.* 1996;384: 321.

55. Hansin JW. Incidence of conjoined twinning. *Lancet.* 1975; ii: 1257.

56. Edmonds LD, Layde PM. Conjoined twins in the United States, 1970–1977. *Teratology.* 1982;25: 301–308.

57. Maymon R, Mendalovic S, Schacher M, Ron-El T, Weinraub Z, Herman A. Diagnosis of conjoined twins before 16 weeks gestation: the four year experience at one medical center. *Prenat Diagn.* 2005;25: 839–843.

58. Pajkrt E, Jauniaux E. First trimester diagnosis of conjoined twins. *Prenat Diagn.* 2005;25: 820–826.

59. Hoyle RM. Surgical separation of conjoined twins. *Surg Gynecol Obstet.* 1990;170: 549–562.

60. Mackenzie TC, Crombleholme TM, Johnson MP, Schaufer L, Flake AW, Hedrick HL et al. The natural history of prenatally diagnosed conjoined twins. *J Pediatr Surg.* 2002;37: 303–309.

61. Barth RA, Filly RA, Goldberg JD, Moore P, Silverman NH. Conjoined twins: prenatal diagnosis and assessment of associated malformations. *Radiology.* 1990;177: 201–207.

62. Bearn JG. The association of sirenomelia with Potter's syndrome. *Arch Dis Child.* 1960;35:254–258.

63. Guidera KJ, Raney E, Ogden JA, Highhouse M, Habal M. Caudal regression: a review of seven cases, including the Mermaid Syndrome. *J Pediatr Orthoped.* 1991;11:743–747.

64. St. Hilaire, G. *Histoire des anomalies.* Traite Teratol; Paris; 1836: 239.

65. Kampmeier OF. On sireniform monsters, with a consideration of the causation and the predominance of the male sex among them. *Anat Rec.* 1927;34:365–389.

66. Stevenson RE, Jones KL, Phelan MC, Jones MC, Barr M, Clericuzio C et al. Vascular steal: the pathogenic mechanism producing sirenomelia and associated defects of the viscera and soft tissues. *Pediatrics.* 1986;78:451–457.

67. Perez-Aytes A, Montero L, Gomez J, Paya A. Single aberrant umbilical artery in a fetus with severe caudal defects: sirenomelia or caudal dysgenesis. *Am J Med Genet.* 1997;69: 409–412.

68. Duhamel B. From the mermaid to anal imperforation: the syndrome of caudal regression. *Arch Dis Childh.* 1961;36: 152–155.

69. Duesterhoeft SM, Ernst LM, Siebert JR, Kapur RP. Five cases of caudal regression with an aberrant abdominal umbilical artery: Further support for a caudal regression-sirenomelia spectrum. *Am J Med Genet Part A.* 2007;143A:3175–3184.

70. Davies J, Chazen E, Nance WE. Symmelia in one of monozygotic twins. *Teratology.* 1971;4:367–378.

71. Stocker JT, Heifetz SA. Sirenomelia. A morphological study of 33 cases and review of the literature. *Perspect Pediatr Pathol.* 1987;10:7–50.

72. Kohler HG. An unusual case of sirenomelia. *Teratology.* 1972; 6:295–301.

73. Kapur RP, Mahony BS, Nyberg DA, Resta RG, Shepard TH. Sirenomelia associated with a "vanishing twin." *Teratology.* 1991;43:103–108.

74. Valenzano M, Paoletti R, Rossi A, Farinini D, Gorlaschi G, Fulcheri E. Sirenomelia, Pathological features, antenatal ultrasonographic clues and a review of current embryogenic theories. *Human Reprod Update.* 1999;5:82–86.

75. Patel S, Suchet I. The role of color and power Doppler ultrasound in the prenatal diagnosis of sirenomelia. *Ultrasound Obstet Gynecol.* 2004;24:684–691.

76. Kjaer KW, Keeling JW, Opitz JM, Gilbert-Barness E, Hartling U, Hansen BF, Kjaer I. Sirenomelia sequence according to the distance between the first sacral vertebra and the ilia. *Am J Med Genet.* 2003;120A:503–508.

77. Schwaibold H, Oehler U, Helpap B, Böhm N. Sirenomelia and anencephaly in one of dizygotic twins. *Teratology.* 1986;34: 243–247.

78. Halder A, Pahi J, Chaddha V, Agarwal SS. Sirenomelia sequence associated with craniorachischisis totalis, limb reduction and primitive heart. *Indian Pediatrics.* 2001;38:1041–1045.

79. Källén B, Castilla EE, Lancaster PA, Mutchinick O, Knudsen L, Martínez-Frías ML et al. The cyclops and the mermaid: an epidemiological study of two types of rare malformation. *J Med Genet.* 1992;29:30–35.

80. Oğuz A, Gökalp A, Gültekin A, Örsal M. A case of sirenomelia in one of a pair of identical twins, and in association with exomphalos. *Turkish J Pediatr.* 1986;28:205–210.

81. Young ID, O'Reilly KM, Kendall CH. Etiological heterogeneity in sirenomelia. *Pediatric Pathology.* 1986;5:31–43.

82. Dias MS, Walker ML. The embryogenesis of complex dysraphic malformations: a disorder of gastrulation? *Pediatr Neurosurg.* 1992;18:229–253.

83. Smith DW, Bartlett C, Harrah LM. Monozygotic twinning and the Duhamel anomalad (imperforate anus to sirenomelia): a nonrandom association between two aberrations in morphogenesis. *Birth Defects*. 1976;12(5):53–63.

84. Schreiner CA, Hoornbeek FK. Developmental aspects of sirenomelia in the mouse. *J Morph*. 1973;141:345–358.

85. Zakin L, Reversade B, Kuroda H, Lyons KM, De Robertis EM. Sirenomelia in Bmp7 and Tsg compound mutant mice: requirement for Bmp signaling in the development of ventral posterior mesoderm. *Development*. 2005;132:2489–2499.

86. Malinger G, Treschan O, Rosen N, Zakut A. Sirenomelia in a twelve week abortus. *Early Human Develop*. 1987;15:217–220.

87. Fantel AG, Shepard TH, Vadheim-Roth C, Stephens TD, Coleman C. Embryonic and fetal phenotypes: Prevalence and other associated factors in a large study of spontaneous abortion. In: Porter IH, Hook EM, eds. *Human Embryonic and Fetal Death*. New York: Academic Press; 1980: p. 7.

88. Stevenson AC, Johnson HA, Stewart MI, Golding DR. Congenital malformations; a report of a study of series of consecutive births in 24 centres. *Bull World Health Organ*. 1996;34(Suppl 1):9–127.

89. Murphy JJ, Fraser GC, Blair GK. Sirenomelia: case of the surviving mermaid. *J Pediatr Surg*. 1992;27:1265–1268.

90. Stanton MP, Penington EC, Hutson JM. A surviving infant with sirenomelia (Mermaid syndrome) associated with absent bladder. *J Pediatr Surg*. 2003;38:1266–1268.

91. Pinette MG, Hand M, Hunt RC, Blackstone J, Wax JR, Cartin A. Surviving sirenomelia. *J Ultrasound Med*. 2005;24:1555–1559.

92. Akbiyik F, Balci S, Akkoyun I, Aktaş D, Çakmak Ö. Type 1 sirenomelia in one of male twins, with imperforate anus in the other male twin. *Clin Dysmorph*. 2000;9:227–229.

93. Rudd NL, Klimek ML. Familial caudal dysgenesis: evidence for a major dominant gene. *Clin Genet*. 1990;38:170–175.

94. Selig AM, Benacerraf B, Greene MF, Garber MF, Genest DR. Renal dysplasia, megalocystis and sirenomelia in four siblings. *Teratology*. 1993;47:65–71.

95. Lynch SA, Wright C. Sirenomelia, limb reduction defects, cardiovascular malformation, renal agenesis in an infant born to a diabetic mother. *Clin Dysmorphol*. 1997;6:75–80.

96. Assimakopoulos E, Athanasiadis A, Zarakas M, Dragoumis K, Bontis J. Caudal regression syndrome and sirenomelia in only one twin in two diabetic pregnancies. *Clin Exp Obst Gyn*. 2004;31:151–153.

97. Passarge E, Lenz W. Syndrome of caudal regression in infants of diabetic mothers: observations of further cases. *Pediatrics*. 1966;37:672–675.

98. Kučera J. Rate and type of congenital anomalies among offspring of diabetic women. *J Reprod Med*. 1971;7:61–70.

99. Mills JL, Baker L, Goldman AS. Malformations in infants of diabetic mothers occur before the seventh gestational week: implications for treatment. *Diabetes*. 1979;28:292–293.

100. Sarpong S, Headings V. Sirenomelia accompanying exposure of the embryo to cocaine. *S Med J*. 1992;85:545–547.

101. Castilla EE, Mastroiacovo P, López-Camelo JS, Saldarriaga W, Isaza C, Orioli IM. Sirenomelia and cyclopia cluster in Cali, Colombia. *Am J Med Genet Part A*. 2008;146:2626–2636.

102. Opitz JM, Gilbert EF. Editorial comment on the papers by Wilson and Hayden and Wilson and Baird on renal agenesis. *Am J Med Genet*. 1985;21:167–169.

103. Sepulveda W, Corral E, Sanchez J, Carstens E, Schnapp C. Sirenomelia sequence versus renal agenesis: prenatal differentiation with power Doppler ultrasound. *Ultrasound Obstet Gynecol*. 1998;11:445–449.

104. Sepulveda W, Romero R, Pryde PG, Wolfe HM, Addis JR, Cotton OB. Prenatal diagnosis if sirenomelus with color Doppler ultrasonography. *Am J Obst Gynecol*. 1994;170:1377–1379.

105. Van Zalen-Sprock MM, Van Vugt JMG, Van Der Harten JJ, Van Geun HP. Early second-trimester diagnosis of sirenomelia. *Prenat Diag*. 1995;15:171–177.

106. Schinzel AAGL, Smith DW, Miller JR. Monozygotic twinning and structural defects. *J Pediatr*. 1979;95:921–930.

107. Mastroiacovo P, Castilla EE, Arpino C, Botting B, Cocchi G, Goujard J et al. Congenital malformations in twins: an international study. *Am J Med Genet*. 1999;83:117–124.

108. Pharoah POD, Adi Y. Consequences of in-utero death in a twin pregnancy. *Lancet*. 2000;355:1597–1602.

109. Williams K, Hennessy E, Alberman E. Cerebral palsy: effects of twinning, birthweight, and gestational age. *Arch Dis Child Fetal Neonatal Ed*. 1996;75:F178–F182.

110. Sebire NJ, Snijders RJ, Hughes E, Sepulveda W, Nocolaides KH. The hidden mortality of monochorionic twin pregnancies. *Br J Obstet Gynecol*. 1997;104:1203–1207.

111. Brennan J, Diwarn RV, Rosen MG, Bella EM. Fetofatal transfusion syndrome: prenatal ultrasonographic diagnosis. *Radiology*. 1982;143:535–536.

112. Taylor MJO, Denbow ML, Duncan KR, Overton TG, Fisk NM. Antenatal factors at diagnosis that predict outcome in twin-twin transfusion syndrome. *Am J Obstet Gynecol*. 2000;183:1023–1028.

113. Senat MV, Deprest J, Boulvain M, Paupe A, Winer N, Ville Y. Bar Endoscopic laser surgery versus serial amnioreduction for severe twin-to-twin transfusion syndrome. *N Engl J Med*. 2004;351:136–144.

114. Dickinson JE, Evans SF. Obstetric and perinatal outcomes from the Australian and New Zealand twin-twin transfusion syndrome registry. *Am J Gynecol*. 2000;182:706–712.

115. Mari G, Roberts A, Detti L, Koranci E, Stefos T, Bahado-Singh RO et al. Perinatal morbidity and mortality rates in severe twin-twin transfusion syndrome: results of an International Amnioreduction Registry. *Am J Obstet Gynecol*. 2001;185:708–715.

116. David TJ. Vascular basis for malformations in a twin. *Arch Dis Childh*. 1985;60:166–167.

117. Karageyim Karsidag AY, Kars B, Dansuk R, Api O, Unal O, Turan MC. Brain damage to the survivor within 30 min of co-twin demise in monochorionic twins. *Fetal Diag Ther*. 2005;20:91–95.

118. Okumura A, Hayakawa F, Kato T, Tsuji T, Negoro T, Watanabe K. Brain malformation of the surviving twin of intrauterine co-twin demise. *J Child Neurol*. 2007;22:85–88.

119. Larroche JC, Droulle P, Delezoide AL, Narcy F, Nessmann C. Brain damage in monozygous twins. *Biol Neonate*. 1990;57:261–278.

120. Olson LM, Flom LS, Kierney CM, Shermeta DW. Identical twins with malrotation and type IV jejunal atresia. *J Pediatr*. 1987;22:1015–1016.

121. Komuro H, Amagai T, Hori T, Hirai M, Matoba K, Wantanabe M, Kaneki M. Placental vascular compromise in jejunal stresia. *J Pediatr Surg*. 2004;39:1701–1705.

122. Askur WE, Wong R. Gangrene of the extremities in the newborn infant. Report of two cases. *J Pediatrics*. 1952;40:588–598.

123. Gilbert EF, Hogan GR, Stevenson MM, Suzuki H. Gangrene of an extremity in the newborn. *Pediatrics*. 1970;45:469–472.

124. Hecher K, Ville Y, Nicolaides K. Umbilical artery steal syndrome and distal gangrene in a case of twin-twin transfusion syndrome. *Obstet Gynecol*. 1994;83:862–865.

125. Lundvall L, Skibsted L, Graem N. Limb necrosis associated with twin-twin transfusion syndrome treated with YAG-laser coagulation. *Acta Obstet Gynecol Scand*. 1999;78:349–352.

126. Hoyme HE, Jones KL, Van Allen MI, Saunders BS, Benrschke K. Vascular pathogenesis of transverse limb reduction defects. *J Pediatr*. 1982;101:839–843.

127. Van Allen MI, Siegel-Bartelt J, Dixon J, Zuker RM, Clarke HM, Toi A. Constriction bands and limb reduction defects in two newborns with fetal ultrasound evidence for vascular disruption. *Am J Med Genet.* 1992;44:598–604.

128. Winer N, Salomon LJ, Essaoui M, Nasr B, Bernard JP, Ville Y. Pseudoamniotic band syndrome: a rare complication of monochorionic twins with fetofetal transfusion syndrome treated by laser coagulation. *Am J Obstet Gynecol.* 2008;198: 393.e1–5.

129. Dawkins RR, Marshal TL, Rogers MS. Prenatal gangrene in association with twin-twin transfusion syndrome. *Am J Obst Gynecol.* 1995;172:1055–1057.

130. Luks FT, Carr SP, Tracy TF Jr. Limb defects in twin-to-twin transfusion (Letter-to-the-editor). *J Pediatr Surg.* 2001;36: 1105–1106.

131. Galea P, Barigye O, Wee L, Jain V, Sullivan M, Fisk NM. The placenta contributes to activation of the renin angiotensin system in twin-twin transfusion syndrome. *Placenta.* 2008;29: 734–742.

132. Blickstein I. Reflections on the hypothesis for the etiology of spastic cerebral palsy caused by the "vanishing twin" syndrome. *Develop Med Child Neurol.* 1998;40: 358.

133. Norton ME. Evaluation and management of twin-twin transfusion syndrome: still a challenge. *Am J Obstet Gynecol.* 2007; 196:419–420.

134. Roberts D, Gates S, Kilby M, Neilson JP. Interventions for twin-twin transfusion syndrome: Cochrane review. *Ultrasound Obstet Gynecol.* 2008;31:701–711.

135. Gonsoulin W, Moise KJ Jr, Kirshon B, Cotton DB, Wheeler JM, Carpenter RJ Jr. Outcome of twin-twin transfusion diagnosed before 28 weeks of gestation. *Obstet Gynecol.* 1990;75: 214–216.

136. Pharoah PO, Cook RW. A hypothesis for the aetiology of spastic cerebral palsy—the vanishing twin. *Develop Med Child Neurol.* 1997;39:292–296.

137. Lenclen R, Paupe A, Ciarlo G, Couderc S, Castela F, Ortqvist L et al. Neonatal outcome in preterm monochorionic twins with twin-to-twin transfusion syndrome after intrauterine treatment with amnioreduction or fetoscopic laser surgery: comparison with dichorionic twins. *Am J Obstet Gynecol.* 2007;196:450e1–7.

138. Quintero RA, Dickinson JE, Morales WJ, Bornick PW, Bermúdez C, Cincotta R et al. Stage-based treatment of twin-twin transfusion syndrome. *Am J Obstet Gynecol.* 2003;188: 1333–1340.

139. Rychik J, Tian Z, Bebbington M, Xu F, McCann M, Mann S et al. The twin-twin transfusion syndrome: spectrum of cardiovascular abnormality and development of a cardiovascular score to assess severity of disease. *Am J Obstet Gynecol.* 2007;197:392.e1–8.

Chapter 25

Minor Anomalies/Normal Variations

MINOR ANOMALIES & NORMAL VARIATIONS

One of the first things many mothers do is to undress her newborn infant and look him or her over very thoroughly. She wants to be certain that everything looks the way it should. In this process, mothers (and fathers) often find minor physical features with which they are not familiar. Some mothers ask the pediatrician about each one; others may wait for the pediatrician to mention finding them.

By being familiar with minor anomalies and normal variations, the physician can inspect the features of concern and, usually, reassure the parents that the feature in question, by itself, occurs in many healthy newborns and has no medical significance. This ability requires that the physician be familiar with the spectrum of common minor anomalies, normal variations, and racial differences. He/she should also know which minor features rarely have medical significance (Table 25-1) and which ones are a significant high risk finding (Table 25-2).

He/she should also be familiar with racial differences that are common among the ethnic/racial groups of his/her patients.

Most infants with one or more minor physical features are healthy. The challenge for a busy clinician is to recognize the infant who is "dysmorphic" and could have a significant multiple anomaly syndrome.

BACKGROUND

During the past 40 years, interest in and awareness of syndromes that include minor anomalies as significant findings has increased among clinicians who take care of newborns, beginning with the seminal study published in 1964 by Philip Marden, David Smith, and Michael McDonald (1). Since this early report, hundreds of "new" malformation syndromes have been described in medical books and journals. These reports describe both the major and minor physical abnormalities. Clinicians have had to become familiar with terms like synophris, anteverted nostrils, prominent nose, clinodactyly, and tibial dimple. These descriptions have prompted questions about the range of normal for minor anomalies and normal variations and the need for guidelines for the busy practitioner (2–14).

Definition

A minor anomaly has been defined, arbitrarily, as a physical feature that has no surgical, medical, or cosmetic importance and occurs in less than 4% of infants of the same race and sex. This definition distinguishes these minor physical features from major malformations, which have surgical, medical, or cosmetic importance.

The term "normal variation" has been used for minor physical features that are similar to minor anomalies, except they occur more frequently, specifically above 4%. One example is an umbilical hernia in an African American infant.

Many alternative terms and definitions have been proposed. Karoly Méhes (2, 3) noted that minor physical defects are, in themselves, harmless phenomena that may also occur in completely healthy individuals, but their frequency is much higher in infants with congenital disorders.

John Opitz (4) noted that "mild malformations are defects of organogenesis, minor anomalies are defects of phenogenesis (defined as all morphogenetic events after organogenesis) . . . mild malformations, minor anomalies, dysplasias and deformities are not synonymous. . . . Developmentally and anatomically, minor anomalies and normal variants are identical but causally have totally different implications, the former being the most common effects of aneuploidy, each of which individually may also occur in the normal populations."

Paul Merlob (5,6) defined minor congenital malformations as "anatomic (structural) defects due to errors of organogenesis; generally not of surgical or medical significance to the patient; at times, can cause cosmetic concern; are rarely responsible for complications; do not disappear by themselves." Minor variants were defined as "phenotypic variations, not present in a malformation syndrome; often present in the family; often present in the patients ethnic group." He suggested the term "mild errors of morphogenesis," as had been recommended by the International Working Group (7).

John Carey (8) pointed out that some minor anomalies are "mild" malformations and others are graded, continuous features. He suggested that "most [minor anomalies] represent previously undescribed syndromes, unrecognized polytopic field defects or coincidence." Jaime Frias and John Carey (9) supported the use of the term "mild errors of morphogenesis" as encompassing "both the errors of organogenesis, including mild malformations, disruptions and dysplasias and the errors of phenogenesis, or minor anomalies."

Leonard Pinksy (10) noted that "the word 'anomaly' denotes a departure from normality . . .; however, most minor congenital anomalies constitute part of the normal range, both qualitatively (subjectively) and in terms of frequency (objectively). Indeed, many are sufficiently common to be considered polymorphisms (in the monogenic sense)." He suggested the term "informative morphogenetic variant" as a new definition for minor congenital anomaly, defined as a clinically/cosmetically insignificant developmental deviation from usual (model) morphological form that has a prenatal origin.

Kenneth Lyons Jones (11) defined minor anomalies as "unusual morphologic features that are of no serious medical or cosmetic consequence to the patient. The value of their recognition is that they may serve as indicators of altered morphogenesis in a general sense or may constitute valuable clues in the diagnosis of a specific pattern of malformation."

Both Gene Hoyme (12) and Michael Cohen (13) noted that minor anomalies may be malformations, deformities, disruptions, or dysplasias.

Incidence/Prevalence Rate

Among four studies (1, 3, 5, 14, 15) in which at least 3,700 infants were examined for 40 or more features, 14.1%, 16.5%, 20.7%, and 39.9%, respectively, of the infants had one or more minor anomalies. Each of these studies used the same definition of a minor anomaly. The lowest frequency of minor physical features was identified in the one study (1) in which an examination protocol was not used.

Unfortunately, many studies of infants for the presence of minor physical features have not used the same list of features (or definitions) to be looked for. The use of an examination protocol, which prompts the examiner to look for specific features, makes it likely that a greater number would be identified. In addition, the subjective nature of many physical features decreases the inter-rater reproducibility in the determination that a specific feature is present or absent. Because of the variations in the methodology from study to study, the frequencies of minor anomalies in populations have varied significantly.

Ernest Hook and Petry (16) and Hook et al. (17) noted that the frequencies of minor anomalies in their own study and that of Marden et al. (1) fit a Poisson distribution. They suggested that each minor anomaly was the result of a single "hit," i.e., teratogenic insult, during development, and that multiple causal events would produce multiple minor anomalies. The distribution of the frequency of all the minor physical features looked for in the systematic examinations in one study in Boston (15, 16) showed that 4% was an arbitrary print on the progressive decrease in rate of occurrence (Figure 25-1, 25-2 and 25-3).

While arbitrary, using less than 4% as a hallmark has become a customary part of the definition.

Race/Ethnicity

Several minor anomalies show marked differences in prevalence in infants from different racial/ethnic groups.

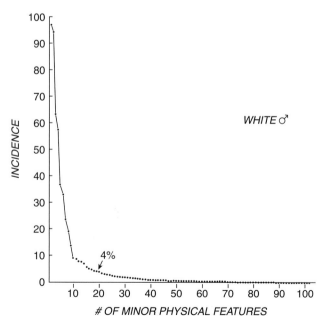

FIGURE 25.1 Shows the distribution of the frequency of the minor anomalies and normal variations in newborn white males examined in a systematic study in Boston (14). Note that the frequency of 4% is not associated with a significant change in the distribution curve

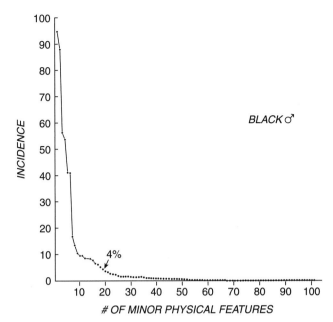

FIGURE 25.2 The distribution of the frequency of the same minor features in newborn black males in the same study (14).

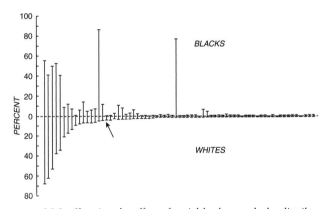

FIGURE 25.3 Showing the effect of racial background, the distribution of the same minor features in black and white newborns. Some features are much more common in one race than in the other. The 4% frequency is marked by the arrow.

For example, preauricular sinus (Table 25-8) and accessory nipple (Table 25-13) were more common in black infants and Brushfield spots (Table 25-5) and bifid xiphoid (Table 25-13) were more common in white infants (14).

Focused Studies: Ear Shape, Variation, and Anomalies

When clinicians focus on defining the range of normal for a specific structure, significant and helpful details are developed. This has occurred in the analysis of ear shape by Jaffe (18) in Boston, by Merlob, Bader, Grun, and their associates in Tel Aviv (19, 20), and by Hunter and Yotsuyanagi in Ottawa (21). This focus leads to better illustrations, definitions, and the delineation of significant shapes, such as the satyr ear and the Beals ear (21).

Sex Differences

Differences in the frequencies among male and female infants of the same race are less dramatic than differences between infants of different racial groups. For example, there were small differences between males and females for syndactyly of toes 2-3 (Table 25-18), transverse palmar crease (Table 25-17), and preauricular sinus (Table 25-8).

Inheritance

Several families have been reported in which several members had the same minor anomaly or normal variation, including clinodactyly of the fifth finger (22), ear lobe sinuses (23), free ear lobes (24), lop ears (25), scalp defects (26), acromial dimples (27) and inverted nipples (28) and flat umbilicus (29). In addition, the presence of specific minor physical features in a parent makes its occurrence more likely in his/her child. For example, in examining 466 newborn infants, Dar et al (30) found that if the mother had a simian crease or variants, 23.8% of her newborns also had this feature, a significant increase (p<0.025).

ASSOCIATION OF MINOR ANOMALIES WITH MAJOR MEDICAL PROBLEMS

Association with Major Malformations

Several studies (1–3, 14) have shown that the infant with three or more minor anomalies has an increased risk for having an associated major malformation. However, the specific risks have varied with the methodology used. Marden, Smith, and McDonald (1) reported that the infant with three or more minor anomalies had a 90% chance of having a major malformation. In contrast, two other studies of similar size showed that only 26% and 19.6%, respectively, (4, 14) of the infants with 3 or more minor anomalies had a major malformation.

One of these studies (14) used an examination protocol, which listed 74 minor anomalies to be looked for, instead of the 40 listed by Marden et al (1). The difference in the findings remained when the comparison was restricted to the same list of features. One possible explanation for the much higher correlations of 3 or more minor anomalies with major malformations was the fact that an examination protocol was not used, which could have promoted more consistency in the findings by each examiner. Instead, there was the opportunity for a more intense search for minor features in the examination, with no examination protocol, of all infants with major malformations by David Smith, the senior investigator. The examinations of the infants with no major malformations were carried out by Philip Marden, who was a fourth-year medical student.

Several associations between the presence of specific minor anomalies and the occurrence of major malformations have been postulated.

    i) <u>extra nipples and renal anomalies.</u> The increased frequency of renal anomalies among infants with supernumerary nipples has been identified in some systematic studies (3, 31, 32), but not others (33, 34). Both extra nipples and genitourinary anomalies are common physical features. A large prospective study with a concurrent comparison group will be needed to determine whether or not this association is valid.

    ii) <u>single umbilical artery (SUA) and major malformations.</u> Several case series have shown that the infant with a single umbilical artery had an increased frequency of major malformations (35). Specifically, there are several major malformations that involve abnormalities of the aorta and renal arteries, such as bilateral renal agenesis and sirenomelia, that are associated with SUA. However, it should be noted that systematic studies by Blackburn, an experienced student of the placenta and umbilical cord (36) have shown that the presence of SUA cannot be established by simple inspection of the end of the umbilical cord. Serial sections are needed.

    On a practical level, a clinical examination is the most efficient way to determine whether an infant is dysmorphic, sick, or both, and whether further diagnostic studies are indicated. On the first day of life, with experience, the presence of enlarged kidney or the absence of the normal kidney can be suspected by deep palpation (37). A controlled prospective study is needed to determine whether the infant with SUA has an increased frequency of major malformations and, in particular, the cost-effectiveness of abdominal screening by ultrasound in this clinical setting.

    iii) <u>preauricular tags and urinary tract abnormalities.</u> Like many postulated associations, some studies have been positive (38) and some negative (39). In a sample of 70 consecutive infants with isolated preauricular tags, ultrasonography identified urinary tract abnormalities in 6 (8.6%) infants, including five with hydronephrosis and one with a horseshoe kidney). The comparison group of 69 infants had no renal anomalies. The negative study, for comparison, was 23 infants with preauricular tags and pits, none of whom had abnormalities of the urinary tract abnormalities (39).

    iv) <u>sacral dimples and intraspinal abnormalities:</u> It is important to differentiate between a sacral dimple and a midline lumbar patch of hair, lipoma, and capillary hemangiomas, which warrant screening for occult spinal dysraphism (40, 41). This association was tested in a systematic study of 50 consecutive infants and children. The sacral skin dimple was defined as an invagination of the skin in the middle of the sacrum. Two of the 50 infants had hairy patch and were

excluded. None of the other 48 infants was found by ultrasonography to have an intraspinal lesion (42).

Association with Mental Deficiency or Illness

Studies of American (43), British (44), Japanese (23), and Hungarian (45) children with mental retardation of unknown etiology have shown they are much more likely to have three or more minor anomalies than children of normal intelligence. Smith and Boston (43) reported that 32% of individuals with unexplained mental retardation had three or more minor anomalies in comparison to 0% of 100 controls. Arima and associates (23) found that 33.1% of mentally retarded Japanese children had three or more minor anomalies in contrast to 9.5% of controls. The reason why more normal (control) children had three or more minor anomalies in the latter study (23) was not clear, since similar definitions were used.

    In another study of this association (44), in which 246 mentally retarded institutionalized children (IQ between 37 and 67) were examined, the frequency of minor anomalies was highest in children with Down Syndrome (3.38/patient), next highest in genetic disorders (2.0), lower for mentally retarded of unknown cause (0.88), and lowest for those retarded by environmental factors, e.g., perinatal asphyxia, meningitis, 0.37.

    VanOverloop et al. (46) tested the hypothesis of an association between the number of minor anomalies and the frequency of cognitive dysfunction. The cognitive function of 98 children, who had been found at birth to have three or more minor anomalies (14), was evaluated between ages 4 and 8 years. This evaluation showed that their full scale, verbal, and performance IQs were normal (118.2 ± 11.9, 117.1 ± 12.2, and 115.6 ± 11.8, respectively).

Association with Hyperactive Behavior

Several investigators have suggested that infants with multiple anomalies are more likely to be hyperactive when older (47—50). Waldrop and associates (47) examined 30 newborn males for the presence of 16 minor physical anomalies*, all of which are phenotypic features of Down Syndrome. They found that the number of minor anomalies correlated with the presence of a short attention span, peer aggression, and impulsivity at age three years. Waldrop and Halverson (48) showed in

---

* The 16 minor anomalies were: head circumference out of normal range, more than one hair whorl, epicanthus, hypertelorism, malformed ears, low-set ears, asymmetrical ears, soft pliable ears, no ear lobes, high steepled palate, furrowed tongue, curved little finger, single palmar crease, wide gap between first and second toes, partial syndactyly of toes, and third toe longer than second (47).

older children that the presence of minor anomalies at 2.5 years predicted hyperactive behavior at 7.5 years.

Other studies have not confirmed this correlation between the presence of minor anomalies and behavior. In an evaluation of 99 children in a normal primary school (50), there was no correlation between the number of minor anomalies and performance IQ, motor ability, and classroom behavior. There was an inverse relationship between the number of minor anomalies and verbal performance. In a study in which 123 infants were examined at birth and followed for one year, the anomaly score was not found to be a single measure that was predictive of abnormal behavior (51).

The identification of physical features that, when present at birth, are predictive of subsequent behavior would provide an opportunity for early intervention. One problem with the studies cited above is the subjective nature of some of the features looked for, such as malformed ears, soft pliable ears, high steepled palate, and wide gap between first and second toes. In studies that look for such features, it is essential to establish the degree of agreement between two examiners of the same child and the incidence of the same features in a control sample of the same social background. Examinations should be done by masked examiners.

Association with Autism

Dissociation and hypoplasia of the dermal ridges on the palms have been found to be significantly more common among children with autism than among unexposed controls (52). In an epidemiologic study of autism in Nova Scotia (53), the children with autism were significantly more likely to have posterior rotation of the ears in comparison to other developmentally disabled children and controls. They did not differ in ear size, position, or configuration.

Association with Schizophrenia

The examination of individuals with schizophrenia and their non-psychotic parents for 41 items, adopted in part from the Waldrop Scale, showed that they had an increased frequency of facial asymmetry, cleft palate, hair whorls, and abnormal palmar creases (54). The presence of "neurological soft signs" and the minor anomaly score classified 71% of the nonpsychotic parents as either "carriers" or "non-carriers" of the genetic predisposition to schizophrenia.

Association with Low Birth Weight

Several studies (55, 56) have shown that minor anomalies are more common in infants of low birth weight, regardless of whether they are born prematurely or are small for their gestational age. Hook et al. (17), in re-analyzing the findings in the study of 4,412 white newborn infants (1), found that the incidence of minor defects was increased slightly for low-birth weight infants, but the increase was not significant. Dar and associates (30) reported that the incidence of simian crease variants was increased among small-for-gestational-age infants, but not simian crease.

Association with Stillbirth

Hook et al. (17) observed that the relative risk for having a single minor defect was higher for stillbirths (RR 2.26) than for low weight infants (RR 1.19), but these differences were not significant statistically.

Association with Twinning

The 373 monozygous twins examined in the Perinatal Collaborative Study of 56,000 pregnant women had twice as many minor anomalies as the 617 dizygous twins (57). Deformed ear pinna and preauricular skin tag were two minor malformations that were more common to a significant degree in monozygous (identical) twins in comparison to dizygous twins.

Minor Anomalies as a Phenotypic Effect of Teratogens

Most reports of the phenotypic features of infants exposed to drugs or teratogenic conditions, such as excessive alcohol exposure, describe an increase in both major and minor anomalies. For example, Ouellette and her associates (58) noted that both major and minor anomalies were three to four times more common in infants whose mothers had chronic alcoholism during the pregnancy. They did not list the specific minor defects noted. Clarren and Smith (59) noted that over half of the infants with the fetal alcohol syndrome had a short, upturned nose, hypoplastic philtrum, and thinned upper vermilion.

Infants of insulin-dependent diabetic mothers (IDM) have been reported in several studies (60–62) to have a higher frequency of minor anomalies. In one study (61) hip dysplasia and polydactyly were considered "minor" malformations, features that were considered more significant malformations in another systematic study of IDM (60). The analysis of the physical features of IDM and unexposed control of infants in the Multicenter Diabetes in Early Pregnancy Study showed marked variation in the frequency of several minor anomalies among the primary examiners at several of the five centers (62). This occurred in spite of several efforts to make the examinations uniform: the examiners had reviewed and agreed to the set of definitions used for determining the presence of specific minor physical features and these features were listed in an examination protocol. The differences in findings appeared to reflect different sensitivities to the presence of a feature, particularly those defined subjectively.

Midface hypoplasia is a common minor physical feature of the anticonvulsant embryopathy, identified in 13.2%, 15.2%, and 5.3% of infants exposed to phenytoin, phenobarbital, and carbamazepine, respectively, in one study of newborn infants with masked examiners who used an examination protocol (63). In that study, the infants with midface and digit hypoplasia were significantly more likely to have major malformations, microcephaly, and growth restriction, the more severe, but less common features of the anticonvulsant embryopathy (64). There was also a marked variation in the frequency of the features identified by trained research assistants who knew the exposure status of the infants being examined (65). When one of the primary study physicians knew that the likelihood the child being examined was drug-exposed, during an interim period with no funding, the likelihood that the examiner would identify the features of drug-related features, such as short nose with anteverted nostrils and nail hypoplasia, was increased, but the frequency of features not attributed to drug exposure were not (66). This increased frequency, considered observer bias, disappeared when the likelihood that the infant was exposed to an anticonvulsant drug decreased.

Minor Anomalies Associated with Malignancy

The association of major malformations and cancers has been observed in several disorders (67), including Down Syndrome with acute lymphocytic leukemia, skeletal anomalies, pancytopenia and malignancies in the Fanconi Anemia (MIM #227650), and Wilms tumor with the chromosome 11 deletion syndrome aniridia-Wilms tumor.

Systematic examinations of 106 children with malignancies by Méhes and his associates (68) showed that 69.2% had one or more minor anomalies in comparison to 63% of their sibs and 34.6% of 100 controls. Among 100 children with acute lymphoblastic leukemia (69) these investigators found a similar increase of more minor anomalies (from a list of 55) among 100 affected children compared to each of their parents and unrelated controls. There was no specific "mild errors of morphogenesis" associated with the occurrence of leukemia. The coexistence of the increased frequency of minor anomalies and normal variation with malignancies was interpreted as evidence of "genetic instability" in the affected individuals (70).

LIMITATIONS OF USING MINOR ANOMALIES IN RESEARCH STUDIES: A CRITIQUE

The frequency of minor anomalies and normal variations, their increased frequency after exposure to several environmental factors, and their correlation with abnormal behaviors has made the identification of minor physical features an attractive option in clinical studies. However, poor reproducibility, observer bias, and context bias limit significantly the usefulness of a search for minor anomalies in clinical studies.

Reproducibility

Most minor anomalies and normal variations are defined subjectively. This means that the determination that a feature is present reflects the perception of the examiner. This makes it possible, indeed very likely, that there will be a significant variation in the findings of two examiners of the same infant, even when they are using the same definitions and the same examination protocol.

In one study (15) in which a study examiner with medical training and a study physician examined the same 444 infants, there was poor agreement on the presence or absence of very subjective features, like anteverted nostrils and prominent heel. There was better agreement on more specific features, such as coronal hypospadias, transverse palmar (simian) crease, and skin tag. The relative infrequency of specific minor features in this sample of 444 infants made the Kappa statistic a more severe measure of agreement and disagreement. Log-linear modeling techniques were considered a better approach (65).

The presumed objectivity of measurements is not free from bias. In one study the findings in two measurements, specifically length of nose and upper lip, by two physicians following the same directions, showed very different results (71). This experience emphasizes the need for regular comparisons between examiners in a study to identify significant differences in technique, so that corrections could be made while the study is underway.

Another measure of reproducibility was a comparison of the physical findings in alcohol-exposed children at birth and again at age 4 years (74). 75 children were evaluated at birth by one physician examiner and at age 4 years by another physician examiner for the presence of dysmorphic features. At each age, the examiner predicted whether or not each child had fetal alcohol effects. The two examiners had received similar training in the same fellowship program by the same mentor. 8 of 10 infants considered at birth to have fetal alcohol effects had the same diagnosis at age 4 years. 12% of 65 infants considered unaffected at birth were considered to be affected at age 4 years.

Wide differences in the frequency of a specific feature in two different groups of infants of similar racial/ethnic background have also been documented. The frequency of sacral dimple and upward eye slant were 1.2 and 3% in the examination of Méhes (5), but only 0.02 and less than 1% for Marden (1). In the Diabetes in Early Pregnancy Study (62) in which there were experienced examiners who used the same definitions and detailed

TABLE 25-1 *Minor anomalies with low predictive value*

FEATURES
Epicanthal folds
Anteverted nostrils
Preauricular sinus
Preauricular tags
Transverse palmar (simian) crease
Clinodactyly of fifth finger
Syndactyly of toes 2-3

TABLE 25-2 *Minor anomalies with high predictive value*

FEATURES	EXAMPLE
Hypoplastic alae Nasi	Johansson – Blizzard syndrome (MIM #243800)
Preauricular skin or tag and branchial cleft sinus	Branchio–Oto–Renal Syndrome (MIN #113650)
Lip pits on lower lip	Van der Woude Syndrome (MIM #119300)
Single flexion crease on fifth finger	No specific disorder
Dermal sinus in midline of nose or upper lip	No specific disorder

examination protocol, the frequency of anteverted nostrils was 58% among study infants in Chicago, but 6% in Seattle, and 18% in Boston. For redundant skin folds on the neck, the frequencies were 0%, 20%, and 2%, respectively, in those same three study sites.

Bias

Observer bias and context bias are also factors in the examination of newborn infants for the presence/absence of specific minor features. For example, in a study of the features of children exposed in utero to anticonvulsant drugs the study physicians will be looking carefully for the presence of the depressed bridge of the nose, short nose, anteverted nostrils, and long upper lip. As a result, due to this context bias (73), the frequency of these features in both drug-exposed and unexposed controls will be higher than in a study in which the same examiners were not focusing on these features (14). If, however, the examiner becomes aware of a greater likelihood that the infant being examined has been exposed to an anticonvulsant drug, he/she will be more likely to "see" the facial features being looked for, an example of observer bias (66).

CLINICAL GUIDELINES

Many minor anomalies have a low predictive value (Table 25-1). These anomalies occur primarily in healthy children, and are only occasionally a feature of a serious disorder. These include epicanthal folds, anteverted nostrils, preauricular sinus or tag, transverse palmar (simian) crease, clinodactyly of the fifth finger, and syndactyly of toes 2-3. As an example, the transverse palmar crease occurs in one hand of 2% of newborn infants. It is also a well-known feature of Down Syndrome, a condition with a frequency of 1:1,000 with 30% of affected infants having a transverse palmar crease on one hand (67). Based on these frequencies, the presence of a single transverse palmar crease is much more more common in healthy infants. This means that the infant with a transverse palmar crease is much more likely to be a healthy infant than an infant with Down Syndrome. If an infant has a transverse palmar crease, the examination of the infant for the more significant features of Down Syndrome (74), such as hypotonia, heart defects, and the distinctive facial features, should be the basis for suggesting this diagnosis, *not* the presence of a transverse palmar crease on one hand.

However, there are also several rare minor physical features that have been identified which are often associated with either a specific serious disorder or a non-specific marker of conditions associated with mental retardation or chromosome abnormalities (Table 25-2). These are findings in a physical examination to which the examining pediatrician should be sensitized; when present, careful evaluations are needed as soon as possible. The welfare of the infant and the perception of his/her parents depend on this early recognition of these minor physical features and their potential medical significance.

SPECIFIC MINOR PHYSICAL FEATURES

HEAD

Frontal bossing: In profile view the brow is strikingly prominent relative to the lower portion of the face.

Keel-shaped brow: This is pointed vertically in the midline and concave at the edges, as in the keel of a boat.

Flat brow: In the profile view, the brow is very flat beginning at the base of the nose and associated with a recessed appearance of the brow.

Prominent occiput: In the profile view, the occiput projects posteriorly to a striking degree.

Flat occiput: In the profile view, the occiput is flattened and has less than the normal amount of projection.

Metopic suture palpable: This is a vertical line easily palpable in the middle of the brow that runs from the most anterior edge of the anterior fontanel to the base of the nose (Figure 25.4).

Metopic suture open to glabella: An opening is easily palpable from the base of the nose up to the anterior fontanel.

TABLE 25-3 *Incidence of minor physical features among 7,157 newborn infants*

Physical Feature	All Races	White		Black		Latin		Mixed Racial	
		Males	Females	Male	Female	Male	Female	Male	Female
HEAD									
Frontal bossing	0.4% 25/7112	0.3% 7/2191	0.4% 9/2091	0.2% 1/469	0.5% 2/443	0.5% 1/223	0.5% 1/188	0 0/691	0.6% 4/659
Keel-shaped brow	0.01 1/7110	0 0/2192	0 0/2089	0 0/469	0 0/443	0 0/223	0.5 1/188	0 0/619	0 0/658
Flat brow	0.01 1/7114	0.05 1/2191	0 0/2090	0 0/469	0 0/443	0 0/223	0 0/189	0 0/619	0 0/661
Prominent occiput	3.4 246/7148	3.9 86/2199	3.4 71/2100	3.2 15/470	2.9 13/447	2.7 6/224	1.6 3/189	4.3 27/623	3.3 22/666
Flat occiput	0.1 7/7112	0.05 1/2189	0.1 3/2091	0 4/469	0 0/442	0 0/223	0.5 1/189	0.2 0/619	0 0/661
Metopic suture palpable	59.8 4072/6813	63.7 1340/2105	65.3 1319/2020	41.7 187/449	43.4 183/422	53.3 112/210	46.1 83/180	58.6 340/580	60.3 377/625
Metopic suture open to glabella	1.0 71/6856	1.0 21/2120	0.4 8/2030	1.8 8/451	3.5 15/424	1.0 2/210	1.7 3/182	0.7 4/584	1.3 8/632
Metopic fontanel	0.2 13/6809	0.3 6/2099	0.3 5/2024	0 0/450	0 0/420	0.5 1/210	0 0/181	0 0/579	0.2 1/625
Third sagittal fontanel	6.0 306/5122	4.0 65/1616	4.9 79/1542	13.6 48/352	13.8 40/290	7.8 13/167	6.5 9/139	3.6 15/413	7.0 30/430
Scalp defect	0.06 4/7110	0.05 1/2189	0.1 2/2090	0 0/469	0 0/443	0 0/220	0.5 1/189	0 0/619	0 0/660
Double whorl of hair	7.4 523/7111	7.4 161/2190	7.0 140/2089	6.2 29/469	6.1 27/443	10.8 24/222	10.6 20/189	8.4 52/619	7.9 52/661
Triple whorl of hair	0.4 19/4833	0.3 5/1534	0.2 3/1456	0.6 2/338	0 0/275	0.6 1/159	2.2 3/134	0.5 2/379	0.8 3/395
Absent whorl	0.9 43/4826	0 0/1531	0 0/1455	5.3 18/337	8.4 23/275	0 0/159	0 0/134	0 0/378	0.3 1/394

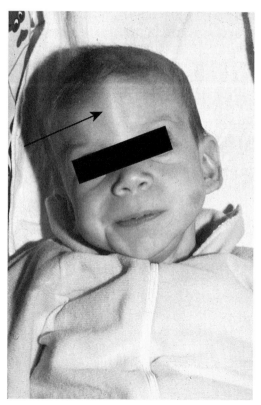

FIGURE 25.4 Metopic suture palpable. (arrow)

Metopic fontanel: Not a true fontanel, but a distinct and localized widening of the metopic suture.

Third sagittal fontanel: Not a true fontanel, but a distinct and localized widening along the sagittal suture; usually located about two centimeters anterior to the posterior fontanel.

Scalp defect: A small area (usually 1 to 2 centimeters in diameter) in which there is no hair or skin, but a reddened base of a "punched-out" lesion; usually at the vertex of the head (Figures 25.5 and 25.6).

Double whorl of hair: Two circular patterns of hair, usually located at the vertex of the head; also includes infants with one whorl on upper brow and one whorl on vertex (Figures 25.7 and 25.8).

Triple whorl of hair: Three circular patterns of scalp hair, usually two on the vertex of the head and one on the brow.

Absent whorl: No circular whorls of hair in scalp.

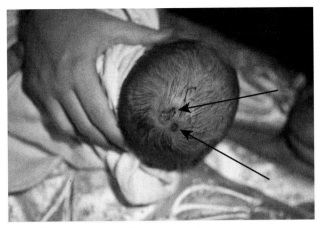

FIGURE 25.5   Scalp defects (2) on crown of head. (arrow)

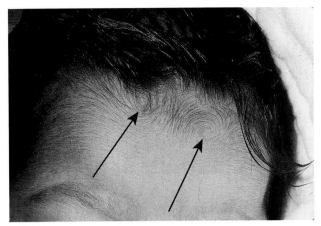

FIGURE 25.7   Double hair whorl on brow, near hair line. (arrow)

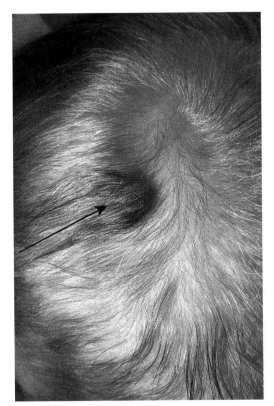

FIGURE 25.6   Scalp defect with surrounding ring of dark hair ("hair collar sign"). (arrow)

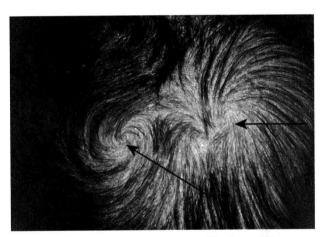

FIGURE 25.8   Double hair whorl on crown of head. (arrow)

FACE

Supraorbital ridge palpable: An elevation of the upper edge of each bony orbit, ususaly plpable over the medial porion of the orbit.

Eyebrows confluent: Meet in midline; not lanugo hair.

Flat bridge of nose: Greater degree of flattening at root or base of nose than is normal for a newborn infant (Figure 25.11).

Prominent bridge of nose: Root of nose lacks normal depression, extends straight from glabella to nose (Figure 25.9).

Nostrils anteverted: Nostrils seen in frontal view; usually nose is short (Figure 25.10 to 25.11).

Long nasal septum: Septum extends below outer edge of nostrils when viewed from side (Figure 25.12).

Epicanthal fold: Extra fold of skin extends across inner canthus and prevents the examinier from seeing the inner canthus (Figures 25-13 and 25-14).

TABLE 25-4 *Face*

Physical Feature	All Races	White		Black		Latin		Mixed Racial	
		Males	Females	Male	Female	Male	Female	Male	Female
Supraorbital ridge palbable									
Left	52.5 3745/7134	57.4 1261/2196	48.6 1091/2096	56.4 265/470	48.9 218/446	53.3 126/224	40.4 76/188	56.6 351/620	51.7 344/665
Right	47.3 3371/7129	52.1 1145/2197	42.7 894/2096	49.9 233/468	45.1 201/446	51.4 114/222	37.4 70/187	50.8 351/620	47.1 313/664
Both	44.4 3163/7126	48.5 1066/2196	40.1 840/2095	48.1 225/468	42.4 189/446	48.2 107/222	35.3 66/187	48.8 302/169	44.3 294/664
Eybrows confluent	0.2 12/7122	0.1 3/2192	0 0/2096	0.2 1/469	0.7 3/444	0.5 1/224	0.5 1/187	0.2 1/618	0.2 1/663
Flat bridge Of nose	2.9 138/4835	1.7 26/1534	1.4 20/1459	8.0 27/336	8.0 22/275	1.9 3/160	6.0 8/134	1.9 7/378	2.5 10/396
Prominent bridge of nose	2.1 101/4836	2.5 39/1533	2.7 39/1460	0.6 2/337	0.4 1/275	1.3 2/160	1.5 2/134	1.3 5/378	2.0 8/396
Nostrils anteverted	2.4 170/7124	2.6 57/2194	2.6 55/2097	1.7 8/467	2.3 10/445	2.7 6/225	1.1 2/185	1.9 12/618	2.3 15/664
Long nasal septum	2.5 175/7094	1.9 42/2187	2.0 42/2087	2.6 12/466	3.6 16/441	1.8 4/224	4.8 9/186	4.1 25/615	2.9 19/660
Epicanthal fold									
Left	3.5 248/7118	2.2 48/2193	2.8 58/2093	1.3 6/469	1.4 6/444	1.8 4/224	2.1 4/188	3.1 19/620	5.2 34/657
Right	3.2 227/7123	2.0 44/2194	2.2 45/2091	1.3 6/469	1.1 5/445	0.9 2/224	2.1 4/188	2.6 16/620	5.4 36/662
Both	2.5 181/7113	1.3 29/2192	1.6 33/2091	0.9 4/469	1.1 5/444	0.9 2/223	1.6 3/188	2.1 13/619	4.0 26/657

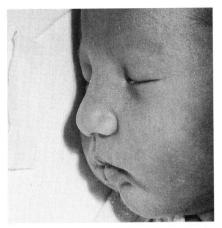

FIGURE 25.9   Prominent bridge of nose.

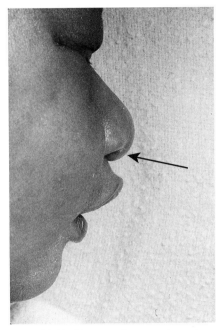

FIGURE 25.12   Long nasal septum. (arrow).

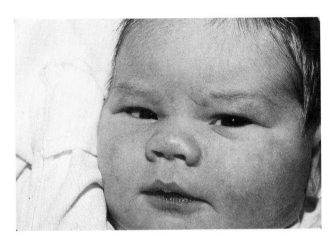

FIGURE 25.10   Anteverted nostrils—frontal view.

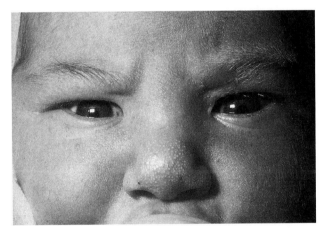

FIGURE 25.13   Epicanthal folds, both eyes.

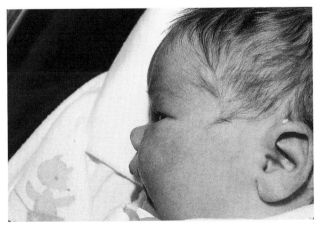

FIGURE 25.11   Lateral view shows depressed bridge of nose and upturned tip of nose.

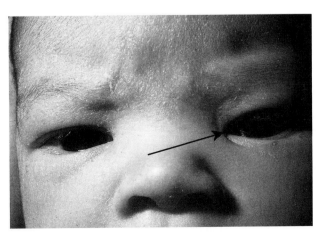

FIGURE 25.14   Epicanthal fold, Left eye. (arrow)

EYES

Ptosis: When the eyes are open voluntarily, the upper eyelid covers some of upper part of the pupil of the eye.

Brushfield spots: Clumps of white-yellow stroma; most often at 3 o'clock and 9 o'clock; should be at least 3 clumps present.

Iris stroma visible: Can identify iris separate from the lens.

Iris freckles: Brown discoloration on the surface iris (Figures 25-15 and 25-16).

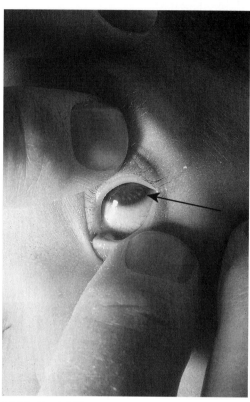

FIGURE 25.15   Brushfield spots. (arrow)

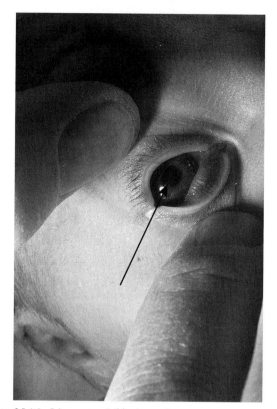

FIGURE 25.16   Iris stroma visible. (arrow)

TABLE 25-5 *Eyes*

Physical Feature	All Races	White		Black		Latin		Mixed Racial	
		Males	Females	Male	Female	Male	Female	Male	Female
Eyes Ptosis -									
Left	.04% 3/6835	0.5% 1/2123	0.5% 0/2028	0 0/452	0 0/415	0 0/209	0 0/179	0.2% 1/585	0 0/631
Right	.07 5/6832	0 0/2120	0.1 2/2023	0 0/449	0.2 0/418	0.5 1/207	0 0/179	0.2 1/588	0 0/628
Both	.03 2/6816	0 0/2116	0 0/2026	0 0/449	0.2 1/414	0 0/207	0 0/179	0.2 1/584	0 0/628
Brushfield Spots -									
Left	5.3% 370/7039	7.9% 171/2178	7.1% 148/2075	0 0/467	0.2% 1/433	1.4% 3/219	3.3% 6/183	3.8% 23/604	2.1% 14/658
Right	5.2 368/7022	7.8 169/2173	7.2 149/2071	0 0/464	0.2 1/435	1.4 3/217	3.3 6/182	4.0 24/605	1.8 12/653
Both	5.1 360/7009	7.7 166/2169	7.1 146/2069	0 0/464	0.2 1/432	1.4 3/217	3.3 6/182	3.7 22/602	1.8 12/652
Iris stroma visible	93.6 4488/4795	94.7 1450/1531	96.5 1391/1442	88.3 294/333	84.8 229/270	91.9 147/160	92.4 122/132	91.0 342/376	94.1 369/392
Iris freckles -									
Left	0.06% 3/4775	0.07% 1/1523	0.07% 1/1435	0 0/333	0 0/267	0 0/159	0.8% 0/132	0 0/373	0 0/392
Right	0.02 4/4757	0.07 1/1578	0 0/1431	0 0/330	0 0/269	0 0/157	0 0/131	0 0/373	0 0/388
Both	0.02 4/4757	0.07 1/1515	0 0/1429	0 0/330	0 0/266	0 0/157	0 0/131	0 0/372	0 0/388

MOUTH

Cleft lip microform: Scar on upper lip that extends from vermillion border of upper lip up toward nostril, which is same site as the most common type of cleft lip; the microform is a mild expression of the unilateral cleft lip deformity (Figure 25-17).

Cleft gum: A cleft up to at least the middle of the gum; always in middle of upper gum (Figure 25-18).

Cleft uvula: Midline cleft of uvula; this is difficult to see in a newborn, as the uvula is retracted upward when the infant cries.

Prominent gum: A subjective impression that the gum is much wider and taller than average.

Broad alveolar ridge: The palate tissue adjacent to the gum is wide, making the palate appear to be narrow and high.

Small chin: Size significantly less than the normal, small chin of newborn infants (Figures 25-19–25-21).

TABLE 25-6 *Mouth*

Physical Feature	All Races	White Males	White Females	Black Male	Black Female	Latin Male	Latin Female	Mixed Racial Male	Mixed Racial Female
Cleft lip microform	0.03% 2/7074	0 0/2176	0.05% 1/2085	0 0/464	0.2% 1/441	0 0/221	0 0/187	0 0/618	0 0/655
Cleft gum	0.2 11/4841	0.1 2/1538	0.1 2/1460	0 0/337	1.1 3/274	0 0/162	0 0/134	0 0/379	1.0 4/395
Cleft uvula	0.5 29/6137	0.5 10/1905	0.4 7/1788	0.8 3/398	0.5 2/387	0.5 1/190	0 0/170	0.6 3/535	0.4 2/563
Prominent gum	0.4 30/6927	0.6 13/2202	0.1 3/2102	1.0 5/470	0.2 1/449	0.9 2/225	0 0/189	0.5 3/624	0.5 3/666
Broad alveolar ridge	0.4 3/6927	0.05 1/2202	0.1 2/2102	0 0/470	0 0/449	0 0/225	0 0/189	0 0/624	0 0/666
Small chin	0.02 12/6927	0.3 7/220	0.2 4/2102	0 0/470	0 0/449	0 0/225	0 0/189	0.2 1/624	0 0/666

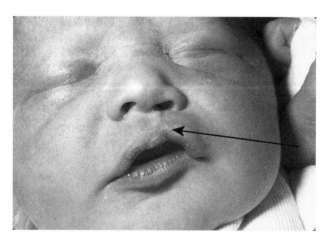

FIGURE 25.17 Cleft lip microform with deformity of left nostril. (arrow)

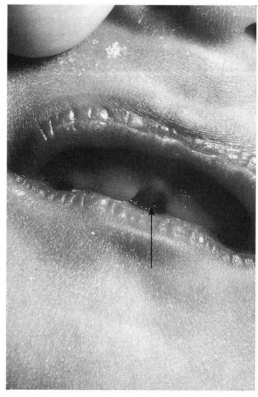

FIGURE 25.18 Cleft gum (upper) (arrow)

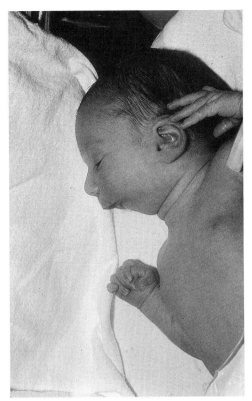

FIGURE 25.19   Small chin—severe.

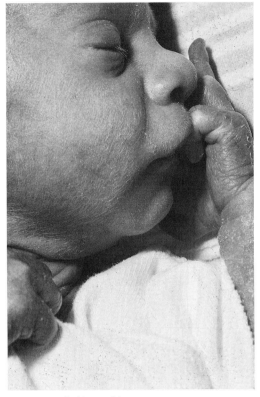

FIGURE 25.21   Small chin—mild.

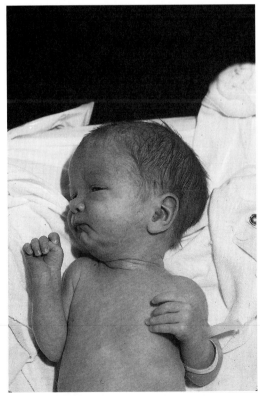

FIGURE 25.20   Small chin—moderate severity.

EAR

Preauricular skin tag: A skin-colored appendage located a few millimeters in front of or just above the tragus of the ear (Figure 25-22 and 25-23).

Skin tag on ear lobe: The appendage is located on the lobe itself (Figure 25-24 and 25-25).

Skin tags elsewhere: These tags occur most often on the face, primarily on the cheek along a line between the corner of the mouth and the tragus of the ear.

Preauricular sinus: A tiny (1to 2 mm diameter) round opening without any associated redness or exudate;

ends blindly; usually located on most anterior end of helix, near site of attachment to scalp.

Darwinian tubercle: Firm, discrete, skin-colored nodule protruding posteriorly at upper posterior edge of helix; usually a 3 to 4 mm wide (Figure 25-30A and 25-30B).

Darwinian point: A point in the helical fold directed anteriorly and located usually at junction of the upper and middle thirds of the helix (Figure 25-25).

TABLE 25-7 *Ear*

Physical Feature	All Races	White		Black		Latin		Mixed Racial	
		Males	Females	Male	Female	Male	Female	Male	Female
Preauricular skin tag									
Left	0.5% 32/7149	0.3% 6/2201	0.4% 8/2099	0.6% 3/469	0.7% 3/448	0.4% 1/225	1.1% 2/189	1.0% 6/622	0.3% 2/666
Right	0.4 31/7152	0.2 5/2201	0.7 15/2101	0 0/470	0.2 1/448	0 0/225	0.5 1/189	0.6 4/623	0.2 1/665
Both	0.07 5/7147	0.05 1/2200	0.1 2/2099	0 0/469	0 0/448	0 0/225	0 0/189	0.2 1/622	0 0/665
Skin tag on ear lobe									
Left	0.2 12/6820	0.3 6/2103	0.1 2/2024	0 0/449	0.2 1/423	0 0/212	0 0/181	0.2 1/580	0 0/625
Right	0.2 11/6819	0.3 6/2103	0.1 2/2023	0 0/450	0.2 1/423	0 0/212	0 0/181	0.2 1/580	0 0/625
Both	0.07 5/6818	0.1 3/2103	0 0/2023	0 0/449	0.2 1/423	0 0/212	0 0/181	0.2 1/580	0 0/625
Skin tags elsewhere									
Left	0.4 25/6821	0.5 10/2102	0.4 9/2025	0 0/450	0.5 2/423	0 0/212	0 0/181	0.2 1/581	0.2 1/625
Right	0.2 10/6821	0.3 6/2103	0.2 3/2025	0 0/450	0 0/423	0 0/212	0 0/181	0.2 1/580	0 0/625
Both	0.04 3/6820	0.1 2/2102	0.05 1/2025	0 0/450	0 0/423	0 0/212	0 0/181	0 0/580	0 0/625

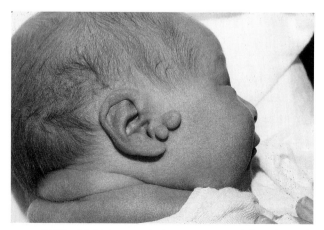

FIGURE 25.22 Multiple preauricular tags in same infant shown in Figure 25.23.

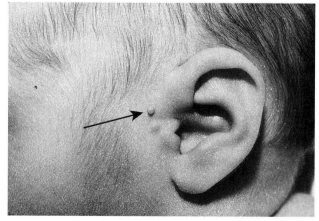

FIGURE 25.23 Single preauricular tag (arrow) in the same infant shown in Figure 25.22.

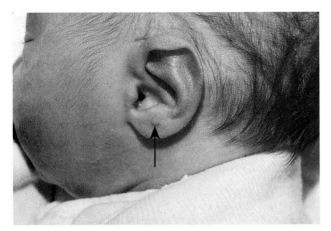

FIGURE 25.24   Skin tag on ear lobe (arrow).

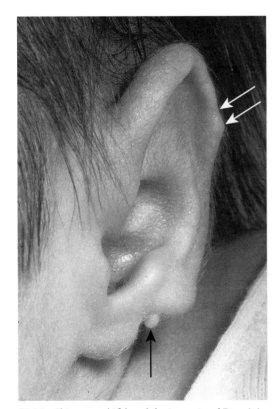

FIGURE 25.25   Skin tag on bifid ear lobe (arrow) and Darwinian point on helix (double arrow).

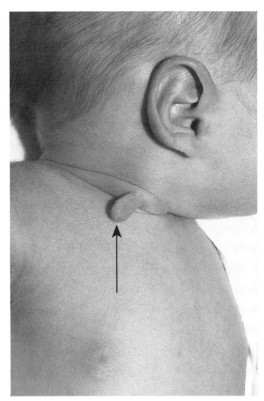

FIGURE 25.26   Skin tag on neck (arrow).

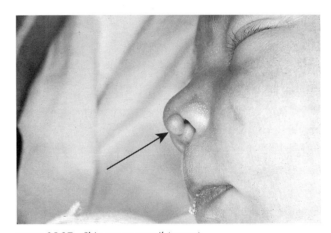

FIGURE 25.27   Skin tag on nostril (arrow).

TABLE 25-8 *Ear*

Physical Feature	All Races	White		Black		Latin		Mixed Racial	
		Males	Females	Male	Female	Male	Female	Male	Female
Preauricular Sinus									
Left	0.9% 61/7149	0.1% 3/2201	0.5% 11/2099	2.8% 13/470	2.5% 11/447	0.9% 2/225	0.5% 1/189	1.8% 11/622	1.1% 7/666
Right	1.0 68/7152	0.3 6/2202	0.7 14/2101	2.3 11/470	3.6 16/447	0.9 2/225	1.6 3/189	1.0 6/623	1.4 9/665
Both	0.4 27/7148	0.05 1/2201	0.2 4/2099	1.1 5/470	1.3 6/447	0.4 1/225	0.5 1/189	0.8 5/622	0.5 3/665
Darwinian Tubercle									
Left	0.3 18/7119	0.2 5/2193	0.2 4/2093	0 0/469	0 0/442	0.9 2/224	0 0/189	0.3 2/620	0.6 4/660
Right	0.4 31/7117	0.6 14/2194	0.6 13/2090	0 0/468	0.2 1/442	0.5 1/224	0 0/189	0 0/620	0.3 2/661
Both	0.03 2/7114	0.05 1/2193	0 0/2090	0 0/468	0 0/492	0 0/224	0 0/189	0 0/620	0 0/659
Darwinian Point									
Left	0.9 54/6162	1.3 24/1927	0.8 15/1842	0 0/409	1.0 0/361	1.0 2/196	0.6 1/164	1.0 5/518	0.6 3/546
Right	1.1 66/6157	1.8 35/1927	0.7 12/1840	0 0/409	0 0/360	1.0 2/195	0.6 1/164	1.4 7/518	0.9 5/545
Both	0.1 8/6157	0.2 4/1927	0.05 1/1840	0 0/409	0 0/360	0 0/195	0 0/164	0.4 2/518	0 0/545

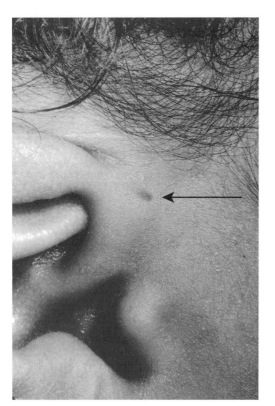

FIGURE 25.28   Preauricular sinus (arrow), black infant.

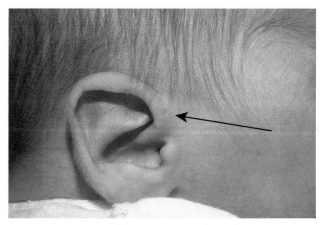

FIGURE 25.29   Preauricular sinus (arrow), white infant.

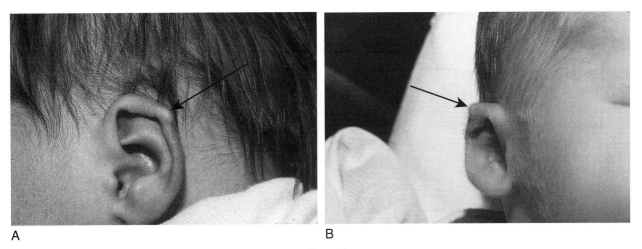

A B

FIGURE 25.30A & 25-30B   Darwinian tubercle (arrow) in two newborn infants.

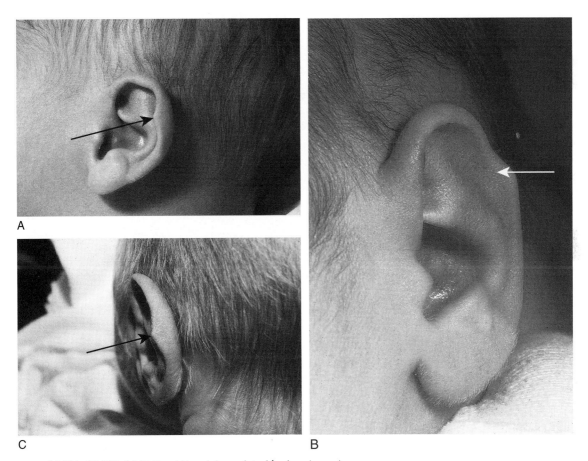

A

C B

FIGURE 25.31A, 25-31B, 25-31C   a) Darwinian point, side view. (arrow)
b) Darwinian point, frontal view. (arrow)
c) Darwinian point, posterior view. (three different infants) (arrow)

EAR

Helix overfolded: Top of ear has helical fold bent down, often with fold crease at upper corner of helix (Figures 25-32 and 25-33) .

Excess helix tissue folded over: Involves upper portion of helix (Figures 25-34 and 25-35).

Elf ear: Ear has pointed shape at upper corner of helix, the junction between the upper (horizontal) and vertical portions of helix (Figures 25-36–25-37).

Lack of helical fold: No turning over of edge of helix (Figures 25-38 and 25-39).

Lack of helical fold on top only: The fold of helix is present along vertical portion of helix, but not at top of helix (Figures 25-40).

Interrupted helical fold: No fold of helix at junction between upper and vertical portions of helix (Figures 25-41 and 25-42).

Lack of helical fold opposite tragus: No fold of helix in lower part of vertical portion of helix, an area at same level as the tragus of the ear (Figure 25-43).

TABLE 25-9 *Ear*

Physical Feature	All Races	White		Black		Latin		Mixed Racial	
		Males	Females	Male	Female	Male	Female	Male	Female
Helix Overfolded									
Left	39.9% 2856/7150	36.6% 810/2200	39.1% 822/2101	53.8% 253/470	48.2% 215/446	41.3% 93/225	41.5% 78/188	38.5% 240/624	38.7% 258/666
Right	36.3 2597/7148	34.3 754/2201	35.4 743/2099	48.9 230/470	45.3 202/446	32.9 74/225	30.9 58/188	35.0 218/623	35.3 235/666
Both	29.5 2107/7146	27.0 549/2200	28.6 599/2098	43.2 203/470	39.5 176/446	28.0 63/225	25.0 47/188	27.9 174/623	28.0 188/666
Excess helix tissue, folded over	0.01 1/7152	0 0/2202	0.05 1/2102	0 0/470	0 0/449	0 0/225	0 0/189	0 0/625	0 0/660
ELF EAR									
Left	0.3 13/5129	0.3 5/1619	0.06 1/1540	1.1 4/352	0.3 1/292	0 0/168	0 0/139	0 0/414	0.2 1/432
Right	0.2 8/5130	0.6 1/1619	0.2 3/1540	0.9 3/352	0 0/292	0 0/168	0 0/139	0 0/415	0 1/432
Both	0.04 2/5129	0 0/1619	0.6 1/1540	0 0/352	0 0/292	0 0/168	0 0/139	0 0/414	0 0/432

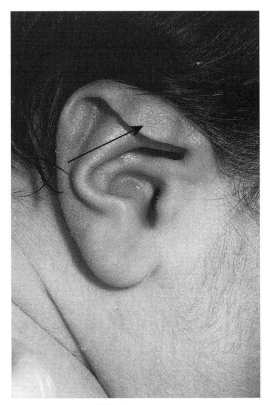

FIGURE 25.32   Helix overfolded (arrow).

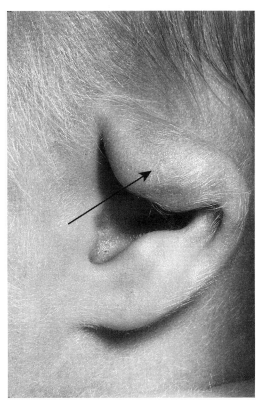

FIGURE 25.34   Excess helical tissue folded over (arrow).

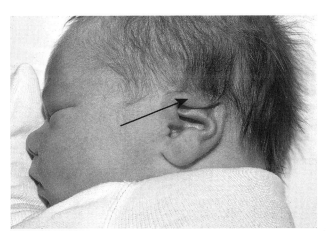

FIGURE 25.33   Helix overfolded (arrow).

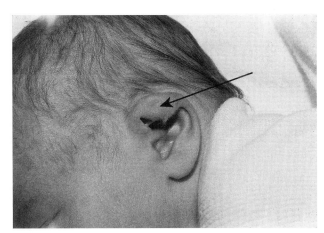

FIGURE 25.35   Excess helical tissue folded over (arrow).

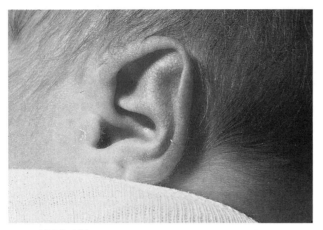

FIGURE 25.36 Elf ear.

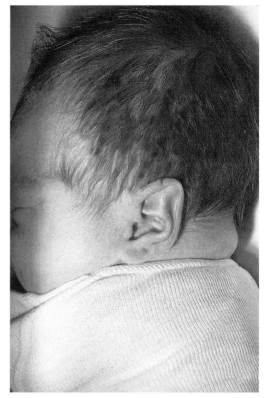

FIGURE 25.37 Elf ear.

TABLE 25-10 *Ear*

		White		Black		Latin		Mixed Racial	
Physical Feature	All Races	Males	Females	Male	Female	Male	Female	Male	Female
Lack of helical fold									
Left	0.3	0.4	0.3	0	0.3	0	0	0	0.5
	14/5142	6/1626	5/1543	0/353	1/291	0/170	0/139	0/414	2/432
Right	0.3	0.4	0.2	0.3	0.3	0.6	0	0	0.5
	15/1549	7/1629	3/1545	1/353	1/292	1/170	0/139	0/414	2/433
Both	0.2	0.3	0.1	0	0.3	0	0	0	0.5
	10/5142	5/1626	2/1543	0/353	1/291	0/170	0/139	0/414	2/432
Lack of helical fold on top only									
Left	1.8	1.8	1.6	1.7	0.9	3.6	1.6	1.9	1.5
	125/7138	39/2196	34/2100	8/469	4/447	8/223	3/188	12/624	10/661
Right	1.5	2.0	0.8	0.9	1.1	4.0	0.5	2.9	1.1
	108/7138	43/2197	17/2096	4/469	5/447	9/223	1/188	18/624	7/664
Both	0.9	1.1	0.6	0.4	0.2	3.1	0.5	1.1	0.6
	63/7132	25/2196	13/2095	2/469	1/447	7/223	1/188	7/624	4/660
Interrupted helical fold									
Left	8.5	8.8	7.3	10.4	8.4	11/3	12/5	9.5	7.9
	412/4834	135/1533	107/1458	35/336	23/274	18/160	17/136	36/379	31/395
Right	6.4	7.4	5.5	5.4	6.9	7.5	8.8	6.6	4.8
	307/4837	114/1532	80/1461	18/336	19/274	12/160	12/136	25/379	19/396
Both	3.0	3.2	2.6	3.0	4.0	3.8	5.9	2.9	2.3
	144/4833	49/1532	38/1458	10/336	11/274	6/160	8/136	11/379	9/395
Lack of helical fold opposite tragus									
Left	4.7	4.1	5.5	3.6	5.2	5.0	3.7	5.3	5.0
	335/7101	89/2186	144/2090	17/469	23/442	11/222	7/189	33/620	33/660
Right	3.1	2.7	3.1	2.1	3.4	5.4	3.2	4.0	3.3
	220/7109	58/2187	65/2090	10/468	15/442	12/222	6/189	25/620	22/662
Both	1.7	1.2	1.9	0.9	2.0	2.3	2.1	2.4	2.1
	120/7103	26/2185	39/2088	4/468	9/442	5/222	4/189	15/620	14/660

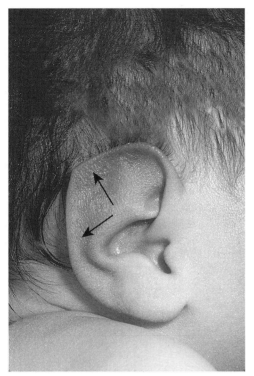

FIGURE 25.38 Lack of helical fold (arrow).

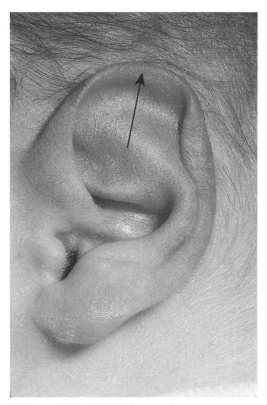

FIGURE 25.40 Lack of helical fold at top of ear (arrow).

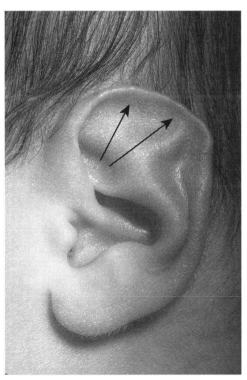

FIGURE 25.39 Lack of helical fold at top of ear (arrow).

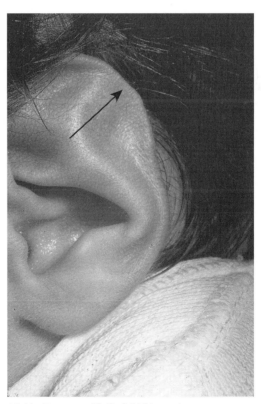

FIGURE 25.41 Interrupted helical fold (arrow).

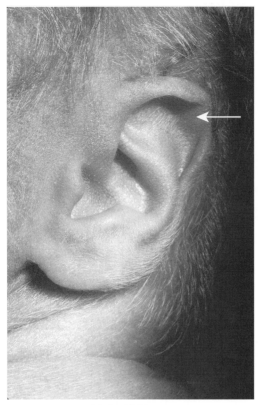

FIGURE 25.42   Interrupted helical fold (arrow).

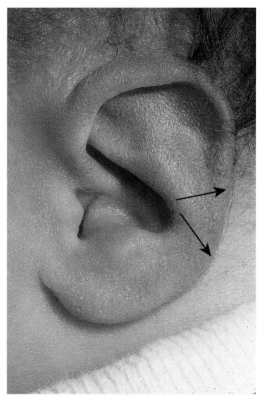

FIGURE 25.43   Lack of helical fold opposite tragus (arrows).

Ear lobe notched: Lobe interrupted; tissue missing (Figure 25-44).

Ear lobe cleft: Cleft in lobe (Figures 25-45 and 25-46).

Sinus on ear lobe: Has same appearance as preauricular sinus (Figures 25-47 and 25-48).

Sinus on back of helix: Tiny opening(s) without swelling (Figures 25-49).

Lop ear: Prominent ear with outward protrusion of the upper and lower portions of the pinna(or helix) (Figures 25-50 and 25-51).

Cup-shaped ear: An outward protrusion of the pinna with the upper and lower ends appearing to be squeezed toward each other (Figures 25-52 and 25-53).

Helix attached to scalp: An additional point of attachment with the upper edge of the helix (Figures 25-54).

TABLE 25-11 *Ear*

Physical Feature	All Races	White Males	Females	Black Male	Female	Latin Male	Female	Mixed Racial Male	Female
Ear lobe Notched									
Left	0.2% 9/4842	0 0/1538	0.3% 4/1458	0 0/337	0.4% 1/277	0.6% 1/160	0.8% 1/134	0 0/380	0.3% 1/395
Right	0.1 6/4842	0 0/1537	0.3 0/1459	0.3 1/337	0 0/277	0 0/160	0 0/134	0.3 1/380	0 0/395
Both	0 0/4841	0 0/1537	0 0/1458	0 0/337	0 0/277	0 0/160	0 0/134	0 0/380	0 0/395
Ear lobe Cleft	0.3 2/7152	1/2202	/2102	0 0/470	0 0/449	0 0/225	0 0/189	0 0/625	0 0/660
Sinus on ear lobe	0.06 4/7152	0. 2/2202	/2102	1/470	/449	1/225	/189	0 0/625	0 0/660
Sinus on back of helix	0.01 1/7152	1/2202	/2102	0 0/470	0 0/449	0 0/225	0 0/189	0 0/625	0 0/660
Lop ear									
Left	0.3 22/7111	0.2 5/2187	0.6 12/2093	0 0/468	0 0/443	0.5 1/222	0 0/189	0.2 1/620	0.3 2/660
Right	0.3 18/7111	0.2 5/2187	0.5 11/2093	0 0/468	0 443	0.5 1/222	0 0/189	0 0/620	0 0/660
Both	0.2 11/7110	0.1 3/2186	0.3 7/2093	0 0/468	0 0/443	0 0/222	0/189	0/620	0/660
Cup-shaped									
Left	0.2 12/6822	0.1 1/2104	0.3 5/2026	0.4 2/450	0.2 1/423	0 0/212	0 1/181	0 1/580	0.2 1/624
Right	0.1 6/6821	0.1 2/2103	0.2 3/2026	0.2 1/450	0 0/423	0 0/212	0 0/181	0 1/580	0 1/624
Both	0.4 3/6821	0 0/2103	0.1 2/2024	0.2 1/450	0 0/423	0 0/212	0 0/181	0 0/580	0 0/624
Helix attached to scalp	.01 1/7152	/2202	2102	0 0/470	0 0/449	0 0/225	0 0/189	0 0/625	0 0/660

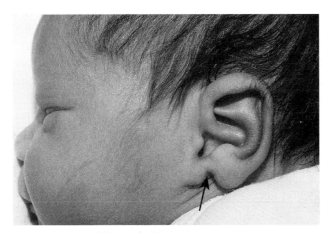

FIGURE 25.44   Ear lobe notched (arrow).

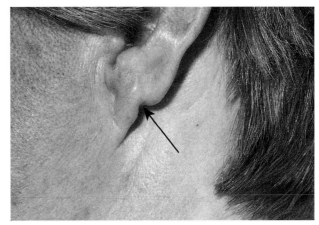

FIGURE 25.45   Ear lobe cleft (arrow).

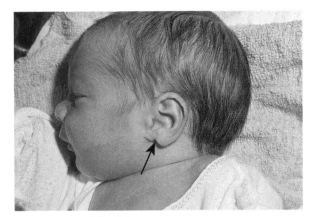

FIGURE 25.46   Ear lobe cleft (arrow).

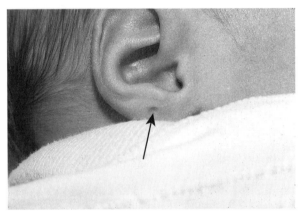

FIGURE 25.47   Sinus on lower portion of helix (arrow).

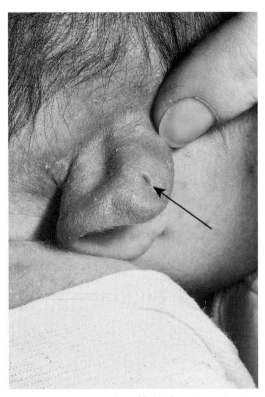

FIGURE 25.49   Sinus edge of behind ear (arrow).

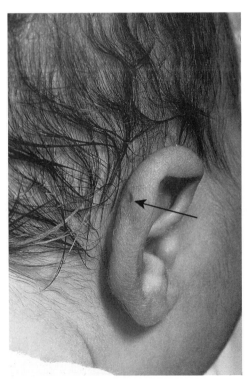

FIGURE 25.48   Sinus on edge of helix (arrow).

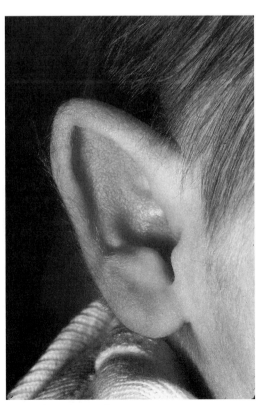

FIGURE 25.50   Prominent or lop ear.

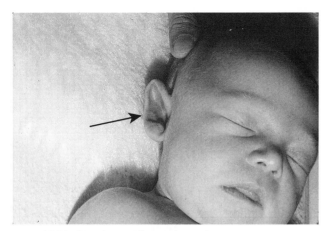

FIGURE 25.51 Prominent or lop ear (arrow).

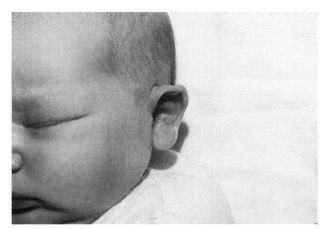

FIGURE 25.52 Cup-shaped ear.

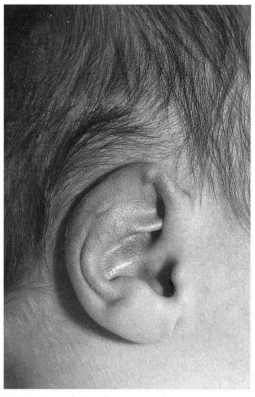

FIGURE 25.54 Upper helix adherent to scalp.

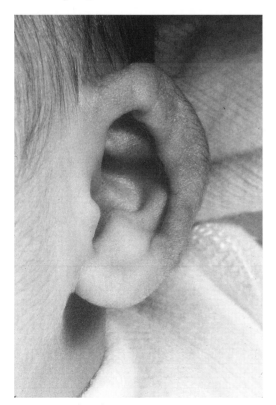

FIGURE 25.53 Cup-shaped ear.

Bridged concha: The bridge higher than normal and up to the level of the anterior portion of the helix (Figures 25-55 and 25-56).

Tragus absent: Not present.

Tragus bifid: The tragus is bifurcated or split in the middle.

Ear lobe present: The soft tissue falls below the lower point of attachment of the helix.

Ear lobe crease: A deep linear groove, not a fold or dent.

TABLE 25-12 *Ear*

Physical Feature	All Races	White		Black		Latin		Mixed Racial	
		Males	Females	Male	Female	Male	Female	Male	Female
Bridged Concha									
Left	0.7% 35/4830	0.7% 11/1533	0.4% 6/1455	1.5% 5/335	1.1% 3/275	0.6% 1/161	0 0/134	1.1% 4/379	0.3% 1/395
Right	1.1 52/4830	1.0 15/1532	1.0 14/1457	1.5 5/337	0.7 2/274	1.3 2/160	1.5 2/134	1.9 7/379	0.3 1/394
Both	0.3 15/4825	0.3 4/1531	0.1 2/1455	0.3 1/335	0.7 2/274	0.6 1/160	0 0/134	0.8 3/379	0.3 1/394
Tragus absent	.01 1/7152	1/2202	0/2102	0 0/470	0 0/499	0 0/225	0 0/189	0 0/625	0 0/660
Tragus bifid	.01 1/7152	1/2202	/2102	0 0/470	0 0/419	0 0/225	0 0/189	0 0/625	0 0/660
Ear lobe Absent									
Left	96.3 6890/7152	97.1 2136/2200	96.2 2022/2102	95.1 446/469	96.2 431/448	98.2 221/225	96.8 183/189	96.3 600/623	94.9 631/665
Right	96.3 6872/7138	96.9 2132/2200	96.4 2022/2097	94.9 445/469	95.3 425/446	98.7 222/225	95.7 180/188	96.0 597/622	94.9 627/661
Both	95.5 6814/7135	96.2 2115/2199	95.5 2002/2097	94.4 442/468	94.6 422/446	98.2 221/225	94.7 178/188	95.5 593/621	94.1 622/611
Ear lobe Crease									
Left	0.5 37/7117	0.6 14/2194	0.4 9/2092	0.4 2/469	0.9 4/443	0.5 1/224	0 0/188	0.7 4/618	0.3 2/660
Right	0.9 65/7116	0.9 20/2193	1.0 21/2092	0.6 3/469	0.9 4/443	0.5 1/224	1.6 3/188	1.1 7/618	0.5 3/660
Both	0.3 19/7116	0.3 6/2193	0.2 4/2092	0.2 1/469	0.5 2/443	0 0/224	0 0/188	0.7 4/618	0.2 1/660

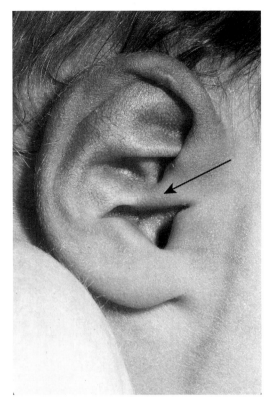

FIGURE 25.55   Bridged concha (arrow).

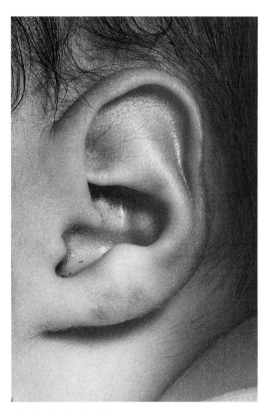

FIGURE 25.57   Lack of ear lobe.

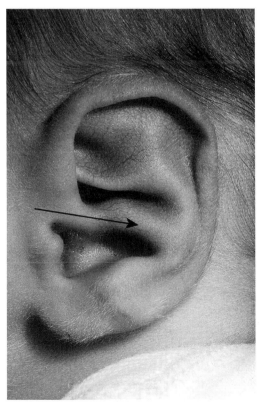

FIGURE 25.56   Bridged concha (arrow).

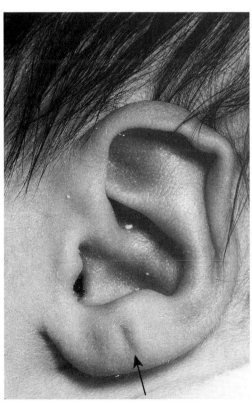

FIGURE 25.58   Dent in ear lobe (arrow).

NECK/CHEST

Webbed neck: Taunt, readily visible ridge of skin that follows the course of the trapezius muscle (Figures 25-59).

Excess neck folds: Redundant folds, significantly more than occurs in the normal infant (Figures 25-60).

Branchial sinus: 1 millimeter sinus opening, usually along anterior edge of sternocleidomastoid muscle on either or both sides of the neck (Figures 25-61).

Extra nipples: Darkly pigmented, elevated tissue; usually not swollen in response to maternal estrogen stimulation; located along the "nipple line "from axilla to groin (Figures 25-63).

Areolar skin tag: Appendage 3–4 millimeters long and 1–2 millimeters wide on areola (Figures 25-64 and 25-65).

Xiphoid bifid: Two separate tips of the xiphoid process are palpable.

Xiphoid not palpable: Not felt when palpating in the region of xiphoid at the lwer end of the sternum.

ABDOMEN

Diastasis recti: A midline protrusion of skin that can be seen with crying (Figure 25-66).

Single umbilical artery: Only two vessels can be seen (1 artery, 1 vein).

Umbilical hernia: A significant protrusion around the umbilical cord (Figures 25-67 and 25-68).

TABLE 25-13 *Neck, Chest and Abdomen*

Physical Feature	All Races	White		Black		Latin		Mixed Racial	
		Males	Females	Male	Female	Male	Female	Male	Female
NECK									
Webbed	0.08% 6/7131	0.05% 1/2916	0.1% 2/2098	0.2% 1/466	0.2% 1/447	0 0/222	0 0/188	0 0/621	0.2% 1/664
Excess neck folds	0.6 39/7142	0.6 13/2202	0.7 14/2100	0.2 1/467	0.7 3/447	0.4 1/225	0 0/188	0.5 3/621	0.6 4/663
Branchial sinus	0.3 2/7112	0 0/2194	0 0/2092	0 0/466	0 2/443	0 0/224	0 0/188	0.2 1/617	0 0/660
CHEST									
Extra nipples									
Left	0.5 34/7144	0.1 2/2202	0.3 6/2099	1.5 7/467	2.5 11/447	0.9 2/225	0 0/188	0.2 1/622	0.5 3/665
Right	0.6 40/7140	0.5 10/2200	0.1 2/2098	2.6 12/466	2.2 10/447	0.9 2/225	0.5 1/188	0.3 2/622	0.2 1/665
Both	0.1 7/7140	0.05 1/2200	0.05 1/2098	0.2 1/466	0.7 3/447	0.4 1/225	0 0/188	0 0/622	0 0/665
Areolar skin Tag									
Left	0.3 20/6820	0.2 4/2103	0.4 8/2025	0.4 2/450	0 0/423	1.4 3/212	0.6 1/181	0.3 2/580	0 0/624
Right	0.3 20/6820	0.3 7/2103	0.2 3/2025	0 0/450	0 0/423	0.5 1/212	0 0/181	0.3 2/580	0.2 1/624
Both	0 0/6820	0 0/2103	0 0/2025	0 0/450	0 0/423	0 0/212	0 0/181	0 0/580	0 0/624
Xiphoid bifid	19.6 1199/6261	19.2 375/1955	22.4 422/1882	6.6 27/411	13.4 50/374	13.2 26/197	22.0 36/164	19.4 101/521	22.6 126/558
Xiphoid not palpable	0.8 55/6815	1.0 20/2111	0.6 13/2055	0.5 2/447	0.5 2/422	0.5 1/211	1.7 3/180	1.0 6/578	1.0 6/620
ABDOMEN									
Diastasis	34.1 2405/7054	33.2 726/2187	32.9 683/2074	41.3 190/460	39.7 174/438	35.8 78/218	30.5 57/187	34.2 209/613	35.9 234/652
Single umbilical artery	0.3 17/5523	0.2 4/1740	0.3 4/1599	0.3 1/371	0 0/328	0 0/177	0.7 1/143	0.8 4/485	0.4 2/511
Umbilical hernia	1.7 117/6759	0.3 7/2096	1.2 23/1996	4.3 19/440	8.8 37/420	0.9 2/214	2.2 4/180	1.6 9/579	2.3 14/620

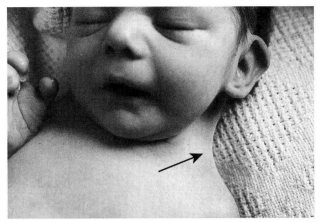

FIGURE 25.59 Webbed neck (arrow) in infant with 45,X (Turner) Syndrome.

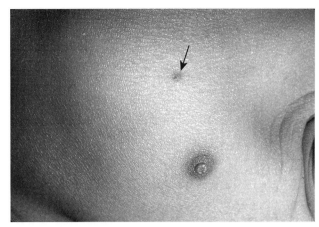

FIGURE 25.62 Accessory nipple (arrow).

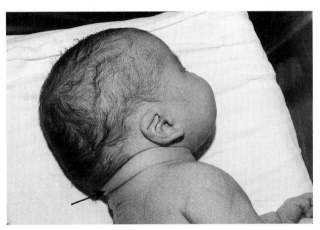

FIGURE 25.60 Excess skin folds on neck (arrow).

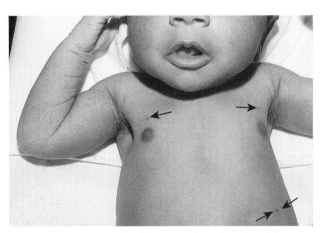

FIGURE 25.63 Extra nipples above normal nipple and in abdomen.

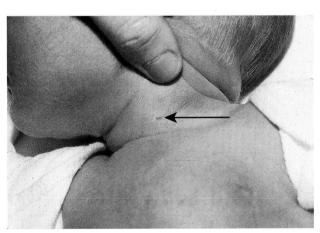

FIGURE 25.61 Branchial cleft sinus in neck. (arrow)

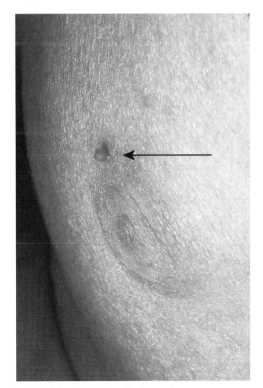

FIGURE 25.64 Skin tag near areola. (arrow)

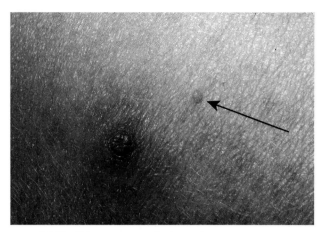

FIGURE 25.65   Skin tag near areola. (arrow)

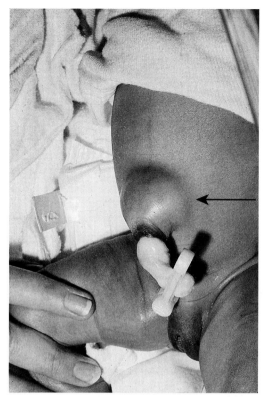

FIGURE 25.67   Umbilical hernia. (arrow)

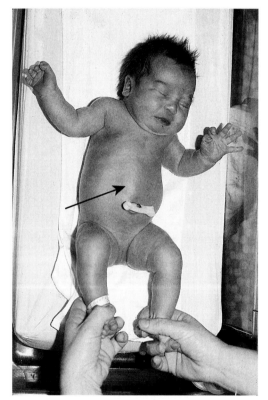

FIGURE 25.66   Protrusion of skin over diastasis in abdominal muscles. (arrow)

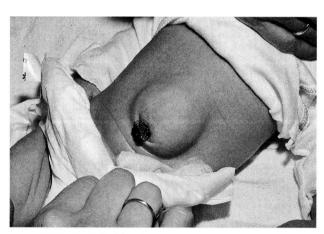

FIGURE 25.68   Umbilical hernia.

GENITALS—MALE

Testis in scrotum: Palpable in the scrotum.

Testis in groin: Palpable in upper portion of the scrotum.

Hypospadias, coronal (first degree; 1°): Urethra located at lower edge of glans penis, at "six o'clock" (Figures 25-69 and 25-70).

Hypospadias, penis (second degree; 2°): Urethral opening in midline along underside of shaft. (This is obviously not a minor anomaly but is included here for comparison.)

Chordee: Abnormal degree of downward curve and fixation of penis caused by excessive band of tissue along midline (Figures 25-71).

Epispadias: Urethral opening at upper edge of glans penis, at "12 o'clock".

Scrotum -up-on-penis: Skin of scrotum attaches to penis further along shaft than normal (Figures 25-72 and 25-73).

GENITALS—FEMALE

Labia majora divided: Separation between the upper ends of the labia at the attachment to mons pubis.

Labia minora prominent: More easily seen than normal, especially when labia majora small.

Vaginal tag: An accessory piece of tissue from the mucosa of the vagina.

TABLE 25-14 *Genitals – Male and Female*

Physical Feature	All Races	White		Black		Latin		Mixed Racial	
		Males	Females	Male	Female	Male	Female	Male	Female
GENITALS–MALE									
Testis in Scrotum									
Left	91.9% 3304/3596	92.1% 2004/2176	-	91.6% 428/469	-	90.6% 203/224	-	92.2% 567/615	-
Right	92.0 3306/3595	92.2 2006/2175	-	90.8 426/469	-	90.2 202/224	-	92.7 570/615	
Both									
Testis in groin									
Left	5.8 141/2448	5.4 85/1511	-	8.4 28/335	-	8.8 14/160	-	2.7 10/368	-
Right	5.5 135/2447	5.2 79/1510	-	8.1 27/335	-	8.8 14/160	-	2.2 8/368	-
Both									
Hypospadias, Coronal (1°)	.7 23/3383	0.6 13/2022	-	0.5 2/449	-	0.5 1/218	-	0.9 5/584	-
Chordee	.5 17/3202	0.5 9/1918	-	0.7 3/430	-	0 0/206	-	0.9 5/541	-
Epispadias	.06 2/3203	0.00 1/1922	-	0.2 1/429	-	0 0/205	-	0 0/540	
Scrotum-up-on-penis	2.8 94/3412	3.0 62/2039	-	0.9 4/453	-	1.4 3/218	-	3.1 18/590	
Saddle scotum	8.9 29/327	10.8 24/223	-	4.2 2/47	-	2.9 1/35	-	9.0 2/22	
GENITALS-FEMALE									
Labia majora divided	15.5 365/2354	-	13.2 192/1459	-	26.6 68/276	-	22.4 30/134	-	13.9 55/396
Labia minora prominent	7.2 250/3492	-	6.0 126/2088	-	12.0 53/422	-	7.9 15/189	-	6.9 45/657
Vaginal tag	4.0 141/3494	-	3.3 68/2088	-	5.2 23/443	-	5.3 10/189	-	4.4 29/658

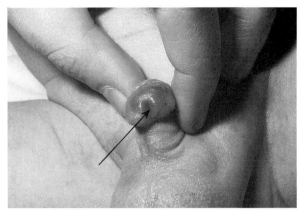

FIGURE 25.69   Glandular hypospadias with opening of urethra at lower edge of glans penis.

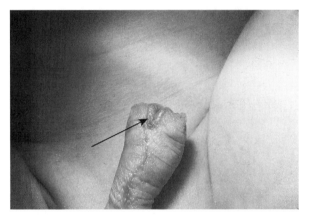

FIGURE 25.70   Glandular hypospadias with opening of urethra at lower edge of glans penis.

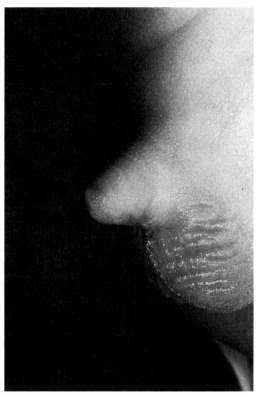

FIGURE 25.72   Scrotum-up-on-penis.

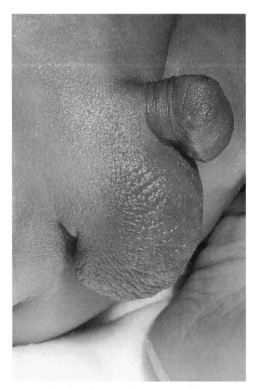

FIGURE 25.71   Chordee; downward curvature of penis.

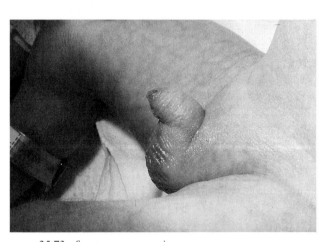

FIGURE 25.73   Scrotum-up-on-penis.

BACK

Sacral dimple: Not a sinus tract, but a midline depression in the skin and bone over upper sacrum; not the same as dimple over sacrum.

Pilonidal sinus: A pinpoint tract in the midline; the bottom cannot be seen.

Dimple over sacrum: A pinpoint depression, usually bilateral and on each side of the midline, typically at the level of the iliac crest (Figures 25-74–25-76).

TABLE 25-15 *Back*

| Physical Feature | All Races | White | | Black | | Latin | | Mixed Racial | |
		Males	Females	Male	Female	Male	Female	Male	Female
Sacral dimple	4.4%	4.9%	5%	1.5%	0.7%	3.2%	2.7%	4.7%	5.5%
	313/7108	108/2189	105/2092	7/465	3/444	7/222	5/188	29/620	36/658
Pilonidal sinus	0.4	0.8	0.1	0	0.2	0	0	0.9	0.2
	26/6825	17/2106	2/2024	0/451	1/424	0/215	0/181	5/579	1/623

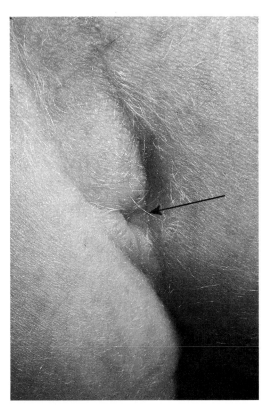

FIGURE 25.74   Sacral dimple (arrow).

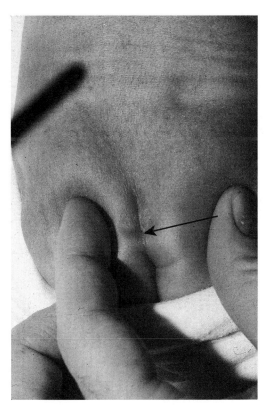

FIGURE 25.75   Sacral dimple (arrow).

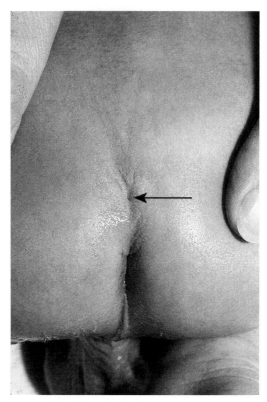

FIGURE 25.76   Pilonidal sinus (arrow).

ARM

Cubitus valgus: With the elbow fully extended, the forearm deviates laterally to a significant degree from the center of the upper arm.

Clinodactyly: Inward (radial) curvature of significant degree, which when measured is three to four degrees from midline of the third finger (Figures 25-77 and 25-78).

Thumb retroflexible: The distal phalanx of the thumb can be extended to an unusual degree at the interphalangeal joint.

Tapered fingers: Marked and progressive proximal-to-distal decrease in size of fingers (Figures 25-79).

Overlapping fingers: With the hand at rest, one finger crosses over another (Figures 25-79–25-81).

Fingernails hypoplastic: Nails much smaller than average size (Figures 25-80 and 25-81).

Fingernails hyperconvex: Nails have a downward extension at each edge and a more convex shape when viewed from the tip (Figures 25-82 and 25-83).

Dimple over bone: Pinpoint depression in soft tissue; not a sinus tract (Figures 25-84 and 25-85).

TABLE 25-16 *Arm, Hand and Dimples*

Physical Feature	All Races	White		Black		Latin		Mixed Racial	
		Males	Females	Male	Female	Male	Female	Male	Female
ARM									
Cubitus valgus	0.1% 8/6588	0.05% 1/2045	0.05% 1/1959	0.2% 1/431	0.8% 3/394	0 0/207	0 0/176	0 0/566	0 2/602
HAND									
Clinodactyly fifth finger									
Left	8.0 571/7140	9.1 201/2198	7.1 149/2100	8.5 40/469	5.8 26/445	11.6 26/224	5.3 10/189	7.9 49/621	8.0 53/665
Right	6.3 452/7137	7.5 165/2198	5.2 109/2100	6.2 29/467	4.3 19/445	9.3 21/225	6.4 12/189	6.1 38/621	7.1 47/664
Both	5.4 384/7135	6.2 137/2198	4.6 97/2100	5.1 24/467	3.6 16/444	8.5 19/224	4.2 8/189	5.2 32/621	5.9 39/664
Thumb retro-flexible									
Left	22.4 1526/6829	23.5 495/2108	21.5 436/2024	17.6 79/450	19.1 81/425	27.5 58/211	24.2 44/182	25.6 148/578	22.6 142/628
Right	21.0 1436/6827	22.2 467/2107	19.8 401/2024	16.5 74/449	22.1 85/424	25.9 55/212	21.2 40/182	25.1 142/578	21.0 132/628
Both	19.3 1319/6825	20.3 427/2107	18.3 370/2023	14.7 66/449	17.5 74/424	24.6 52/211	20.9 38/182	22.8 132/578	22.2 127/628
Tapered fingers	0.4 27/7142	0.3 7/2198	0.4 9/2100	0.2 1/469	0.2 1/446	0.4 1/225	0 0/189	0.8 5/621	0.5 3/665
Overlapping fingers									
Left	0.06 4/7112	0 0/2193	0 0/2091	0 0/469	0.22 1/442	0 0/223	0.5 1/189	0 0/617	0.2 1/660
Right	0.07 5/7108	0 0/2192	0.1 0/2091	0 0/467	0.23 1/441	0 0/224	0.5 1/189	0 0/617	0.2 1/660
Both	0.06 4/7107	0 0/2192	0 0/2091	0 0/467	0.5 2/441	0 0/223	0.5 1/189	0 0/617	0.2 1/660
Fingernails hypoplastic	0.3 20/7112	0.2 5/2192	0.3 7/2092	0.2 1/468	0.5 2/442	0 0/224	0 0/189	0.5 3/617	0.3 2/660
Fingernails hyperconvex	1.2 87/7110	1.5 33/2191	0.8 17/2092	1.7 8/468	0.9 4/442	2.2 5/224	2.7 5/189	1.0 6/617	0.8 5/660
DIMPLE									
Over bone	0.2 16/7144	0.3 7/2098	0.2 4/2100	0.2 1/469	0.2 1/446	0 0/225	0 0/189	0.32 2/622	0.2 1/666
On shoulder	0.04 3/7147	0.05 1/2200	0.05 1/2102	0 0/468	0.2 1/446	0 0/225	0 0/189	0 0/622	0 0/666
Over sacrum	0.7 5/7149	0.1 3/2201	0.05 1/2102	0 0/469	0 0/446	0 0/225	0 0/189	0.16 1/622	0 0/666
Other location	0.11 8/7147	0.14 3/2200	0.09 2/2101	0.21 1/469	0 0/446	0 0/225	0 0/189	0.16 1/622	0.2 1/666

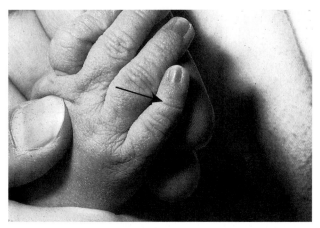

FIGURE 25.77   Clinocactyly, fifth finger, marked degree (arrow).

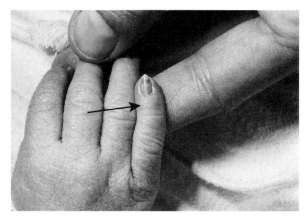

FIGURE 25.78   Clinodactyly, fifth finger, mild degree (arrow).

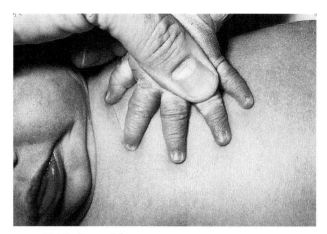

FIGURE 25.79   Tapered fingers.

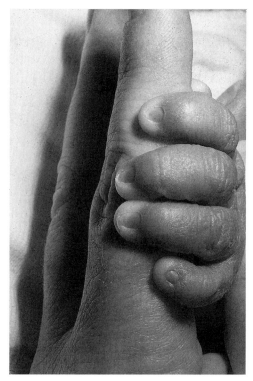

FIGURE 25.80   Hypoplastic fingernails.

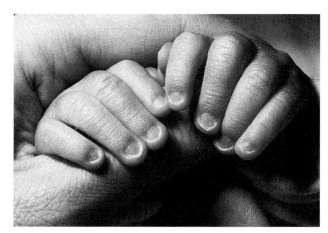

FIGURE 25.81   Hypoplastic fingernails.

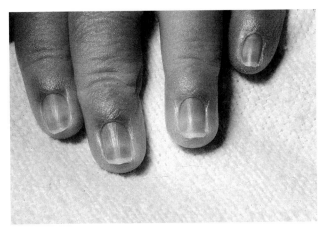

FIGURE 25.82   Hyperconvex fingernails.

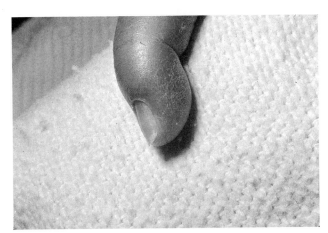

FIGURE 25.83   Hyperconvex fingernails.

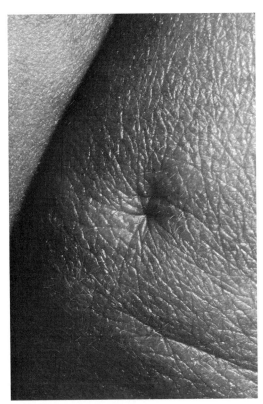

FIGURE 25.85   Dimple over shoulder.

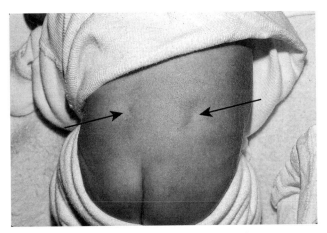

FIGURE 25.84   Dimples over sacroiliac joint. (arrows)

HAND

Simian crease: Transverse palmar crease; single straight line across palm at approximate level of metacarpal-phalangeal joint (Figure 25-86).

Bridged simian crease: A single straight line across palm made up of two or three connected lines (Figure 25-87).

Simian-transitional normal: A line across palm made up of two or three interconnected lines; not a straight line Figure 25-88.

Sydney line: A line across the palm that begins on radial side at or just below level of simian crease, crosses palm at angle and exits on ulnar side about midway between base of fifth finger and wrist crease; must cross entire palm; many infants have a line that stops at hypothenar eminence, a line not considered a Sydney line (Figures 25-89).

Fifth finger, single crease: A single flexion crease on fifth finger instead of the customary two creases that are located over an interphalangeal joint; usually associated with marked clinodactyly and a small, wedge-shaped middle phalanx.

Fifth finger, extra crease: A third flexion crease, usually located between the two creases over interphalangeal joints (Figures 25-90–25-91).

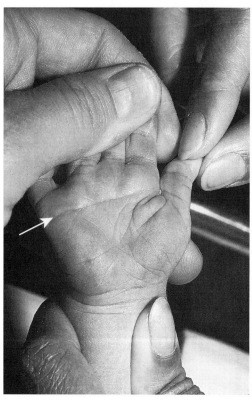

FIGURE 25.86   Transverse palmar (simian) crease.

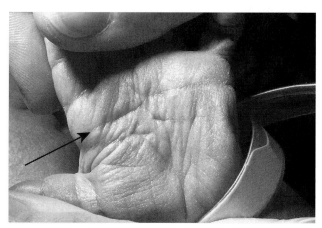

FIGURE 25.88   Simian—transitional normal: made up of interconnected lines. (arrow)

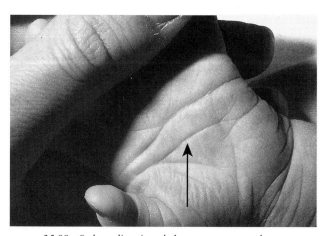

FIGURE 25.89   Sydney line just below transverse palmar crease. (arrow)

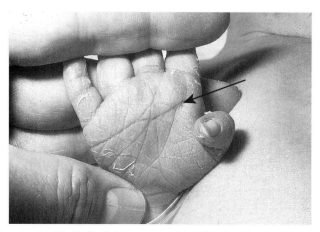

FIGURE 25.87   Bridged simian crease. (arrow)

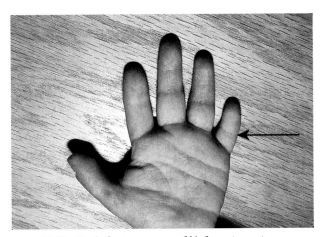

FIGURE 25.90   Single flexion crease on fifth finger (arrow).

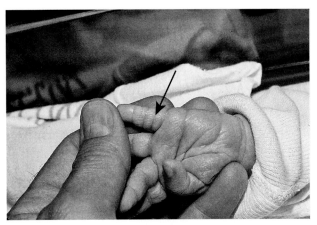

FIGURE 25.91   Extra proximal flexion crease on fifth finger (arrow).

TABLE 25-17 *Hand*

Physical Feature	All Races	White		Black		Latin		Mixed Racial	
		Males	Females	Male	Female	Male	Female	Male	Female
Dermal Patterns									
Simian crease*									
Left	2.1% 149/7143	2.9% 63/2200	1.5% 31/2101	1.7% 8/468	0.9% 4/446	2.2% 5/224	0 0/189	2.6% 16/621	1.7% 11/665
Right	1.8 125/7142	2.2 49/2201	1.2 26/2100	1.7 8/468	1.1 5/445	1.8 4/225	0.5 1/189	1.8 11/621	1.8 12/66
Both	0.6 46/7139	0.9 20/2200	0.4 8/2100	0.6 3/467	0.5 2/445	0.5 1/224	0 0/189	0.6 4/621	0.6 4/665
Bridged simian									
Left	1.3 94/7134	1.4 31/2196	1.0 20/2099	0.6 3/468	1.4 6/445	0.9 2/224	0.5 1/189	1.3 8/620	2.3 15/665
Right	1.2 83/7183	1.7 38/2198	0.8 16/2101	0.9 4/466	0.7 3/445	2.7 6/225	0 0/189	1.5 9/621	0.8 5/665
Both	0.3 20/7129	0.4 8/2195	0.2 5/2099	0 0/465	0.2 1/444	0.5 1/224	0 0/189	0.5 3/620	0.2 1/665
Simian transitional normal									
Left	2.7 132/4827	2.9 44/1531	2.3 34/1458	1.8 6/336	1.8 5/275	2.5 4/160	3.7 5/134	3.5 13/376	2.5 10/394
Right	1.7 84/4832	2.1 32/1531	1.2 18/1460	0.9 3/336	0.7 2/276	3.1 5/160	1.5 2/134	2.1 8/378	0.8 3/394
Both	0.7 32/4825	0.7 10/1531	0.5 7/1457	0.6 2/335	0 0/275	1.3 2/160	0.8 1/134	0.8 3/376	0.8 3/394
Sydney line									
Left	13.0 927/7142	13.8 303/2201	14.2 299/2101	9.6 45/467	7.4 33/446	11.2 25/224	12.2 23/189	13.2 82/620	13.1 87/665
Right	12.7 908/7140	13.8 304/2201	12.7 266/2101	7.1 33/465	5.9 26/444	16.4 37/225	15.9 30/189	13.9 86/621	14.3 95/665
Both	6.5 466/7138	7.1 157/2201	6.9 145/2101	3.9 18/465	3.4 15/444	7.1 16/224	4.8 9/189	7.9 49/620	6.6 44/665
Fifth finger									
Single crease									
Left	0.1 9/7133	0.05 1/2194	0.1 2/2097	0.2 1/469	0 0/446	0.5 1/223	0 0/189	0.6 4/621	0 0/665
Right	0.1 8/7133	0.09 2/2196	0.05 1/2096	0. 0/468	0.2 1/446	0.5 1/223	0 0/189	0.3 2/621	0.1 1/665
Both	0.04 3/7131	0 0/2194	0 0/2096	0 0/468	0 0/446	0.5 1/223	0 0/189	0.3 2/621	0 0/665
Fifth finger									
Extra crease									
Left	1.0 48/4827	0.8 12/1532	0.8 11/1456	2.7 9/336	2.2 6/275	0.6 1/160	1.5 2/134	0.3 1/377	1.0 4/394
Right	1.2 60/4824	0.9 13/1533	0.8 12/1455	4.2 14/333	3.3 9/275	1.3 2/160	0 0/134	0.5 2/377	1.8 7/394
Both	0.4 20/4823	0.3 5/1532	0.4 6/1455	1.2 4/333	1.5 4/275	0.6 1/160	0 0/134	0 0/377	0 0/394

Legend: * similar crease = transverse palmer crease.

FEET

Increased space between toes 1-2: This judgment should be made when foot is at rest and not after plantar stimulation (Figure 25-92).

Syndactyly of toes 2-3: Soft tissue webbing extending further along toes than occurs between other toes; subdivided arbitrarily into three groups, depending on whether the syndactyly extends to the proximal interphalangeal (I-P) joint, to the middle I-P joint or to the tip of the two toes (Figures 25-93, 25-94 and 25-95).

Overlapping toes: When the foot is relaxed, one toe extending over another (Figures 25-96 and 25-97).

TABLE 25-18 *Feet*

		White		Black		Latin		Mixed Racial	
Physical Feature	All Races	Males	Females	Male	Female	Male	Female	Male	Female
Increased space between toes 1-2									
Left	1.5% 105/7149	1.9% 41/2201	1.3% 38/2101	0 0/468	0.5% 2/448	3.1% 7/225	2.7% 5/189	1.4% 9/623	1.7% 11/666
Right	1.3 90/7149	1.6 36/2201	1.1 24/2101	0 0/468	0.7 3/448	2.7 6/225	2.7 5/189	1.1 7/623	1.2 8/666
Both	1.2 85/7149	1.6 36/2201	1.0 21/2101	0 0/468	0.5 2/448	2.7 6/225	2.7 5/189	1.1 7/623	1.1 7/666
Syndactyly of toes 2-3 to first interphalangeal joint									
Left	0.6 41/7151	0.9 19/2201	0.3 7/2101	0.6 3/469	0.5 2/448	0.4 1/225	0 0/189	0.8 5/623	0.6 4/666
Right	0.6 41/7152	0.8 18/2202	0.4 9/2101	0.6 3/470	0.7 3/448	0.5 1/224	0 0/189	0.6 4/623	0.5 3/666
Both	0.5 33/7150	0.6 13/2201	0.3 7/2101	0.6 3/469	0.5 2/448	0.5 1/224	0 0/189	0.6 4/623	0.5 3/666
Syndactyly of toes 2-3 to second inter-phalangeal joint									
Left	0.1 8/7151	0.2 5/2201	0.1 2/2100	0 0/470	0 0/448	0 0/225	0 0/189	0 0/623	0 0/666
Right	0.1 9/7154	0.2 5/2202	0.1 2/2102	0 0/469	0 0/448	0 0/225	0 0/189	0.2 1/623	0 0/666
Both	0.6 4/7150	0.1 3/2201	0 0/2100	0 0/469	0 1/448	0 0/225	0 0/189	0 0/623	0 0/666
Syndactyly of toes 2-3 to end of toes									
Left	0 0/7155	0 0/2202	0 0/2102	0 0/470	0 0/448	0 0/225	0 0/189	0 0/623	0 0/666
Right	0.01 1/7152	0.05 1/2201	0 0/2102	0 0/469	0 0/448	0 0/225	0 0/189	0 0/623	0 0/666
Both	0 0/7152	0 0/2201	0 0/2102	0 0/469	0 0/448	0 0/225	0 0/189	0 0/623	0 0/666
Overlapping toes, fifth over fourth									
Left	0.9 62/7152	0.8 18/2201	0.9 18/2102	0.9 4/470	1.3 6/447	2.7 6/225	0.5 1/189	0.6 4/623	0.8 5/666
Right	0.9 65/7151	0.9 19/2201	1.1 22/2102	0.9 4/469	1.1 5/447	2.2 5/225	0.5 1/189	0.5 3/623	0.8 5/666
Both	0.4 31/7151	0.4 8/2201	0.4 8/2102	0.4 2/469	0.7 3/447	1.8 4/225	1.05 1/189	0.2 1/623	0.6 4/666
Overlapping toes, other									
Left	1.4% 101/7152	1.2% 27/2201	1.5% 32/2102	1.5% 7/469	2.2% 10/448	0.9% 2/225	2.1% 4/189	0.8% 5/623	1.7% 11/666
Right	1.4 101/7152	1.1 25/2201	1.7 35/2102	1.7 8/469	2.2 10/448	0.9 2/225	2.1 4/189	0.5 3/623	1.7 11/666
Both	0.9 66/7152	0.8 17/2201	0 0/2101	1.1 5/469	1.3 6/448	0.9 2/225	1.6 3/189	0.3 2/623	1.2 8/666

Continued

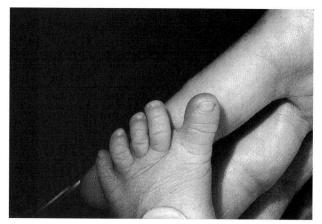

FIGURE 25.92   Increased space between toes 1 and 2.

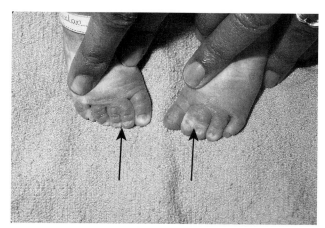

FIGURE 25.95   Syndactyly of toes 2-3, almost to tip of toes. (arrows)

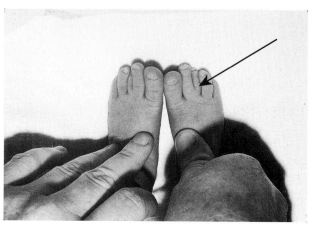

FIGURE 25.93   Syndactyly of toes 2-3 out to first inter-phalangeal joint. (arrow)

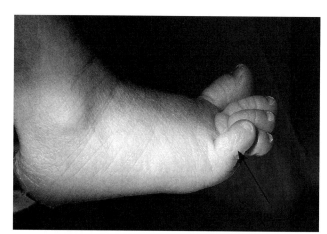

FIGURE 25.96   Fifth toes overlapping 4th toes (arrow).

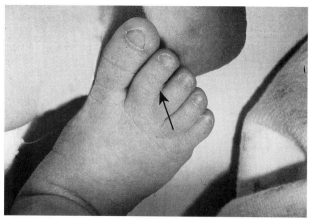

FIGURE 25.94   Syndactyly of toes 2-3 out to second inter-phalangeal joint. (arrow)

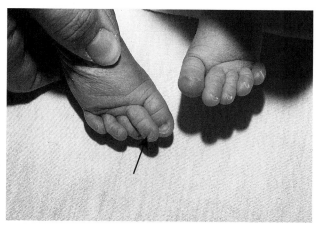

FIGURE 25.97   Second toe overlapping first toe (arrow).

Recessed fourth toe: When the first interphalangeal joint of the fourth toe is proximal to the origin (the metatarsal-phalangeal joint) of the third toe.

Recessed fifth toe: When the first interphalangeal joint of the fifth toe is proximal to the origin (the metatarsal-phalangeal joint) of the fourth toe (Figures 25-98 and 25-99).

Toenails hypoplastic: Nails definitely smaller than average; remember that toenails are normally very small (Figures 25-100 and 25-101).

Toenails hyperconvex: Nails have a downward extension at each edge and a more convex shape when viewed from the tip.

Heel prominent: A protrusion posteriorly of the calcaneous showing prominently the lowest portion of the heel (Figure 25-102).

Sole crease: A deep crease in soft tissue that extends upward between the first and second toes (Figure 25-103).

TABLE 25-18 *Feet* *(Continued)*

Physical Feature	All Races	White Males	White Female	Black Males	Black Female	Latin Males	Latin Female	Mixed Racial Males	Mixed Racial Female
Recessed fourth toe									
Left	0.04% 3/7107	0.05% 1/2187	0.05% 1/2089	0 0/467	0.2% 1/444	0 0/221	0 0/189	0 0/620	0 0/661
Right	0.07 5/7109	0.09 2/2187	0.05 1/2090	0 0/468	0.2 1/444	0 0/221	0 0/189	0 0/620	0.2 1/661
Both	.04 3/7107	0.05 1/2187	0.05 1/2089	0 0/467	0.2 1/444	0 0221	0 0/189	0 0/620	0 0/661
Recessed fifth toe									
Left	0.9 63/7112	0.9 20/2187	0.9 18/2092	1.3 6/468	1.1 5/444	1.4 3/222	0.5 1/189	1.3 8/620	0 0/661
Right	0.7 47/7112	0.7 16/2187	0.8 16/2092	0.9 4/468	0.2 1/444	1.4 3/222	0.5 1/189	0.5 3/620	0.2 1/661
Both	0.5 35/7112	0.5 11/2187	0.6 12/2092	0.6 3/468	0.2 1/444	1.4 3/222	0 0/189	0.5 3/620	0 0/661
Toenails hypoplastic	7.5 532/7120	7.8 172/2195	8.4 175/2092	8.3 39/469	5.4 24/444	4.5 10/224	5.3 10/189	7.0 43/619	7.1 47/661
Toenails hyperconvex	0.4 27/7120	0.4 9/2195	0.4 8/2092	0.2 1/469	0.2 1/444	1.3 3/224	1.1 2/189	0.2 1/619	0 0/661
Heel prominent									
Left	5.6 401/7116	4.6 101/2193	3.6 76/2090	9.6 45/468	10.6 47/444	6.7 15/223	6.9 13/189	6.6 41/619	7.9 52/661
Right	5.4 389/7119	4.6 101/2194	3.7 77/2092	9.0 42/468	9.9 44/444	6.3 14/223	6.4 12/189	6.0 37/619	7.4 49/661
Both	5.3 377/7116	4.5 98/2193	3.5 73/2090	8.8 41/468	9.9 44/444	6.3 14/223	6.4 12/189	6.0 37/619	7.3 48/661
Sole crease									
Left	2.8 198/7150	2.8 61/2199	2.4 51/2102	1.9 9/470	2.5 11/447	4.0 9/225	4.2 8/189	3.4 21/624	3.9 26/665
Right	2.7 195/7149	2.2 48/2200	2.5 52/2101	2.8 13/470	3.6 16/447	3.6 8/225	2.7 5/189	4 25/623	3.6 24/665
Both	1.9 136/7148	1.8 39/2199	1.5 31/2101	1.7 8/470	2.0 9/447	3.1 7/225	2.7 5/189	3.1 19/623	2.6 17/665

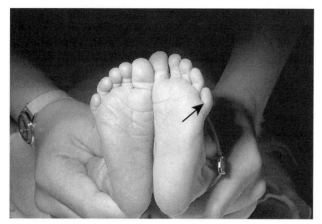

FIGURE 25.98   Recessed fifth toe (arrow).

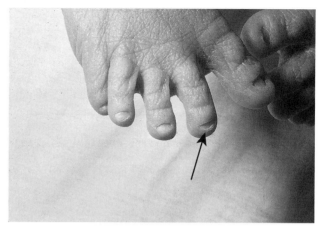

FIGURE 25.101   Hypoplasia of toenails (arrow).

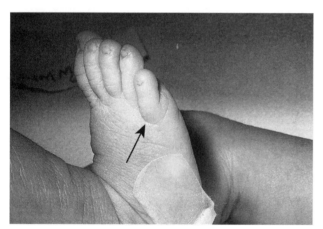

FIGURE 25.99   Recessed fifth toe (arrow).

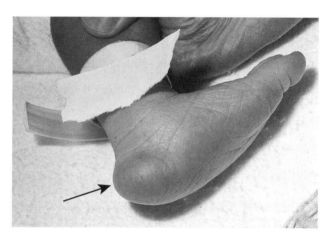

FIGURE 25.102   Prominent heel (arrow).

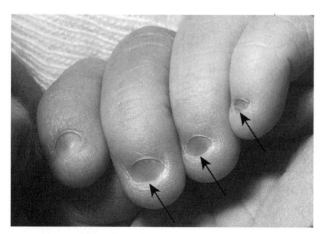

FIGURE 25.100   Hypoplasia of toenails (arrows).

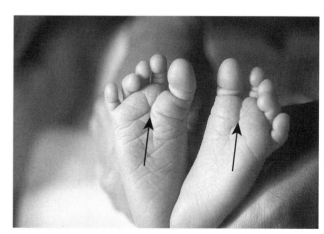

FIGURE 25.103   Sole creases in both feet (arrows).

REFERENCES

1. Marden PM, Smith DW, McDonald MJ. Congenital anomalies in the newborn infant, including minor variations. *J Pediatr.* 1964;64:357–371.

2. Méhes K, Mestyan J, Knoch V, Vinceller M. Minor malformations in the neonate. *Helv Paediatr Acta.* 1973;28:477–483.

3. Méhes K. Minor malformations in the neonate. Budapest: Akademia Kiado; 1983.

4. Opitz JM. Invited editorial comment: Study of minor anomalies in childhood malignancy. *Eur J Pediatr.* 1985;144:252–254.

5. Merlob P. Mild errors of morphogenesis: one of the most controversial subjects in dysmorphology. *Issues Rev Terato.* 1994;7: 57–102.

6. Merlob P, Atkin I. Time trends (1980–1987) of ten selected informative morphogenetic variants in a newborn population. *Clin Genet.* 1990;38:33–37.

7. Spranger J, Bernischeke K, Hall JG, Lenz W, Lowry RB, Opitz JM, Pinsky L, Schwarzacher HG, Smith DW. Errors of morphogenesis: concepts and terms. Recommendations of an International Working Group. *J Pediatr.* 1982;100:160–165.

8. Carey JC. Invited editorial comments: Study of minor anomalies in childhood malignancy. *Eur J Pediatr.* 1985;144:250–251.

9. Frias JF, Carey JC. Mild errors of morphogenesis. *Adv Pediatr.* 1996;43:27–75.

10. Pinsky L. Informative morphogenetic variants; minor congenital anomalies revisited. In: Kalter H, ed. *Issues and Reviews in Teratology.* New York: Plenum Press; 1985: 135–170.

11. Jones KL, Smith S. *Recognizable Patterns of Human Malformation.* 5th ed. Philadelphia: WB Saunders; 1997:727–746.

12. Hoyme HE. Minor malformations. Significant or insignificant? *Am J Dis Child.* 1987; 141:947.

13. Cohen MM Jr. *The Child with Multiple Birth Defects.* New York: Raven Press; 1982: 1–26.

14. Leppig KA, Werler MM, Cann CI, Cook CA, Holmes LB. Predictive value of minor anomalies in association with major malformations. *J Pediatr.* 1987;110:531–537.

15. Holmes LB, Kleiner BC, Leppig KA, Cann CI, Munoz A, Polk BF. Predictive value of minor anomalies: II use in cohort studies to identify teratogens. *Teratology.* 1987;36:291–297.

16. Hook EB, Petry JJ. Single hit aetiology of human minor congenital malformations unassociated with major congenital malformations. *Nature.* 1970;227:846–848.

17. Hook EB, Marden PM, Reiss NP, Smith DW. Some aspects of the epidemiology of human minor birth defects and morphological variants in a completely ascertained newborn population (Madison Study). *Teratology.* 1976;13:47–55.

18. Jaffe F. Deformities of the external ear associated with middle ear, inner ear, or distant malformations. *Clinics in Plastic Surgery.* 1978;5:413–418.

19. Grun M, Merlob P, Grunfeld A, Abend M, Chystiakov I, Riskin-Mashiah S, Bader D. auricular mild eras of morphogenesis: epidemiological study with application of a targeted computer program. *Ann Genet.* 2002;45:207–212.

20. Bader D, Grun M, Riskin S, Greenfeld A, Chystiakov I, Merlob P. Auricular mild errors of morphogenesis: epidemiological analysis, local correlations and clinical significance. *Ann Genet.* 2004;47:225–234.

21. Hunter AGW, Yotsuyanagi T. The external ear: more attention to detail may aid syndrome diagnosis and contribute answers to embryological questions. *Am J Med Genet.* 2005;135A:237–250.

22. Stewart AL, Keay AJ, Smith PG. Congenital malformations: a detailed study of 2,500 liveborn infants. *Ann Hum Genet.* 1969;32:353–360.

23. Arima M, Komiay K, Ono K, Hisada K. Congenital minor anomalies in mentally retarded children. *Proc Aust Assoc Neurol.* 1968;5:177–182.

24. Powell EF, Whitney DD. Ear lobe inheritance. An unusual three-generation photographic pedigree-chart. *J Hered.* 1937;28:185–186.

25. Leung AKC, Kong AYF, Robson WLM, McLeod DR. Dominantly-inherited lop ears. *Am J Med Genet Part A.* 2007;143A:2330–2333.

26. Weippl G, Ader H. Kongenitaler Skalp-Defekt in vier Generationen. *Klin Paediatr.* 1975;187:84–86.

27. Bianchine JW. Acromial dimples: a benign familial trait. *Am J Hum Genet.* 1974;26:412–413.

28. Shafir R, Bonne-Tamir B, Ashbel S, Tsur H, Goodman RM. Genetic studies in a family with inverted nipples (mammillae invertita). *Clin Genet.* 1979;15:346–350.

29. Leung AKC, McLeod DR. Autosomal dominant flat umbilicus. *Am J Med Gen.* 2004;131A:307–309.

30. Dar H, Schmidt R, Nitowsky HM. Palmar crease variants and their clinical significance: a study of newborns at risk. *Pediatr Res.* 1977;11:103–108.

31. Hersh JH, Bloom AS, Craner AO et al. Does a supernumerary nipple/renal field defect exist? *Am J Dis Child.* 1987;141:989–991.

32. Varsano IB, Jaber L, Garty B-Z, Mukamel MM, Gurnebaum M. Urinary tract abnormalities in children with supernumerary nipples. *Pediatrics.* 1984;73:103–105.

33. Rahbar F. Clinical significance of supernumerary nipples in black neonates. *Clini Pediatr.* 1982;21:46–47.

34. Kenney RD, Flippo JL, Black EB. Supernumerary nipples and renal anomalies in neonates. *Am J Dis Child.* 1987;141:987–988.

35. Bryan EM, Kohler HG. The missing umbilical artery: I. Prospective study based on a maternity unit. *Arch Dis Child.* 1974;49: 844–851. II. Pediatric follow up. *Arch Dis Child.* 1975;50: 714–718.

36. Blackburn W. The umbilical cord. In: Stevenson RE, Hall JG, Goodman RM, eds. *Human Malformations and Related Anomalies.* 2nd ed. New York: Oxford University Press; 2006: 1413–1472.

37. Museles M, Gaudry CL Jr, Bason WM. Renal anomalies in the newborn found by deep palpation. *Pediatrics.* 1971;47:97–100.

38. Kohelet D, Arbel E. A prospective search for urinary tract abnormalities in infants with isolated preauricular tags. *Pediatrics.* 2000;105:e61. (http://www.pediatrics.org/cgi/content/full/105/5/e61)

39. Kugelman A, Hadad B, Ben-David J, Podoshin L, Borochowitz Z, Bader D. Preauricular tags and pits in the newborn: the role of hearing tests. *Acta Paediatr.* 1997;86:170–172.

40. Guggisberg D, Hadj-Rabia S, Viney C, Bodemer C, Brunelle F, Zerah M et al. Skin markers of occult spinal dysraphism in children. A review of 54 cases. *Arch Dermatol.* 2004;140:1109–1115.

41. Allen RM, Sandquist MA, Piatt JH Jr, Selden NR. Ultrasonographic screening in infants with isolated spinal strawberry nevi. *J Neurosurg (Spine).* 2003;98:247–250.

42. Abu Sneineh AK, Gabos PG, Keller MS, Bowen JR. Ultrasonography of the spine in neonates and young infants with a sacral skin dimple. *J Pediatr Orthop.* 2002;22:761–762.

43. Smith DW, Bostian KE. Congenital anomalies associated with idiopathic mental retardation. *J Pediatr.* 1964;65:189–196.

44. Daryn E. Problem of children with "diffuse brain damage." *Arch Gen Psychiatry.* 1961;4:105–112.

45. Meggyessy V, Révhelyi M, Méhes K. Minor malformations in mental retardation of various etiology. *Acta Paediatr Acad Sci Hung.* 1980;21:175–180.

46. VanOverloop D, Schnell RR, Harvey EA, Holmes LB. The effects of prenatal exposure to phenytoin and other anticonvulsants on intellectual function at 4 to 8 years. *Neurotoxicol Teratol.* 1992; 14:329–335.

47. Waldrop MF, Bell RQ, McLaughlin B, Halverson CF Jr. Newborn minor physical anomalies predict short attention span, per aggression and impulsivity at age 3. *Science.* 1978;199:563–565.

48. Waldrop MF, Halverson CF Jr. Minor physical anomalies and hyperactive behavior in young children. In: Smart RC, Smart MS, eds. *Readings in Development and Relationships.* New York: Macmillan; 1972: 146.

49. Quinn PO, Rapoport JL. Minor physical anomalies and neurologic status in hyperactive boys. *Pediatrics.* 1974;53:742–747.

50. Rosenberg JB, Weller GM. Minor physical anomalies and academic performance in young school children. *Devel Med Child Neurol.* 1973;15:131–135.

51. Burg C, Quinn PQ, Rapoport JL. Clinical evaluation of one year old infants: possible predictors of risk for the "hyperactivity syndrome". *J Ped Psychol.* 1978;3:164.

52. Arricta I, Martinez B, Criado B, Lobato N. Ridge hypoplasia and ridge dissociation: minor physical anomalies in autistic children. *Clinical Genetics.* 1993;43:1–2.

53. Rodier PM, Bryson SE, Welch JP. Minor malformations and physical measurements in autism: data from Nova Scotia. *Teratology.* 1997; 55(5):319–325.

54. Gurion DG, Goldberger CG, Krebs MOK. Facial asymmetry in patients with schizophrenia and their biological relatives: an informative phenotype? *Am J Med Gen.* 2004;1303:10.

55. Crichton JU, Dunn HG, McBurney K, Robertson A, Fredger E. Minor congenital defects in children of low birth weight. *J Pediatr.* 1972;80:830–832.

56. Drillien CM. The small-for-date infant: etiology and prognosis. *Ped Clin N Amer.* 1970;17:9–24.

57. Myrianthopoulos NC. *Congenital Malformation in Twins: Epidemiologic Survey.* New York: Stratton Intercontinental Medical Book Corp; 1975.

58. Ouellette EM, Rosett HL, Rosman NP, Weiner L. Adverse effects on offspring of maternal alcohol abuse during pregnancy. *N Engl J Med.* 1977;297:528–530.

59. Clarren SK, Smith DW. The fetal alcohol syndrome. *N Engl J Med.* 1978;298:1063–1067.

60. Hod M, Merlob P, Friedman S, Litwin A, Mor N, Rusecki Y, Schoenfeld A, Ovadia J. Prevalence of minor congenital anomalies in newborns of diabetic mothers. *Eur J Obstet Gyn Reprod Bio.* 1992;44(2):111–116.

61. Kitzmiller JL, Cloherty JP, Younger MD, Tabatabaii A, Rothschild SB, Sosenko I, Epstein MF, Singh S, Neff RK. Diabetic pregnancy and perinatal morbidity. *Am J Obstet Gynecol.* 1978;131: 560–580.

62. Holmes LB. Major malformations and minor anomalies identified in the Multicenter Diabetes in Early Pregnancy (DIEP) Study. *Proc Greenwood Genetics Ctr.* 1991;10:67.

63. Holmes LB, Harvey EA, Coull BA, Huntington KB, Khoshbin S, Hayes AM, Ryan LM. The teratogenicity of anticonvulsant drugs. *N Engl J Med.* 2001;344:1132–1138.

64. Holmes LB, Coull BA, Harvey EA, Hayes AM. Major malformations in anticonvulsant exposed children: association or coincidence. (In Spanish) *Boletin Del ECEMC: Revisto de Dismorfologia y Epidemiologia.* 2001;Series IV, 6:31–34.

65. Carlin JB, Ryan LM, Harvey EA, Holmes LB. Anticonvulsant teratogenesis 4: Inter-rater agreement in assessing minor physical features related to anticonvulsant therapy. *Teratology.* 2000;62: 406–412.

66. Harvey EA, Coull BA, Holmes LA. Anticonvulsant teratogenesis 5: observer bias in a cohort study. *Birth Defects Res (Part A): Clin Mol Teratol.* 2003;67(6):452–456.

67. Friedman JM. Genetics and epidemiology, congenital anomalies and cancer. *Am J Hum Genet.* 1997;60(3):469–473.

68. Méhes K, Signer E, Pluss HJ, Muller HJ, Stalder G. Increased prevalence of minor anomalies in childhood malignancy. *Eur J Pediatr.* 1985;144(3):243–254.

69. Méhes K, Kajtar P, Sandor G, Scheel-Walter M, Niethammer D. Excess of mild errors of morphogenesis in childhood lymhoblastic leukemia. *Am J Med Genet.* 1998;75(1):22–7.

70. Méhes K, Kosztolanyi G. Clinical manifestations of genetic instability overlap one another. *Pathol Oncol Res.* 2004;10(1): 12–16.

71. Harvey EA, Hayes, AM, Holmes LB. Lessons on objectivity in clinical studies. *Am J Med Genet.* 1994;53(1):19–20.

72. Graham JM Jr, Hanson JW, Darby BL, Barr HM, Streissguth AP. Independent dysmorphology evaluations at birth and 4 years of age for children exposed to varying amounts of alcohol in utero. *Pediatrics.* 1988;81(6):772–778.

73. Egglin TK, Feinstein AR. Contex bias: a problem in diagnostic radiology. *JAMA.* 1996;276:172–1755.

74. Lee LG, Jackson JF. Diagnosis of Down's syndrome: clinical vs. laboratory. *Clin Pediatr.* 1972;11(6):353–356.

Chapter 26

Birth Marks

AUTHORS: DANIELA KROSHINSKY, JOSEPH C. ALPER, AND LEWIS B. HOLMES

NEVUS SIMPLEX (SALMON PATCH)

Definition

A capillary malformation and macular stain that is present at birth. Also referred to as "angel kiss" and "stork bite."

ICD-9:	757.380	(flammeus nevus or port wine stain)
ICD-10:	Q82.5	(congenital non-neoplastic naevus, includes naevus flammeus)
Mendelian Inheritance in Man:	%163100	(nevus flammeus of nape of neck)

Historical Note

The earliest report of nevas flammeus nuchae ("stork bite"), according to K. L. Tan (1), was in 1880 (2). For many years this nevus was referred to as a capillary hemangioma. The underlying histologic features were an excessive number of mature or relatively mature, well-formed vessels of capillary caliber (3).

In 1982, Mulliken and Glowacki (4) suggested that vascular anomalies be subdivided into tumors and malformations, based on the underlying endothelial cell mitotic activity. The term capillary hemangiomas, which had been used for a variety of nevi, was considered more appropriate for "true errors in vascular morphogenesis" (5). It was suggested that the term capillary hemangiomas was an "overly generic term" and that more precise, biologically based terms should be used.

Appearance

These lesions are usually isolated. This nevus is a flat, dull, pink macule with an irregular shape (Figures 26-1–26-3).

The salmon patch on the glabella or eyelids has been referred to as an "angel kiss" (Figure 26-1); on the nape of the neck, it has been called a "stork bite."

Histologic Features

The histologic features of this macular stain have not been studied well. One description is that the red color reflects the presence of an excessive number of mature or relatively mature well-formed capillaries (3).

Location

This nevus is usually isolated and located on the face, in general, and on the glabella, nape of neck, or the crown

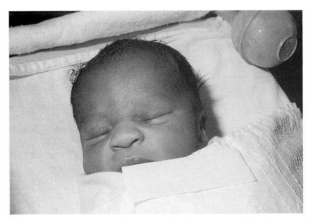

FIGURE 26.1 Shows macular stain on both upper eyelids (the "angel kiss").

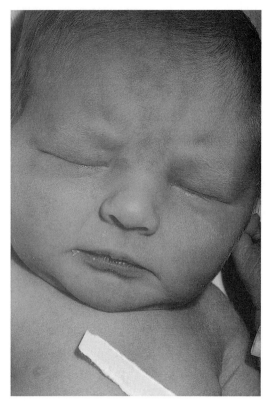

FIGURE 26.2 A macular stain on the forehead.

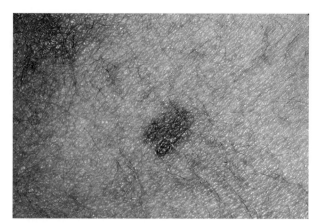

FIGURE 26.3 A macular stain on the abdomen.

of the head, in particular (Figures 26-1, 26-2; Tables 26-1 and 26-2).

Frequency

The prevalence rates of salmon patches identified in newborn infants have varied among the several studies (1, 6–12). In the surface examination of 7,157 newborn infants in Boston (13), 68.6% had at least one macule.

In comparing the frequency of these nevi at specific sites in different studies, Jacobs and Walton (8) identified the salmon patch on the glabella in 33.1% of 1,058 newborns, whereas Pratt (6) identified this nevus at that site in 5%.

Size

No systematic measurements have been reported. Usually this macule is 1 to 3 centimeters in greatest width. Occasionally, they are much larger (greater than 10 cm in diameter).

Racial/Ethnic Differences

In Singapore (1), this macule was present in 26.6% of 2,901 newborn infants with either Chinese, Malay, or Indian ancestry. In the surface exam of another group of 3,345 Chinese newborns, 22.6% had a salmon patch (12). By comparison, Jacobs and Walton (8) identified

TABLE 26-1 *Frequency and anatomic location of salmon patch in newborn infants–Boston*

In this study:	All races	Whites	Blacks	Hispanics	Mixed	Other
All locations	68.6%	70.3%	59.2%	67.9%	70.1%	66.8%
	4885/7122*	3912/4275	540/912	281/414	899/1282	153/229
Face	51.1%	51.8%	47.4%	51.3%	52.7%	41.9%
	3628/7101	2215/4277	431/909	212/413	674/1279	96/229
Nape of Neck	51.1%	52.6%	41.2%	53.65	51.9%	52.8%
	3637/7121	2253/4285	376/912	222/414	665/1281	121/229
Crown of Head	13.1%	15.0%	4.1%	13.2%	13.3%	9.9%
	629/4821	447/2987	25/609	39/296	102/768	16/161
Other locations	41.1%	4.9%	1.9%	2.2%	4.0%	3.1%
	292/7086	209/4269	17/905	9/412	51/1273	7/227

Legends: *Findings in surface examination of 7,157 newborn infants examined between birth and five days of age at Boston Lying-In Hospital (1972–1974) [13].
  Racial/ethnic origin: based on the mother's report of the racial origin of the four grandparents of the infant.
  Mixed ancestry: More than one racial/ethnic group in the ancestry of the four grandparents.

TABLE 26-2 *Frequency and anatomic location of salmon patch–other studies*

Other Studies:	Pratt (6)				Tan (4)					Jacobs & Walton (5)
Number of Infants	1096				2901					1058
Total Affected	43.5%				26.6%					40. 3%
Location	White	Black	Chinese		Malay		Indian		All races	
			M	F	M	F	M	F		
Glabella	5%	6%	4.2%	6.3%	5.2%	8.5%	4.5%	9.1%	33.1%	
Upper eyelid	11%	10%	1.4	3.9	1.7	3.7	2.7	3.7	45.1	
Nuchal	48%	31%	2.1	27.8	1.9	29.4	9.9	19.3	81.2	
All locations	48%	39%	23.2	31.8	21.1	32.1	14.1	27.3	40.3	

this macule in 40.3% of 1,055 newborn infants, most of whom were Caucasian.

While differences in the frequency of these macules are apparent in a comparison of the findings in different racial/ethnic groups, these differences could also reflect differences in the definitions used and the methods of examination.

Sex Ratio

The male:female ratio in the surface examination at St. Bartholomew's Hospital in London was 42 females:32 males (14).

Management

These lesions are not considered an abnormality.

These patches or macular stains fade in intensity during the first year of life. The macules on the eyelid and glabella are barely visible by 6 to 12 months of age, although they may become more intense with crying and straining, even in adolescence (14). The "stork bite" on the neck fades in intensity more slowly and is often visible in adults.

This benign capillary malformation must be distinguished from the darker, more extensive capillary hemangiomas that are a feature of the Sturge-Weber Syndrome and the Klippel-Trenaunay-Weber Syndrome (15), two disorders with major associated medical problems.

The presence of a salmon patch rarely has any medical significance. One exception is the presence of this capillary malformation in the midline over a lipoma and the lumbar vertebrae. This finding can reflect the presence of spinal dysraphism and would warrant further clinical studies (16).

Genetic Counseling

This macule is not medically significant. Since it is very common, it would be expected that several close relatives would be affected, as has been reported (17).

INFANTILE HEMANGIOMA

Definition

An infantile hemangioma is a vascular tumor that is not present at birth and becomes visible in the early weeks of life and involutes spontaneously by age 5 to 7 years.

ICD-9:	228.010	(hemangioma)
ICD-10:	Q82.5	(congenital non-neoplastic nalvus, includes strawberry)
Mendelian Inheritance in Man:	#602089	(hemangioma, capillary infantile)

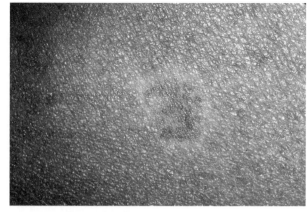

FIGURE 26.5   Shows white halo around lesion expected to develop an infantile hemangioma.

Appearance

Infantile hemangiomas are often difficult to identify in newborn infants. In the first days of life they are ill-defined, flat, and may have a <u>faint blue color</u> or be hypopigmented (Figure 26-4).

Some have fine telangiectases. When this area is rubbed vigorously, a hypopigmented halo will often develop around the lesion, making it easier to see [Figures 26-4 to 26-6] (18, 19).

Most of these hemangiomas are localized and seem to grow from a single focal point (Figure 26-7).

The other distributions are segmental (clusters which correspond to a developmental segment) and multifocal (such as the presence of ten or more cutaneous hemangiomas) [Figure 26-8].

In one multicenter study by pediatric dermatologists (20), 66.8% of 1,530 hemangiomas were localized, 13.1% were segmental, 16.5% were indeterminate and 3.6% were multifocal.

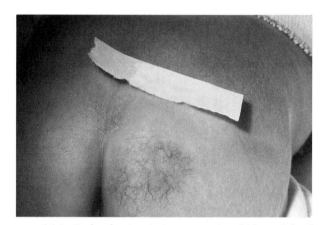

FIGURE 26.6   Dark telangietasia in an area in which an infantile hemangioma will develop.

Histologic Features

These benign vascular proliferations are composed of densely packed capillaries that contain endothelial cells and pericytes. Histologically, there is endothelial cell hyperplasia and an increased number of mast cells (18). The process of involution is characterized by apoptosis and disappearance of capillaries, with replacement by loose fibrous or fatty tissue (21). Endothelial cells from these hemangiomas express many genes. The expression of the gene *erythrocyte-type glucose transport protein* (GLUT1) was one of the first distinctive molecular findings in infantile hemangiomas (22).

One hypothesized etiology is the clonal proliferation of endothelial cells from a single progenitor cell. Another postulated cause is somatic mutations in one or more genes that regulate the growth of endothelial cells in the infantile hemangiomas (23). For example, somatic mutations in the kinase domain of the VEGFR2 (FLK1/KDR) gene and the VEGFR3 (FLT4) gene have been identified in proliferating infantile hemangiomas (24).

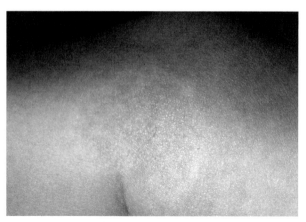

FIGURE 26.4   An area of decreased pigmentation in which an infantile hemangioma will develop.

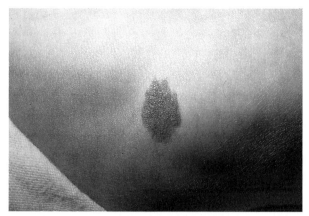

FIGURE 26.7   A white halo around a hemangioma in a newborn infant.

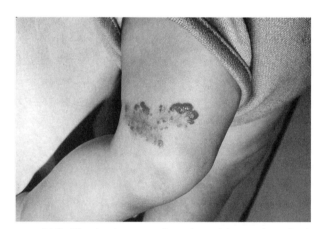

FIGURE 26.8   The development of an elevated hemangioma in the weeks and months after birth.

Prevalence

The incidence of visible infantile hemangiomas at birth is 1 to 2% (Table 26-3) [25–29] and 9 to 10% by age 1 year (30, 31).

In the surface examination of a systematic sample of 4,641 newborn infants in the Boston Lying-In Hospital (1972–1974), 59 had infantile hemangiomas for a prevalence rate of 1.3% (26). In another study, the prevalence rate was 15.6% among infants below 1,500 grams and 22.9% among infants below 1,000 grams birth weight (32, 33).

Location

Several studies (18, 20, 21, 25, 26) have shown that infantile hemangiomas are most common in the face, head and neck (Table 26-4).

In a survey of 1,915 hemangiomas in 1,058 children age 12 or younger by pediatric dermatologists (2002–2003), 41.2% of the hemangiomas were located on the face, 21%

on the head and neck, 23.3% on the trunk, 21% on the extremities, and 6.1% in the perineum (20).

Size

In the systematic examination of 4,641 newborn infants, the average length was 1.5 cm and the width 1.0 cm (Figure 26-7) [26].

Sex Ratio

Several studies have shown significantly that there are more affected females than males (34, 35).

Race/Ethnicity

No significant differences in the frequency of infantile hemangiomas have been identified in studies of white, black, and Japanese newborns (25, 26, 28).

TABLE 26-3 *Prevalence rates of infantile hemangiomas at birth by race in four studies.*

	Japan (25) (n= 2,168)	Jacobs & Walton (31) (n=1,058)	Pratt (28) (n=1,096)	Boston (26) (n=4,641)
All races		2.6%	1.1%	1.3%
Whites			1.1%	1.7%
Blacks			1.3%	0.6%
Asians	0.9 %			
Hispanic				0.4%
Mixed				0.8%
Other				1.4%

TABLE 26-4 *Location of infantile hemangiomas*

	Boston Lying-In Hospital (26) 1972–1974			Japan (25) (n=19)
	Males* (n=16)	Females (n=24)	Normal Surface Area Distribution	
Scalp	13%	4%	12%	10%
Face	6	21	7	11
Chest	19	4	5	5
Back	6	4	13	32
Buttock	0	25	3	5
Abdomen	19	17	8	0
Arms	6	4	19	5
Legs	3	17	30	16
Other locations	19	4	3	26
	101%	100%	100%	100%

Legends: *Findings in the surface examination of 7,157 newborn infants who were evaluated in a systematic study between birth and 5 days of age at the Boston Lying-In Hospital in the years 1972–1974 (27).

Twins

In a study of 118 twin pairs, the likelihood that both twins would be affected was 32% among 40 identical pairs and 20% among 78 non-identical twins, an insignificant difference (p = 0.5) [34].

Environmental Factors

Infantile hemangiomas are more common in infants whose mothers have had pre-eclampsia or placenta previa (34), but the causative factors are not known.

This type of hemangioma is also more common in infants whose mothers have had the prenatal diagnosis procedure chorionic villus sampling (CVS) (36). One hypothesis for the cause after CVS is that injury to the placenta leads to the embolization of angioblasts from the placenta to the skin. After birth, these cells develop rapidly in the first days and weeks of life to form an infantile hemangioma (37).

Differential Diagnosis

Infantile hemangiomas are to be distinguished from the much less common "congenital hemangiomas," which have been shown by ultrasound to be fully formed and grow during pregnancy and are usually visible at birth. The congenital hemangiomas differ from the infantile hemangioma in that the immunohistochemical staining is negative for the expression of the gene GLUT1 (38).

Clinical Course and Management

The life cycle of infantile hemangiomas has been shown to have three stages: proliferative phase, a plateau phase, and an involutional phase (39). The first phase of proliferation is between birth and the first birthday. The most rapid growth is during the first six months of life.

The process of involuting occurs, often, between 1 and 7 years of age. During that time, the skin over the hemangioma becomes pale and the texture of the skin becomes softer (38). The rate of involution has been estimated to be 10% a year (18, 40), with 50% involuted by age 5 years. The patient may be left with atrophy, fibrofatty changes, or telangiectases in these areas.

The treatment of an infantile hemangioma is affected by its size, location, rate of growth, presence of ulceration, the potential for disfigurement, and the age of the infant (40, 41). Most of these hemangiomas can be managed with "active-non-intervention," which includes documentation in photographs, clinical observation, and a series of re-examinations.

The lesions with the highest risk for disfigurement are those in areas prone to trauma, large plaque-like lesions, and those on the lip, nose, and ear (39).

Serious complications in one study included ulceration (16%), threat to vision (5.6%), airway obstruction (1.4%), auditory canal obstruction (0.6%), and compromise of heart function (0.4%) [20].

Treatments are initiated carefully after the treating physician and parents have agreed to a timeline and the justification and have discussed the options. Treatment approaches vary with the lesions and include propranolol or steroids (systemic, intralesional, or topical), pulsed due laser therapy, and surgical excision (40, 41).

PORTWINE STAIN

Definition

A vascular birth mark present at birth with pink, red, or purple discoloration of the skin. This is also known as nevus flammeus.

ICD-9:	757.380	(flammeus nevus or portwine stain)
ICD-10:	Q82.5	(congenital non-neoplastic nevus, including nevus flammeus)
Mendelian Inheritance in Man:	%163000	(capillary malformations, congenital, 1; CMC1; nevi flammei familial multiple; port-wine stain)

Appearance

At birth, the portwine stain has a lighter pink color (Figure 26-9).

Over time, it darkens to be red, then purple and becomes elevated. The boundaries of the portwine stain are demarcated sharply (Figures 26-10 and 26-11).

This nevus blanches with pressure (42, 43).

Occasionally, a portwine stain is not visible at birth, but becomes visible within a few hours or days.

The portwine stain is usually an isolated lesion, confined to one area. However, in some affected infants the distribution is over several areas, such as face, neck, chest, arm and buttocks (Figures 26-11 to 26-14).

Histology

Biopsies show a normal epidermis overlying an abnormal plexus of dilated capillary-like vessels, located as a

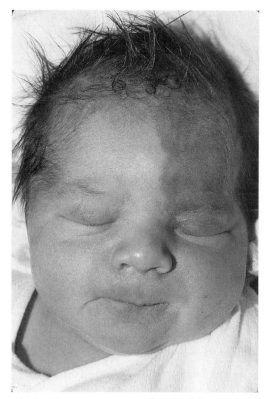

FIGURE 26.10   The portwine stain on the side of the face that involves the upper eyelid and upper lip.

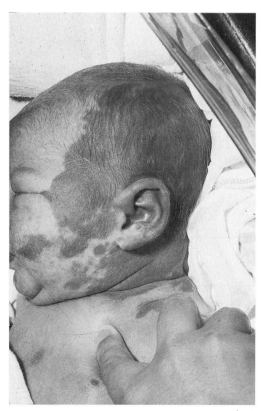

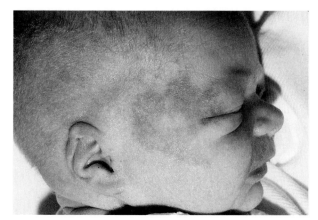

FIGURE 26.9   Shows portwine stain that stops at the midline and includes the upper eyelid.

FIGURE 26.11   A portwine stain that extends through the scalp and down the neck.

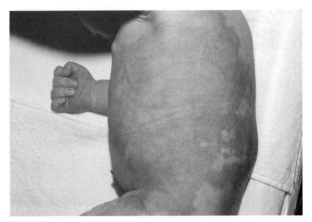

FIGURE 26.12   The portwine stain on the chest and abdomen.

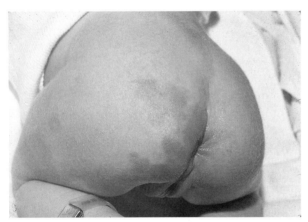

FIGURE 26.13   A portwine stain on the buttocks.

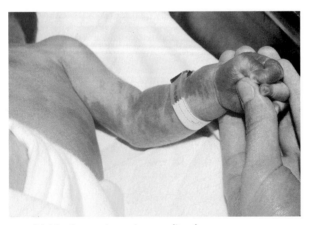

FIGURE 26.14   A portwine stain extending down one arm.

layer of the upper dermis (42–44). The portwine stain is located in the papillary and superficial reticular dermis. The depth varies from 100 to 1,000 µm (mean depth 460 µm) and blood vessel diameter from 10 to 300 µm (45).

The ectatic dermal capillaries of the portwine stain have been postulated to represent the persistence of

fetal circulatory patterns in the skin (42, 46). The endothelial cells and vascular walls of these capillary malformations have a normal appearance, in analysis by immunochemistry (45,47). However, the neuronal marking is decreased significantly, suggesting that a lack of innervation could be a cause of dilatation of the cutaneous capillaries in a portwine stain (48).

Prevalence

In the examination of 1,058 newborn infants under 72 hours of age in California, three (0.3% or 3/1,000) had a portwine stain (49).

0.4% of 3,345 newborn Chinese infants less than 48 hours of age in Taiwan (1990–1991) had a portwine stain (50).

In the systematic surface examination of 7,157 newborn infants in Boston (1972–1974) [51,52], four infants were identified for a prevalence rate of 0.56/1,000 or 1:1,789.

Location

The portwine stain can be present on any part of the body, but are most common on the face and neck (49–52). For example, among the 7,157 newborn infants in Boston (51, 52), four had a portwine stain: 3 on one side of the forehead, including the eyelids (Figures 26-10 and 26-11) and in one infant the portwine stain was located on the face, scalp, back, chest, buttocks and one arm (Figures 26-11 to 26-14).

Size

Most portwine stains occur as an isolated, single birth mark. The size varies from an irregular stain a few centimeters in size to one which covers most of one or both sides of the face and neck or a large area of the chest, back or arm.

No measurements of the size in newborn infants have been published. The portwine stain grows commensurately with the child (53).

Race/Ethnicity

In the Boston study (51, 52), the four affected newborn infants identified were Caucasian. In this racial group the prevalence rate was 0.6/1,000 or 1:644 births. The prevalence rates in other racial and ethnic groups have not been established.

Genetic Factors

Multiple individuals with portwine stains have been reported in a few families (54–57). In these families autosomal dominant inheritance was postulated.

Gene linkage studies have suggested that the CMC1 locus was on chromosome 5 at 5q13-22 (56, 57). However, locus heterogeneity seems likely (43).

Environmental Factors

No exposures in pregnancy, known to be a teratogen in humans, has been shown to produce portwine stains.

Management

Portwine stains are low-flow vascular malformations. Treatment of the cosmetic burden of this birth mark became more positive and effective after the seminal presentation of the use of photothermolysis by laser, described by Anderson and Parrish in 1983 (58). Since 1983, several light devices have been used, but lasers have been the modality of choice (44). The most effective blanching of the portwine stains have been with pulsed-dye laser in conjunction with epidermal cooling. Experience has shown that this treatment does not achieve complete resolution. Some regions of the portwine stain respond only minimally (44).

Unfortunately, follow-up studies over a period of 10 years have shown a significant occurrence of darkening in about one-third of the individuals since the initial blanching by pulsed-dye-laser therapy (59) Further refinements of the laser treatment modalities are expected to address this issue.

The infant with a portwine stain should be evaluated, also, for the possible association of two more serious disorders: the Sturge-Weber Syndrome (MIM: 185300) and the Klippel-Trenaunay-Weber Syndrome (MIM: %149000) [60].

The Sturge-Weber Syndrome is defined as a capillary malformation that involves the leptomeninges over the cerebral cortex, the choroid, and the skin of the face on the same side of the body. The common associated complications, epilepsy and glaucoma, were described by Sturge in 1879 (61, 62).

As to the pattern of the portwine stain that is associated with the Sturge-Weber Syndrome: the stain involves the upper eyelid and the ipsilateral eye (with glaucoma). A broader axiom is that the Sturge-Weber Syndrome is characterized by a portwine stain that involves the distribution of the first branch (ophthalmic) of the trigeminal nerve. A follow-up study of individuals with the portwine stain showed that 91% of those with associated ocular and CNS abnormalities had the stain in both the upper and lower eyelids in comparison to only 9% having the stain on the lower eyelid alone (64). Experience has shown, further, that the associated leptomeningeal vascular malformation in individuals with the Sturge-Weber Syndrome is more often over the occipital lobes, but not the frontal lobe near the stain on the forehead (65). While a lot has been learned about the spectrum of problems associated with the Sturge-Weber Syndrome, the frequency of this syndrome in a newborn infant with the portwine stain has not been determined.

The Klippel-Trenaunay-Weber Syndrome is characterized by a superficial vascular stain, like a portwine stain, anomalies of deep veins, arteriovenous shunting in the affected limb, and overgrowth of part or all of an extremity (62). The legs are involved in 95% of affected individuals, the arms in 5%, and both arms and legs in about 15% (60). Cohen has noted that no individual with the Klippel-Trenaunay Syndrome "has capillary malformations involving the face or craniofacial region" (60). This means that the portwine stain of the Klippel-Trenaunay Syndrome does not have the facial stain that is a characteristic of the Sturge-Weber Syndrome.

CONGENITAL NEVI

Definition

A light to dark brown nevus, present at birth, with increased skin markings in comparison to the surrounding skin.

ICD-9:   216.900   (pigmented mole)

ICD-10:   D22   (melanocytic naevi)

Mendelian   NONE
Inheritance in Man:

Appearance

At birth this nevus may be flat or raised. The color spectrum is tan, brown, or dark brown (Figures 26-15–26-20).

Some contain speckles of dark brown pigment in the periphery of the nevus (Figure 26-16) [66]. The markings in the surrounding skin do not extend into the congenital nevus, in contrast to the café-au-lait spot.

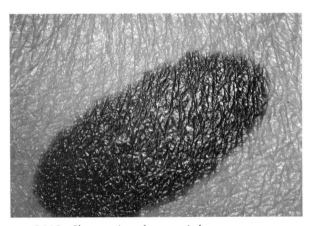

FIGURE 26.15   Close-up view of a congenital nevus.

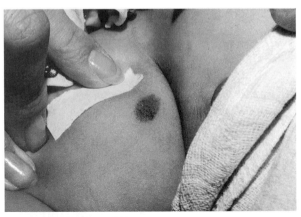

FIGURE 26.16   Shows speckling.

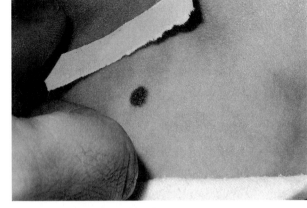

FIGURE 26.17   A small congenital nevus.

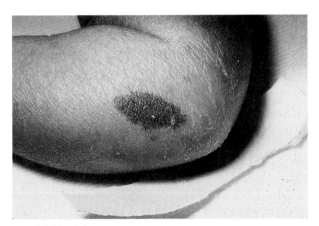

FIGURE 26.18   A larger nevus.

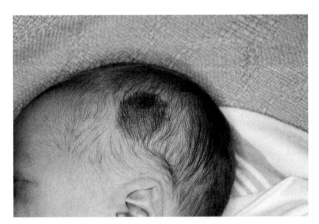

FIGURE 26.19   A congenital nevus in the scalp.

Histology

The expected features, developed by an NIH Consensus Conference (67), are nevus cells in the lower two-thirds of the dermis, between collagen bundles distributed as single cells and in the lower two-thirds of the reticular dermis or subcutis, associated with blood vessels and nerves. These characteristics had been established initially

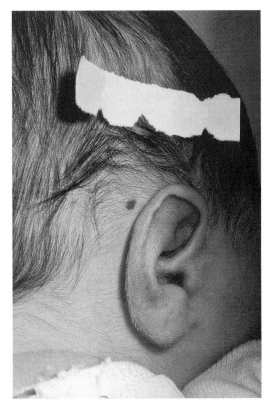

FIGURE 26.20   A small congenital nevus behind the ear.

Most of the nevi were not biopsied, so the diagnoses were based on the appearance of the nevus. Since the diagnostic criteria were not provided, and most nevi were not biopsied, the prevalence rates and potential racial differences have not been established. However, the findings in the studies of newborn infants (70–75) [Table 26-5] suggest that congenital nevi are more common in black infants than in white infants.

An epidemiologic survey of 531,831 liveborn infants in 59 maternity hospitals in several South American countries identified 989 infants with pigmented nevi. No biopsies were obtained to confirm that these were congenital nevi. However, these nevi were significantly more common in black infants, in comparison to white infants and Native Indians (76).

Location

Congenital nevi may occur on any part of the body.

Size

In the studies of newborn infants (Table 26-5), the average size is 0.5 to 1.5 cm in diameter.

Twinning

In the epidemiologic survey of 531,831 newborn infants in several South American hospitals (76), 12 sets of twins were identified. Among the five like-sex twins, only one twin had a pigmented nevus.

Genetic Factors

Mole counts in identical twins have been very similar, suggesting a role of genetic factors (77). However, the concordance of the biopsy-proven congenital nevi in identical twin newborns has not been established.

by Mark and his colleagues (68). Later, an analysis of 39 congenital nevi showed that these histologic patterns were observed primarily in larger congenital nevi over 3 cm in size (69). The smaller (less than 1.5 cm) congenital nevi did not have all of these histologic findings.

Prevalence Rate/Race/Ethnicity

The findings in newborn infants have been described for several racial and ethnic groups (Table 26-5).

TABLE 26-5 *Prevalence rates, ethnic groups and sizes of congenital nevi in several countries.*

Location	Ref.	Sample Size	Race/ethnic group	Number affected	Prevalence rate	Size
Australia, Sydney and Camperdown	(5)	420	Mixed	9	2.1%	0.5 cm median (0.1–3. cm range)
Denmark, Copenhagen	(6)	314	97% Caucasian 3% Other	2*	0.6%	Pt. 1: 1. x 1.2 cm Pt. 2: 1.7 x 07. cm
United States 1) Boston	(7)	4,641	2,682 Caucasian (51.8%) 492 Black (10.6%) 250 Hispanic (5.4%) 1,058 Mixed (15.2%) 89 Other (11%)	27 9 2 8 0	1.0% 1.8% 0.8% 0.8% 0	0.7 x 0.4 (average)
2) Stanford and Modesto	(8)	1,058	846 Caucasian (80%) 63 Black (6%) Hispanic (11%) Asian (3%)	21* 13 4 1	2.4% 19.7% 3.4% 3.1%	1.2 x 0.9 1.6 x 0.7 0.6 x 0.4 0.7 x 0.3
3) Washington	(9)	1,000	Black	57	5.7%	0.3 x 0.8
Japan, Tokyo	(10)	5,387	Asian (100%)	148	2.7%	Less than 1.0 cm

Family studies are needed to determine the empiric likelihood that the infant of an affected parent (or the sibling of an affected infant) will be affected.

Management

In the 1970s and 1980s, it was often recommended that all congenital nevi, including those less than 3 cm in diameter, be removed (66, 78). One reason was that studies of individuals with melanoma had shown that this malignancy had developed from a congenital nevus that was present at birth (79). Another reason was that the scar from removal at a young age will be small when this individual is older.

However, at this time (80, 81), there is much less enthusiasm for the removal of small congenital nevi. There seems to be no increased risk of melanoma arising in small congenital nevi. Follow-up observation is recommended with removal of lesion recommended, if there are changes in appearance.

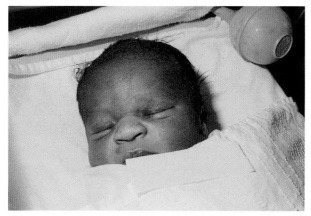

FIGURE 26.1 Shows macular stain (Nevus Simplex) on both upper eyelids (the "angel kiss").

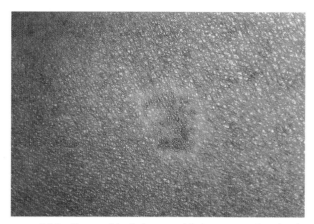

FIGURES 26.5 Shows white halo around lesion expected to develop an infantile hemangioma.

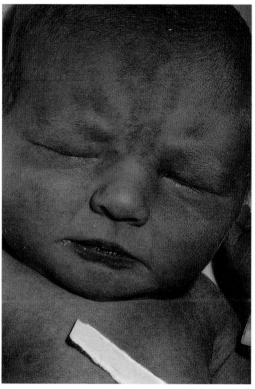

FIGURE 26.2 A macular stain on the forehead (Nevus Simplex).

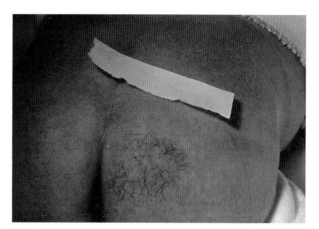

FIGURE 26.6 Dark telangietasia in an area in which an infantile hemangioma will develop.

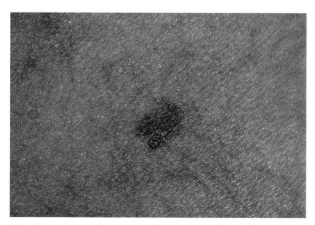

FIGURE 26.3 A macular stain on the abdomen (Nevus Simplex).

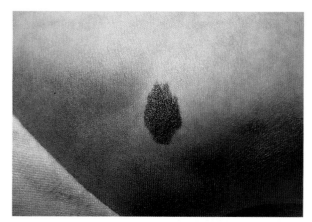

FIGURES 26.7 A white halo around a hemangioma in a newborn infant.

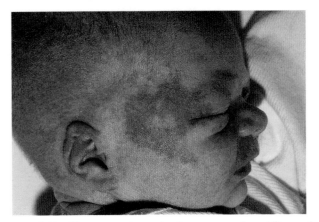

FIGURE 26.9 Shows portwine stain that stops at the midline and includes the upper eyelid.

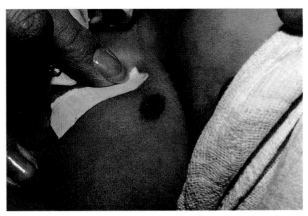

FIGURE 26.16 Shows speckling in congenital nevus.

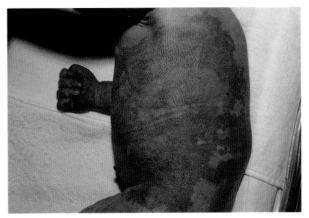

FIGURE 26.12 The portwine stain on the chest and abdomen.

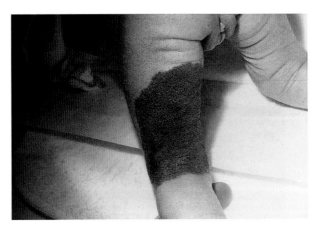

FIGURE 26.21 Giant hairy nevus on back of one leg.

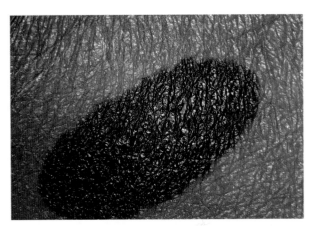

FIGURE 26.15 Close-up view of a congenital nevus.

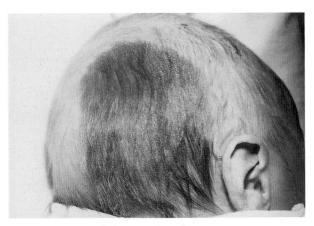

FIGURES 26.22 Giant hairy nevus in scalp.

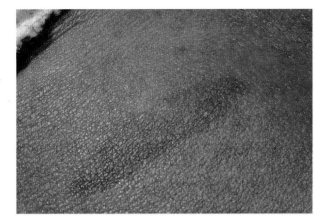

FIGURE 26.27   Café au lait spots on the chest.

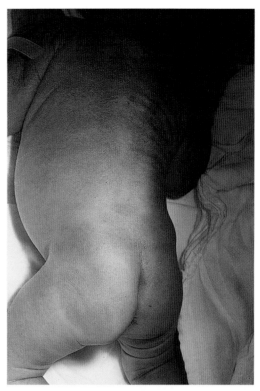

FIGURES 26.31   A typical large mongolian spot on buttocks and lower back.

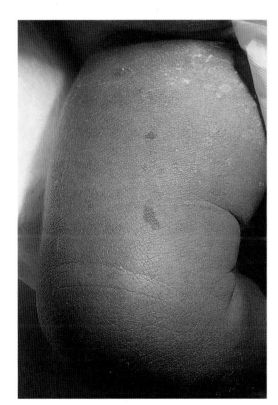

FIGURE 26.28   Café au lait spots on one leg.

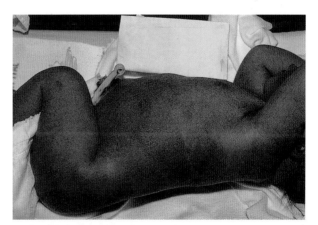

FIGURE 26.32   Located on back, chest, and one leg.

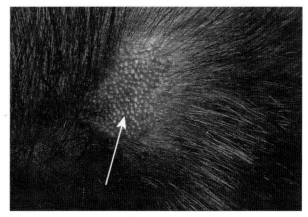

FIGURES 26.37   Sebaceous nevus in scalp (arrow).

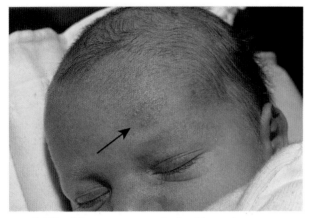

FIGURE 26.39   Sebaceous nevus on forehead (arrow).

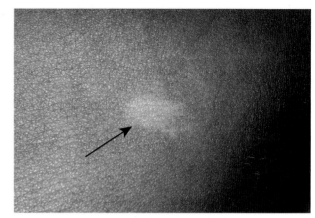

FIGURE 26.45   Depigmented nevus on back (arrow).

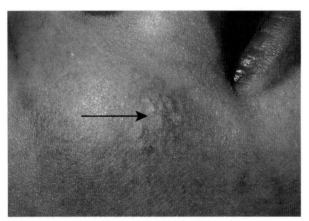

FIGURE 26.42   Sebaceous nevus next to mouth (arrow).

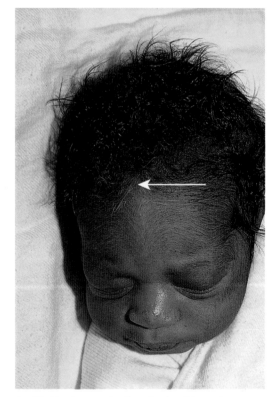

FIGURE 26.47   Depigmented tuft on forehead (arrow).

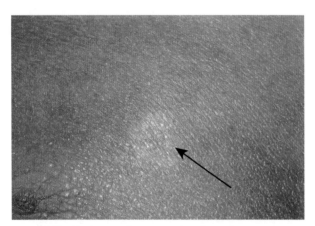

FIGURE 26.44   Depigmented nevus on chest (arrow).

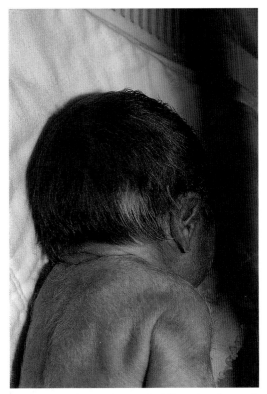

FIGURE 26.49 A newborn infant with vitiligo, showing on face and patches of hair. The infant's father also had vitiligo.

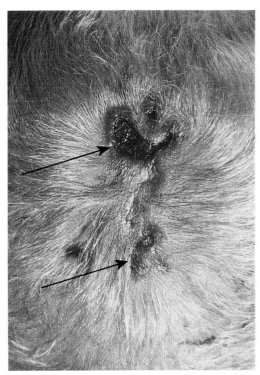

FIGURE 26.53 Multiple scalp defects in an infant with trisomy 13.

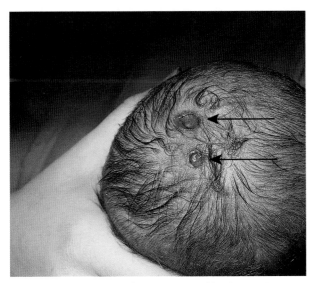

FIGURE 26.52 Two scalp defects on crown of head (arrow).

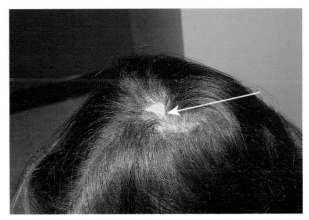

FIGURES 26.55 The healed, hairless scar (arrow) in the scalp of the mother of the infant shown in Figure 26.54.

GIANT HAIRY NEVUS

Definition

A raised, darkly pigmented and hairy nevus that is typically large and visible at birth.

ICD-9:   216.920   (hairy nevus)

ICD-10:   216.920   (melanocytic naevi, includes hairy nevus)

Mendelian   137550   (giant pigmented hairy
Inheritance   nevus [GPHN])
in Man:

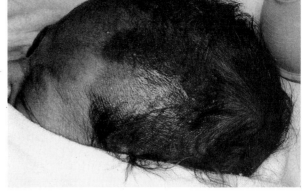

FIGURE 26.23   Nevi in scalp.

Appearance

The term "giant" was proposed by Pilney, Broadbent, and Woolf (82) in 1967 because this nevus was so large that it could not be excised completely. Because of their distribution, they have been referred to, also, as glove-like, coat-like, swimming trunk, or garment nevi.

These large nevi are easily distinguished from the surrounding skin because they are dark and appear raised (Figures 26-21–26-24).

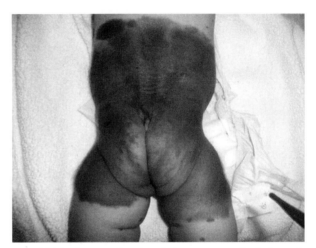

FIGURE 26.24   An extensive giant hairy nevus over back, buttocks, and legs. (Courtesy of Daniela Kroshinsky, M.D., Massachusetts General Hospital, Boston, MA.)

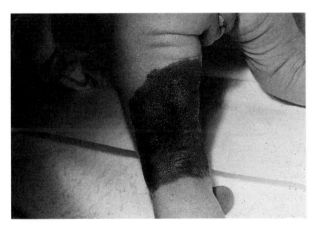

FIGURE 26.21   On back of one leg.

Most are hairy. The pigmentation is not always uniform; some are dark in the center of the nevus and light in the periphery. There may be several additional pigmented satellite nevi in other areas with or without hair (83–86).

Appearance

The presence of satellite nevi increases the risk of leptomeningeal involvement, especially when located in the midline of the trunk or on the head (87). When the nevus cells are present within the leptomeninges, there can be increased intracranial pressure, hydrocephalus, seizures, and neurologic deficits.

Histology

In biopsies of giant pigmented hairy nevi (GPHN), the dermal portions contained primarily moderate sized to small nevus cells with uniform ovoid nuclei, which were

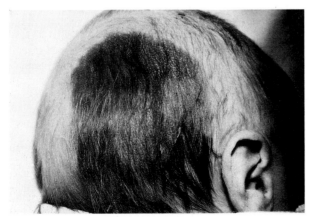

FIGURE 26.22   Nevi in scalp.

thought to represent immature melanocytic cells (88). Similar cells, smaller and more elongated, extended to the deepest portion of the dermis. Multiple long hair follicles were also present.

Prevalence

In the systematic examination of 4,641 newborn infants in Boston, 4 infants had a giant pigmented hairy nevus for a prevalence rate of 0.9/1,000 or 1 in 1,160 (Figures 26-21 and 26-22) [85].

Location

Among the 54 affected individuals enrolled in an international registry (89), the most common locations of the giant hairy nevi were: back (33.3%), scalp (20.4%), legs (18.5%), and bathing trunk area (18.5%). The minimum size for enrollment was 20 cm or more in diameter.

Size

The average size of four giant hairy nevi identified in the systematic examination of 4,641 newborn infants (Figures 26-21 and 26-22) in Boston was 12.2 x 9.1 cm (85). Only one of the four infants had a nevus with a diameter of 20 cm or more (Figure 26-24).

Sex Ratio

In the registry of 54 individuals with giant hairy nevi (89), 56% were female and 44% were males.

Race/Ethnicity

The prevalence rates in different racial and ethnic groups has not been established.

Twinning

The findings in a population-based study of an unselected series of identical twins have not been published. In one set of identical twins (90), only one had a giant hairy nevus.

Genetic Factors

Affected relatives have been described in a few families: two cousins in one (91); in three other families, relatives of the individuals with GPHN had multiple small pigmented nevi (92).

Gene expression profiles were evaluated in tissue from three patients with GPHN. The microarray showed increased expression of 22 genes and decreased expression of 73 genes in the nevi. In the nearly unaffected normal skin there was increased expression of 36 genes and decreased expression of five genes. The strongest increases in gene expression were in the melanoma associated gene *SPARCL1* (87).

Environmental Factors

No exposures during pregnancy have been shown to increase the frequency of giant hairy nevi.

Management

The significant risk for melanoma is well-established, but the specific rate has differed among studies (86, 89). In a follow-up study for up to 60 years in Sweden, the rate was 4% (93). In a follow-up of 47 affected individuals for a mean duration of 53 months, one (2.1%) developed melanoma. Other follow-up studies in the 1960s and 1970s showed rates of 6.9 to 31.1%. A 6 to 8% estimate has been used for counseling the parents of affected infants (89).

Two philosophies of management have developed— the surgical and the non-surgical approaches. Rhodes and his colleagues (86) analyzed the finding in follow-up studies and estimated the lifetime risk for developing melanoma was 6.3%, a 17-fold increase in comparison to the general population. They noted that the melanomas arise before age 10, often before age 5 years. They recommended excision as soon as the affected infant was healthy. They noted that the excision should go down to muscle fascia or deeper if nevus cells extend further.

One disadvantage of the surgical approach is the huge scars and the morbidity of surgical procedures. The non-surgical approach is to carry out examinations of the nevi every six months. When imaging studies identify neural melanosis, removal of the nevus is not realistic.

It is important for the parents of the affected infant to learn about the advantages and disadvantages of each approach.

CAFÉ-AU-LAIT SPOTS

Definition

Uniform tan-brown round, oval, or polygonal flat, evenly pigmented macules with distinct margins and irregular contour.

ICD-9:	757.390	(café-au-lait spots)
ICD-10:	L81.3	(café-au-lait spots)
Mendelian Inheritance in Man:	114030	(multiple café-au-lait spots)

Appearance

These flat light to dark brown uniform lesions can be visible at birth or soon thereafter (95, 96) [Figures 26-25–26-28].

A distinctive characteristic of the café-au-lait spot is the fact that the skin markings in the macule continue uninterrupted into the surrounding skin (97, 98). This is in contrast to the features of the nevocellular nevus, in which the skin markings in the surrounding skin do not continue into the nevus. The borders of the café-au-lait spot are distinct.

Café-au-lait spots can occur on any part of the body.

Histology

These macules have an increased amount of epidermal melanin in both melanocytes and keratinocytes. There is no proliferation of melanocytes, which distinguishes a café-au-lait spot from a nevocellular nevus (95, 97, 98). In one early study (99), giant pigmented granules in the melanocytes were present in biopsies of the café-au-lait spot and in the normal skin separated by several centimeters.

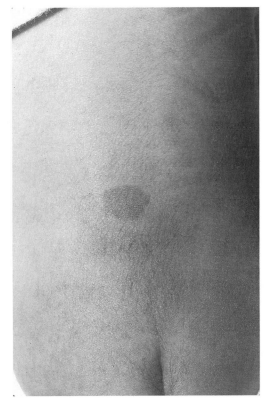

FIGURE 26.26   Café au lait spots on the lower back.

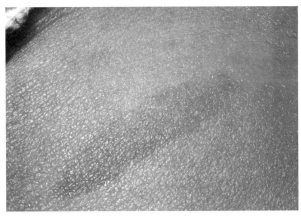

FIGURE 26.27   Café au lait spots on the chest.

Size

In the systematic surface examination of 4,641 newborn infants in Boston (97), 124 infants were identified who had one or more café-au-lait spots. The range in the sizes was 0.2 to 4.0 cm in length and 0.2 to 3.5 cm in width.

In the examination of 3,345 Chinese infants under 48 hours of age, 14 (0.4%) had café-au-lait spots with the average size: 0.6 x 1.1 cm (100).

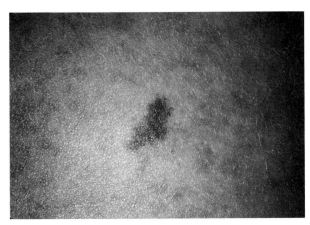

FIGURE 26.25   Café au lait spots on the abdomen.

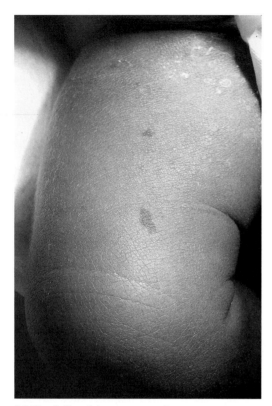

FIGURE 26.28   Café au lait spots on one leg.

Prevalence Rate

Frequencies of occurrence in newborn infants have been reported in several populations, but the definitions used were not presented in most studies. The frequency of one or more café-au-lait spots have included: Boston, 2.7% [several racial groups] (97), Japan, 1.7% (101), and Taiwan 0.4% (100).

Location

In the Boston study (97), the café-au-lait spots were in many areas of the body. A large number were on the buttocks and very few on the scalp.

Race/Ethnicity

In Boston (97), racial designation was based on the information provided by the mother concerning the racial origin of each of the four grandparents of the infant. There were differences in frequency for the two major racial groups: 0.3% of 2,682 white infants had one or more café-au-lait spots and 2.7% of 492 black infants. A higher frequency of café-au-lait spots was also established in examinations of African American school children in comparison to Caucasian children (102).

Environmental Factors

No exposures to teratogens have been shown to be associated with the occurrence of café-au-lait spots.

Management

Most infants with a café-au-lait spot have no other medical problems and are healthy. Café-au-lait spots increase in size proportionally, as the infant grows. They persist into the adult years and do not fade over time.

Multiple café-au-lait spots are much more common among black than white infants and are not likely to have any medical significance.

The clinician who identifies several café-au-lait spots in a newborn infant has several issues to consider:

1. The presence of multiple café-au-lait spots does not mean the infant has neurofibromatosis, type I.
2. It is important to distinguish multiple café-au-lait spots from multiple lentigines (Figures 26-29 and 26-30). These are evenly pigmented, sharply defined light to dark brown macules, which vary in size (3 to 15 mm) and are numerous. These are located most often on the face, back, and buttocks. These macules are unchanged by exposure to the sun. They fade over time in children.
3. Café-au-lait spots occur in many disorders, including:

Neurofibromatosis, type I:	(MIM +162200)
McCune Albright Syndrome:	(MIM #174800)
Noonan Syndrome:	(MIM #163950)
Costello Syndrome:	(MIM #218040)
Fanconi Anemia:	(MIM #227650)
Watson Syndrome:	(MIM 193520)
Russell Silver Syndrome:	(MIM 180860)

The clinician can look for additional signs of these phenotypes in the newborn infant with multiple cafe-au-lait spots. Since many of these associated features develop over time, follow-up reevaluations

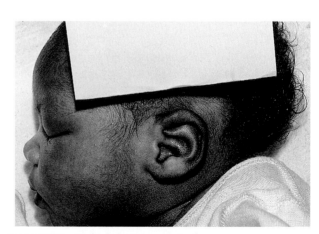

FIGURE 26.29   Multiple lentigines on the face.

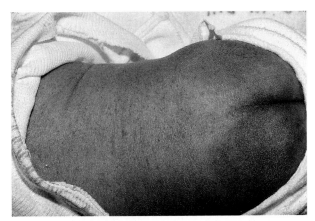

FIGURE 26.30 Multiple lentigines on an infant's back and a mongolian spot on the buttocks.

are essential to establishing the clinical phenotype and selecting disease-specific diagnostic testing.

4. There is high awareness among pediatricians of the fact that multiple café-au-lait spots are a common feature of neurofibromatosis, type I. The café-au-lait spots associated with NF1 can be present at birth. However, the predictive value of the number (or the size) of café-au-lait spots in newborn infants has not been established. Nevertheless, the presence of multiple café-au-lait spots in newborn infants is an important potential marker. The affected infant should be reevaluated periodically for additional features of NF1, including axillary freckling. Lisch nodules in the irides and subcutaneous neurofibromatosis can develop over time and their presence is helpful in establishing the diagnosis (103).

5. Multiple café-au-lait spots have also been identified as a separate genetic disorder (MIM 114030) [104,105]. The phenotype includes multiple café-au-lait spots, pectus deformity, and learning disabilities. An associated mutation in the SPRED1 gene has been identified (105). If a parent of the infant being evaluated also has multiple café-au-lait spots and no signs of any of the genetic disorders with associated café-au-lait spots, this diagnosis will warrant consideration.

MONGOLIAN SPOT

Definition

A large flat macule that is present at birth and has no medical significance.

ICD-9:	757.386	(mongolian spots)
ICD-10:	Q82.5	(congenital non-neoplastic naevus)
Mendelian Inheritance in Man:	None	

Historical Note

The term "mongolian spot" is archaic and inaccurate, but well-established. It is more common in newborns in Asia, but not all Asians are descended from Mongolian tribes (106, 108). Alternative terms have been suggested, such as ink-blot macules (107) and blue-gray macule in infancy (106). Regrettably, none has "caught on."

Appearance

These are patches with indistinct margins. The color varies from brown-black to blue-black to grey. An infant may have one or several of these spots (Figures 26-31–26-36) [106,107,110–119].

Size

The size varies from a few centimeters to more than 10 centimeters.

Location

The mongolian spot is most often on the sacrum and the buttocks (Table 26-6).

In a systematic examination of 437 full-term newborn infants in Jackson, Mississippi (112), 80% of the mongolian spots were in the sacro-gluteal area, 23% on shoulders, 14% of lumbar area, 6% on the dorsum of hand, and 0.6% on the forehead.

Prevalence Rate

In a systematic surface examination of 7,157 newborn infants from several racial/ethnic groups in the Boston Lying-In Hospital (1972–1974), 25.5% of the infants examined had one or more mongolian spots. The highest prevalence rate was among the 915 African American infants (88.7%) and the 412 Hispanic infants (6.5%). The lowest rate was among the 4,289 Caucasian infants (4.8%) [113,114].

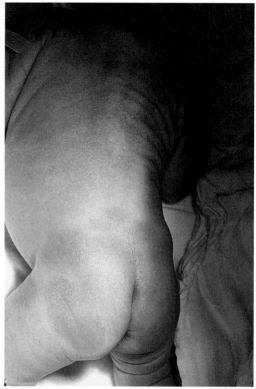

FIGURE 26.31   A typical large mongolian spot on buttocks and lower back.

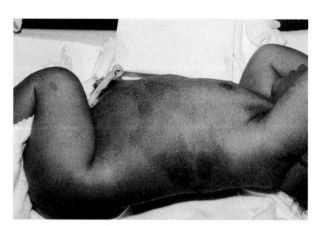

FIGURE 26.32   Located on back, chest, and one leg.

In two other studies (110,111) of newborn infants, the prevalence rates were 8.5% and 9.6%, respectively, among Caucasian infants and 60% and 95.5% among black infants.

In the systematic examination of 437 consecutive newborns in Jackson (112), marked differences in the frequency were observed in the predominant racial groups: 96% of African American infants, 46.3% of Hispanics, and 9.5% of Caucasian infants.

In Nigeria (117), 74.8% of 369 neonates had a mongolian spot and 13.6% of 381 children between 1 month

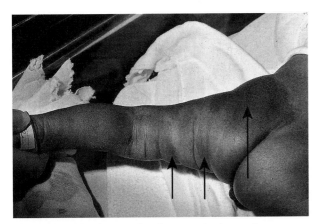

FIGURE 26.33   Macule extending down one leg (arrows).

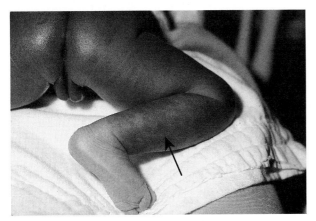

FIGURE 26.34   Macule extending down one leg (arrow).

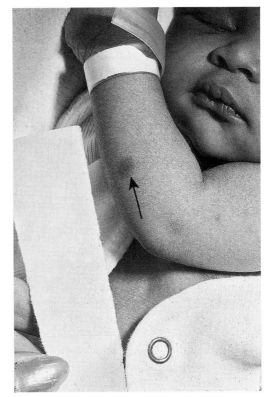

FIGURE 26.35   Smaller macule on forearm (arrow).

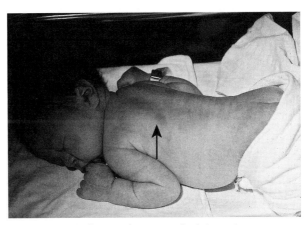

FIGURE 26.36   Smaller macule on upper back (arrow).

and 14 years had a mongolian spot. No child over age 6 was found to have a mongolian spot.

Among 500 newborn infants in Taiwan (118), 61.6% had a mongolian spot.

Histology

This lesion is caused by the presence of spindle-shaped melanocytes in the lower dermis, instead of their normal location in the epidermis (106, 107). The blue or black color is caused by the Tyndall effect of blue-indigo-violet light-scattering in the dermal melanocytes.

Clinical Management

A mongolian spot has no medical significance. Each fades in intensity during childhood (106, 107, 112, 117, 120).

Mongolian spots have been classified in durability into those which fade over time and those which are persistent. In the examination of 800 adults with a mean age of 45 years, 2.9% had mongolian spots, defined as "persistent" (120).

The mongolian spot is well-known, but the extensive distribution that occurs is not. One potential consequence is the misinterpretation that these nevi are bruises, with potential misinterpretation of being a sign of abuse (121).

The mongolian spot is to be distinguished from the nevus of Ito and the nevus of Ota. The nevus of Ota is distributed along the first and second divisions of the trigeminal nerve (106, 107). These nevi are often, but not always, present at birth. There can also be increased pigmentation of the sclera and oral mucosa. The nevus of Ota is more common in individuals of Asian ancestry

TABLE 26-6 *Frequency of "Mongolian spot" in newborn infants.*

In this study*:	All races	Whites	Blacks	Hispanics	Mixed	Other
All locations	25.5%	4.8%	88.7%	65.1%	29.0%	69.6%
	1819/7132	206/4289	812/915	268/412	373/1286	160/230
Sacrum	25.0%	4.7%	87.4%	63.6%	27.9%	68.3%
	1780/7133	202/4290	800/915	262/412	359/1286	157/230
Buttocks	20.3%	2.7%	78.8%	48.7%	22.0%	55.7%
	1448/7133	116/4291	721/915	200/411	283/1286	128/230
Back	4.4%	0.4%	22.0%	9.0%	3.0%	10.0%
	314/7136	15/4292	201/914	37/412	38/1288	23/230
Shoulders	3.7%	0.1%	20.7%	5.8%	2.4%	6.1%
	261/7135	3/4291	189/914	24/412	31/1288	14/230
Other sites	3.7%	0.05%	19.7%	5.6%	2.6%	10.0%
	261/7132	2/4289	180/914	23/421	33/1288	23/229

Legends: *Findings in the surface examination of 7,157 newborn infants examined between birth and five days of age at Boston Lying-In Hospital (1972–1974) [113, 114].

Race designation: Based on the mother's report of the racial origin of the four grandparents of the infant.

Mixed ancestry: More than one racial/ethnic group represented by the four grandparents of the infant of interest.

and more darkly pigmented racial/ethnic groups and females. The biopsy shows changes similar to those in a mongolian spot, but the melanocytes are more numerous and are located more superficially. Unlike the mongolian spot, the nevus of Ota does not lighten over time. Another difference from a mongolian spot is that it may increase in size and intensity of color over time, usually beginning in puberty.

The nevus of Ito has similar coloration to the nevus of Ota and the mongolian spot. It is located primarily on the shoulders, neck, upper arm, scapula, and deltoid regions. Like the nevus of Ota, the elongated dendritic melanocytes are usually more numerous and superficial than in mongolian spots. It is usually a benign condition, but can be associated rarely with transformation into melanoma.

SEBACEOUS NEVUS OF JADASSOHN

Definition

A yellow-tan or yellow-orange plaque on the face or scalp, which is present at birth.

ICD-9:   None

ICD-10:   None

Mendelian Inheritance in Man: None

Appearance

An oval or linear, elevated plaque, which is visible at birth and usually located on the scalp (Figures 26-37–26-39), face, or neck (Figures 26-40–26-42).

This nevus has a pebble-like, or velvety appearance. Typically this is a single or solitary nevus (122–129).

Histologic Features

Proliferation of the sebaceous glands in the mid to upper dermis, enlargement of the apocrine glands in the lower dermis, and papillomatosis of the epidermis.

Size

0.5 cm to 1 cm in 13 infants identified at birth (124).

Location

These lesions occur where pilosebaceous and epocrine glands are prominent, primarily on the scalp and face. In a systematic examination (124) of 4,461 newborns in Boston (1972–1974), the locations of the sebaceous nevus in 13 affected infants were: face (8/13; 62%), scalp (4; 31%) and sternum (1; 7%).

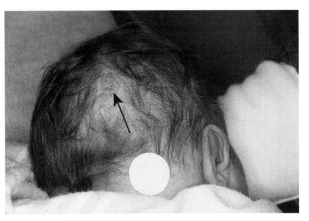

FIGURE 26.38   Sebaceous nevus in scalp (arrow).

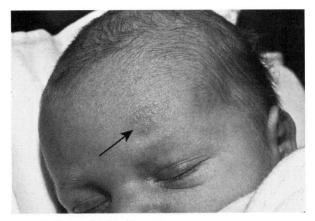

FIGURE 26.39   On forehead (arrow).

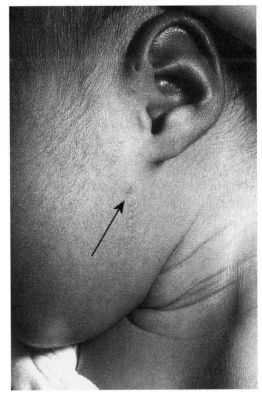

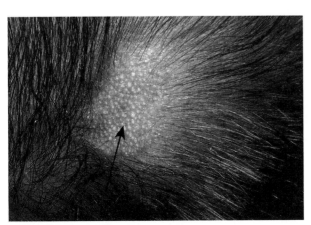

FIGURE 26.37   Sebaceous nevus in scalp (arrow).

FIGURE 26.40   On cheek in front of ear (arrow).

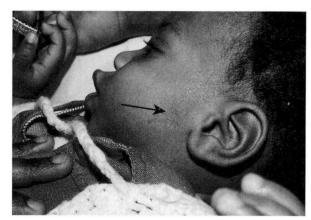

FIGURE 26.41   On cheek in front of ear (arrow).

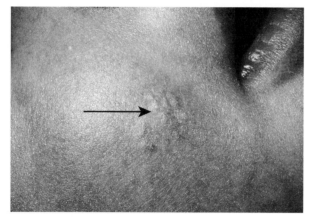

FIGURE 26.42   Next to mouth (arrow).

Prevalence Risk

The presence of sebaceous nevus in newborn infants has been reported in several clinical studies (124–126). The overall prevalence rates were 0.3% in two (124, 125) and 0.1% in the third (126). The prevalence rates have been similar in three racial/ethnic groups: Caucasian, 0.4% (124), Japanese, 0.3% (125), and Chinese newborns, 0.1% (126).

Genetic Factors

Several instances of familial sebaceous nevus have been reported (130–132), although the pattern of inheritance has not been established.

An affected parent and child were reported with the lesions confined to the scalp (130), and autosomal dominant inheritance was postulated.

Two affected siblings with affected parents were reported (132) and the authors postulated paradominant inheritance. In this mechanism, the mutation is present in a mosaic form; if normal cells were not present, the mutation would be lethal. The heterozygous carrier would be clinically unaffected and would pass the mutation along to his/her child. When a mutation leads to loss of the healthy allele during embryogenesis, a clone of mutant cells will arise. The severity of the phenotype would vary with the stage of embryogenesis in which the mutation occurs.

Management

Sebaceous nevi become smaller in the months after birth, which gives the parents and the infant's pediatrician a false reassurance that the nevus will not be a problem. However, during adolescence the same nevi undergo verrucous hyperplasia. After puberty the proliferation of both sebaceous and apocrine glands becomes marked (133). Since most are located on the face or scalp, they can have a serious cosmetic effect.

The sebaceous nevus can also be the site of trichoblastomas, syringocystadenoma papilliforum, and basal cell (low) carcinomas (133–135)

Because of this risk of verrucous hyperplasia at puberty and the development of benign and malignant tumors in the adult, the removal of sebaceous nevi has been recommended. One practical advantage of early removal is that the scar produced will be smaller when the infant is older. However, in the retrospective analysis of 757 affected individuals age 16 or younger, none had had a basal cell carcinoma identified. This raised the question as to whether prophylatic surgical removal is indicated.

The nevus sebaceous of Jadassohn appears to be usually isolated and is not associated with other abnormalities or developmental delay.

However, two rare syndromes in which there is a sebaceous nevus of the face or scalp and other abnormalities have been delineated (136):

1. Linear sebaceous syndrome: Schimmelpenning-Feirstein-Mims Syndrome (MIM: %163200). The affected infants have CNS abnormalities, ocular anomalies including coloboma, skeletal defects, as well as sebaceous nevus. A dominant gene mutation has been postulated as the cause.
2. Sebaceous nevus syndrome and hemimegalencephaly (MIM: 601359). The affected individuals have had, also, ipsilateral defects of the brain, eye, and connective tissue.

NEVUS DEPIGMENTOSUS (NEVUS ACHROMICUS)

Definition

Hypopigmented lesions that are present at birth and remain stable over time.

ICD-9:   NONE

ICD-10:   L81.5   (leukoderma)

Mendelian Inheritance
in Man:

Appearance

The nevus depigmentosus is usually a solitary lesion. These nevi are well-demarcated, often have irregular borders, and are lighter than the surrounding skin (137,138).

Under Wood's lamp, these lesions have an off-white coloration without fluorescence (138).

Three patterns of this nevus have been described (139): 1) an isolated patch, either circular or irregular in shape and size in a small segment of the body; 2) a streak or band along Blaschko's lines; 3) a systemic type with multiple whorls or streaks. The systemic type appears to be very rare (138).

While the nevus depigmentosus may be present at birth, it has developed in the first year or two of life. In general, this diagnosis is restricted to hypopigmented macules that develop "at an early age" (137), meaning less than age 3 (140).

Histology

The histologic studies have shown no special characteristics. With electron microscopy, there is a significant reduction in the number of melanosomes in melanocytes of this nevus in comparison to normal skin.

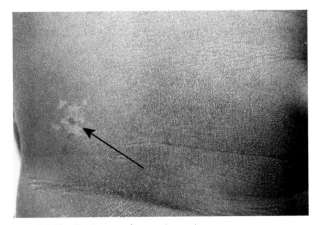

FIGURE 26.43   Depigmented nevus (arrow).

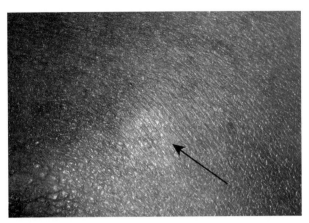

FIGURE 26.44   Depigmented nevus on chest (arrow).

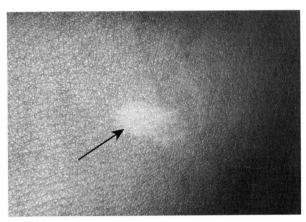

FIGURE 26.45   Depigmented nevus on back (arrow).

Aggregated melanosomes are also observed in keratinocytes (137, 140).

Prevalence

The prevalence rate of hypopigmented nevi in newborn infants has been determined in several studies (141–143). In the examination of 1,000 newborns by Kennedy and Kalish (141), using a long-wave ultraviolet light, four had hypopigmented macular lesions (0.4%), one solitary and the others multiple. In the examination of 9,737 newborn infants in Paris (142), 60 (0.6%) had one depigmented nevus, eight (0.08%) had two, and three (0.03%) had three or more.

In Boston, the systematic study examination of 4,641 infants for all types of birth marks, 35 infants (0.8%) were found to have depigmented nevi[143].

Location

These nevi are usually present on the trunk (137, 138).

Size

In the study in Boston, the greatest diameter varied, but was typically 1 to 2 centimeters.

Race/Ethnicity

The information available is from relatively small numbers of infants, so clear differences between major racial groups have not been established.

Twinning

The likelihood that one or both identical twins will have a depigmented nevus has not been determined.

Genetic Factors

There have been no studies of the occurrence of depigmented nevi in siblings or offspring of affected individuals.

Environmental Factors

Exposure to human teratogens has been shown to increase the frequency of depigmented nevi.

Management

The nevus depigmentosus has no medical significance.

The challenge for the clinician evaluating the infant with a nevus depigmentosus is to make certain the infant does not have a more serious medical condition, such as:

1. tuberous sclerosis (MIM: #191100): an autosomal dominant condition; most affected individuals have depigmented nevi at birth; there are often several depigmented nevi; other features like the chagrin patch may be present at birth; other features, such as periungal fibromas and angiofibromas, may develop over the next 5 to 10 years.
2. piebaldism (MIM: #172800): an autosomal dominant condition; there are more extensive patches of depigmentation, as well as white patches of hair.
3. Waardenburg Syndrome, type I (MIM: #193500): an autosomal dominant condition; the features in the affected newborn include patches of depigmented skin, a white forelock, dystopia canthorum; a broad nasal root; and congenital deafness.
4. hypomelanosis of Ito (MIM: #300337): the skin lesions are more extensive, such as whorl or linear white spots; the depigmented areas may not be present at birth.

It had been proposed by Fitzpatrick and his associates (144) that the presence of multiple depigmented nevi in a newborn infant made it more likely that the affected infant had tuberous sclerosis. However, the follow-up studies of affected infants by Alper et al. (143) identified newborn infants with multiple depigmented nevi that were no longer present at 6 months of age. Several parents, contacted by telephone, reported that a depigmented nevus identified at birth was no longer visible later in the first year of life.

The probability that a nevus depigmentosus, present at birth, is benign or has serious medical significance must be established by a prospective study of affected newborn infants.

HYPOPIGMENTED TUFT OF HAIR

Definition

A tuft of light blonde hair.

ICD-9:   None

ICD-10:   L67.1   (poliosis)

Mendelian Inheritance in Man: None

Appearance

This tuft of light blonde hair may be present in any region of the scalp. The hypopigmented hair has the same appearance as the adjacent scalp hair.

Histology

The shafts of hair are normal.

The hair follicles in two affected infants were analyzed and found to have tyrosinase activity.

Prevalence

The prevalence rate has not been established. In a systematic examination of 4,641 newborn infants in Boston (145, 146), fifteen infants were identified with a hypopigmented tuft of hair: 3.2/1,000 or 1:309. Information is needed from additional studies of newborn infants.

Location

In the study in Boston, the location of the light tuft of hair was recorded in 11 infants: parietal region in 5, along midline on top of head in 5, and along forehead (Figures 26-46–26-48).

Size

The average size was two by one centimeter in 12 affected infants.

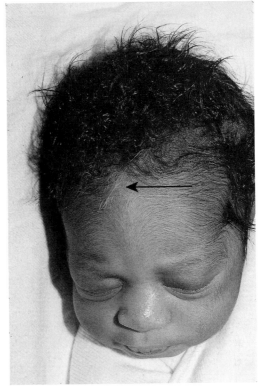

FIGURE 26.47   Depigmented tuft of hair in upper brow (arrow).

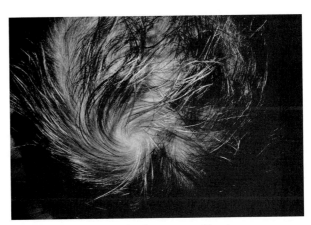

FIGURE 26.48   Depigmented tuft on crown of head.

Sex Ratio

In the small sample of 15 infants, there were 6 affected males and 9 females.

Race/Ethnicity

In the sample of 4,641 infants examined, 12 of 2,682 (1:223) Caucasian infants were affected. There were too few affected infants to establish prevalence rates in any other racial group.

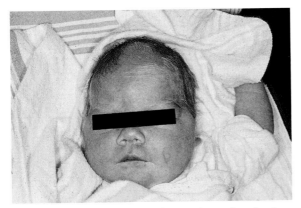

FIGURE 26.46   Depigmented tuft on brow at front edge of scalp.

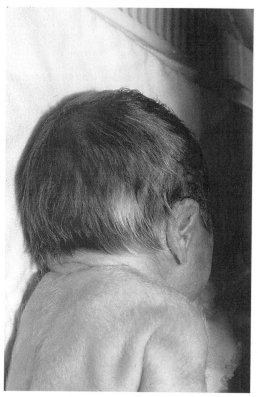

FIGURE 26.49   A newborn infant with vitiligo, showing on face and patches of hair. The infant's father also had vitiligo.

Environmental Factors

None have been associated with the occurrence of a hypopigmented tuft of hair.

Differential Diagnosis

Theoretically, the hypopigmented tuft of hair, like a nevus depigmentosus, is associated with tuberous sclerosis. However, this association has not been established in any systematic study.

Management

The hypopigmented tuft of hair appears to have no medical significance. It would be helpful to confirm that there is no association with tuberous sclerosis or important other causes of decreased pigment in hair.

In follow-up interviews with parents of 11 affected infants several months after their birth, the hypopigmented tuft of hair was still present in 9 (82%).

Genetic Counseling

Six of the parents of 11 infants interviewed reported that close relatives had, also, a hypopigmented tuft of hair.

The examining clinician should evaluate the infant for signs of other causes of poliosis, that is, a decreased pigment in the hair. The conditions to consider include:

1. vitiligo (Mendelian Inheritance in Man: #193200); see Figure 26-49, which shows decreased pigmentation in the skin and hair;
2. Waardenburg Syndrome (MIM: #193500), which can be associated with a white forelock, and distinctive facial features, such as telecanthus.
3. tuberous sclerosis (MIM: #191100): an autosomal dominant condition; most affected individuals have depigmented nevi at birth; there are often several depigmented nevi; other features, such as periungal fibromas and angio fibromas, may develop over the last 5 to 10 years."

APLASIA CUTIS CONGENITA (SCALP DEFECTS)

Definition

A defect in the skin, present at birth, which is characterized by absence of the epidermis, dermis, and sometimes underlying subcutaneous tissues.

ICD-9:	757.800	(scalp defect)
ICD-10:		None
Mendelian Inheritance in Man:	%107600	(aplasia/cutis congenital, nonsyndromic, ACC)

Appearance

These are sharply demarcated defects in the skin occurring either as single (Figures 26-50 and 26-51) or multiple (Figures 26-52 and 26-53) defects. They are circular or oval in shape. Typically they have a red base of exposed subcutaneous tissue (147, 148). In the newborn infant, they can be oozing, granulating or ulcerated. Once healed, the base of this skin defect is a scar without hair.

A less common type of aplasia cutis is called "membranous aplasia cutis," which has a translucent, glistening membrane. These can be fluid-filled beneath the membrane (149).

The "hair collar sign" is a ring of long dark hair that surrounds the circular skin defect. These are usually located on the vertex of the scalp or in the parietal region (149, 150) [Figure 26-51].

Histologic Features

There is a loss of the epidermis, often with loss of dermis as well. The skin defect is demarcated clearly from surrounding skin (147).

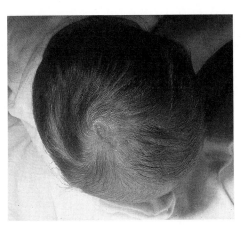

FIGURE 26.50   A single scalp defect at crown of head.

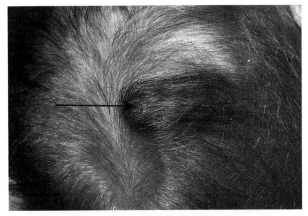

FIGURE 26.51   A small scalp defect with the "hair collar sign," which is a ring of long dark hair. (arrow)

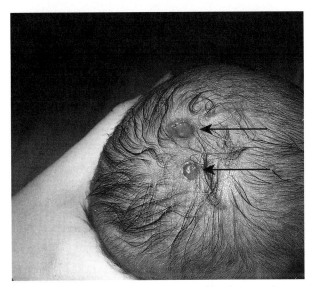

FIGURE 26.52   Two scalp defects on crown of head. (arrows)

The skin defect in the scalp will heal with a scar over the base and lack of hair (Figure 26-54).

Size/Number

Usually the size is one to two centimeters in diameter.

Most (70%) of these are a single, isolated skin defect (151).

Location

Most often these are scalp defects over the crown of the head, near the normal location of the hair whorl (148).

They may occur, especially in twin-twin transfusion syndrome, as defects in skin over knees and lateral aspects of abdomen (152, 153).

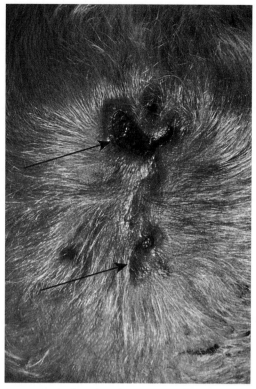

FIGURE 26.53   Multiple scalp defects in an infant with trisomy 13.

Midline aplasia cutis in the lumbar region is an occasional manifestation of an underlying posterior vertebral defect with an associated fibrous tract that may enter the spinal canal and be connected to the filum terminate, causing tethering of the spinal cord [154].

Prevalence Rate

Not established.

One infant with aplasia cutis in midline of lumbar region was found in a systematic examination of 4, 641 newborn infants (151).

Management

The isolated aplasia cutis skin defect is usually on the scalp. Typically it heals and forms a scar without treatment. However, large single or multiple scalp defects may require surgical repair.

The scalp defect associated with a ring of dark hair (the "hair collar sign") [Figure 26-51] should be evaluated by imaging studies for associated skull defects and brain and cardiovascular anomalies (149, 155).

Environmental Factors

Exposure during pregnancy to two drugs, methimazole (156) and misoprostol (157, 158), have been associated

with the occurrence of scalp defects. Methimazole and carbimazole are medications used to treat hyperthyroidism. Scalp defects were first reported in methimazole-exposed pregnancies by Milham and Elledge in 1972 (156).

More recently it has been suggested that the methimazole-exposed infant may have a specific embryopathy, which includes choanal atresia and esophageal atresia (157).

Misoprostol is a prostaglandin E_1 analogue that has been used as an illegal abortifacient in communities in Central and South America. Extensive scalp defects, including a deficiency of the underlying cranium, were described by Fonseca and his associates in 1993 (158). However, scalp defects have not been a common finding in subsequent case series. Möebius Syndrome (due to cranial nerve deficiencies), limb deficiencies, arthrogryposis, and hemifacial microsomia have been the most common misoprostol-associated defects all of that have been attributed to vascular disruption (159).

Genetic Counseling

The isolated scalp defect may occur as a familial condition (Figures 26-54 and 26-55).

It has been considered an autosomal dominant condition (MIM %107600) with parent to child transmission. However, affected half brothers with unaffected parents (160) suggest other patterns of inheritance, as well.

The infant with a membranous scalp defect, including a hair collar sign, should be evaluated for an underlying atretic encephalocele (149, 150, 155).

The infant with a midline skin defect in the lumbosacral region should be evaluated for spinal dysraphism, with an associated posterior defect of the underlying vertebrae and tethering of the spinal cord (154).

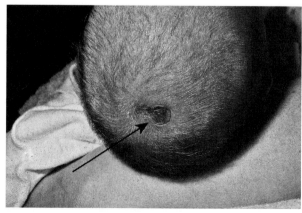

FIGURE 26.54   A scalp defect (arrow) in a newborn infant whose mother (Figure 26.55) has a healed, hairless scar in the same area.

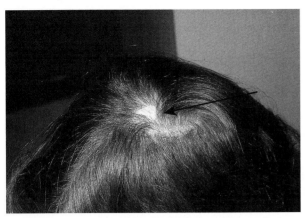

FIGURE 26.55 The healed, hairless scar (arrow) in the scalp of the mother of the infant shown in Figure 26.54.

Congenital scalp defects occur in association with several syndromes (161), including:

1. Adams-Oliver Syndrome (MIM %100300), features of which are scalp defects, skull defect below the scalp defect, heart defects, and terminal transverse limb defects.

2. Skin defects are produced by emboli from the deceased co-twin in the twin-twin transfusion syndrome (150). These can be caused also when the co-twin is a "fetus papyraceous" (150, 152). Presumably, the aplasia of the skin is an effect of embolization of necrotic tissue in the surviving twin.

3. Chromosome 13 trisomy, in which there are often multiple scalp defects.

REFERENCES

1. Tan KL. Nevus flammeus of the nape, glabella and eyelids. A clinical study of frequency racial distribution, and association with congenital anomalies. *Clin Pediatr.* 1972;11:112–118.
2. Bossard K. Die blassen Feuermale der Kinder. *Jahrb f. Kinderh.* 1918;88:204.
3. Margileth AM, Museles M. Current concepts in diagnosis and management of congenital cutaneous hemangiomas. *Pediatrics.* 1965;36:410–416.
4. Mulliken JB, Glowacki J. Hemangiomas and vascular malformations in infants and children: classification based on endothelial characteristics. *Plast Reconstr Surg.* 1982;69:412–422.
5. North PE, Waner M, Buckmiller L, James CA, Mihm MC Jr. Vascular tumors of infancy and childhood: beyond capillary hemangioma. *Cardiovascular Pathology.* 2006;15:303–317.
6. Pratt AG. Birthmarks in infants. *Arch Dermatol.* 1953;67:302–305.
7. Selmanowitz VJ. Nevus flammeus of the forehead. *J Pediatr.* 1968;73:755–757.
8. Jacobs AH, Walton RG. The incidence of birthmarks in the neonate. *Pediatric.* 1976;58:218–222.
9. Alper JC, Holmes LB. The incidence and significance of birthmarks in a cohort of 4,641 newborns. *J Pediatr Derm.* 1983;1:58–68.
10. Osburn K, Schosser RH, Everett MA. Congenital pigmented and vascular lesions in newborn infants. *J Am Acad Dermatol.* 1987; 16:788–792.
11. Rivers JK, Frederiksen PC, Dibdin C. A prevalence survey of dermatoses in the Australian neonate. *J Am Acad Dermatol.* 1990; 23:77–81.
12. Tsai F-J, Tsai C-H. Birthmarks and congenital skin lesions in Chinese newborns. *J Formos Med Assoc.* 1993;92:838–841.
13. Leppig KA, Werler MM, Cann CI, Cook CA, Holmes LB. Predictive value of minor anomalies in association with major malformations. *J Pediatr.* 1987;110:531–537.
14. Smith MA, Manfield PA. The natural history of salmon patches in the first year of life. *Brit J Dermatol.* 1962;73:31–33.
15. Garzon MC, Huang JT, Enjolras O, Frieden IJ. Vascular malformations. Part II. Associated syndromes. *J Am Acad Dermatol.* 2007;56:541–564.
16. Tubbs RS, Wellons JC III, Iskandar BJ, Oakes WJ. Isolated flat capillary midline lumbosacral hemangiomas as indicators of occult spinal dysraphism. *J Neurosurg (Pediatrics 2).* 2004;100:86–89.
17. Selmanowitz VJ. Nevus flammeus of the forehead. *J Pediatr.* 1968;73:755–757.
18. Finn MC, Glowacki J, Mulliken JB. Congenital vascular lesions: clinical application of a new classification. *J Pediatr Surg.* 1983; 18:894–900.
19. Enjoras O, Garzon MC. Vascular stains, malformations, and tumors. In: Eichenfield LF, Frieden IJ, Esterly NB, eds. *Textbook of Neonatal Dermatology.* Philadelphia: Saunders; 2001: 324–346.
20. Haggstrom AN, Drolet BA, Baselga E, Chamlin SL, Garzon MC, Horeii KA et al. Prospective study of infantile hemangiomas: clinical characteristics predicting complications and treatment. *Pediatrics.* 2006;118:882–887.
21. Dudras SS, North PE, Bertoncini J, Mihm MC, Detmar M. Infantile hemangiomas are arrested in an early developmental vascular differentiation state. *Modern Pathology.* 2004;17: 1068–1079.
22. North PE, Waner M, Mizeracki A, Mihm MC Jr. GLUT1: a newly discovered immunohistochemical marker for juvenile hemangiomas. *Hum Pathol.* 2000;31:11–22.
23. Baschoff J. Monoclonal expansion of endothelial cells in hemangiomas? *Trends Cardiovas Med.* 2002;12:220–224.
24. Walter JW, North PE, Wander M, Mizeracki A, Blei F, Walker JWT et al. Somatic mutation of vascular endothelial growth factor receptors in juvenile hemangioma. *Genes Chromosomes Cancer.* 2002;33:295–303.
25. Hidano A, Nakajim S. Earliest features of the strawberry mark in the newborn. *Brit J Dermatol.* 1972;87:138–144.
26. Alper JC, Holmes LB. Incidence and significance of birthmarks in a cohort of 4,641 newborns. *J Pediatr Derm.* 1983;1:58–68.
27. Leppig KA, Werler MM, Cann CI, Cook CA, Holmes LB. Predictive value of minor anomalies in association with major malformations. *J Pediatr.* 1987;110:531–537.
28. Pratt AG. Birthmarks in infants. *Arch Dermatol.* 1953;67: 302–305.
29. Jacobs AH, Walton RG. The incidence of birthmarks in the neonate. *Pediatrics.* 1976;58:218–222.
30. Bivings L. Spontaneous regression of angiomas in children. 22 years observation covering 236 cases. *J Pediatr.* 1954;45: 643–647.
31. Jacobs AH. Strawberry hemangiomas. The natural history of the untreated lesion. *Calif Med.* 1957;86:8–10.
32. Amir J, Metzker A, Krikler R, Reisner SH. Strawberry hemangioma in preterm infants. *Pediatr Dermatol.* 1986;3:331–332.
33. Drolet BA, Frieden IJ. Infantile hemangiomas: an emerging health issue linked to an increasing rate of low birth weight infants in the United States. *J Pediatr.* 2008;153:712–715.
34. Cheung DSM, Warman ML, Mulliken JB. Hemangiomas in twins. *Ann Plast Surg.* 1997;38:269–274.
35. Haggstrom AN, Drolet BA, Baselga E, Chamlin SL, Garzon MC, Horii KA et al. Prospective study of infantile hemangiomas:

demographic, prenatal, and perinatal characteristics. *J Pediatr.* 2007;150:291–294.

36. Burton BK, Schulz CJ, Angle B, Burd LI. An increased incidence of haemangiomas in infants born following chorionic villus sampling (CVS). *Prenat Diagn.* 1995;15:209–214.

37. North PE, Waner M, Brodsky MC. Are infantile hemangiomas of placental origin? *Ophthalmology.* 2002;109:633–634.

38. Mulliken JB, Enjolras O. Congenital hemangiomas and infantile hemangiomas: missing links. *J Am Acad Dermatol.* 2004;50: 875–882.

39. Marler JJ, Mulliken JB. Current management of hemangiomas and vascular malformations. *Clin Plast Surg.* 2005;32:99–116.

40. Higuera S, Gordley K, Metry DW, Stal S. Management of hemangiomas and pediatric vascular malformations. *J Craniofac Surg.* 2006;17:783–789.

41. Frieden IJ. Which hemangiomas to treat and how? *Arch Dermatol.* 1997;133:1593–1595.

42. Mulliken JB, Young AE. *Vascular Birthmarks: Hemangiomas and Malformations.* Philadelphia: WB Saunders, 1988.

43. Brouillard P, Vikkula M. Vascular malformations: localized defects in vascular morphogenesis. *Clin Genet.* 2003;63:340–351.

44. Kelly KM, Choi B, McFarlane S, Motosue A, Jung B, Khan MH et al. Description and analysis of treatments for port-wine stain birthmarks. *Arch Facial Plast Surg.* 2005;7:287–294.

45. Barsky SH, Rosen S, Geer DE, Noe JM. The nature and evolution of port wine stains: a computer-assisted study. *J Invest Dermatol.* 1980;74:154–157.

46. Leung AKC. The nature of naevus flammeus. *Eur J Pediatr.* 2003;162:816.

47. Neumann R, Leonhartsberger H, Knobler R, Honigsmann H. Immunohistochemistry of portwine stains and normal skin with endothelium-specific antibodies PAL-E, anti-ICAM-1, anti-ELAM-1, and anti-factor VIIIrAg. *Arch Dermatol.* 1994;130:879–883.

48. Smoller BR, Rosen S. Port-wine stains. A disease of altered neuronal modulation of blood vessels? *Arch Dermatol.* 1986;122: 177–179.

49. Jacobs AH, Walton RG. The incidence of birthmarks in the neonate. *Pediatrics.* 1976;58:218–222.

50. Tsai F-J, Tsai C-L. Birthmarks and congenital skin lesions in Chinese newborns. *J Formos Med Assoc.* 1993;92:838–841.

51. Alper JC, Holmes LB. The incidence and significance of birthmarks in a cohort of 4,641 newborns. *Pediatr Dermatol.* 1983;1: 58–66.

52. Leppig KA, Werler MM, Cann CI, Cook CA, Holmes LB. Predictive value of minor anomalies: I. Association with major malformations. *J Pediatr.* 1987;110:531–537.

53. Azizkhan RG. Laser surgery: new applications for pediatric skin and airway lesions. *Current Opin Pediatr.* 2003;15:243–247.

54. Berg JN, Quaba AA, Georgantopoulou A, Porteous ME. A family with hereditary portwine stain. *J Med Genet.* 2000;37:E12.

55. Redondo P, Vazquez-Doval FJ. Familial multiple nevi flammei. *J Am Acad Dermatol.* 1996;35:769–770.

56. Eerola I, Boon LM, Watanabe S, Grynberg H, Mulliken JB, Vikkula M. Locus for susceptibility for familial capillary malformation ('port-wine stain') maps to 5q. *Eur J Hum Genet.* 2002; 10:375–380.

57. Breugem CC, Alders M, Salieb-Beugelaar GB, Mannens MM, Van der Horst CM, Hennekam RC. A locus for hereditary capillary malformations mapped on chromosome 5q. *Hum Genet.* 2002;110:343–347.

58. Anderson RR, Parrish J. Selective photothermolysis: precise microsurgery by selective absorption of pulsed radiation. *Science.* 1983;220:524–529.

59. Huikeshoven M, Koster PHL, de Boyie CAJM, Beek JF, van Gemert MJC, van der Horst CMAM. Redarkening of port-wine stains 10 years after pulsed-dye-laser treatment. *N Engl J Med.* 2007;356:1235–1240.

60. Cohen MM Jr. Vascular update: morphogenesis, tumors, malformations, and molecular dimensions. *Am J Med Genet Part A.* 2006;140A:2013–2038.

61. Sturge WA. A case of partial epilepsy apparently due to a lesion of one of the vasomotor centers of the brain. *Clin Soc Trans.* 1879;12:162–167.

62. Garzon MC, Huang JT, Enjolras D, Frieden IJ. Vascular malformations Part II. Associated syndromes. *J Am Acad Dermatol.* 2007;56:541–564.

63. Anderson JR. *Hydrophthalmia or Congenital Glaucoma, Its Causes, Treatments, and Outlook.* London: Cambridge University Press; 1939: 180.

64. Tallman B, Tan OT, Morelli JG, Piepenbrink J, Stafford TJ, Trainer S et al. Location of port-wine stains and the likelihood of ophthalmic and/or central nervous system complications. *Pediatrics.* 1991;87:323–327.

65. Enjolras O, Riche MC, Merland JJ. Facial portwine stains and the Sturge-Weber Syndrome. *Pediatrics.* 1985;76:48–51.

66. Alper JC, Holmes LB, Mihm MC Jr. Birthmarks with serious medical significance: nevocellular nevi, sebaceous nevi and multiple café au lait spots. *J Pediatr.* 1979;95:696–700.

67. National Institutes of Health Consensus Development Conference. Precursors to malignant melanoma. *J Am Acad Dermatol.* 1984; 10:683–688.

68. Mark GJ, Mihm MC Jr, Liteplo MG, Reed RJ, Clark WH. Congenital melanocytic nevi of the small and garmant type. *Hum Pathol.* 1973;4:395–418.

69. Everett MA. Histopathology of congenital pigmenti nevi. *Am J Dermatopath.* 1989;11:11–12.

70. Rivers JK, Frederiksen PC, Dibdin C. A prevalence survey of dermatoses in the Australian neonate. *J Am Acad Dermatol.* 1990; 23:77–81.

71. Kroon S, Clemmenson OJ, Hastrup N. Incidence of congenital melanocytic nevi in newborn babies in Denmark. *J Am Acad Dermatol.* 1987;17:422–426.

72. Alper JC, Holmes LB. The incidence and significance of birthmarks in a cohort of 4,641 newborns. *Pediatr Dermatol.* 1983; 1:58–66.

73. Jacobs AH, Walton RG. The incidence of birthmarks in the neonate. *Pediatrics.* 1976;58:218–222.

74. Saraçli T, Kenney JA Jr, Scott RB. Common skin disorders in the newborn Negro infant. *J Pediatr.* 1963;62:358–363.

75. Hidano A, Purwoko R, Jitsukawa K. Statistical survey of skin changes in Japanese neonates. *Pediatr Dermatol.* 1986;3: 140–144.

76. Castilla EE, DaGraca Dutra M, Orioli-Parreiras IM. Epidemiology of congenital pigmented naevi: incidence rates and relative frequencies. *Brit J Dermatol.* 1981;104:307–315.

77. Easton DF, Cox GM, MacDonald AM, Ponder BAJ. Genetic susceptibility to naevi: a twin study. *Br J Cancer.* 1991;64:1164–1167.

78. Alper JC. Congenital nevi. The controversy rages on. *Arch Dermatol.* 1985;121:734–735.

79. Mackie RM, Watt D, Doherty V, Aitchison T. Malignant melanoma occurring in those under 30 in the west of Scotland 1976–1986: a study of incidence, clinical features, pathologic features and survival. *Br J Dermatol.* 1991;124:560–564.

80. Makkar HS, Frieden IJ. Congenital melanocytic nevi: an update for the pediatrician. *Current Opin Pediatr.* 2002;14:397–402.

81. Paller AS, Mancini AJ. *Hurwitz Clinical Pediatric Dermatology.* Philadelphia: Elsevier Saunders; 2006: 208–211.

82. Pilney FT, Broadbent TR, Woolf RM. Giant pigmented nevus of the face. *Plast Reconstr Surg.* 1967;40:469–474.

83. Walton RG, Jacobs AH, Cox AJ. Pigmented lesions in newborn infants. *Brit J Dermatol.* 1976;95:389–396.

84. Lavier VC, Pickrell KL, Georgiade NG. Congenital giant nevi: clinical and pathological considerations. *Plast Reconstr Surg.* 1976;58:48–54.

85. Alper J, Holmes LB, Mihm MC Jr. Birthmarks with serious medical significance: nevocellular nevi, sebaceous nevi, and multiple café-au-lait spots. *J Pediatr.* 1979;95:676–700.

86. Rhodes AR, Wood WC, Sobert AJ, Mihm MC Jr. Nonepidermal origin of malignant melanoma associated with a giant congenital nevocellular nevus. *Plast Reconstr Surg.* 1981;67:782–790.

87. Amer A, Fischer H. Giant congenital melanocytic nevi. *Clin Pediatr.* 2008;47:824–826.

88. Dasu MRK, Barrow RE, Hawkins HK, McCauley RL. Gene expression profiles of giant hairy naevi. *J Clin Pathol.* 2004;57: 849–855.

89. Gari LM, Rivers JK, Kopf AW. Melanomas arising in large congenital nevocytic nevi: a prospective study. *Pediatr Dermatol.* 1988;5:151–158.

90. Castilla EE, Da Graca Dutra M, Orioli-Parreiras IM. Epidemiology of congenital pigmented naevi: incidence rates, and relative frequencies. *Brit J Dermatol.* 1981;104:307–315.

91. Cantu JM, Urrusti J, Hernandez A, Del Castillo V, Macotela-Rutz E. Discordance for giant pigmented nevi in monozygotic twins. *Ann Genet.* 1973;16:289–292.

92. Hecht F, La Canne KM, Carroll DB. Inheritance of giant pigmented hairy nevus of the scalp. *Am J Med Genet.* 1981;9: 177–178.

93. Goodman RM, Caren J, Ziprkowski M, Padeh B, Ziprkowski L, Cohen BE. Genetic considerations in giant pigmented hairy naevus. *Brit J Derm.* 1971;85:150–157.

94. Lorentzen M, Pers M, Bretteville-Jenson G. The incidence of malignant transformation in giant pigmented nevi. *Scand J Plast Reconstr Surg.* 1977;11:163–167.

95. Eichenfield F, Frieden IJ, Esterly NB. *Textbook of Neonatal Dermatology.* Philadelphia: Saunders/Elsevier;2001: 370–373, 451–454.

96. Paller AS, Mancini AJ. *Hurwitz Clinical Pediatric Dermatology. A Textbook of Skin Disorders of Childhood and Adolescence.* 3rd ed. Philadelphia: Saunders/Elsevier; 2006; 287–290.

97. Alper JC, Holmes LB. The incidence and significance of birthmarks in a cohort of 4,461 newborns. *Pediatr Dermatol.* 1983; 1:58–68.

98. Taïeb A, Boralevi F. Hypermelanoses of the newborn and of the infant. *Dermatol Clin.* 2007;25:327–336.

99. Benedict PH, Szabo G, Fitzpatrick TB, Sinesi SJ. Melanotic macules in Albright's syndrome and in neurofibromatosis. *JAMA.* 1968;205:618–628.

100. Tsai F-J, Tsai C-L. Birthmarks and congenital skin lesions in Chinese newborns. *J Formos Med Assoc.* 1993;92:838–841.

101. Hidano A, Purwoko R, Jitsukawa K. Statistical survey of skin changes in Japanese neonates. *Pediatr Dermatol.* 1986;3: 140–144.

102. Whitehouse D. Diagnostic value of the café-au-lait spot in children. *Arch Dis Child.* 1966;41:316–319.

103. Riccardi VM. Pathophysiology of neurofibromatosis. IV. Dermatologic insights into heterogeneity and pathogenesis. *J Am Acad Dermatol.* 1980;3:157–166.

104. Abeliovich D, Gelman-Kohan Z, Silverstein S. Familial café-au-lait spots: a variant of neurofibromatosis type 1. *J Med Genet.* 1995;32:985–986.

105. Brems H, Chmara M, Sahbatou M, Denayer E, Taniguchi K, Kato R et al. Germline loss of function mutations in SPRED1 cause a neurofibromatosis 1-like phenotype. *Nat Genet.* 2007; 39:1120–1126.

106. Eichenfield LF, Frieden IJ, Esterly NB, eds. *Textbook of Neonatal Dermatology.* Philadelphia: Saunders; 2001.

107. Paller AS, Mancini AJ. *Hurwitz Clinical Pediatric Dermatology. A Textbook of Skin Disorders of Childhood and Adolescence.* 3rd ed. Philadelphia: Elsevier Saunders, 2005.

108. Lin AE, Feingold M. Out, out damn spot or the demise of the Mongolian spot. *Am J Dis Child.* 1993;147:714.

109. Kaplan RE. Ink-blot macules: an alternative to "Mongolian spots." *Pediatr Dermatol.* 1984;2:86.

110. Pratt AG. Birthmarks of infants. *Arch Dermat.* 1953;67: 302–305.

111. Jacobs AH, Walton RG. The incidence of birthmarks in the neonate. *Pediatrics.* 1976;58:218–222.

112. Cordova A. The Mongolian Spot: a study of ethnic differences and a literature review. *Clin Pediatr.* 1981;20:714–719.

113. Alper JC, Holmes LB. Incidence and significance of birthmarks in a cohort of 4,641 newborns. *J Pediatr Derm.* 1983;1:58–68.

114. Leppig KA, Werler MM, Cann CI, Cook CA, Holmes LB. Predictive value of minor anomalies in association with major malformations. *J Pediatr.* 1987;110:531–537.

115. Rivers JK, Frederiksen PC, Dibdin C. A prevalence survey of dermatoses in the Australian neonate. *J Am Acad Dermatol.* 1990;23:77–81.

116. Moosavi Z, Hosseini T. One-year survey of cutaneous lesions in 1,000 consecutive Iranian newborns. *Pediat Dermatol.* 2006;23: 61–63.

117. Onayemi O, Adejuyigbe EA, Torimiro SE, Oyelami O, Jegede OA. Prevalence of Mongolian spots in Nigerian children in Ile-Ife, Nigeria. *Niger J Med.* 2001;10:121–123.

118. Shih I-H, Lin J-Y, Chen C-H, Hong H-S. A birthmark survey in 500 newborns: clinical observation in two northern Taiwan medical center nurseries. *Chang Gung Med J.* 2007;30:220–224.

119. Boccardi D, Menni S, Ferraroni M, Stival G, Bernardo L, La Vecchia C, Decarli A. Birthmarks and transient skin lesions in newborns and their relationship to maternal factors: a preliminary report from northern Italy. *Dermatology.* 2007;215:53–58.

120. Kikuchi I, Inoue S. Natural history of the Mongolian spot. *J Dermatol.* 1980;7:449–450.

121. Asnes RS. Buttock bruises—Mongolian Spot. *Pediatrics.* 1984; 74:321.

122. Jadassohn J. Il Bemerrkungen zur Histologie der systematisierten Naevi und uiter Talgdueson-Naevi. *Arch Dermat Syph.* 1895;33:355–394.

123. Solomon LM, Esterly NB. Epidermal and other congenital nevi. *Curr Probl Pediatr.* 1975;6:1–56.

124. Alper J, Holmes LB, Mihm MC Jr. Birthmark with serious medical significance: nevocellular nevi sebaceous nevi; and multiple café au lait spots. *J Pediatr.* 1979;79:696–700.

125. Hidano A, Purwoko R, Jitsukawa K. Statistical survey of skin changes in Japanese neonates. *Pediatr Dermat.* 1986;3: 140–144.

126. Tsai F-J, Tsai C-I. Birth marks and congenital skin lesions in Chinese newborns. *J Formosan Med Assoc.* 1993;92:838–841.

127. van de Warrenburg BPC, van Gulik S, Remier WO, Lammeus M, Doelman JC. The linear naevus sebaceous syndrome. *Clin Neurol Neurosurg.* 1998;100:126–132.

128. Labbe D, Badix Modini B, Petit F. Sebaceous nevus of Jadassohn. Apropos of 62 surgically treated cases and review of the literature. *Rev Stomatol Chir Maxillo Fac.* 1999;100:175–179.

129. Weiss G, Shemer A, Trau H. Yellowish, verrucous lesions on the scalp. *Am Fam Physician.* 2005;71:961–962.

130. Sahl WJ Jr. Familial nevus sebaceous of Jadassohn: occurrence in the generations. *J Am Acad Dermatol.* 1990;22:853–854.

131. Happle R, Konig A. Familial nevus sebaceous may be explained by paradominant transmission. *Br J Dermatol.* 1999;141:377.

132. Laimo L, Steensel AM Innocenzi D, Camplone G. Familial occurrence of nevus sebaceous of Jadassohn: another case of paradominant inheritance? *Eur J Dermatol.* 2001;11:97–98.

133. Morioka S. The natural history of nevus sebaceous. *J Cutaneous Pathology.* 1985;12:200–213.

134. Santibanez-Gallerami AM, Marshall D, Duarte AM, Melnick SJ, Thaller S. Should nevus sebaceous of Jadassohn in children be excised? A study of 757 cases, and literature review. *J Craniofac Surg.* 2003;14:658–660.

135. Miller CJ, Ioffreda MD, Billingsley EM. Sebaceous carcinoma, basal cell carcinoma, trichoadenoma, trichoblastoma, and syringocystadenoma papilliferum arising within a nevus sebaceus. *Dermatol Surg.* 2004;30:1546–1549.

136. Happle R. How many epidermal nevus syndromes exist? A clinicogenetic classification. *J Am Acad Dermatol.* 1991;25:550–556.

137. Xu A-E, Huang B, Li Y-W, Wang P, Shen H. Clinical, histopathological and ultrastructural characteristics of naevus depigmentosus. *Clin Exper Dermatol.* 2008;33:400–405.

138. Ruiz-Maldonado R. Hypomelanotic conditions of the newborn and infant. *Dermatol Clin.* 2007;25:373–382.

139. Bolognia JL, Pawelek JM. Biology of hypopigmentation. *J Am Acad Dermatol.* 1988;19:217–255.

140. Lee HS, Chun YS, Hann SK. Nevus depigmentosus: clinical features and histopathologic characteristics in 67 patients. *J Am Acad Dermatol.* 1999;40:21–26.

141. Kennedy JL Jr, Kalish GH. Incidence of depigmented nevi in 1000 healthy term newborns. *Pediatr Res.* 1972;6:411.

142. Debard A, Richardet JM. Signification des taches achromiques chez le nourisson. *Nouv Presse Med.* 1975;4:20.

143. Alper JC, Holmes LB. The incidence and significance of birthmarks in a cohort of 4,641 newborns. *Pediatr Dermatol.* 1983;1:58–68.

144. Fitzpatrick TB, Szabo G, Hori Y, Simone AA, Reed WB, Greenberg MH. White leaf-shaped macules; earliest visible sign of tuberous sclerosis. *Arch Determatol.* 1968;98:1–6.

145. Alper JC, Holmes LB. The incidence and significance of birthmarks in a cohort of 4,641 newborns. *Pediatr Dermatol.* 1983;1:58–68.

146. Alper J, Holmes LB, Mihm MC Jr. Birthmarks with serious medical significance: nevocellular nevi, sebaceous nevi and multiple café au lait spots. *J Pediatr.* 1979;95:696–700.

147. Eichenfield LF, Frieden IJ, Esterly NB. *Textbook of Neonatal Dermatology.* Philadelphia: Saunders; 2001: 5, 39, 126–130.

148. Paller AS, Mancini AJ. *Hurwitz Clinical Pediatric Dermatology. A Textbook of Skin Disorders of Childhood and Adolescence.* 3rd ed. Philadelphia: Elsevier Saunders; 2006: 31, 32.

149. Drolet B, Prendiville J, Golden J, Enjolras O, Esterly NB. 'Membranous aplasia cutis' with hair collars. Congenital absence of skin or neurocutaneous defect? *Arch Dermatol.* 1995;131:1427–1431.

150. Stevens CA, Galen W. The hair collar sign. *Am J Med Genet Part A.* 2008;146A:484–487.

151. Alper JC, Holmes LB. The incidence and significance of birth marks in a cohort of 4,641 newborns. *Pediat Dermat.* 1983; 1:58–68.

152. Lemke RP, Machin G, Muttitt, S, Bamforth F, Rao S, Welch R. A case of aplasia cutis congenital in dizygotic twins. *J Perinatol.* 1993;13:22–27.

153. Verhelle NA, Heymans O, Deleuze JP, Fabre G, Vranckx, JJ, Van den hof B. Abdominal aplasia cutis congenital: case report and review of the literature. *Pediatr Surg.* 2004;39:237–239.

154. Higginbottom MC, Jones KL, James HE, Bruce DA, Schut L. Aplasia cutis congenital: a cutaneous marker of occult spinal dysraphism. *J Pediatr.* 1980;96:687–689.

155. Drolet BA, Clowry L Jr, McTigue MK, Esterly NB. The hair collar sign: marker for cranial dysraphism. *Pediatrics.* 1995;96 (2 pt 1):209–213.

156. Milham S, Elledge W. Maternal methimazole and congenital defects in children. *Teratology.* 1972;5:125.

157. Clementi M, Di Gianantonio E, Pelo E, Mammi I, Basile RT, Tenconi R. Methimazole embryopathy: delineation of the phenotype. *Am J Med Genet.* 1999;83:43–46.

158. Fonseca W, alencar AJC, Pereira RMM, Misago C. Congenital malformation of the scalp and cranium after failed first trimester abortion attempt with misoprostol. *Clin Dysmorphol.* 1993; 2:76–80.

159. Vargas FR, Schuler-Faccini L, Brunoni D, Kim C, Meloni VFA, Sugayama SMM et al. Prenatal exposure to misoprostol and vascular disruption defects: a case-control study. *Am J Med Gen.* 2000;95:302–306.

160. Elliott AM, Teebi AS. Further examples of autosomal dominant transmission of nonsyndromic aplasia cutis congenita. *Am J Med Genet.* 1997;73:495–496.

161. Evers ME, Steijlen PM, Hamel BC. Aplasia cutis congenital and associated disorders: an update. *Clin Genet.* 1995;47:295–301.

Chapter 27

Anthropologic Measurements

INTRODUCTION

In evaluating the physical features of a newborn infant, those which are considered "too long," "too short," "too wide," or "too narrow" can be evaluated more precisely with measurements. With measurements, a finding that is two standard deviations above or below the mean value for infants of the same race, sex, and gestational age can be used as a definition of "significant."

Fortunately, the published measurements in infants, children, and adults have been published by Hall, Allanson, Gripp, and Slavotinek in *Handbook of Physical Measurements* (1). This chapter adds to these published measurements in newborns with values specific for white and black infants and for gestational ages from 30 weeks to 42 weeks.

Measurements are not a magic solution. For example, in a study of anticonvulsant drug-exposed infants, documenting the shortened nose and the length or height of the upper lip was needed to establish the presence of a short nose, a significant finding in these children (2). A comparison of the findings in infants examined and measured by the two study physicians showed significant differences in the range of the measurements (3). The reason for the differences in findings were that the two physicians were actually making measurements in different ways, even though they thought they were following the same protocol. This finding emphasized the need for different examiners to compare findings periodically in duplicate evaluations of the same infants. For the busy clinician, this variation in the findings by two study physicians emphasizes the need to repeat measurements if a significant abnormality has been identified.

Several instruments can be used to make measurements. We have used for the data presented here, as often as possible, two instruments that a physician could be expected to have: a flat plastic ruler and a tape measure.

We found that taping pieces of two plastic rulers together would create a ruler with a 90-degree angle, which makes it easier to measure ear level and rotation and eye slant. The spreading caliper was considered more reliable for some measurements, such as width of palpebral fissures. However, spreading calipers are not available to most clinicians. A small, plastic spreading caliper was used for many short measurements, while the larger, more expensive steel spreading caliper was used to measure longer distances, such as the length of the foot and the length and width of the head.

We have learned the value of using rulers and tape measures subdivided into millimeters. This lesson is relevant to the fact that many nurseries for newborns provide a paper tape measure subdivided only by centimeters and half a centimeter. In a comparison of the measurements of head size made using these two types of tape measures, we found that the examiner using the disposable paper tape was more likely to record 0, 0.2, 0.5, 0.8 cm fractions (3). By comparison, when a tape measure subdivided by millimeters was used, there was an equal distribution to all lengths: 0, 0.1, 0.2, 0.3, 0.4, 0.5, 0.6, 0.7, 0.8 and 0.9 cm.

Between February 16, 1972, and June 30, 1974, we examined a systematic sample of 7,742 infants of at least 20 weeks gestation born at the Boston Lying-In Hospital (now part of Brigham and Women's Hospital). One purpose was to define the range of normal for minor physical features, including minor anomalies (4), birthmarks (5), and anthropologic measurements. A second goal was to determine the frequency of major malformations in a sample of newborn infants examined by study personnel.

The 7,742 infants were selected systematically (e.g., every infant, every other infant, or every sixth infant), depending on the examination planned. The anthropologic measurements took much more time than the surface examination, so only 1,500 of the 7,742 infants were measured. After the infants were selected from the delivery room logbook, informed consent for study participation was obtained from the mother. Infants were included regardless of birth status (liveborn, stillborn, or neonatal death), but only if they were at least 20 weeks gestational age, calculated from the mother's last menstrual period. If the mother agreed to participate, a family history, pregnancy history, and demographic information were obtained. The race of each infant was based on the country of origin of the four grandparents, as reported by the mother.

A physical examination, using a written protocol, was performed by one of two examiners (C.I.C. and L.B.H., a non-physician(but former medical student) and physician, respectively) within the first 4 days of the infant's birth and before discharge from the hospital. For the measurements presented here, the instruments and the methods used are described for each.

The measurements were recorded on an optical scan form for data entry. The findings were subdivided by gestational age (based on the reported last menstrual period), sex, and race. We present here the distribution of the measurements made, subdivided into the percentiles 97, 90, 75, 50, 25, 10, and 3, plus the mean and standard deviation.

REFERENCES

1. Hall JG, Allanson JE, Gripp KW, Slavotinek AM. *Handbook of Physical Measurements*. 2nd ed. New York: Oxford University Press; 2007.
2. Holmes LB, Coull BA, Dorfman J, Rosenberger PB. The correlation of deficits in IQ with midface and digit hypoplasia in children exposed in utero to anticonvulsant drugs. *J Pediatr.* 2005;146:118–122.
3. Harvey EA, Hayes AM, Holmes LB. Lessons on objectivity in clinical studies. *Am J Med Genet.* 1994;50:74–79.
4. Leppig KA, Werler MM, Cann CI, Cook CA, Holmes LB. Predictive value of minor anomalies. I. Association with major malformations. *J Pediatr.* 1987;110:530–537.
5. Alper JC, Holmes LB. The incidence and significance of birthmarks in a cohort of 4,641 newborns. *Pediatr Dermatol.* 1983;1:58–68.

HEAD SIZE

TABLE 27-1 *Distributions for Head Circumference: centimeters(cm): Both Sexes*

Gestational Age	Race	Number of Infants	Mean	Standard Deviation	Percentiles						
					97	90	75	50	25	10	3
30-34	All	38	32.4816	2.3129	36.57	35.67	33.95	32.80	30.00	29.54	27.75
35-36	All	46	33.6957	2.4578	42.54	36.06	34.50	33.35	32.37	31.56	29.70
37-38	White	93	34.0118	1.0354	36.04	35.50	34.70	34.00	33.35	32.50	32.06
	Black	27	33.6074	1.4673	36.90	35.90	34.40	33.50	32.80	31.60	30.50
	Mixed	38	33.9211	1.3429	38.39	35.53	34.80	33.75	33.00	32.27	31.83
	All	168	33.9071	1.1842	36.20	35.50	34.67	33.90	33.00	32.39	31.81
39	White	136	34.4963	1.2262	36.50	35.93	35.50	34.50	33.82	32.80	32.00
	Black	36	34.1861	1.4588	37.44	36.65	35.00	34.00	33.00	32.30	32.02
	Mixed	54	34.3352	1.1699	36.41	35.90	35.00	34.40	33.67	32.45	31.68
	All	239	34.4414	1.2589	36.96	36.00	35.30	34.50	33.70	32.60	32.00
40	White	204	34.8539	1.3563	36.98	36.50	35.97	34.95	34.00	33.00	32.06
	Black	44	34.4136	1.2216	36.60	35.90	35.37	34.50	33.52	33.00	31.32
	Mixed	74	34.7041	1.2287	37.00	36.30	35.55	34.80	33.70	33.00	32.22
	All	330	34.7521	1.3054	36.91	36.40	35.70	34.80	34.00	33.00	32.29
41	White	140	35.1336	1.1470	37.15	36.80	35.87	35.05	34.30	33.51	32.80
	Black	23	34.5783	1.1782	37.00	36.26	35.40	34.50	34.00	32.88	32.40
	Mixed	56	35.0357	1.0688	36.92	36.26	35.80	35.35	34.40	33.51	32.47
	All	230	35.0483	1.1593	37.01	36.60	35.80	35.00	34.30	33.50	32.80
42-43	White	125	35.2192	1.2978	38.09	37.00	35.85	35.30	34.45	33.50	32.80
	Black	19	34.6842	0.9605	36.70	36.20	35.50	34.60	34.00	33.20	33.20
	Mixed	38	35.2605	1.2725	38.41	36.91	36.20	35.00	34.40	33.77	32.47
	All	188	35.1415	1.2674	37.87	36.81	35.80	35.00	34.40	33.50	32.80

Head circumference: Using a tape measure marked in millimeters, the examiner measures the circumference at the maximum point in the mid-forehead and over the occiput.

TABLE 27-2 *Distributions for Head Length (cm): Both Sexes*

Gestational Age	Race	Number of Infants	Mean	Standard Deviation	Percentiles						
					97	90	75	50	25	10	3
30-34	All	37	11.1135	0.7804	12.59	12.24	11.65	11.20	10.45	9.88	9.61
35-36	All	41	11.3732	0.7075	12.87	12.30	11.75	11.40	10.90	10.34	9.73
37-38	White	92	11.5739	0.4116	12.42	12.00	11.80	11.60	11.30	11.10	10.74
	Black	27	11.3370	0.5422	12.40	12.32	11.70	11.30	10.90	10.76	10.50
	Mixed	37	11.4730	0.5961	12.66	12.32	11.80	11.50	11.20	10.40	10.31
	All	166	11.4982	0.4839	12.40	12.10	11.80	11.50	11.27	10.80	10.40
39	White	134	11.7269	0.5070	12.60	12.35	12.10	11.80	11.40	10.90	10.70
	Black	34	11.6118	0.5656	13.09	12.45	11.82	11.50	11.20	11.00	10.61
	Mixed	51	11.7392	0.5024	12.74	12.40	12.00	11.70	11.40	11.04	10.57
	All	232	11.7310	0.5217	12.80	12.40	12.10	11.80	11.40	11.00	10.70
40	White	197	11.8888	0.5175	12.80	12.52	12.20	11.90	11.60	11.20	10.79
	Black	46	11.7370	0.4949	12.46	12.40	12.20	11.80	11.30	11.20	10.62
	Mixed	69	11.7551	0.5855	12.70	12.60	12.15	11.80	11.40	11.10	10.22
	All	320	11.8347	0.5274	12.80	12.49	12.20	11.80	11.50	11.20	10.70
41	White	136	11.9250	0.4671	12.98	12.53	12.20	11.80	11.70	11.40	11.01
	Black	20	11.7550	0.4979	12.90	12.39	12.07	11.80	11.45	11.01	10.90
	Mixed	58	11.9293	0.4272	12.70	12.40	12.30	12.00	11.67	11.38	10.98
	All	224	11.9174	0.4710	12.80	12.50	12.20	11.90	11.62	11.35	10.97
42-43	White	120	11.9567	0.5185	13.00	12.79	12.30	11.90	11.62	11.40	10.90
	Black	19	11.7000	0.5175	12.90	12.40	11.80	11.70	11.40	10.90	10.60
	Mixed	38	11.9316	0.4479	12.78	12.42	12.32	11.90	11.60	11.40	10.85
	All	183	11.9104	0.5166	12.90	12.60	12.30	11.80	11.60	11.34	10.85

Head length: Using spreading calipers, measure the length from the mid-forehead to the most posterior point over occiput.

TABLE 27-3 *Distributions for Biparietal Head Width (cm): Both Sexes*

Gestational Age	Race	Number of Infants	Mean	Standard Deviation	Percentiles						
					97	90	75	50	25	10	3
30-34	All	39	8.6615	0.7383	9.80	9.60	9.30	8.70	8.00	7.70	7.06
35-36	All	41	9.0220	0.5452	10.25	9.80	9.40	8.90	8.60	8.40	8.00
37-38	White	91	9.1703	0.3889	10.10	9.58	9.40	9.20	8.90	8.70	8.30
	Black	27	8.9519	0.6762	9.80	9.62	9.30	9.10	8.80	8.28	6.20
	Mixed	36	9.1861	0.4051	10.34	9.80	9.47	9.10	8.90	8.77	8.51
	All	164	9.1390	0.4514	10.00	9.60	9.40	9.20	8.90	8.70	8.30
39	White	134	9.2724	0.3632	9.80	9.80	9.50	9.30	9.00	8.80	8.50
	Black	35	9.1914	0.4189	9.98	9.74	9.50	9.20	8.90	8.58	8.30
	Mixed	53	9.2283	0.4087	10.00	9.80	9.50	9.20	9.00	8.68	8.12
	All	235	9.2515	0.3831	9.89	9.80	9.50	9.30	9.00	8.80	8.31
40	White	205	9.3956	0.4002	10.10	9.90	9.70	9.40	9.20	8.80	8.70
	Black	45	9.2533	0.3609	9.96	9.70	9.50	9.30	9.10	8.80	8.31
	Mixed	72	9.3556	0.3911	10.00	9.80	9.67	9.40	9.10	8.83	8.44
	All	330	9.3639	0.3934	10.00	9.80	9.60	9.40	9.10	8.80	8.59
41	White	138	9.4703	0.3526	10.08	9.90	9.72	9.40	9.30	9.00	8.80
	Black	21	9.3524	0.3473	10.30	9.86	9.50	9.30	9.05	8.90	8.90
	Mixed	59	9.5085	0.3223	10.20	10.00	9.80	9.40	9.30	9.00	8.86
	All	228	9.4640	0.3509	10.11	9.90	9.70	9.40	9.30	9.00	8.80
42-43	White	126	9.5325	0.4014	10.36	10.00	9.80	9.50	9.30	9.00	8.80
	Black	19	9.4053	0.3763	10.50	9.80	9.60	9.40	9.20	8.90	8.90
	Mixed	40	9.4800	0.4046	10.28	10.16	9.70	9.45	9.20	8.91	8.49
	All	191	9.5084	0.3971	10.30	10.00	9.80	9.40	9.30	9.00	8.80

Biparietal head width: Using spreading calipers, measure the width of the head at a point on side of head one inch above each ear.

LENGTH

TABLE 27-4 *Distributions for Length (cm): Males*

Gestational Age	Race	Number of Infants	Mean	Standard Deviation	Percentiles						
					97	90	75	50	25	10	3
30-34	All	20	48.2850	4.6224	57.00	54.18	51.00	49.20	44.82	40.06	39.50
35-36	All	21	49.9333	2.1437	54.00	53.00	51.00	50.50	48.45	46.60	46.20
37-38	White	41	51.9244	2.4300	56.55	55.40	53.75	52.00	49.80	49.00	46.65
	Black	15	51.2733	2.0721	56.00	54.50	52.80	51.00	50.00	48.00	48.00
	Mixed	15	51.0800	1.8432	55.80	54.12	52.00	50.80	50.10	48.70	47.50
	All	73	51.5822	2.2232	56.38	54.76	53.00	51.00	50.00	49.00	47.61
39	White	67	52.6328	1.8959	55.40	55.00	54.00	53.00	51.20	49.74	48.71
	Black	16	52.1562	2.4991	55.60	55.53	54.00	52.75	49.88	48.20	47.50
	Mixed	26	52.0462	1.9198	55.60	54.45	53.22	52.00	51.00	49.35	46.70
	All	118	52.5042	1.9829	55.54	55.00	54.00	53.00	51.00	49.50	48.28
40	White	113	53.1389	2.1998	56.79	56.00	54.80	53.40	51.50	50.00	49.00
	Black	20	52.0300	1.8134	55.30	54.95	53.52	52.00	50.85	49.53	49.00
	Mixed	31	53.5194	1.5800	56.60	55.00	54.50	53.60	52.50	51.50	48.80
	All	170	53.0429	2.0833	56.49	55.50	54.50	53.35	51.50	50.02	49.00
41	White	64	53.6203	2.1781	57.81	56.75	55.00	53.50	52.00	50.40	49.42
	Black	10	52.8700	1.6826	55.00	54.93	54.07	53.30	51.95	49.28	49.00
	Mixed	31	52.9548	2.0263	56.80	56.24	54.00	52.60	52.00	50.18	49.00
	All	111	53.3637	2.0696	57.45	56.24	55.00	53.20	52.00	50.56	49.00
42-43	White	62	53.7613	2.0904	58.02	56.67	55.42	53.65	52.27	51.00	49.94
	Black	11	52.6182	2.6653	58.00	57.40	55.00	52.50	51.00	48.50	48.00
	Mixed	20	53.3450	1.8588	56.70	55.81	54.90	53.00	52.50	50.20	49.00
	All	96	53.4937	2.1276	58.00	56.53	55.00	53.15	52.20	50.85	49.45

Body length: Using a tape measure marked in millimeters, measure from bottom of one foot to top of head. To establish the top of head, the examiner looks down at 90 degree angle.

TABLE 27-5 *Distributions for Length (cm): Females*

Gestational Age	Race	Number of Infants	Mean	Standard Deviation	Percentiles						
					97	90	75	50	25	10	3
30-34	All	20	47.5150	4.2502	54.50	53.45	51.00	48.00	44.30	41.15	39.00
35-36	All	24	49.4542	3.0477	55.00	53.30	51.27	49.55	48.00	45.50	41.00
37-38	White	50	50.2920	2.6818	54.52	52.97	52.00	50.50	49.00	47.55	42.14
	Black	12	50.7083	2.9460	56.20	55.54	53.50	50.55	48.13	46.80	46.50
	Mixed	23	50.8783	2.2899	54.30	54.12	53.00	51.30	49.50	47.40	46.00
	All	93	50.5000	2.5415	54.44	53.62	52.00	50.50	49.00	47.50	46.41
39	White	71	51.4606	2.2395	55.94	54.00	53.00	52.00	50.00	48.00	47.00
	Black	21	50.6190	2.4480	55.50	54.50	52.50	50.50	48.35	47.50	47.00
	Mixed	28	50.8536	2.2215	54.50	53.55	52.50	50.75	49.25	47.41	46.50
	All	124	51.2040	2.2797	55.52	54.00	53.00	51.55	49.50	48.00	46.90
40	White	91	52.1165	2.1671	56.57	54.78	53.40	52.00	51.00	20.00	46.52
	Black	25	51.9120	2.3127	56.20	54.88	53.30	52.00	50.75	48.20	46.80
	Mixed	43	51.6581	1.8208	54.84	53.92	53.00	52.00	50.50	49.00	46.94
	All	161	51.9460	2.0906	56.23	54.46	53.05	52.00	51.00	49.50	46.97
41	White	77	52.4519	1.9948	55.90	55.08	54.00	52.60	51.00	49.96	48.34
	Black	13	51.5615	1.8324	55.00	54.60	52.75	51.50	50.50	48.70	48.50
	Mixed	27	52.5704	1.9592	55.00	55.00	54.00	53.00	50.50	49.50	49.00
	All	121	52.3760	2.0029	55.63	55.00	54.00	52.50	51.00	49.56	48.33
42-43	White	60	52.7650	1.9523	56.75	55.49	54.60	52.30	51.50	20.23	49.50
	Black	8	51.9375	1.5910	54.00	54.00	53.00	52.25	50.75	49.00	49.00
	Mixed	19	53.1368	2.4293	59.00	58.00	54.00	53.00	51.50	51.00	49.80
	All	90	52.7089	2.0672	57.63	55.49	54.00	52.30	51.50	50.23	49.36

BIRTH WEIGHT

TABLE 27-6 *Distributions for Weight (kg): Males*

Gestational Age	Race	Number of Infants	Mean	Standard Deviation	Percentiles						
					97	90	75	50	25	10	3
30-34	White	21	2.4952	0.7959	3.90	3.76	3.30	2.20	1.85	1.46	1.40
	All	39	2.3538	0.7953	3.88	3.50	3.10	2.20	1.80	1.30	0.96
35-36	White	16	2.8562	0.3098	3.40	3.40	3.07	2.80	2.70	2.44	2.30
	All	40	2.8575	0.3876	3.65	3.40	3.10	2.85	1.60	2.41	1.76
37-38	White	90	3.2189	0.4434	4.10	3.80	3.52	3.30	2.90	2.60	2.40
	Black	24	2.9375	0.4292	3.70	3.55	3.27	3.00	2.60	2.35	2.10
	Mixed	20	2.9350	0.4082	3.80	3.50	3.20	2.90	2.70	2.51	2.00
	All	143	3.1399	0.5618	4.07	3.70	3.50	3.20	2.80	2.54	2.23
39	White	136	3.3434	0.4001	4.00	3.90	3.60	3.30	3.10	2.90	2.60
	Black	33	3.2152	0.44651	4.19	3.70	3.50	3.30	2.95	2.64	1.90
	Mixed	48	3.2417	0.3724	4.01	3.71	3.50	3.20	3.10	2.78	2.35
	All	236	3.3102	0.4087	4.00	3.80	3.60	3.30	3.10	2.87	2.40
40	White	212	3.4840	0.7635	4.50	4.00	3.80	3.40	3.20	2.90	2.6o
	Black	48	3.3500	0.3519	4.01	3.81	3.60	3.30	3.10	2.89	2.65
	Mixed	50	3.4720	0.4281	4.45	4.10	3.70	3.50	3.20	2.90	2.65
	All	327	3.4609	0.6570	4.40	3.90	3.70	3.40	3.20	2.90	2.60
41	White	161	3.5925	0.6638	4.50	4.08	3.85	3.60	3.25	3.10	2.70
	Black	27	3.5395	0.4585	4.10	4.02	3.70	3.30	3.00	2.68	2.50
	Mixed	43	3.5329	0.4072	4.60	4.06	3.70	3.50	3.30	3.10	2.73
	All	243		0.6316	4.47	4.00	3.80	3.50	3.20	3.00	2.70
42-43	White	136	3.5750	0.4495	4.49	4.10	3.90	3.50	3.30	3.00	2.71
	Black	24	3.4625	0.4372	4.70	4.15	3.67	3.40	3.20	3.00	2.80
	Mixed	28	3.4714	0.3770	4.20	4.00	3.70	3.50	3.22	3.08	2.48
	All	196	3.5439	0.4432	4.50	4.10	3.60	3.50	3.30	3.00	2.79

Weight: The weight in grams/kilograms was obtained without clothes on the scale in the hospital nursery.

TABLE 27-7 *Distributions for Birth Weight (kg): Females*

Gestational Age	Race	Number of Infants	Mean	Standard Deviation	Percentiles						
					97	90	75	50	25	10	3
30-34	All	22	2.4227	0.8129	4.30	3.64	2.92	2.30	1.67	1.50	1.30
35-36	All	45	2.6667	0.5081	3.95	3.34	2.95	2.60	2.40	1.96	1.59
37-38	White	90	2.9956	0.4467	4.13	3.59	3.20	3.00	2.77	2.40	2.17
	Black	19	3.0474	0.5295	4.30	3.70	3.40	3.00	2.50	2.30	2.30
	Mixed	32	3.0594	0.4055	3.90	3.67	3.30	3.05	2.70	2.53	2.30
	All	156	3.0154	0.4424	4.03	3.60	3.30	3.00	2.70	2.40	2.27
39	White	136	3.2037	0.4702	4.36	3.73	3.50	3.20	2.90	2.60	2.31
	Black	35	3.0686	0.4457	3.90	3.74	3.30	3.00	2.80	2.56	2.12
	Mixed	38	3.1316	0.4627	4.15	3.71	3.50	3.20	2.70	2.50	2.23
	All	220	3.1673	0.4612	4.00	3.70	3.50	3.20	2.82	2.60	2.36
40	White	184	3.2783	0.5534	4.24	3.85	3.60	3.30	3.00	2.80	2.35
	Black	51	3.2059	0.4125	4.03	3.88	3.50	3.20	3.00	2.62	2.26
	Mixed	73	3.2726	0.5308	4.08	3.80	3.60	3.30	3.00	2.74	2.62
	All	319	3.2624	0.5193	4.14	3.80	3.50	3.20	3.00	2.80	2.40
41	White	143	3.4063	0.4491	4.20	3.90	3.70	3.40	3.10	2.84	2.60
	Black	22	3.3136	0.3468	3.90	3.80	3.62	3.30	3.07	2.80	2.70
	Mixed	53	3.3585	0.6084	4.41	4.06	3.70	3.30	3.10	2.80	1.79
	All	228	3.3846	0.4790	4.30	3.90	3.70	3.40	3.10	2.80	2.60
42-43	White	112	3.4366	0.4893	4.42	4.07	3.70	3.40	3.10	2.73	2.54
	Black	11	3.2455	0.2734	3.70	3.68	3.50	3.20	3.10	2.84	2.80
	Mixed	40	3.3775	0.3971	4.38	3.89	3.60	3.40	3.20	2.81	2.49
	All	170	3.4012	0.4543	4.30	3.99	3.70	3.40	3.10	2.80	2.60

FACE

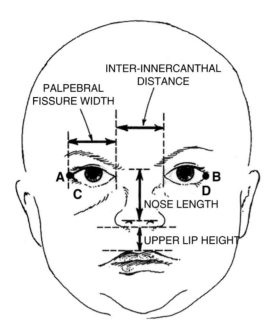

OUTER ORBITAL WIDTH = DISTANCE FROM A to B
(examiner palpates the outer edge of boney orbit just beyond the outer canthus of eye)

OUTER CANTHAL WIDTH = DISTANCE FROM C to D

FIGURE 27.1 Measurements of inner and outer canthus, length of palpebral fissures, length of nose and height of upper lip.

TABLE 27-8 *Distributions for Inter-Inner Canthal Distance (cm): Both Sexes*

Gestational Age	Race	Number of Infants	Mean	Standard Deviation	Percentiles						
					97	90	75	50	25	10	3
30-34	All	38	1.9553	0.2565	2.48	2.21	2.12	2.00	1.77	1.50	1.50
35-36	All	46	2.0130	0.2166	2.56	2.20	2.12	2.00	1.90	1.67	1.54
37-38	White	93	2.0613	0.1668	2.40	2.30	2.20	2.10	2.00	1.80	1.76
	Black	27	2.0556	0.1888	2.50	2.30	2.10	2.10	2.00	1.78	1.60
	Mixed	39	2.0333	0.1528	2.38	2.20	2.10	2.00	2.00	1.80	1.72
	All	168	2.0548	0.1652	2.40	2.30	2.20	2.10	2.00	1.80	1.71
39	White	140	2.0736	0.1594	2.40	2.30	2.20	2.10	2.00	1.81	1.80
	Black	36	2.0556	0.1629	2.39	2.30	2.20	2.05	1.92	1.80	1.71
	Mixed	54	2.0944	0.1698	2.50	2.30	2.20	2.10	2.00	1.85	1.80
	All	243	2.0774	0.1619	2.40	2.30	2.20	2.10	2.00	1.90	1.80
40	White	205	2.1302	0.1635	2.40	2.34	2.20	2.10	2.20	1.96	1.80
	Black	45	2.1089	0.1893	2.50	2.40	2.20	2.10	2.20	1.86	1.74
	Mixed	76	2.1487	0.1661	2.50	2.40	2.20	2.10	2.20	2.00	1.80
	All	334	2.1308	0.1670	2.50	2.40	2.20	2.10	2.20	1.90	1.80
41	White	143	2.1231	0.1630	2.50	2.30	2.20	2.10	2.00	1.90	1.80
	Black	23	2.1261	0.2240	2.60	2.46	2.30	2.10	2.00	1.80	1.70
	Mixed	60	2.1383	0.1842	2.55	2.40	2.20	2.10	2.00	2.00	1.77
	All	237	2.1287	0.1733	2.50	2.40	2.20	2.10	2.00	1.90	1.80
42-43	White	129	2.1450	0.1625	2.50	2.40	2.25	2.10	2.00	2.00	1.80
	Black	19	2.1526	0.1744	2.40	2.40	2.30	2.20	2.00	1.90	1.80
	Mixed	41	2.1439	0.1379	2.47	2.30	2.20	2.20	2.00	2.00	1.93
	All	195	2.1436	0.1573	2.50	2.40	2.20	2.10	2.00	2.00	1.80

Inter-innercanthal distance: See Figure 27-1

Spreading calipers were used to measure the distance between the inner canthi of each eye. This measurement requires that the eyes be open voluntarily.

A plastic ruler in millimeters placed over the nose is used to measure from the base of the nose (established by palpation) to the tip of the nose (judged by the examiner in lateral view of the nose as lateral edge of the alae nasi).

TABLE 27-9 *Distributions for Outercanthal Width (cm): Both Sexes*

Gestational Age	Race	Number of Infants	Mean	Standard Deviation	Percentiles						
					97	90	75	50	25	10	3
30-34	All	9	5.8333	0.4717	6.70	6.70	6.10	5.80	5.50	5.20	5.20
35-36	White	4	5.5500	0.3786	5.80	5.80	5.80	5.70	5.15	5.00	5.00
	All	5	5.4600	0.3847	5.80	5.80	5.80	5.60	5.05	5.00	5.00
37-38	White	23	6.3130	0.4320	7.10	6.86	6.60	6.40	6.00	5.64	5.40
	All	33	6.2848	0.4273	7.10	6.86	6.55	6.40	5.95	5.64	5.40
39	White	24	6.2458	0.4201	7.10	6.90	6.50	6.25	5.85	5.75	5.40
	All	49	6.3224	0.4053	7.20	6.80	6.60	6.30	6.05	5.80	5.50
40	White	53	6.3132	0.5065	7.24	6.90	6.80	6.30	6.00	5.54	5.30
	All	85	6.3318	0.4683	7.24	6.90	6.75	6.30	6.00	5.66	5.36
41	White	32	6.3937	0.3741	7.30	6.87	6.60	6.40	6.22	5.83	5.40
	All	48	6.4125	0.3912	7.16	6.81	6.60	6.40	6.22	5.79	5.45
42-43	White	34	6.3529	0.3863	7.00	6.85	6.62	6.40	6.10	5.80	5.42
	All	44	6.3523	0.3837	7.06	6.85	6.60	6.40	6.10	5.80	5.54

Outercanthal width: See Figure 27-1.
Spreading calipers were used to measure the distance between the left and right outer canthi.

TABLE 27-10 *Distributions for Outer Orbital Distance (cm): Both Sexes*

Gestational Age	Race	Number of Infants	Mean	Standard Deviation	Percentiles						
					97	90	75	50	25	10	3
30-34	White	17	6.4294	0.7338	7.80	7.48	6.85	6.70	5.75	5.40	5.40
	Black	12	6.6750	0.6355	7.90	7.69	7.07	6.80	6.10	5.73	5.70
	Mixed	5	6.9800	0.6760	7.80	7.80	7.55	7.20	6.30	6.10	6.10
	All	40	6.5650	0.6762	7.88	7.39	7.07	6.65	6.00	5.70	5.40
35-36	White	17	6.6353	0.3622	7.20	7.12	6.80	6.70	6.40	6.00	6.00
	Black	17	6.7118	0.5255	7.50	7.34	7.20	6.70	6.30	5.86	5.70
	Mixed	10	6.8600	0.5700	7.50	7.48	7.30	7.05	6.40	5.83	5.80
	All	45	6.7178	0.4711	7.50	7.30	7.15	6.80	6.35	6.00	5.74
37-38	White	91	6.9308	0.3761	7.52	7.40	7.20	6.90	6.70	6.40	6.15
	Black	27	7.0852	0.5593	9.20	7.52	7.40	7.00	6.70	6.48	6.20
	Mixed	36	6.8000	0.4678	7.60	7.40	7.17	6.80	6.50	6.25	5.70
	All	163	6.9313	0.4374	7.60	7.40	7.20	6.90	6.70	6.40	6.00
39	White	139	7.0194	0.4210	7.80	7.60	7.30	7.10	6.70	6.50	6.12
	Black	37	6.9892	0.4795	7.99	7.72	7.35	6.90	6.65	6.30	6.20
	Mixed	54	7.0352	0.3939	7.80	7.60	7.32	7.00	6.80	6.40	6.40
	All	243	7.0243	0.4237	7.80	7.60	7.30	7.00	6.70	6.44	6.20
40	White	207	7.0865	0.4520	7.98	7.60	7.40	7.10	6.80	6.50	6.30
	Black	45	7.1222	0.4134	7.80	7.70	7.35	7.20	6.95	6.46	6.14
	Mixed	74	7.0554	0.4000	7.80	7.60	7.30	7.05	6.80	6.60	6.12
	All	334	7.0859	0.4327	7.80	7.60	7.40	7.10	6.80	6.55	6.20
41	White	142	7.1197	0.3956	7.87	7.60	7.40	7.10	6.80	6.60	6.40
	Black	23	7.0478	0.4252	7.70	7.66	7.40	7.10	6.70	6.36	6.20
	Mixed	59	7.1593	0.3996	7.82	7.70	7.40	7.20	6.80	6.70	6.16
	All	235	7.1234	0.4040	7.80	7.60	7.40	7.10	6.80	6.60	6.30
42-43	White	128	7.1844	0.4081	8.00	7.80	7.40	7.20	6.90	6.59	6.40
	Black	19	7.1947	0.4143	8.00	7.80	7.50	7.30	7.00	6.60	6.30
	Mixed	41	7.2073	0.3888	8.02	7.80	7.45	7.20	6.90	6.80	6.43
	All	194	7.1747	0.4117	8.00	7.80	7.40	7.20	6.90	6.60	6.38

Outer orbital distance: Using sliding calipers, measure the distance between ridges of the outer edge of the boney orbit of each eye.

TABLE 27-11 *Distributions for Palpebral Fissure (cm) [Left]: Both Sexes*

Gestational Age	Race	Number of Infants	Mean	Standard Deviation	Percentiles						
					97	90	75	50	25	10	3
30-34	All	8	1.8125	0.1553	2.00	2.00	1.97	1.80	1.65	1.60	1.60
35-36	All	8	1.7875	0.1126	1.90	1.90	1.90	1.80	1.70	1.60	1.60
37-38	All	40	1.8725	0.1768	2.20	2.20	2.00	1.80	1.70	1.70	1.62
39	White	32	1.9156	0.1780	2.20	2.17	2.10	1.90	1.80	1.70	1.50
	Black	12	1.9500	0.1931	2.30	2.30	2.07	1.90	1.80	1.73	1.70
	Mixed	16	1.9375	0.1628	2.20	2.20	2.07	1.90	1.82	1.70	1.70
	All	64	1.9328	0.1737	2.30	2.20	2.10	1.90	1.80	1.70	1.69
40	White	73	1.9260	0.2211	2.30	2.20	2.10	2.00	1.70	1.70	1.50
	Black	14	2.1000	0.1664	2.40	2.35	2.30	2.00	2.00	1.90	1.90
	Mixed	24	1.9167	0.1523	2.30	2.10	2.00	1.90	1.80	1.70	1.60
	All	116	1.9422	0.2111	2.30	2.20	2.10	2.00	1.80	1.70	1.55
41	White	45	1.9467	0.1779	2.30	2.20	2.10	1.90	1.80	1.76	1.60
	All	65	1.9431	0.2015	2.30	2.24	2.10	1.90	1.80	1.70	1.59
42-43	White	43	1.9605	0.1720	2.30	2.20	2.10	2.00	1.80	1.74	1.63
	All	57	1.9649	0.1674	2.30	2.20	2.10	2.00	1.80	1.78	1.67

Palpebral fissures: See Figure 27-1.
Spreading calipers were used to measure the width between the medial and lateral corners of each palpebral fissure.

TABLE 27-12 *Distributions for Palpebral Fissure (cm) [Right]: Both Sexes*

Gestational Age	Race	Number of Infants	Mean	Standard Deviation	Percentiles						
					97	90	75	50	25	10	3
30-34	All	8	1.8375	0.1408	2.10	2.10	1.90	1.85	1.70	1.70	1.70
35-36	All	8	1.8000	0.1309	2.00	2.00	1.90	1.80	1.70	1.60	1.60
37-38	White	30	1.8567	0.1654	2.20	2.10	1.92	1.80	1.70	1.70	1.60
	All	40	1.8575	0.1738	2.28	2.10	1.97	1.80	1.70	1.70	1.60
39	White	31	1.9129	0.1765	2.20	2.20	2.00	1.90	1.80	1.70	1.50
	All	64	1.9172	0.1658	2.20	2.20	2.00	1.90	1.80	1.70	1.59
40	White	73	1.9192	0.2059	2.30	2.20	2.10	1.90	1.80	1.70	1.52
	Mixed	24	1.9208	0.1474	2.20	2.15	2.00	1.90	1.80	1.70	1.70
	All	115	1.9339	0.1969	2.30	2.20	2.10	1.90	1.80	1.70	1.55
41	White	44	1.9477	0.1705	2.30	2.20	2.07	1.90	1.80	1.80	1.70
	All	63	1.9413	0.1738	2.30	2.20	2.10	1.90	1.80	1.80	1.68
42-43	White	43	1.9279	0.1667	2.30	2.16	2.00	1.90	1.80	1.70	1.56
	All	57	1.9351	0.1653	2.30	2.20	2.00	1.90	1.80	1.70	1.57

Palpebral fissures: See Figure 27-1.
Spreading calipers are used to measure in millimeters the width of the palpebral fissure and the inter-innercanthal distance. The lateral and medial corner of the palpebral fissures with voluntary opening of the eyes are the landmarks for measuring.

TABLE 27-13 *Distributions for Left Eye Slant(mm): Both Sexes*

Gestational Age	Race	Number of Infants	Mean	Standard Deviation	Percentiles						
					97	90	75	50	25	10	3
30-34	All	35	-0.3143	1.6409	3.00	2.00	1.00	-1.00	-1.00	-2.00	-3.92
35-36	All	42	-0.4048	1.7116	3.71	2.00	1.25	-1.00	-1.25	-2.00	-3.00
37-38	White	87	-0.2874	1.1504	2.00	1.00	1.00	-1.00	-1.00	-1.00	-2.00
	Black	23	0.2174	1.7044	3.00	3.00	2.00	0.00	-1.00	-2.00	-2.00
	Mixed	34	-0.6471	1.1250	1.95	1.00	0.00	-1.00	-1.00	-2.00	-2.95
	All	153	-0.2288	1.3402	2.38	2.00	1.00	-1.00	-1.00	-2.00	-2.00
39	White	127	0.1165	1.5184	3.00	2.00	1.00	0.00	-1.00	-2.00	-2.00
	Black	34	-0.0588	1.7742	2.95	2.00	2.00	-1.00	-1.00	-2.50	-3.00
	Mixed	53	0.0943	1.5224	3.38	2.00	1.50	-1.00	-1.00	-1.00	-2.38
	All	227	0.0828	1.5410	3.00	2.00	1.00	-1.00	-1.00	-2.00	-2.00
40	White	195	-0.0154	1.4835	3.00	2.00	1.00	-1.00	-1.00	-2.00	-2.00
	Black	41	-0.4146	1.5488	2.74	2.00	1.00	-1.00	-2.00	-2.00	-2.74
	Mixed	73	0.0274	1.4997	2.00	2.00	1.00	0.00	-1.00	-2.00	-2.00
	All	316	-0.0538	1.4908	2.00	2.00	1.00	-1.00	-1.00	-2.00	-2.00
41	White	130	-0.0231	1.6587	3.00	2.00	2.00	-1.00	-1.00	-2.00	-3.00
	Black	19	0.3158	1.5653	2.00	2.00	2.00	1.00	-1.00	-2.00	-2.00
	Mixed	54	0.1481	1.4973	2.35	2.00	2.00	-1.00	-1.00	-1.00	-2.00
	All	212	0.0142	1.5893	3.00	2.00	2.00	-1.00	-1.00	-2.00	-2.00
42-43	White	116	-0.1121	1.5647	3.00	2.00	1.00	-1.00	-1.00	-2.00	-2.00
	Black	16	0.5000	1.5916	2.00	2.00	2.00	1.00	-1.00	-2.30	-3.00
	Mixed	37	0.0270	1.7076	2.86	2.00	2.00	-1.00	-1.00	-2.00	-3.72
	All	175	0.0114	1.6188	3.00	2.00	2.00	-1.00	-1.00	-2.00	-2.00

Eye slant: Using a plastic ruler, establish the horizontal line through the inner canthus of each eye. At the outer canthus of each eye, measure the distance above or below the horizontal line in millimeters. The eyes should be open voluntarily.

TABLE 27-14 *Distributions for Right Eye Slant (mm): Both Sexes*

Gestational Age	Race	Number of Infants	Mean	Standard Deviation	Percentiles						
					97	90	75	50	25	10	3
30-34	All	36	-0.3611	1.5703	3.00	2.00	1.00	-1.00	-1.75	-2.00	-2.89
35-36	All	42	-0.5476	1.6704	2.00	2.00	1.25	-1.00	-2.00	-2.70	-3.00
37-38	White	87	-0.4483	1.1690	2.00	1.00	1.00	-1.00	-1.00	-2.00	-2.00
	Black	23	-0.0870	1.5642	3.00	2.00	1.00	0.00	-1.00	-2.00	-2.00
	Mixed	33	-0.7879	1.1390	1.98	1.00	0.00	-1.00	-1.50	-2.00	-2.98
	All	152	-0.4079	1.2937	2.00	1.00	1.00	-1.00	-1.00	-2.00	-2.00
39	White	127	0.0079	1.5249	3.00	2.00	1.00	-1.00	-1.00	-2.00	-2.00
	Black	34	-0.0588	1.8413	3.00	2.00	2.00	-1.00	-1.25	-2.50	-3.00
	Mixed	53	-0.0755	1.5298	3.00	2.00	1.00	-1.00	-1.00	-2.00	-2.38
	All	227	-0.0264	1.5626	3.00	2.00	1.00	-1.00	-1.00	-2.00	-2.16
40	White	195	-0.1077	1.4480	2.00	2.00	1.00	-1.00	-1.00	-2.00	-2.00
	Black	41	-0.5366	1.5827	2.00	2.00	1.00	-1.00	-2.00	-2.00	-3.00
	Mixed	74	-0.0541	1.4228	2.00	2.00	1.00	-1.00	-1.00	-2.00	-2.00
	All	317	-0.1451	1.4575	2.00	2.00	1.00	-1.00	-1.00	-2.00	-2.00
41	White	129	-0.2481	1.6251	3.00	2.00	1.00	-1.00	-1.00	-2.00	-3.00
	Black	19	0.1053	1.4868	2.00	2.00	2.00	-1.00	-1.00	-2.00	-2.00
	Mixed	54	-0.1296	1.4927	2.00	2.00	1.00	-1.00	-1.00	-2.00	-2.70
	All	211	-0.2133	1.5544	2.00	2.00	1.00	-1.00	-1.00	-2.00	-2.00
42-43	White	118	-0.2288	1.5382	3.00	2.00	1.00	-1.00	-1.00	-2.00	-2.00
	Black	16	0.0000	1.5492	2.00	2.00	1.00	0.00	-1.00	-2.30	-3.00
	Mixed	37	0.1081	1.5948	2.86	2.00	2.00	-1.00	-1.00	-2.00	-2.00
	All	177	-0.1077	1.5634	3.00	2.00	1.00	-1.00	-1.00	-2.00	-2.00

Eye slant: Using a plastic ruler, establish the horizontal line through the inner canthus of each eye. At the outer canthus of each eye, measure the distance above or below the horizontal line in millimeters. The eyes should be open voluntarily.

TABLE 27-15 *Distributions for Nose Length (cm): Both Sexes*

Gestational Age	Race	Number of Infants	Mean	Standard Deviation	Percentiles						
					97	90	75	50	25	10	3
30-34	White	14	1.9500	0.1743	2.30	2.25	2.05	1.90	1.80	1.80	1.80
	Black	12	2.0083	0.1730	2.30	2.27	2.17	2.00	1.90	1.73	1.70
	Mixed	5	1.9800	0.2168	2.20	2.20	2.15	2.10	1.75	1.70	1.70
	All	37	1.9757	0.1657	2.30	2.20	2.10	2.00	1.80	1.80	1.70
35-36	White	17	2.0000	0.1458	2.30	2.22	2.10	2.00	1.85	1.80	1.80
	Black	17	2.0235	0.2016	2.30	2.30	2.20	2.10	1.80	1.78	1.70
	Mixed	11	2.1182	0.1328	2.30	2.28	2.20	2.10	2.10	1.84	1.80
	All	46	2.0391	0.1680	2.30	2.23	2.20	2.10	1.87	1.80	1.74
37-38	White	93	2.0344	0.1748	2.30	2.30	2.20	2.00	1.90	1.80	1.68
	Black	27	2.0963	0.1224	2.30	2.22	2.20	2.10	2.00	1.90	1.90
	Mixed	39	2.1179	0.1652	2.40	2.30	2.30	2.10	2.00	1.80	1.80
	All	169	2.0651	0.1666	2.30	2.30	2.20	2.10	2.00	1.80	1.70
39	White	137	2.1175	0.1350	2.30	2.30	2.20	2.10	2.00	2.00	1.80
	Black	36	2.1222	0.1476	2.39	2.30	2.20	2.10	2.00	1.90	1.80
	Mixed	54	2.1019	0.1407	2.33	2.30	2.20	2.10	2.00	1.90	1.80
	All	240	2.1196	0.1390	2.30	2.30	2.20	2.10	2.00	2.00	1.80
40	White	206	2.1466	0.1447	2.40	2.30	2.30	2.20	2.10	2.00	1.80
	Black	46	2.1109	0.1494	2.30	2.30	2.20	2.10	2.00	1.90	1.78
	Mixed	71	2.1254	0.1471	2.40	2.30	2.20	2.10	2.00	1.92	1.90
	All	331	2.1372	0.1447	2.40	2.30	2.20	2.10	2.00	2.00	1.80
41	White	140	2.1564	0.1369	2.40	2.30	2.27	2.20	2.02	2.00	1.90
	Black	23	2.1087	0.1443	2.30	2.30	2.20	2.10	2.00	1.94	1.80
	Mixed	59	2.1559	0.1611	2.50	2.30	2.30	2.20	2.10	2.00	1.76
	All	232	2.1513	0.1441	2.40	2.30	2.30	2.20	2.00	2.00	1.90
42-43	White	128	2.1289	0.1517	2.40	2.30	2.20	2.10	2.00	1.99	1.80
	Black	19	2.0895	0.1729	2.40	2.30	2.20	2.00	2.00	1.80	1.80
	Mixed	38	2.1632	0.1496	2.50	2.31	2.30	2.20	2.00	2.00	1.90
	All	191	2.1335	0.1547	2.40	2.30	2.20	2.10	2.00	2.00	1.80

Nose length: (See Figure 27-1)
A plastic ruler placed over the nose was used to measure from the base of the nose (established by palpation) to the tip of the nose, defined as the lateral edge of the alae nasi (judged by inspection).

TABLE 27-16 *Distributions for Length(Height) of Upper Lip (cm): Both Sexes*

Gestational Age	Race	Number of Infants	Mean	Standard Deviation	Percentiles						
					97	90	75	50	25	10	3
30-34	All	38	0.8184	0.1411	1.08	1.00	0.90	0.80	0.70	0.60	0.52
35-36	All	46	0.8913	0.1458	1.22	1.10	1.00	0.90	0.80	0.67	0.60
37-38	All	168	0.9060	0.1334	1.19	1.10	1.00	0.90	0.80	0.70	0.60
39	All	237	0.9152	0.1219	1.10	1.10	1.00	0.90	0.80	0.80	0.61
40	White	203	0.9296	0.1263	1.20	1.10	1.00	0.90	0.80	0.80	0.70
	Black	44	0.9682	0.1410	1.26	1.15	1.07	1.00	0.90	0.80	0.70
	Mixed	74	0.9284	0.1319	1.20	1.10	1.00	0.90	0.80	0.75	0.70
	All	329	0.9337	0.1304	1.20	1.10	1.00	0.90	0.80	0.80	0.70
41	White	139	0.9115	0.1077	1.10	1.00	1.00	0.90	0.80	0.80	0.70
	Black	22	1.0273	0.1316	1.30	1.20	1.12	1.00	0.90	0.90	0.80
	Mixed	57	0.8982	0.1232	1.13	1.10	1.00	0.90	0.80	0.70	0.67
	All	229	0.9231	0.1190	1.20	1.10	1.00	0.90	0.80	0.80	0.70
42-43	White	127	0.9512	0.1259	1.20	1.10	1.00	1.00	0.90	0.80	0.70
	Black	18	0.9667	0.2058	1.40	1.22	1.10	1.00	0.87	0.59	0.50
	Mixed	38	0.9526	0.1428	1.28	1.11	1.00	1.00	0.90	0.79	0.62
	All	189	0.9550	0.1381	1.20	1.10	1.00	1.00	0.90	0.80	0.67

Height of lip: See Figure 27-1.
The upper lip height or length is measured in the midline between the nasal septum (columella) to the upper edge of the vermilion of the upper lip.

SKULL: FONTANELS

TABLE 27-17 *Distributions for Anterior Fontanel: Length (cm): Both Sexes*

Gestational Age	Race	Number of Infants	Mean	Standard Deviation	*Percentiles*						
					97	90	75	50	25	10	3
30-34	All	35	2.3486	0.9001	5.29	3.52	3.00	2.10	1.70	1.42	0.56
35-36	All	48	2.7542	1.3473	6.21	5.08	3.37	2.50	1.80	1.38	0.79
37-38	White	96	2.1896	0.9624	4.05	3.53	2.80	2.05	1.30	1.00	0.89
	Black	26	2.8192	1.2110	6.20	4.51	3.27	2.60	1.95	1.40	1.10
	Mixed	37	2.6405	1.0487	5.23	4.00	3.55	2.40	2.00	1.30	1.00
	All	171	2.4140	1.0526	4.77	3.80	3.20	2.30	1.60	1.20	0.90
39	White	144	2.3090	0.9315	4.70	3.65	2.70	2.20	1.62	1.25	0.90
	Black	37	2.9919	1.1410	5.87	4.56	3.75	2.90	2.15	1.56	0.87
	Mixed	51	2.5451	0.9530	4.73	4.00	3.00	2.50	2.00	1.22	0.81
	All	246	2.5150	1.0615	4.80	4.00	3.00	2.30	1.80	1.30	0.90
40	White	212	2.3986	0.9321	4.26	3.60	3.10	2.30	1.70	1.20	0.90
	Black	43	3.2977	1.1869	6.27	5.00	3.80	3.00	2.60	2.04	1.12
	Mixed	76	2.3539	1.0546	5.08	4.03	3.00	2.25	1.60	1.21	0.76
	All	341	2.4988	1.0398	4.70	3.80	3.20	2.40	1.70	1.30	0.90
41	White	146	2.4349	1.0055	4.92	4.00	3.00	2.30	1.70	1.17	0.84
	Black	23	3.4261	1.0813	5.30	5.06	4.30	3.40	2.50	2.04	1.80
	Mixed	61	2.5377	1.0732	5.03	4.20	3.30	2.30	1.70	1.32	0.97
	All	242	2.5769	1.0940	5.00	4.20	3.20	2.40	1.80	1.30	0.90
42-43	White	130	2.4046	1.0506	4.81	4.00	3.00	2.20	1.70	1.20	0.89
	Black	20	3.2400	1.1736	5.20	4.92	4.17	3.40	2.37	1.61	0.90
	Mixed	40	2.6600	0.9647	4.98	3.58	3.10	2.90	2.00	1.50	0.97
	All	196	2.5561	1.0689	5.00	4.10	3.20	2.40	1.80	1.20	0.90

Anterior fontanel length: Using a plastic ruler in millimeters, the examiner palpates the most anterior and most posterior points of the anterior fontanel and measures the distance between these points.

TABLE 27-18 *Distributions for Anterior Fontanel: Width (cm): Both Sexes*

Gestational Age	Race	Number of Infants	Mean	Standard Deviation	*Percentiles*						
					97	90	75	50	25	10	3
30-34	All	35	2.2343	0.7308	3.97	3.32	2.80	2.00	1.80	1.60	0.37
35-36	All	47	2.5106	1.0759	5.20	4.16	3.00	2.30	1.70	1.36	0.65
37-38	White	93	1.9914	0.8058	3.62	3.16	2.55	2.00	1.35	1.00	0.63
	Black	26	2.7615	0.9575	5.20	4.33	3.12	2.60	2.10	1.47	1.30
	Mixed	37	2.3784	0.9721	5.26	3.80	2.95	2.20	1.70	1.18	1.00
	All	167	2.2114	0.9028	4.00	3.32	2.70	2.20	1.50	1.10	0.80
39	White	139	2.1180	0.8053	4.08	3.20	2.60	2.10	1.50	1.10	0.92
	Black	37	2.6649	0.8097	4.00	3.62	3.25	2.80	2.25	1.44	0.67
	Mixed	50	2.2120	0.8314	4.63	3.19	2.55	2.20	1.60	1.30	0.96
	All	239	2.2711	0.8677	4.10	3.30	2.80	2.20	1.60	1.20	1.00
40	White	202	2.2361	0.7935	4.00	3.27	2.80	2.20	1.70	1.20	0.81
	Black	43	2.7349	0.8888	5.36	3.86	3.20	2.70	2.00	1.80	1.26
	Mixed	74	2.1338	0.8265	4.15	3.30	2.60	2.10	1.60	1.10	0.47
	All	327	2.2832	0.8452	4.10	3.32	2.80	2.20	1.80	1.20	0.80
41	White	142	2.2479	0.8190	4.07	3.34	2.70	2.20	1.70	1.20	1.00
	Black	23	2.7217	0.6802	4.80	3.66	3.00	2.70	2.20	2.00	1.70
	Mixed	61	2.3836	0.9349	4.83	3.76	2.90	2.30	1.60	1.32	0.93
	All	237	2.3439	0.8554	4.36	3.50	2.80	2.30	1.80	1.30	1.00
42-43	White	123	2.2228	0.9670	4.16	3.50	3.00	2.00	1.50	1.14	0.74
	Black	19	3.1684	0.9844	5.00	4.60	4.00	3.00	2.30	2.00	1.30
	Mixed	39	2.4103	0.8271	4.84	3.50	3.00	2.20	1.80	1.40	1.32
	All	187	2.3706	0.9795	4.54	3.80	3.00	2.20	1.60	1.28	0.80

Anterior fontanel width: Using a plastic ruler in millimeters, the examiner palpates the most lateral points on the left and right of the fontanel and measures the distance between these points.

TABLE 27-19 *Distributions for Posterior Fontanel: Length (cm): Both Sexes*

Gestational Age	Race	Number of Infants	Mean	Standard Deviation	Percentiles						
					97	90	75	50	25	10	3
30-34	All	13	0.4538	0.5043	1.70	1.50	0.60	0.20	0.20	0.20	0.20
35-36	All	14	0.2643	0.2205	1.00	0.70	0.20	0.20	0.20	0.15	0.10
37-38	White	46	0.2913	0.3189	1.61	0.56	0.20	0.20	0.20	0.17	0.10
	Black	10	0.2800	0.1814	0.70	0.68	0.35	0.20	0.20	0.11	0.10
	Mixed	18	0.3056	0.4235	2.00	0.47	0.20	0.20	0.20	0.20	0.20
	All	83	0.2928	0.3177	1.54	0.56	0.20	0.20	0.20	0.20	0.10
39	White	67	0.2612	0.2504	1.30	0.22	0.20	0.20	0.20	0.20	0.10
	Black	15	0.3933	0.3990	1.50	1.20	0.50	0.20	0.20	0.16	0.10
	Mixed	23	0.2609	0.2445	1.30	0.48	0.20	0.20	0.20	0.14	0.10
	All	109	0.2771	0.2710	1.30	0.50	0.20	0.20	0.20	0.20	0.10
40	White	94	0.3319	0.3122	1.21	0.80	0.22	0.20	0.20	0.20	0.10
	Black	20	0.3800	0.2966	1.00	0.99	0.62	0.20	0.20	0.20	0.20
	Mixed	36	0.2917	0.2310	0.99	0.73	0.20	0.20	0.20	0.20	0.10
	All	156	0.3237	0.2874	1.03	0.80	0.20	0.20	0.20	0.20	0.10
41	White	66	0.3227	0.3262	1.40	0.80	0.20	0.20	0.20	0.20	0.10
	Black	12	0.4667	0.4830	1.60	1.45	0.82	0.20	0.20	0.20	0.20
	Mixed	23	0.2652	0.2166	1.20	0.46	0.20	0.20	0.20	0.20	0.20
	All	105	0.3295	0.3302	1.36	0.84	0.20	0.20	0.20	0.20	0.12
42-43	White	58	0.3017	0.2899	1.26	0.61	0.20	0.20	0.20	0.20	0.10
	Black	13	0.7308	0.5266	2.00	1.72	1.00	0.70	0.20	0.20	0.20
	Mixed	19	0.3684	0.4796	2.20	0.90	0.20	0.20	0.20	0.20	0.10
	All	93	0.3710	0.3950	1.84	0.86	0.35	0.20	0.20	0.20	0.10

Posterior fontanel length: Using a plastic ruler in millimeters, the examiner palpates the most posterior points of the anterior fontanel and measures the distance between these points.

TABLE 27-20 *Distributions for Posterior Fontanel: Width (cm): Both Sexes*

Gestational Age	Race	Number of Infants	Mean	Standard Deviation	Percentiles						
					97	90	75	50	25	10	3
30-34	All	14	0.4000	0.4132	1.60	1.30	0.50	0.20	0.20	0.20	0.20
35-36	All	14	0.2786	0.2723	1.20	0.80	0.20	0.20	0.20	0.15	0.10
37-38	White	46	0.2717	0.2344	1.12	0.56	0.20	0.20	0.20	0.17	0.10
	Black	10	0.2800	0.1814	0.70	0.68	0.35	0.20	0.20	0.11	0.10
	Mixed	18	0.3222	0.4941	2.30	0.50	0.20	0.20	0.20	0.20	0.20
	All	83	0.2916	0.3116	1.20	0.56	0.20	0.20	0.20	0.20	0.10
39	White	67	0.2552	0.2032	1.00	0.30	0.20	0.20	0.20	0.20	0.10
	Black	15	0.3733	0.3432	1.20	1.08	0.50	0.20	0.20	0.16	0.10
	Mixed	23	0.2609	0.2231	1.10	0.56	0.20	0.20	0.20	0.20	0.10
	All	109	0.2706	0.2290	1.07	0.50	0.20	0.20	0.20	0.20	0.10
40	White	93	0.3118	0.2862	1.24	0.60	0.20	0.20	0.20	0.20	0.10
	Black	19	0.3684	0.3465	1.40	1.10	0.40	0.20	0.20	0.20	0.20
	Mixed	36	0.2861	0.2232	1.08	0.66	0.20	0.20	0.20	0.20	0.11
	All	154	0.3084	0.2753	1.13	0.60	0.20	0.20	0.20	0.20	0.10
41	White	65	0.2908	0.2614	1.40	0.60	0.20	0.20	0.20	0.20	0.10
	Black	12	0.4333	0.4677	1.60	1.48	0.45	0.20	0.20	0.20	0.20
	Mixed	23	0.2652	0.2166	1.20	0.46	0.20	0.20	0.20	0.20	0.20
	All	104	0.3029	0.2830	1.37	0.60	0.20	0.20	0.20	0.20	0.11
42-43	White	57	0.2807	0.2199	1.10	0.60	0.20	0.20	0.20	0.20	0.10
	Black	13	0.6923	0.5123	2.00	1.64	1.00	0.60	0.20	0.20	0.20
	Mixed	19	0.3789	0.5224	2.40	0.90	0.20	0.20	0.20	0.20	0.10
	All	92	0.3554	0.3734	1.29	0.87	0.30	0.20	0.20	0.20	0.10

Posterior fontanel width: Using a plastic ruler in millimeters, the examiner palpates the most posterior points of the anterior fontanel and measures the distance between these points.

CHEST

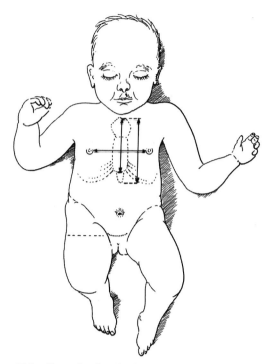

FIGURE 27-2 Shows landmarks for measuring length of sternum including and not including xiphoid process, internipple distance and the top edge of symphysis pubis, for measuring upper segment.

TABLE 27-21 *Distributions for Sternum Length Including Xiphoid (cm): Both Sexes*

Gestational Age	Race	Number of Infants	Mean	Standard Deviation	Percentiles						
					97	90	75	50	25	10	3
30-34	All	39	6.9410	0.7731	8.28	8.00	7.50	7.00	6.30	5.90	5.24
35-36	All	46	7.2304	0.5906	8.38	8.00	7.80	7.20	6.70	6.40	6.24
37-38	White	89	7.3191	0.6094	8.56	8.10	7.65	7.30	7.00	6.60	6.02
	Black	27	7.4519	0.5727	8.90	8.22	7.80	7.40	7.00	6.68	6.40
	Mixed	37	7.2270	0.8329	9.50	8.04	7.75	7.30	6.65	6.28	4.97
	All	163	7.3202	0.6676	8.52	8.10	7.80	7.30	7.00	6.44	6.00
39	White	138	7.4522	0.5594	8.60	8.11	7.80	7.50	7.00	6.70	6.50
	Black	37	7.4676	0.7165	8.59	8.42	8.10	7.40	7.00	6.68	5.34
	Mixed	53	7.5113	0.6603	9.01	8.40	7.95	7.50	7.00	6.64	6.19
	All	240	7.4862	0.6084	8.68	8.29	7.90	7.50	7.00	6.70	6.42
40	White	201	7.6144	0.5899	8.79	8.30	8.00	7.60	7.20	6.92	6.51
	Black	44	7.6477	0.6098	8.70	8.50	8.15	7.65	7.20	6.90	6.50
	Mixed	70	7.6029	0.5934	8.89	8.40	8.00	7.60	7.20	6.81	6.60
	All	323	7.6167	0.5915	8.73	8.40	8.00	7.60	7.20	6.90	6.60
41	White	140	7.6379	1.6213	8.70	8.49	8.00	7.70	7.20	6.81	6.40
	Black	23	7.7696	0.5579	8.90	8.40	8.20	7.80	7.20	7.04	6.80
	Mixed	57	7.6632	0.4894	8.85	8.40	7.95	7.60	7.30	7.10	6.75
	All	231	7.6645	0.5760	8.80	8.40	8.00	7.70	7.30	7.00	6.59
42-43	White	125	7.6944	0.5309	8.80	8.44	8.00	7.70	7.35	7.00	6.80
	Black	19	7.7526	0.5264	8.80	8.50	8.20	7.70	7.40	6.90	6.90
	Mixed	40	7.7625	0.5261	8.65	8.39	8.17	7.80	7.50	7.20	6.08
	All	190	7.7163	0.5244	8.80	8.40	8.00	7.70	7.40	7.01	6.80

Sternum length including xiphoid: See Figure 27-2.
Using a plastic ruler, the examiner palpates the manubrial notch and the lowest end of the xiphoid process at the lower end of the sternum. The distance is measured from the manubrial notch (top of sternum) to the tip of the xiphoid.

TABLE 27-22 *Distributions for Sternum Length Minus Xiphoid (cm): Both Sexes*

Gestational Age	Race	Number of Infants	Mean	Standard Deviation	Percentiles						
					97	90	75	50	25	10	3
30-34	All	14	5.8214	0.8011	7.00	6.85	6.55	5.70	5.20	4.55	4.30
35-36	All	10	5.9300	0.4644	6.70	6.68	6.35	5.80	5.50	5.41	5.40
37-38	White	42	6.2143	0.5707	7.17	6.80	6.50	6.30	5.95	5.53	4.59
	Mixed	10	6.3600	0.6059	7.20	7.19	6.87	6.30	5.75	5.51	5.50
	All	65	6.2385	0.5612	7.20	6.94	6.70	6.30	5.85	5.56	4.79
39	White	53	6.5057	0.5489	7.99	7.20	6.80	6.60	6.00	5.80	5.70
	Black	12	6.4167	0.4668	7.20	7.08	6.80	6.45	6.02	5.80	5.80
	Mixed	19	6.5789	0.7285	8.60	7.60	6.80	6.40	6.20	5.70	5.50
	All	87	6.5172	0.5775	7.98	7.20	6.80	6.50	6.10	5.80	5.70
40	White	91	6.5341	0.5694	7.80	7.20	6.90	6.50	6.20	5.82	5.35
	Black	15	6.6000	0.4826	7.50	7.32	6.80	6.70	6.20	5.92	5.80
	Mixed	32	6.5750	0.5292	7.40	7.40	7.00	6.55	6.30	5.80	5.60
	All	142	6.5472	0.5519	7.50	7.27	6.90	6.50	6.20	5.80	5.53
41	White	46	6.5217	0.5448	7.66	7.23	6.80	6.50	6.17	5.80	5.16
	Mixed	17	6.7588	0.5635	7.90	7.82	6.95	6.80	6.45	5.80	5.80
	All	75	6.6133	0.5539	7.77	7.34	6.90	6.70	6.20	5.92	5.48
42-43	White	58	6.7017	0.5501	8.04	7.40	7.00	6.75	6.30	6.08	5.68
	Mixed	13	6.9308	0.3903	7.60	7.52	7.20	6.80	6.80	6.28	6.00
	All	79	6.7316	0.5185	7.78	7.40	7.00	6.80	6.40	6.20	5.80

Sternum length minus xiphoid: See Figure 27-2.

Using a plastic ruler, the examiner palpates the manubrial notch and the end of the sternum. The ruler measures the distance from the lower edge of the notch to the lowest point on the sternum, with no xiphoid process palpable.

TABLE 27-23 *Distributions for Chest Circumference (cm): Both Sexes*

Gestational Age	Race	Number of Infants	Mean	Standard Deviation	Percentiles						
					97	90	75	50	25	10	3
30-34	All	36	29.7028	2.8501	34.39	33.09	31.72	30.10	28.00	25.70	23.52
35-36	All	44	31.0409	1.8402	34.82	33.50	32.22	30.90	30.00	28.50	26.87
37-38	White	90	31.9044	1.8876	36.00	34.39	33.05	32.00	30.75	29.51	28.00
	Black	24	31.8583	1.6344	35.60	33.50	33.15	32.00	30.50	29.60	28.50
	Mixed	35	31.6171	1.7311	35.33	34.08	33.00	31.50	30.50	29.00	28.82
	All	158	31.8323	1.7882	35.67	34.02	33.00	32.00	30.50	29.50	28.48
39	White	127	32.7488	1.6965	35.66	35.00	34.00	32.80	31.70	30.46	29.50
	Black	37	32.0054	1.5503	34.96	34.12	33.10	32.00	31.00	30.00	28.14
	Mixed	51	32.3706	1.6146	35.13	34.50	33.50	32.70	31.50	29.92	29.28
	All	228	32.5667	1.6594	35.41	34.80	33.80	32.55	31.50	30.00	29.50
40	White	189	33.1497	1.8009	36.15	35.20	34.30	33.30	32.00	30.80	29.35
	Black	42	32.6500	1.5675	34.94	34.64	34.00	33.00	31.37	30.50	29.15
	Mixed	70	33.1386	1.6301	36.77	35.00	34.25	33.00	32.00	31.05	30.41
	All	309	33.0563	1.7254	36.00	35.00	34.20	33.00	32.00	30.80	29.80
41	White	133	33.2789	1.5344	36.00	35.46	34.45	33.40	32.00	31.34	30.40
	Black	22	32.9545	1.3717	35.00	34.64	34.10	33.00	32.17	30.53	30.50
	Mixed	54	33.4315	1.6404	36.52	35.45	34.50	33.70	32.15	31.40	29.63
	All	219	33.2717	1.5469	36.00	35.40	34.40	33.40	32.00	31.30	30.36
42-43	White	118	33.4788	1.6061	36.54	35.50	34.70	33.50	32.40	31.27	30.50
	Black	17	33.1412	1.5855	36.20	36.04	34.45	33.00	31.75	31.24	31.00
	Mixed	38	33.6000	1.3823	36.83	35.32	34.50	33.50	32.95	32.32	29.59
	All	179	33.4430	1.5409	36.42	35.50	34.50	33.50	32.40	31.50	30.54

Chest circumference: Using a tape measure, measure the circumference at the level of the nipple. Measure when the infant is breathing normally.

TABLE 27-24 *Distributions for Internipple Distance (cm): Both Sexes*

Gestational Age	Race	Number of Infants	Mean	Standard Deviation	Percentiles						
					97	90	75	50	25	10	3
30-34	All	38	7.2316	0.7480	8.50	8.23	7.70	7.30	6.77	6.18	5.22
35-36	All	46	7.5652	0.5152	8.46	8.33	8.00	7.70	7.10	6.94	6.52
37-38	White	91	7.7308	0.7012	9.35	8.80	8.10	7.70	7.30	6.90	6.68
	Black	27	7.7407	0.6059	9.60	8.34	8.10	7.70	7.40	6.96	6.60
	Mixed	38	7.5263	0.6488	9.15	8.22	7.92	7.60	7.15	6.50	6.25
	All	166	7.6723	0.6658	9.30	8.50	8.02	7.70	7.27	6.80	6.50
39	White	137	7.8672	0.5759	9.00	8.70	8.20	7.80	7.40	7.10	6.71
	Black	36	7.8417	0.7777	9.59	8.92	8.37	7.90	7.32	6.70	6.61
	Mixed	54	7.8278	0.5708	9.10	8.45	8.20	7.85	7.40	7.00	6.69
	All	240	7.8700	0.6120	9.15	8.70	8.27	7.90	7.40	7.10	6.70
40	White	203	7.9591	0.5922	9.00	8.80	8.30	8.00	7.60	7.20	6.81
	Black	44	7.8386	0.5792	8.80	8.55	8.30	7.85	7.40	7.00	6.44
	Mixed	72	7.9306	0.5349	9.12	8.67	8.20	7.90	7.60	7.33	6.82
	All	327	7.9413	0.5733	9.00	8.70	8.30	8.00	7.60	7.20	6.80
41	White	140	7.9700	0.4875	8.80	8.69	8.30	8.00	7.70	7.40	7.02
	Black	23	8.0652	0.5548	9.00	8.80	8.60	8.00	7.80	7.24	6.90
	Mixed	58	8.0190	0.4799	9.00	8.70	8.32	8.00	7.70	7.30	7.15
	All	232	7.9991	0.4892	9.00	8.70	8.30	8.00	7.70	7.40	7.10
42-43	White	126	8.0254	0.6825	9.36	8.90	8.40	8.00	7.60	7.20	6.70
	Black	19	8.0684	0.6037	9.20	9.00	8.60	8.00	7.60	7.20	7.10
	Mixed	40	8.0750	0.6444	9.20	9.00	8.40	8.05	7.80	7.42	6.18
	All	191	8.0398	0.6589	9.22	8.90	8.40	8.00	7.60	7.20	6.78

Nipple distance: See figure 27-2
A ruler was used to measure the distance between the centers of each normal nipple.

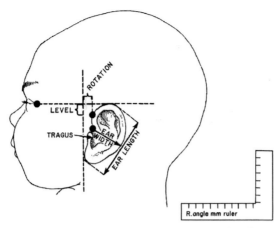

FIGURE 27-3   A vertical line is established at a 90° angle to horizontal line, which intersects with lower point of attachment of ear. The posterior rotation of the ear is the distance of the highest point of attachment of the ear in millimeters behind the vertical line. There were no infants examined who had an anterior rotation of the external ear.

TABLE 27-25 *Distributions for Ear Length (cm) [Right]: Both Sexes*

Gestational Age	Race	Number of Infants	Mean	Standard Deviation	Percentiles						
					97	90	75	50	25	10	3
30-34	All	39	3.4359	0.3528	4.16	3.90	3.70	3.40	3.10	3.00	2.76
35-36	All	46	3.5043	0.3120	4.06	3.93	3.70	3.50	3.20	3.10	3.00
37-38	White	93	3.6097	0.2774	4.12	4.00	3.80	3.60	3.40	3.20	3.10
	Black	27	3.5704	0.2216	4.00	3.82	3.70	3.60	3.40	3.28	3.10
	Mixed	38	3.5711	0.2770	4.17	3.90	3.80	3.60	3.40	3.19	3.02
	All	169	3.5911	0.2681	4.10	3.90	3.80	3.60	3.40	3.20	3.10
39	White	139	3.6511	0.2471	4.08	4.00	3.80	3.70	3.50	3.30	3.10
	Black	35	3.6429	0.2441	4.10	3.90	3.80	3.60	3.50	3.32	3.11
	Mixed	54	3.6685	0.1979	4.00	3.90	3.80	3.70	3.50	3.40	3.20
	All	241	3.6614	0.2367	4.10	3.90	3.80	3.70	3.50	3.40	3.20
40	White	207	3.7000	0.2725	4.20	4.10	3.90	3.70	3.50	3.40	3.20
	Black	44	3.6750	0.2902	4.20	4.00	3.97	3.70	3.40	3.25	3.10
	Mixed	73	3.7233	0.2486	4.10	4.00	3.90	3.70	3.50	3.40	3.20
	All	332	3.7015	0.2700	4.20	4.00	3.90	3.70	3.50	3.40	3.20
41	White	143	3.7210	0.2506	4.20	4.00	3.90	3.70	3.60	3.40	3.20
	Black	23	3.6783	0.2984	4.30	4.12	3.80	3.70	3.50	3.40	2.90
	Mixed	60	3.7217	0.2650	4.32	4.09	3.90	3.70	3.50	3.40	3.27
	All	237	3.7186	0.2586	4.20	4.00	3.90	3.70	3.50	3.40	3.20
42-43	White	128	3.7367	0.2417	4.20	4.00	3.97	3.70	3.60	3.40	3.29
	Black	19	3.7158	0.2814	4.40	4.10	3.80	3.70	3.50	3.30	3.30
	Mixed	40	3.7900	0.2818	4.28	4.20	3.97	3.80	3.70	3.31	3.12
	All	193	3.7472	0.2535	4.20	4.00	3.95	3.70	3.60	3.40	3.20

Ear length: See Figure 27-3. Landmarks for top of ear are shown. The length is the distance from the top of the ear to the bottom of the lobe of ear.

TABLE 27-26 *Distributions for Ear Width (cm) [Right]: Both Sexes*

Gestational Age	Race	Number of Infants	Mean	Standard Deviation	Percentiles						
					97	90	75	50	25	10	3
30-34	All	39	2.0641	0.1828	2.30	2.30	2.20	2.10	1.90	1.80	1.64
35-36	All	45	2.1333	0.1719	2.40	2.34	2.25	2.20	2.00	1.80	1.80
37-38	White	93	2.1398	0.1819	2.60	2.30	2.20	2.20	2.00	1.90	1.78
	Black	26	2.1885	0.1583	2.40	2.40	2.30	2.20	2.10	2.00	1.80
	Mixed	38	2.1395	0.1424	2.48	2.31	2.20	2.10	2.00	2.00	1.83
	All	168	2.1488	0.1720	2.50	2.40	2.20	2.20	2.00	2.00	1.80
39	White	137	2.1686	0.1504	2.49	2.40	2.25	2.20	2.00	2.00	1.90
	Black	35	2.1829	0.1524	2.60	2.40	2.20	2.20	2.10	2.00	2.00
	Mixed	54	2.1648	0.1494	2.40	2.40	2.30	2.20	2.07	2.00	1.83
	All	239	2.1732	0.1493	2.48	2.40	2.30	2.20	2.10	2.00	1.90
40	White	207	2.2029	0.1510	2.50	2.40	2.30	2.20	2.10	2.00	1.90
	Black	44	2.2182	0.1808	2.60	2.50	2.30	2.20	2.10	2.00	1.90
	Mixed	73	2.2151	0.1401	2.50	2.40	2.30	2.20	2.10	2.00	2.00
	All	332	2.2057	0.1533	2.50	2.40	2.30	2.20	2.10	2.00	1.90
41	White	143	2.2280	0.1836	2.60	2.50	2.30	2.20	2.10	2.00	1.90
	Black	23	2.1870	0.2074	2.70	2.50	2.30	2.20	2.00	1.90	1.90
	Mixed	60	2.2100	0.1581	2.60	2.40	2.30	2.20	2.10	2.00	1.88
	All	236	2.2182	0.1793	2.60	2.50	2.30	2.20	2.10	2.00	1.90
42-43	White	128	2.1867	0.1554	2.50	2.40	2.30	2.20	2.10	2.00	1.97
	Black	18	2.2000	0.1495	2.60	2.42	2.30	2.20	2.10	2.00	2.00
	Mixed	40	2.2525	0.1617	2.58	2.49	2.37	2.30	2.20	2.00	2.00
	All	192	2.2021	0.1575	2.50	2.40	2.30	2.20	2.10	2.00	2.00

Ear width: See Figure 27-3. Landmarks for measuring width are shown in figure.)
Using a plastic ruler in millimeters, the distance is measured between a point just above the tragus to the outer edge of the ear.

TABLE 27-27 *Distributions for Ear Level (mm) [Right]: Both Sexes*

Gestational Age	Race	Number of Infants	Mean	Standard Deviation	Percentiles						
					97	90	75	50	25	10	3
30-34	All	39	-2.3077	2.5147	2.80	1.00	0.00	-2.00	-4.00	-6.00	-7.00
35-36	All	45	-3.5556	3.2582	2.00	1.40	-1.00	-4.00	-6.50	-8.00	-9.86
37-38	White	92	-2.9348	2.7528	2.21	2.00	-2.00	-3.00	-4.75	-6.70	-8.00
	Black	27	-3.5926	2.7771	3.00	0.40	-2.00	-4.00	-5.00	-6.20	-10
	Mixed	38	-3.2105	2.4067	2.83	0.00	-2.00	-3.00	-5.00	-6.10	-8.00
	All	168	-3.1548	2.6150	2.00	1.00	-2.00	-3.00	-5.00	-6.00	-8.00
39	White	139	-2.9784	2.4685	2.00	0.00	-2.00	-3.00	-4.00	-6.00	-8.00
	Black	34	-3.1765	3.9425	4.90	2.50	-1.00	-3.00	-5.25	-9.50	-11.9
	Mixed	54	-2.7593	2.9070	4.00	2.00	-2.00	-3.00	-4.00	-6.00	-9.00
	All	240	-3.0000	2.8535	3.00	1.00	-2.00	-3.00	-5.00	-6.00	-9.00
40	White	206	-3.3301	2.7244	2.79	0.00	-2.00	-3.00	-5.00	-7.00	-8.00
	Black	44	-3.5682	3.3229	2.65	1.50	-2.00	-4.00	-5.75	-8.00	-11
	Mixed	73	-3.8356	2.6511	2.00	-1.00	-2.00	-4.00	-6.00	-7.60	-8.78
	All	331	-3.4592	2.7799	2.00	0.00	-2.00	-4.00	-5.00	-7.00	-8.00
41	White	141	-2.9929	3.0036	3.00	1.80	-1.00	-3.00	-5.00	-7.00	-8.00
	Black	23	-2.7826	2.6792	3.00	1.60	-1.00	-3.00	-4.00	-5.60	-9.00
	Mixed	60	-2.9667	3.1621	3.17	2.00	-1.25	-3.00	-5.00	-7.00	-9.17
	All	234	-2.9915	2.9705	3.00	2.00	-1.75	-3.00	-5.00	-7.00	-8.00
42-43	White	126	-3.6746	2.6678	2.00	0.00	-2.00	-4.00	-5.00	-7.00	-9.00
	Black	19	-3.3158	3.2327	5.00	2.00	-2.00	-3.00	-5.00	-8.00	-8.00
	Mixed	40	-3.3250	2.9298	4.31	2.00	-2.00	-3.50	-5.00	-7.00	-8.00
	All	191	-3.5969	2.7644	2.00	0.00	-2.00	-4.00	-5.00	-7.00	-8.24

Ear level: See Figure 27-3.
Using a plastic ruler in millimeters, the line horizontal to the outer canthus is established. The level of the ear is the distance in millimeters between the horizontal line and the upper point of attachment of the external ear to the scalp.

TABLE 27-28 *Distributions for Ear Rotation (mm) [Right]: Both Sexes*

Gestational Age	Race	Number of Infants	Mean	Standard Deviation	Percentiles						
					97	90	75	50	25	10	3
30-34	All	39	-5.9487	1.9728	-2.00	-3.00	-5.00	-6.00	-8.00	-8.00	-9.80
35-36	All	45	-6.2000	3.1738	4.96	-3.60	-5.00	-7.00	-8.00	-9.40	-11
37-38	White	92	-6.0652	2.3290	-1.79	-3.00	-5.00	-6.00	-7.00	-9.00	-11
	Black	27	-7.6667	2.3534	-4.00	-5.00	-5.00	-8.00	-10	-11	-12
	Mixed	39	-6.4359	2.2687	-1.00	-3.00	-5.00	-7.00	-8.00	-9.00	-10.6
	All	169	-6.4201	2.3238	-2.00	-4.00	-5.00	-6.00	-8.00	-9.00	-11
39	White	139	-6.2446	2.3586	-1.00	-4.00	-5.00	-6.00	-7.00	-10	-11
	Black	36	-7.5278	2.7096	-2.22	-4.00	-5.25	-7.00	-10	-11	-12.9
	Mixed	53	-6.3019	2.3986	-1.24	-4.00	-5.00	-6.00	-8.00	-10	-11
	All	241	-6.4606	2.4426	-2.00	-4.00	-5.00	-7.00	-8.00	-10	-11
40	White	206	-6.4660	2.4086	-3.00	-4.00	-5.00	-7.00	-8.00	-9.00	-11
	Black	44	-7.5455	2.8971	-1.35	-4.00	-5.25	-7.50	-10	-11	-13.7
	Mixed	73	-6.1918	2.0993	-2.22	-4.00	-4.50	-6.00	-7.00	-9.00	-10.8
	All	331	-6.5227	2.4362	-2.96	-4.00	-5.00	-7.00	-8.00	-10	-11
41	White	141	-6.2199	2.3877	-0.26	-4.00	-5.00	-7.00	-7.50	-9.00	-11
	Black	23	-6.7826	2.7954	-1.00	-3.00	-5.00	-7.00	-8.00	-11.2	-12
	Mixed	60	-5.9000	2.3194	-0.83	-3.00	-5.00	-6.00	-7.00	-8.00	-11.2
	All	234	-6.2179	2.3998	-1.00	-3.50	-5.00	-6.00	-8.00	-9.00	-11
42-43	White	126	-6.2788	2.4808	0.00	-3.00	-5.00	-7.00	-8.00	-9.00	-11
	Black	19	-8.1053	2.9608	-2.00	-4.00	-7.00	-8.00	-10	-12	-14
	Mixed	40	-6.0000	2.4495	-1.23	-3.00	-4.00	-6.00	-8.00	-9.90	-10.8
	All	191	-6.3455	2.6390	-0.76	-3.00	-5.00	-7.00	-8.00	-10	-11

Ear rotation: (See Figure 27-3)

Using the horizontal line and the point of attachment of the external ear to the scalp.

A vertical line is established at 90° angle to horizontal line, which intersects with lower point of attachment of ear. The posterior rotation of the ear is the distance in millimeters behind the vertical line. There were no infants examined who had an anterior rotation of the external ear.

HANDS

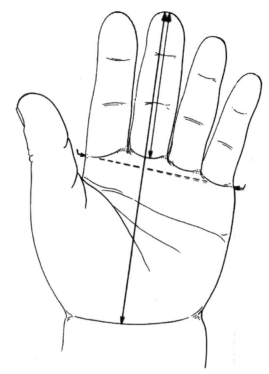

FIGURE 27.4   Measurements of length and width of the hand and the third finger.

TABLE 27-29 *Distributions for Hand Length (cm) [Right]: Both Sexes*

Gestational Age	Race	Number of Infants	Mean	Standard Deviation	Percentiles						
					97	90	75	50	25	10	3
30-34	All	38	6.0895	0.5516	7.08	6.72	6.50	6.20	5.67	5.20	5.12
35-36	All	45	6.2978	0.4093	7.10	6.94	6.50	6.30	6.00	5.80	5.33
37-38	White	91	6.4451	0.4137	7.12	6.98	6.70	6.50	6.20	5.92	5.48
	Black	26	6.6269	0.3317	7.30	7.06	6.82	6.65	6.30	6.17	6.10
	Mixed	37	6.5162	0.3625	7.29	7.02	6.75	6.50	6.20	6.00	5.91
	All	164	6.4866	0.3868	7.20	7.00	6.70	6.50	6.20	6.00	5.79
39	White	138	6.5841	0.3613	7.20	7.00	6.82	6.60	6.30	6.10	5.80
	Black	35	6.6886	0.3261	7.57	7.08	6.90	6.07	6.50	6.20	6.11
	Mixed	53	6.5623	0.3077	7.20	6.90	6.80	6.60	6.30	6.20	5.86
	All	238	6.6055	0.3490	7.20	7.00	6.80	6.60	6.30	6.20	5.90
40	White	202	6.7059	0.3373	7.39	7.20	7.00	6.70	6.50	6.30	6.10
	Black	44	6.8136	0.3296	7.43	7.20	7.00	6.80	6.70	6.30	6.00
	Mixed	73	6.6438	0.3114	7.20	7.06	6.90	6.70	6.40	6.20	5.94
	All	327	6.7070	0.3326	7.30	7.12	7.00	6.70	6.50	6.30	6.08
41	White	142	6.7085	0.3461	7.30	7.20	7.00	6.70	6.50	6.30	6.03
	Black	22	6.8091	0.3663	7.70	7.34	7.00	6.80	6.50	6.33	6.10
	Mixed	59	6.7102	0.3257	7.36	7.10	6.90	6.70	6.40	6.30	6.16
	All	233	6.7245	0.3425	7.30	7.20	7.00	6.70	6.50	6.30	6.10
42-43	White	124	6.6984	0.3586	7.32	7.20	6.90	6.70	6.42	6.30	6.05
	Black	19	6.9053	0.3205	7.40	7.40	7.20	7.00	6.70	6.40	6.30
	Mixed	39	6.7667	0.3644	7.48	7.20	7.00	6.70	6.60	6.30	5.80
	All	188	6.7287	0.3575	7.40	7.20	7.00	6.70	6.50	6.30	6.10

Hand length: See Figure 27-4.

Using a plastic ruler in millimeters, the hand length was measured between the most distal wrist crease and the tip of the third finger, as judged by the examiner on inspection at a 90 degree angle.

TABLE 27-30 *Distributions for Third Finger Length (cm) [Right]: Both Sexes*

Gestational Age	Race	Number of Infants	Mean	Standard Deviation	Percentiles						
					97	90	75	50	25	10	3
30-34	All	38	2.6184	0.2577	3.00	3.00	2.80	2.60	2.40	2.29	2.02
35-36	All	45	2.7400	0.1839	3.06	3.00	2.90	2.70	2.60	2.60	2.19
37-38	White	93	2.8097	0.2059	3.20	3.10	3.00	2.80	2.65	2.60	2.40
	Black	27	2.8889	0.1847	3.30	3.10	3.00	2.90	2.80	2.60	2.50
	Mixed	37	2.8405	0.1907	3.29	3.10	3.00	2.80	2.70	2.60	2.43
	All	167	2.8281	0.1975	3.20	3.10	3.00	2.80	2.70	2.60	2.40
39	White	138	2.8457	0.1903	3.18	3.00	3.00	2.90	2.70	2.60	2.50
	Black	36	2.9167	0.1875	3.40	3.20	3.00	2.90	2.80	2.70	2.60
	Mixed	53	2.8623	0.1547	3.18	3.00	3.00	2.90	2.75	2.60	2.56
	All	239	2.8640	0.1853	3.20	3.00	3.00	2.90	2.70	2.60	2.50
40	White	202	2.9134	0.1926	3.30	3.10	3.00	2.90	2.80	2.70	2.50
	Black	44	2.9591	0.1604	3.26	3.20	3.07	3.00	2.82	2.80	2.57
	Mixed	73	2.8863	0.1548	3.18	3.10	3.00	2.90	2.80	2.70	2.60
	All	327	2.9119	0.1802	3.30	3.10	3.00	2.90	2.80	2.70	2.58
41	White	142	2.9190	0.1879	3.27	3.20	3.00	3.00	2.80	2.70	2.53
	Black	22	2.9318	0.2276	3.70	3.10	3.00	2.90	2.80	2.63	2.50
	Mixed	59	2.9034	0.1564	3.20	3.10	3.00	2.90	2.80	2.70	2.60
	All	233	2.9176	0.1840	3.20	3.20	3.00	2.90	2.80	2.70	2.60
42-43	White	124	2.9234	0.1740	3.30	3.10	3.00	2.90	2.80	2.70	2.60
	Black	19	3.0158	0.1425	3.30	3.20	3.10	3.00	2.90	2.80	2.80
	Mixed	39	2.9179	0.1848	3.36	3.20	3.00	2.90	2.80	2.70	2.52
	All	188	2.9282	0.1743	3.30	3.20	3.00	2.90	2.80	2.70	2.60

Length of third finger: See Figure 27-4.
Using a plastic ruler in millimeters, the length of the third finger was measured from the crease at the base of the finger(above the third metacarpal-phalangeal joint) to the tip of the third finger, as judged by the examiner on inspection at an angle of 90 degrees at the tip.

TABLE 27-31 *Distributions for Hand Width (cm) [Right]: Both Sexes*

Gestational Age	Race	Number of Infants	Mean	Standard Deviation	Percentiles						
					97	90	75	50	25	10	3
30-34	All	40	3.1200	0.3695	3.58	3.50	3.40	3.15	2.92	2.50	2.11
35-36	All	47	3.2553	0.3262	3.76	3.62	3.50	3.30	3.10	2.88	2.33
37-38	White	93	3.3645	0.2689	3.92	3.70	3.50	3.40	3.20	2.94	2.80
	Black	27	3.4333	0.2166	3.80	3.80	3.60	3.40	3.30	3.10	3.00
	Mixed	39	3.3897	0.2125	3.88	3.70	3.50	3.40	3.30	3.10	2.94
	All	169	3.3805	0.2423	3.80	3.70	3.50	3.40	3.30	3.10	2.81
39	White	138	3.4232	0.2242	3.88	3.70	3.60	3.40	3.30	3.19	3.00
	Black	36	3.4361	0.2620	3.90	3.80	3.60	3.40	3.30	3.10	2.73
	Mixed	53	3.4226	0.2016	3.80	3.70	3.50	3.40	3.30	3.14	2.86
	All	240	3.4308	0.2247	3.80	3.70	3.60	3.40	3.30	3.11	3.00
40	White	203	3.4571	0.2122	3.80	3.70	3.60	3.40	3.30	3.20	3.01
	Black	44	3.4909	0.2165	3.96	3.70	3.60	3.50	3.40	3.20	2.90
	Mixed	73	3.4329	0.2102	3.88	3.70	3.60	3.40	3.30	3.14	3.00
	All	328	3.4552	0.2130	3.81	3.70	3.60	3.40	3.30	3.20	3.00
41	White	140	3.4914	0.1876	3.80	3.70	3.60	3.50	3.40	3.21	3.20
	Black	23	3.5043	0.2458	4.10	3.80	3.70	3.50	3.40	3.14	3.00
	Mixed	58	3.5155	0.2050	3.90	3.80	3.70	3.50	3.40	3.29	3.00
	All	233	3.4910	0.2194	3.80	3.80	3.60	3.50	3.40	3.20	3.10
42-43	White	127	3.4811	0.2034	3.90	3.72	3.60	3.50	3.40	3.30	3.00
	Black	19	3.5737	0.1821	4.00	3.90	3.60	3.60	3.50	3.30	3.20
	Mixed	40	3.5175	0.2062	3.90	3.79	3.70	3.55	3.32	3.30	3.05
	All	192	3.4948	0.2020	3.90	3.70	3.60	3.50	3.40	3.30	3.08

Hand width: Figure

Using spreading calipers, the distance was measured between the metacarpal-phalangeal (M-P) joint in the index finger and the M-P joint of the fifth finger.

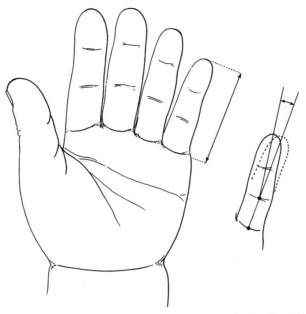

FIGURE 27-5 Shows the landmarks for measuring the length of the fifth finger, as well as the deviation of the distal phalanx from the midline axis, used to measure the degree of curvature in clinodactyly.

TABLE 27-32 *Distributions for Fifth Finger Length (cm) [Right]: Both Sexes*

Gestational Age	Race	Number of Infants	Mean	Standard Deviation	Percentiles						
					97	90	75	50	25	10	3
30-34	All	17	2.1471	0.2601	2.60	2.52	2.30	2.20	1.95	1.70	1.70
35-36	All	35	2.2371	0.1555	2.50	2.44	2.30	2.20	2.10	2.10	1.81
37-38	White	69	2.2420	0.2025	2.60	2.50	2.40	2.20	2.10	2.00	1.81
	Black	15	2.3400	0.2063	2.70	2.70	2.50	2.30	2.20	2.06	2.00
	Mixed	8	2.2625	0.2066	2.50	2.50	2.47	2.25	2.12	1.90	1.90
	All	99	2.2586	0.2010	2.70	2.50	2.40	2.30	2.10	2.00	1.90
39	White	74	2.4014	0.9274	2.77	2.60	2.50	2.40	2.20	2.10	0.65
	Black	26	2.3538	0.1655	2.60	2.53	2.50	2.40	2.30	2.17	1.80
	Mixed	19	2.3000	0.1491	2.60	2.50	2.40	2.30	2.20	2.10	2.00
	All	130	2.3700	0.7076	2.70	2.60	2.50	2.30	2.20	2.10	1.80
40	White	119	2.4723	0.6796	2.70	2.60	2.50	2.40	2.30	2.20	2.10
	Black	48	2.4396	0.3207	3.59	2.61	2.50	2.40	2.30	2.20	2.05
	Mixed	30	2.3800	0.1375	2.80	2.50	2.50	2.40	2.30	2.20	2.20
	All	211	2.4498	0.5370	2.70	2.60	2.50	2.40	2.30	2.20	2.10
41	White	98	2.4122	0.1986	2.80	2.70	2.52	2.45	2.27	2.19	2.00
	Black	21	2.4429	0.1912	2.80	2.70	2.60	2.50	2.30	2.22	2.10
	Mixed	26	2.3500	0.4958	2.90	2.73	2.52	2.40	2.30	2.17	0.10
	All	148	2.4074	0.2723	2.80	2.70	2.60	2.40	2.30	2.20	2.05
42-43	White	74	2.3595	0.2443	2.70	2.60	2.50	2.40	2.30	2.20	2.10
	Black	18	2.4278	0.1904	2.90	2.81	2.50	2.40	2.30	2.20	2.20
	Mixed	20	2.3450	0.1191	2.60	2.58	2.40	2.35	2.22	2.20	2.20
	All	118	2.3703	0.2173	2.74	2.60	2.50	2.40	2.30	2.20	2.10

Length of fifth finger: See figure 27-5

Using plastic ruler, measure the distance from the metacarpal-phalangeal joint crease at the base of the fifth finger to the tip. The end of the finger was judged by inspection by the examiner, looking at a 90 angle.

TABLE 27-33 *Distributions for Fifth Finger Clinodactyly [Right]: Both Sexes*

Gestational Age	Race	Number of Infants	Mean	Standard Deviation	Percentiles						
					97	90	75	50	25	10	3
30-34	All	25	2.4800	1.6862	5.00	5.00	4.00	2.00	1.00	0.00	0.00
35-36	All	44	1.8636	1.6080	5.65	4.00	3.00	1.50	0.25	0.00	0.00
37-38	White	97	2.3608	1.6085	6.00	5.00	3.00	3.00	1.00	0.00	0.00
	Black	20	1.7000	1.0311	3.00	3.00	2.75	2.00	1.00	0.00	0.00
	Mixed	13	1.9231	1.4412	4.00	4.00	3.50	2.00	1.00	0.00	0.00
	All	144	2.2778	1.5440	5.00	4.00	3.00	2.00	1.00	0.00	0.00
39	White	128	2.2422	1.4459	5.13	4.00	3.00	2.00	1.00	0.00	0.00
	Black	35	1.7429	1.4621	6.76	3.40	2.00	2.00	1.00	0.00	0.00
	Mixed	38	2.0263	1.6683	6.83	4.10	3.00	2.00	1.00	0.00	0.00
	All	218	2.1055	1.4851	5.43	4.00	3.00	2.00	1.00	0.00	0.00
40	White	198	1.8939	1.4228	5.00	4.00	3.00	2.00	1.00	0.00	0.00
	Black	58	1.3966	1.3884	5.00	3.10	2.00	1.00	0.00	0.00	0.00
	Mixed	56	1.8929	1.1390	4.29	3.00	3.00	2.00	1.00	0.00	0.00
	All	333	1.7898	1.3920	5.00	3.60	3.00	2.00	1.00	0.00	0.00
41	White	162	2.0062	1.6247	6.00	4.70	3.00	2.00	1.00	0.00	0.00
	Black	28	1.1786	1.0203	3.00	3.00	2.00	1.00	0.00	0.00	0.00
	Mixed	40	2.1500	1.6572	5.77	5.00	3.00	2.00	1.00	0.00	0.00
	All	240	1.9417	1.5728	6.00	4.00	3.00	2.00	1.00	0.00	0.00
42-43	White	129	2.0233	1.5282	6.00	4.00	3.00	2.00	1.00	0.00	0.00
	Black	19	1.2105	0.9763	3.00	3.00	2.00	1.00	0.00	0.00	0.00
	Mixed	30	2.6333	2.0254	8.00	5.90	4.00	2.00	1.00	0.10	0.00
	All	185	2.0324	1.6114	6.00	4.40	3.00	2.00	1.00	0.00	0.00

Fifth finger clinodactyly: See Figure 27-5 (for measuring the angle of curvature in clinodactyly.)

The examiner marks the midpoint of the most proximal metacarpal-phalangeal joint and in the proximal interphalangeal joint. A plastic ruler is placed over these two marks out beyond the tip of the fifth finger. The midpoint of the tip of the fifth finger is determined by inspection. The examiner measures the distance in millimeters between the two lines at the end of the fifth finger.

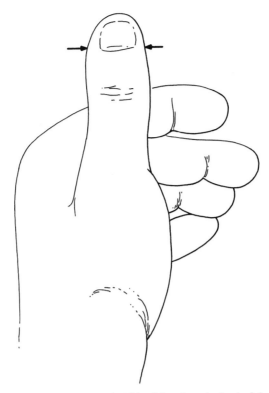

FIGURE 27.6 Measurement of width of thumb at the level of the base of the nail

TABLE 27-34 *Distributions for Thumb Width (cm) [Right]: Males*

Gestational Age	Race	Number of Infants	Mean	Standard Deviation	Percentiles						
					97	90	75	50	25	10	3
30-34	All	4	0.7250	0.1500	0.80	0.80	0.80	0.80	0.57	0.50	0.50
35-36	All	8	0.7625	0.1188	1.00	1.00	0.80	0.75	0.70	0.60	0.60
37-38	White	13	0.8538	0.1266	1.10	1.06	1.00	0.80	0.80	0.70	0.70
	All	17	0.8294	0.1263	1.10	1.02	0.90	0.80	0.80	0.68	0.60
39	White	24	0.8375	0.1013	1.00	1.00	0.95	0.80	0.80	0.70	0.70
	All	40	0.8500	0.1198	1.08	1.00	1.00	0.80	0.80	0.70	0.62
40	White	36	0.8639	0.1150	1.10	1.00	1.00	0.80	0.80	0.77	0.70
	All	57	0.8509	0.1071	1.10	1.00	1.00	0.80	0.80	0.78	0.70
41	White	23	0.8348	0.0935	1.00	1.00	0.80	0.80	0.80	0.74	0.70
	All	36	0.8389	0.0994	1.00	1.00	0.95	0.80	0.80	0.70	0.70
42-43	White	24	0.8625	0.1135	1.00	1.00	1.00	0.80	0.80	0.70	0.70
	All	35	0.8629	0.1285	1.19	1.00	1.00	0.80	0.80	0.70	0.70

Thumb width: See Figure 27-6.
Spreading calipers are used to measure the width of the thumb at the level of the base of the nail.

FEETS

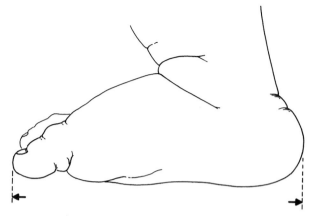

FIGURE 27.7 Shows points of placement of calipers used to measure length of foot

TABLE 27-35 *Distributions for Foot Length (cm) [Right]: Both Sexes*

Gestational Age	Race	Number of Infants	Mean	Standard Deviation	Percentiles						
					97	90	75	50	25	10	3
30-34	White	17	7.1000	0.9158	8.50	8.34	7.85	7.00	6.40	5.70	5.30
	Black	12	7.1000	0.6030	8.30	8.12	7.55	7.15	6.57	6.26	6.20
	Mixed	5	7.4600	0.4159	7.80	7.80	7.75	7.70	7.05	6.80	6.80
	All	40	7.1575	0.7274	8.45	8.00	7.70	7.20	6.62	6.20	5.41
35-36	White	16	7.3937	0.5092	8.00	8.00	7.82	7.45	7.20	6.67	5.90
	Black	17	7.4647	0.4513	8.40	8.00	7.80	7.40	7.20	6.78	6.70
	Mixed	11	7.8182	0.5173	8.70	8.64	8.30	7.80	7.60	7.02	7.00
	All	45	7.5200	0.5048	8.59	8.12	7.90	7.50	7.20	6.92	6.20
37-38	White	90	7.7256	0.5038	8.53	8.30	8.10	7.70	7.40	7.02	6.70
	Black	27	7.8333	0.3961	8.70	8.38	8.00	7.80	7.70	7.20	7.20
	Mixed	37	7.7946	0.3800	8.73	8.30	8.05	7.80	7.60	7.38	6.91
	All	163	7.7577	0.4532	8.60	8.30	8.10	7.80	7.50	7.20	6.79
39	White	132	7.9098	0.3885	8.70	8.40	8.20	7.90	7.70	7.40	7.10
	Black	35	7.8286	0.4315	8.69	8.48	8.00	7.80	7.50	7.40	6.74
	Mixed	53	7.8094	0.3919	8.51	8.30	8.10	7.80	7.60	7.20	6.99
	All	232	7.8789	0.3917	8.60	8.40	8.10	7.90	7.70	7.40	7.10
40	White	203	8.0030	0.4050	8.80	8.60	8.20	8.00	7.70	7.50	7.30
	Black	43	7.8860	0.3944	8.47	8.30	8.20	8.00	7.60	7.40	6.83
	Mixed	69	7.8536	0.2993	8.40	8.20	8.10	7.80	7.70	7.50	7.20
	All	323	7.9526	0.3917	8.70	8.46	8.20	8.00	7.70	7.50	7.20
41	White	137	8.0066	0.4046	8.80	8.50	8.30	8.00	7.75	7.50	7.20
	Black	21	8.0238	0.3859	8.60	8.40	8.30	8.20	7.80	7.32	7.30
	Mixed	58	8.0103	0.3396	8.65	8.50	8.22	8.00	7.80	7.60	7.28
	All	227	8.0154	0.3853	8.72	8.50	8.30	8.00	7.80	7.50	7.28
42-43	White	123	8.0285	0.3398	8.80	8.46	8.20	8.00	7.80	7.60	7.40
	Black	19	7.9737	0.3739	9.00	8.30	8.10	8.00	7.80	7.50	7.30
	Mixed	39	8.1077	0.3505	8.68	8.60	8.40	8.00	7.90	7.70	7.32
	All	187	8.0299	0.3530	8.74	8.60	8.20	8.00	7.80	7.60	7.36

Foot length: See Figure 27-7.
Using spreading calipers, the relaxed foot is measured from the tip of the first toe to the heel at a point one inch above the bottom of the heel.

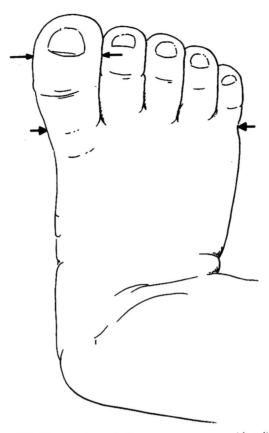

FIGURE 27.8 Shows points of placement to measure with calipers, width at base of first toe and width of foot at metatarsal phalangal point

TABLE 27-36 *Distributions for Foot Width (cm) [Right]: Both Sexes*

Gestational Age	Race	Number of Infants	Mean	Standard Deviation	\multicolumn{7}{c}{Percentiles}						
					97	90	75	50	25	10	3
30-34	All	39	3.0872	0.3541	3.50	3.50	3.40	3.20	2.80	2.60	2.10
35-36	All	44	3.2159	0.2949	3.80	3.60	3.40	3.30	3.00	2.80	2.60
37-38	White	91	3.3604	0.2607	3.90	3.68	3.50	3.40	3.20	3.00	2.80
	Black	27	3.3407	0.1907	3.70	3.60	3.50	3.40	3.20	3.00	3.00
	Mixed	36	3.3333	0.2438	3.88	3.63	3.47	3.40	3.20	3.07	2.71
	All	163	3.3454	0.2442	3.81	3.60	3.50	3.40	3.20	3.00	2.80
39	White	134	3.4172	0.2226	3.89	3.60	3.52	3.40	3.30	3.10	2.90
	Black	35	3.3429	0.2671	3.80	3.70	3.50	3.30	3.10	3.00	2.81
	Mixed	53	3.3698	0.1977	3.74	3.60	3.50	3.40	3.20	3.10	2.92
	All	235	3.4009	0.2270	3.80	3.70	3.50	3.40	3.30	3.10	2.91
40	White	205	3.4337	0.2212	3.80	3.70	3.60	3.40	3.30	3.10	3.00
	Black	44	3.3886	0.2093	3.89	3.65	3.50	3.40	3.30	3.10	2.87
	Mixed	70	3.4357	0.2022	3.80	3.70	3.60	3.40	3.30	3.11	3.10
	All	327	3.4281	0.2172	3.80	3.70	3.60	3.40	3.30	3.10	3.00
41	White	138	3.4659	0.2091	3.90	3.80	3.60	3.40	3.30	3.20	3.10
	Black	21	3.4619	0.2617	4.00	3.78	3.70	3.50	3.20	3.10	3.00
	Mixed	57	3.4965	0.2053	3.80	3.80	3.60	3.50	3.40	3.20	3.00
	All	227	3.4740	0.2124	3.82	3.80	3.60	3.50	3.20	3.20	3.10
42-43	White	126	3.4667	0.2198	3.90	3.80	3.60	3.40	3.30	3.20	3.10
	Black	19	3.5158	0.2062	4.00	3.80	3.70	3.50	3.30	3.30	3.20
	Mixed	39	3.5256	0.2161	4.06	3.80	3.70	3.50	3.40	3.30	3.02
	All	190	3.4821	0.2187	3.90	3.80	3.62	3.50	3.30	3.20	3.10

Foot width: See Figure 27-8.
Using spreading calipers, the relaxed foot was measured from the metatarsal-phalangeal(M-P) joint of the first toe to the M-P joint of the fifth toe.

TABLE 27-37 *Distributions for Toe Width (cm) [Right]: Both Sexes*

Gestational Age	Race	Number of Infants	Mean	Standard Deviation	Percentiles						
					97	90	75	50	25	10	3
30-34	All	17	0.9294	0.1448	1.10	1.10	1.05	0.90	0.85	0.68	0.60
35-36	All	17	1.0235	0.1715	1.40	1.24	1.15	1.00	0.95	0.78	0.70
37-38	White	55	1.0291	0.1242	1.20	1.20	1.10	1.00	0.90	0.90	0.77
	All	81	1.0296	0.1198	1.20	1.20	1.10	1.00	1.00	0.90	0.80
39	White	67	1.0448	0.1158	1.30	1.20	1.10	1.00	1.00	0.90	0.80
	All	108	1.0509	0.1131	1.30	1.20	1.10	1.00	1.00	0.90	0.83
40	White	104	1.0692	0.1071	1.28	1.20	1.10	1.10	1.00	0.90	0.81
	All	164	1.0543	0.1104	1.20	1.20	1.10	1.10	1.00	0.90	0.80
41	White	68	1.0706	0.1107	1.29	1.20	1.10	1.10	1.00	0.90	0.81
	All	102	1.0863	0.1081	1.30	1.20	1.20	1.10	1.00	0.90	0.90
42-43	White	74	1.0595	0.1146	1.20	1.20	1.10	1.10	1.00	0.90	0.80
	All	102	1.0686	0.1266	1.30	1.20	1.10	1.10	1.00	0.90	0.80

Toe (first) width: See Figure 27-8
Spreading calipers are used to measure the width of the first toe at the base of the toenail.

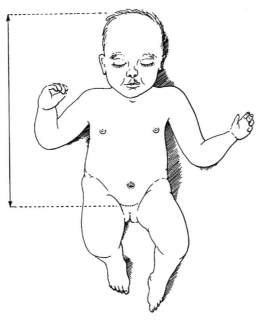

FIGURE 27.9 Anatomic landmarks identified to use in measuring upper segment of body

TABLE 27-38 *Distributions for Upper Segment (cm): Both Sexes*

Gestational Age	Race	Number of Infants	Mean	Standard Deviation	Percentiles						
					97	90	75	50	25	10	3
30-34	All	40	27.3250	2.1569	31.62	30.45	29.00	27.50	25.50	24.50	23.61
35-36	All	46	28.4522	1.5355	31.00	30.43	29.70	28.50	27.00	26.50	25.11
37-38	White	68	28.8341	1.3983	31.50	31.00	29.95	29.00	28.00	27.00	26.33
	Black	27	29.0481	1.5111	31.50	30.70	30.00	29.00	28.00	27.00	25.00
	Mixed	38	28.5368	1.5725	31.00	30.55	29.63	28.75	28.00	26.00	25.08
	All	163	28.8147	1.4726	31.50	30.92	30.00	29.00	28.00	27.00	25.96
39	White	135	29.2415	1.2570	31.00	31.00	30.00	29.00	28.50	27.50	26.50
	Black	37	29.0892	1.2290	31.00	30.60	30.00	29.00	28.00	27.00	26.57
	Mixed	54	28.8741	1.6329	32.10	31.00	30.00	29.00	28.00	26.95	24.65
	All	138	29.2029	1.4169	32.00	31.00	30.00	29.00	28.22	27.50	26.08
40	White	203	29.6291	1.4500	32.00	31.24	30.50	29.50	29.00	28.00	26.56
	Black	43	29.3512	1.1205	31.68	31.00	30.00	29.50	28.50	28.00	27.00
	Mixed	71	29.2465	1.3577	32.00	31.00	30.00	29.00	28.00	27.50	26.50
	All	325	29.4966	1.3859	32.00	31.00	30.00	29.50	28.50	28.00	26.89
41	White	139	29.6719	1.3743	32.80	31.40	30.50	29.80	29.00	28.00	27.00
	Black	23	29.1870	1.1925	31.00	30.80	30.00	29.30	28.50	27.50	26.50
	Mixed	57	29.6035	1.2326	32.26	31.00	30.00	30.00	29.00	28.00	26.87
	All	230	29.6230	1.3145	32.00	31.00	30.50	29.65	29.00	28.00	27.00
42-43	White	127	29.9354	1.2300	32.06	31.52	31.00	30.00	29.00	28.24	27.50
	Black	18	29.4167	1.2748	32.00	31.10	30.13	29.25	28.38	27.90	27.00
	Mixed	39	30.0744	1.0267	32.00	32.00	31.00	30.00	29.00	29.00	28.34
	All	190	29.8984	1.2061	32.00	31.50	31.00	30.00	29.00	28.30	27.50

See Figure 27-9 To measure the upper segment using a tape measure, the examiner measures the distance from the center of the tip of the head to the upper edge of the pelvis. The edge of the pelvis in the center is determined by palpation.

GENITALS-MALES

TABLE 27-39 *Distributions for Penis Length Bottom (cm): Males*

Gestational Age	Race	Number of Infants	Mean	Standard Deviation	Percentiles						
					97	90	75	50	25	10	3
30-34	All	19	2.2684	0.6299	3.40	3.20	2.80	2.10	1.80	1.50	1.40
35-36	All	17	2.1353	0.5207	3.20	2.88	2.40	2.20	1.90	1.24	1.00
37-38	White	35	2.2686	0.4928	3.20	3.00	2.60	2.30	2.00	1.60	1.21
	Black	15	2.6667	0.5627	3.60	3.54	3.20	2.60	2.20	1.92	1.80
	Mixed	10	2.2800	1.0042	3.80	3.75	3.15	2.30	1.40	0.92	0.90
	All	62	2.3597	0.6289	3.62	3.20	2.80	2.30	2.00	1.53	1.08
39	White	67	2.1448	0.5737	3.30	2.90	2.40	2.20	1.80	1.48	0.81
	Black	14	2.4071	0.4393	3.10	3.05	2.70	2.45	2.17	1.65	1.60
	Mixed	25	2.1880	0.7590	4.20	2.96	2.70	2.20	1.80	1.02	0.70
	All	114	2.2184	0.6033	3.30	2.95	2.60	2.25	1.80	1.55	0.84
40	White	94	2.2830	0.4972	3.30	3.05	2.70	2.20	2.00	1.70	1.30
	Black	19	2.5895	0.6073	3.70	3.60	3.20	2.50	2.10	2.00	1.50
	Mixed	30	2.3167	0.3602	3.20	2.80	2.60	2.35	2.00	1.81	1.70
	All	149	2.3248	0.4952	3.35	3.10	2.60	2.20	2.00	1.70	1.40
41	White	52	2.3135	0.4851	3.66	3.00	2.60	2.20	2.00	1.73	1.60
	Black	10	2.8300	0.4762	3.30	3.29	3.20	3.00	2.55	1.86	1.80
	Mixed	27	2.1926	0.5622	3.40	3.20	2.50	2.00	1.80	1.54	1.20
	All	95	2.3505	0.5640	3.51	3.20	2.60	2.30	2.00	1.70	1.48
42-43	White	56	2.2732	0.5591	3.53	2.86	2.70	2.20	1.80	1.60	1.31
	Black	11	2.6727	0.6198	3.80	3.70	3.00	2.70	2.30	1.66	1.60
	Mixed	20	2.4400	0.5906	3.80	3.00	2.87	2.45	2.02	1.80	1.10
	All	90	2.3711	0.5789	3.65	3.00	2.80	2.40	1.97	1.60	1.32

Penis length bottom: Using a plastic ruler, length, underside of penis from based to tip.

TABLE 27-40 *Distributions for Penis Length Top (cm): Males*

Gestational Age	Race	Number of Infants	Mean	Standard Deviation	Percentiles						
					97	90	75	50	25	10	3
30-34	All	19	2.7158	0.6238	4.00	4.00	3.00	2.50	2.30	2.00	1.90
35-36	All	19	2.5421	0.6104	4.00	3.40	2.80	2.50	2.20	1.80	1.20
37-38	White	35	2.6714	0.4430	3.58	3.20	3.00	2.70	2.30	2.00	1.82
	Black	15	3.1533	0.5317	4.20	3.96	3.80	2.90	2.80	2.58	2.40
	Mixed	11	2.6182	0.9075	3.80	3.78	3.60	2.60	1.90	1.32	1.30
	All	63	2.7619	0.6009	3.83	3.66	3.10	2.80	2.40	2.00	1.39
39	White	68	2.5691	0.6124	3.86	3.30	3.00	2.60	2.20	1.80	1.01
	Black	13	2.8769	0.4885	3.90	3.74	3.20	2.80	2.60	2.20	2.00
	Mixed	25	2.6120	0.7293	5.00	3.32	2.90	2.70	2.25	1.72	1.20
	All	114	2.6535	0.6344	3.90	3.40	3.00	2.65	2.30	2.00	1.14
40	White	95	2.6895	0.4666	3.62	3.24	3.00	2.70	2.40	2.00	1.70
	Black	19	2.9842	0.6414	4.20	4.00	3.50	2.80	2.60	2.20	1.80
	Mixed	31	2.6581	0.4217	3.60	3.26	2.80	2.70	2.50	2.00	1.80
	All	151	2.7212	0.4834	3.84	3.30	3.00	2.70	2.40	2.02	1.80
41	White	52	2.7115	0.4805	3.68	3.40	3.15	2.65	2.30	2.13	2.00
	Black	10	3.2200	0.6286	4.00	3.99	3.90	3.20	2.85	2.07	2.00
	Mixed	27	2.6185	0.5248	3.90	3.52	3.00	2.60	2.20	1.96	1.80
	All	95	2.7600	0.5572	3.90	3.60	3.20	2.70	2.30	2.10	1.98
42-43	White	56	2.7536	0.5208	4.06	3.33	3.20	2.70	2.40	2.07	1.77
	Black	11	3.1545	0.6440	4.20	4.12	3.60	3.30	2.70	2.06	2.00
	Mixed	20	2.9200	0.7008	4.40	3.77	3.40	2.85	2.45	2.31	1.00
	All	90	2.8422	0.5829	4.20	3.50	3.20	2.80	2.40	2.20	1.77

Penis length top: Using a plastic ruler, length on top of penis from base to tip.

TABLE 27-41 *Distributions for Testis Length (cm) [Right]: Males*

Gestational Age	Race	Number of Infants	Mean	Standard Deviation	Percentiles						
					97	90	75	50	25	10	3
30-34	All	7	1.8286	0.1704	2.00	2.00	2.00	1.90	1.60	1.60	1.60
35-36	All	7	1.8143	0.1215	2.00	2.00	1.90	1.80	1.80	1.60	1.60
37-38	White	24	1.8833	0.1880	2.20	2.10	2.00	1.90	1.72	1.65	1.40
	All	35	1.8800	0.2041	2.29	2.10	2.00	1.90	1.80	1.56	1.41
39	White	29	1.9448	0.1723	2.30	2.20	2.05	1.90	1.80	1.70	1.70
	All	51	1.9392	0.1981	2.34	2.20	2.10	2.00	1.80	1.70	1.51
40	White	58	1.8741	0.2237	2.30	2.20	2.00	1.80	1.70	1.70	1.30
	All	90	1.8911	0.2075	2.30	2.20	2.00	1.80	1.77	1.70	1.45
41	White	44	1.8932	0.1993	2.33	2.10	2.00	1.90	1.80	1.60	1.43
	All	66	1.8970	0.2353	2.40	2.20	2.10	1.90	1.80	1.60	1.20
42-43	White	31	1.9452	0.2219	2.60	2.20	2.10	1.90	1.80	1.70	1.60
	All	44	1.9386	0.2014	2.53	2.20	2.10	1.90	1.80	1.70	1.63

Testis length: The examiner holds the testis in one hand and uses spreading calipers to measure length of testis.

TABLE 27-42 *Distributions for Testis Width (cm) [Right]: Males*

Gestational Age	Race	Number of Infants	Mean	Standard Deviation	Percentiles						
					97	90	75	50	25	10	3
30-34	All	6	0.8500	0.1643	1.10	1.10	1.02	0.80	0.70	0.70	0.70
35-36	All	6	0.9500	0.1975	1.30	1.30	1.07	0.90	0.80	0.80	0.80
37-38	White	24	0.9250	0.1595	1.30	1.15	1.00	0.90	0.80	0.70	0.70
	All	35	0.9143	0.1458	1.29	1.10	1.00	0.90	0.80	0.70	0.70
39	White	29	0.9552	0.1804	1.40	1.30	1.05	1.00	0.80	0.70	0.70
	All	50	0.9480	0.1681	1.35	1.20	1.00	0.90	0.80	0.80	0.70
40	White	58	0.9017	0.1433	1.12	1.10	1.00	0.90	0.80	0.70	0.68
	All	90	0.9133	0.1463	1.20	1.10	1.00	0.90	0.80	0.70	0.70
41	White	43	0.9326	0.1304	1.10	1.10	1.10	0.90	0.80	0.80	0.70
	All	67	0.9493	0.1407	1.30	1.10	1.10	0.90	0.80	0.80	0.70
42-43	White	31	0.9065	0.1459	1.30	1.08	1.00	0.90	0.80	0.70	0.70
	All	44	0.9273	0.1436	1.26	1.10	1.00	0.90	0.80	0.75	0.70

Testis width: Using spreading calipers, measure width of testis.

GENITALS-MALES

TABLE 27-43 *Anogenital distance (cm)*

Gestational Age	Race	Number of Infants	Mean	Standard Deviation	Percentiles						
					97	90	75	50	25	10	3
30-34	All	17	1.9941	0.4493	2.80	2.72	2.20	2.00	1.70	1.28	1.20
35-36	All	15	2.0200	0.3764	2.40	2.40	2.30	2.10	2.00	1.22	1.10
37-38	White	31	2.2677	0.4969	3.00	3.00	2.50	2.30	2.00	1.72	0.70
	Black	11	2.4455	0.4677	3.30	3.24	2.80	2.40	2.00	1.76	1.70
	Mixed	11	2.2455	0.6170	3.00	2.96	2.70	2.30	2.00	0.96	0.70
	All	54	2.3037	0.5091	3.10	3.00	2.62	2.30	2.00	1.75	0.70
39	White	52	2.3827	0.4484	3.25	3.00	2.67	2.40	2.10	1.86	1.36
	Black	11	2.5545	0.4845	3.30	3.28	3.00	2.50	2.10	2.02	2.00
	Mixed	22	2.4227	0.3878	3.20	3.07	2.72	2.35	2.20	2.00	1.80
	All	92	2.4076	0.4305	3.22	3.00	2.77	2.40	2.10	2.00	1.56
40	White	91	2.4714	0.4072	3.32	3.00	2.80	2.40	2.20	2.00	1.80
	Black	15	2.4333	0.4370	3.20	3.08	2.80	2.40	2.00	1.80	1.80
	Mixed	24	2.4708	0.4196	3.20	3.05	2.80	2.55	2.20	1.85	1.50
	All	134	2.4649	0.4069	3.20	3.00	2.80	2.40	2.20	2.00	1.80
41	White	51	2.4529	0.4496	3.39	3.00	2.80	2.40	2.20	1.92	1.51
	Black	8	2.8000	0.3586	3.40	3.40	3.00	2.80	2.55	2.20	2.20
	Mixed	24	2.5125	0.3882	3.60	3.10	2.65	2.40	2.30	2.10	2.00
	All	89	2.5135	0.4254	3.43	3.00	2.80	2.40	2.20	2.00	1.74
42-43	White	49	2.5388	0.3978	3.30	3.20	2.85	2.50	2.25	2.00	1.85
	Black	7	2.6286	0.5314	3.30	3.30	3.30	2.60	2.20	2.00	2.00
	Mixed	16	2.5875	0.4113	3.20	3.06	2.97	2.60	2.32	1.84	1.70
	All	74	2.5581	0.4058	3.30	3.20	2.90	2.50	2.30	2.00	1.82

Perineum-male: Using a plastic ruler in millimeters, measure distance from center of anal opening to lower edge of scrotum.

GENITALS-FEMALES

TABLE 27-44 *Anogenital distance (cm)*

Gestational Age	Race	Number of Infants	Mean	Standard Deviation	Percentiles						
					97	90	75	50	25	10	3
30-34	All	19	1.2684	0.2907	1.80	1.60	1.50	1.30	1.10	0.80	0.70
35-36	All	23	1.4087	0.4512	2.80	2.10	1.50	1.30	1.20	0.88	0.80
37-38	White	50	1.3080	0.2039	1.75	1.59	1.40	1.30	1.20	1.10	0.80
	Black	11	1.2455	0.1916	1.60	1.56	1.40	1.30	1.00	1.00	1.00
	Mixed	23	1.3826	0.3339	2.30	1.84	1.50	1.30	1.20	1.04	0.60
	All	92	1.3174	0.2402	1.84	1.60	1.47	1.30	1.20	1.00	0.80
39	White	70	1.3386	0.2176	1.80	1.60	1.50	1.30	1.20	1.00	1.00
	Black	21	1.1857	0.1195	1.40	1.38	1.25	1.20	1.10	1.00	1.00
	Mixed	27	1.2370	0.2221	1.70	1.52	1.40	1.20	1.10	0.90	0.80
	All	121	1.2917	0.2170	1.73	1.60	1.40	1.30	1.20	1.00	0.90
40	White	87	1.3126	0.2067	1.80	1.60	1.40	1.30	1.20	1.00	1.00
	Black	25	1.3160	0.2055	1.70	1.64	1.45	1.30	1.15	1.06	0.90
	Mixed	40	1.3100	0.1905	1.70	1.60	1.40	1.30	1.20	1.00	0.92
	All	154	1.3110	0.2005	1.70	1.60	1.40	1.30	1.20	1.00	1.00
41	White	75	1.3587	0.2182	1.87	1.70	1.50	1.30	1.20	1.10	1.00
	Black	13	1.4308	0.1548	1.80	1.72	1.50	1.40	1.30	1.24	1.20
	Mixed	27	1.3593	0.2005	1.80	1.70	1.50	1.30	1.20	1.10	1.10
	All	119	1.3790	0.2557	1.84	1.70	1.50	1.30	1.20	1.10	1.00
42-43	White	58	1.3155	0.1871	1.70	1.51	1.40	1.30	1.20	1.00	0.98
	Black	8	1.4000	0.1690	1.60	1.60	1.57	1.40	1.30	1.10	1.10
	Mixed	18	1.4333	0.1879	1.80	1.62	1.60	1.45	1.30	1.18	1.00
	All	87	1.3575	0.1969	1.74	1.60	1.50	1.40	1.20	1.08	1.00

Perineum-female: Using a plastic ruler in millimeters, measure distance from center of anal opening to lowest edge opening between labia majora.

Index

Note: Page numbers followed by "*f*" and "*t*" denote figures and tables, respectively.